Bullying, Impact on Health, and Beyond

Bullying, Impact on Health, and Beyond

Exploring the Spectrum of Maltreatment

Jorge C. Srabstein, MD

Medical Director, Program for Health Problems Related to Bullying
Children's National Hospital
Clinical Professor of Psychiatry, Behavioral Sciences and Pediatrics
George Washington University School of Medicine and Health Sciences

OXFORD
UNIVERSITY PRESS

OXFORD
UNIVERSITY PRESS

Oxford University Press is a department of the University of Oxford. It furthers the University's objective of excellence in research, scholarship, and education by publishing worldwide. Oxford is a registered trade mark of Oxford University Press in the UK and certain other countries.

Published in the United States of America by Oxford University Press
198 Madison Avenue, New York, NY 10016, United States of America.

CIP data is on file at the Library of Congress

ISBN 978–0–19–937933–0

DOI: 10.1093/med/9780199379330.001.0001

This material is not intended to be, and should not be considered, a substitute for medical or other professional advice. Treatment for the conditions described in this material is highly dependent on the individual circumstances. And, while this material is designed to offer accurate information with respect to the subject matter covered and to be current as of the time it was written, research and knowledge about medical and health issues is constantly evolving and dose schedules for medications are being revised continually, with new side effects recognized and accounted for regularly. Readers must therefore always check the product information and clinical procedures with the most up-to-date published product information and data sheets provided by the manufacturers and the most recent codes of conduct and safety regulation. The publisher and the authors make no representations or warranties to readers, express or implied, as to the accuracy or completeness of this material. Without limiting the foregoing, the publisher and the authors make no representations or warranties as to the accuracy or efficacy of the drug dosages mentioned in the material. The authors and the publisher do not accept, and expressly disclaim, any responsibility for any liability, loss, or risk that may be claimed or incurred as a consequence of the use and/or application of any of the contents of this material.

Printed by Marquis Book Printing, Canada

FSC www.fsc.org MIX Paper from responsible sources FSC® C103567

To my children, grandchildren, and their future generations

מפני תיקון העולם
(mip'nei tikkun ha-olam)
For the sake of repairing the world

From the Mishnah, Gittin 4:2-9

Contents

Preface ix
Acknowledgments xi

1. **The Concept of Bullying** 1
2. **The Prevalence of Bullying** 10
3. **Polyvictimization and Revictimization** 25
4. **Morbidity Associated with Bullying and Other Forms of Victimization** 34
5. **Psychosocial Problems and Risk Behaviors Linked to Bullying and Other Forms of Victimization** 71
6. **Mortality Linked to Bullying and Other Forms of Maltreatment** 84
7. **Prevention of Bullying and Other Forms of Victimization** 100
8. **Detection of Bullying and Other Forms of Victimization** 115
9. **Intervention and Treatment for Bullying and Other Forms of Victimization** 132
10. **National Initiatives for the Prevention of Bullying and Other Forms of Maltreatment** 164
11. **Bullying and Other Forms of Maltreatment in the School Milieu** 211
12. **Workplace Bullying and Other Forms of Maltreatment** 234
13. **Victimization at Home** 263
14. **Bullying and Other Forms of Maltreatment in Cyberspace** 291
15. **Maltreatment in the Neighborhood** 314
16. **Victimization in Adolescent Dating Relationships** 339
17. **Victimization in Competitive Sports** 349
18. **Bullying and Other Forms of Victimization in Tertiary Education** 370
19. **Bullying and Other Forms of Maltreatment in Prisons** 389
20. **Witnessing Bullying and Other Forms of Maltreatment** 406

Epilogue 421
Index 423

Preface

This book is the result and reflection of more than two decades of clinical and advocacy work for the prevention of bullying, across social settings, and treatment of its associated health risks. My interest in this area was generated by global news of suicides linked to bullying, as well as the American Medical Association's recognition in 2002 of the potential serious health consequences of bullying, and the AMA's urging of physicians to detect bullying-related morbidity and to advocate for the development of policies for its prevention.[1]

Initially, this book was intended to raise awareness among health and public health professionals about the evolving understanding of the multifaceted and toxic nature of bullying, which is a psychosocial stressor that has been linked to a wide range of morbidity and is prevalent across social settings, across the life span, and around the world. In this context, the book is primarily aimed at fostering the role of health and public health practitioners in developing strategies for the prevention and detection of bullying and treatment of its associated health risks. During the development of this book, it was recognized that bullying is a type of maltreatment that may be associated with other forms of victimization, and this led me to go beyond the notion of bullying and to explore the spectrum of maltreatment.

Many years were spent in the development of this book, because it required finding free time in the midst of a busy full-time clinical practice to search, to select, and to go through at least 2,000 peer-reviewed studies of bullying and other forms of victimization that were published since 2000. This evolving body of literature has revealed the nature, prevalence, and health/psychosocial risks of bullying and other forms of victimization in different social environments, as well as the strategies developed, thus far, for their prevention, detection, and treatment.

In my research, the bibliographic search tools Google Scholar and PubMed were extremely valuable, as also were immediate and regular access to other databases and complete texts of articles through the Himmelfarb Health Sciences Library at the George Washington University School of Medicine and Health Sciences, where I hold a clinical faculty appointment.

Jorge C. Srabstein
December 30, 2022

Note

1. American Medical Association. Bullying behaviors among children and adolescents H-60.943. https://policysearch.ama-assn.org/policyfinder/detail/H-60.943?uri=%2FAMADoc%2FHOD.xml-0-5037.xml. Accessed September 15, 2023.

Acknowledgments

My interest in, and knowledge of, this field have been fostered through communication with many colleagues around the world. Among them, I want to acknowledge Bennett Leventhal (United States), Young Shin Kim (United States), Andre Sourander (Finland), Anat Brunstein-Klomek (Israel), Dieter Wolke (United Kingdom), Tomas Silber (United States), Joav Merrick (Israel), Debra Pepler (Canada), Dorothy Espelage (United States), Phillip T. Slee (Australia), Ken Rigby (Australia), P. K. Smith (United Kingdom), Jane L. Ireland (United Kingdom), Louise Arsenault (United Kingdom), Loraleigh Keashly (United States), Lucie Laflamme (Sweden), Pernille Due (Denmark), Kirsti Kumpulainen (Finland), Ian Rivers (United Kingdom), Emilia Menesini (Italy), Elizabeth Allan (United States), Marla Eisenberg (United States), Dianne Neumark-Sztainer (United States), Ron White (Australia), David A. Wolfe (Canada), George Holden (United States), Joseph Wright (United States), Edgardo Menvielle (United States), Paramjit Joshi (United States), and Adelaide Robb (United States).

My most sincere gratitude and recognition go to the late Dr. James B. Harris, who encouraged me to take my initial steps in submitting a proposal for this book to Oxford University Press (OUP). Finally, throughout this long journey I have very much valued working with Andrea Knobloch, Lilith Dorko, Emily Hu, and Craig Panner of OUP, who have very strongly supported the book.

Jorge C. Srabstein

1
The Concept of Bullying

Coverage of Bullying in the Media and Scientific Literature

As a start to exploring the evolving understanding of bullying in different contexts, it is appropriate to first examine the prevalent public exposure to the concept. A global review[1] of newspapers from 1990 through 2020 (Figure 1.1) shows an exponentially increasing number of articles and editorials dealing with the subject of bullying, with some of the publications written in languages other than English.[2–4]

Through the first eight and a half decades of the 20th century, there was extremely limited coverage of bullying in the print media. The concept of bullying was used to depict the political use of force by a government, political leader, or organization to intimidate or aggressively dominate its members, citizens, and/or other countries.[5–9] A few isolated articles drew attention to the occurrence of bullying in military institutions and schools.[10–13]

By 1985, the first reports appeared in a long series of accounts underscoring the association of school bullying with suicide attempts.[14–17] By the late 1980s, the media increasingly recognized the serious public health risks linked to this type of maltreatment and the need for its prevention.[18–21] For the past three decades, global awareness of the nature and gravity of bullying has been maintained by ongoing reports of its link to hundreds of deaths[22–26] and the recognition of its prevalence in the school environment.[27–31] Furthermore, the range of news reports about bullying has been significantly widened by the recognition of its occurrence across diverse social settings, including cyberspace[32–35] and the workplace.[36–39]

A broad search[40] of the peer-reviewed medical literature shows that, since 1990, a rapidly growing number of articles have included bullying in their titles and abstracts (Figure 1.2), echoing the pattern of news articles published about the subject during the same period (Figure 1.1).

Understanding the Concept of Bullying

Since the 1990s, the global understanding of the nature and significance of bullying has been evolving. The process was launched by Olweus' pioneering research,[41,42] and it is being shaped by the influence of individual, developmental, cultural, and experiential awareness as well as by the developing body of knowledge about the ecology, prevalence, and public health importance of bullying.

Bullying has been defined as "the abuse and mistreatment of someone vulnerable by someone stronger [and] more powerful."[43] It has also been characterized as "the behavior of a person who hurts or frightens someone smaller or less powerful, often forcing that person to do something they do not want to do."[44]

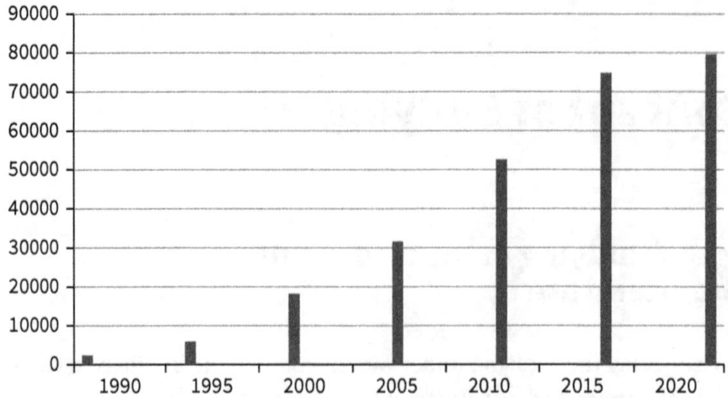

Figure 1.1. Global news coverage of bullying: number of articles every five years from 1990 to 2020.

Olweus first typified the notion of bullying, in the context of students' relations, by explaining it as a student's being "exposed, repeatedly and over time, to negative actions on the part of one or more students."[41] The range of negative actions included physical aggression (hitting, pushing, kicking, pinching), language harassment (teasing, threatening, taunting, name-calling, making faces or dirty gestures), and/or indirect maltreatment (such as ignoring or excluding somebody from a group).[42] Furthermore, it has been specified that the concept of bullying is characterized by intentionality, repetition, and imbalance of power.[45]

Smith and Levan[46] showed that children as young as 6 years old "have a reasonably good understanding of the term bullying" and can recognize indirect as well as physical and verbal forms of it. Yet, children's conception of bullying includes fighting and/or somebody that is nasty and hurtful, without the behavior having to be intentional, repetitive, or occurring within an imbalance of power.

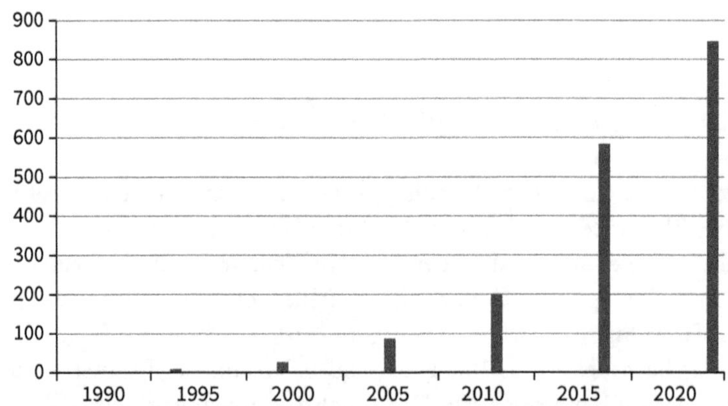

Figure 1.2. Coverage of bullying in the medical literature: number of articles every five years from 1990 to 2020.[40]

Legal Definition of Bullying

A review of school bullying prevention laws[47] enacted in different jurisdictions throughout Canada and the United States shows that there is a moderate difference in the legal definition of bullying in at least 50% of the statutes. Yet, at least 30% to 60% of the laws concur in their description of bullying, intimidation, or harassment as an intentional and/or continuous written, electronic, verbal, or physical act that places the victim in reasonable fear of harm to person or property and/or causes physical hurt and/or emotional distress, physical harm, or damage to property. Furthermore, the actions may interfere with educational performance, opportunities, or benefits; may create an intimidating, threatening, or abusive environment; and may disrupt the orderly operation of the school.

The Notion of Bullying in the Public Health Domain

Documents published by the Public Health Agency of Canada (PHAC)[48] and the Centers for Disease Control and Prevention (CDC)[49] regard bullying as a form of aggression that is repeated and involves an imbalance of power. The CDC's current uniform definition[49] considers that "bullying may inflict harm or distress on the targeted youth, including physical, psychological, social, or educational harm." It includes direct aggressive behaviors that occur in the presence of the targeted youth, but it is not limited to face-to-face interaction and can include harmful written or verbal communication with the target. It also involves "indirect aggressive behaviors that are not directly communicated to the targeted youth," such as spreading false and/or harmful rumors. Furthermore, it encompasses a wide array of types of bullying, such as physical actions (i.e., hitting, kicking, punching, spitting, tripping, and pushing), verbal harassment (taunting, name-calling, threatening or offensive written notes or hand gestures, inappropriate sexual comments, or threats), and a relational mode (spreading false rumors, writing derogatory comments, or posting embarrassing images in a physical or electronic space without the target's permission or knowledge).

A description of what is understood by the term *bullying* can be found in the Health Behavior in School-aged Children (HBSC) survey[50] and the Global School-based Student Health Survey (GSHS).[51] These surveys specify that a student is bullied when bad,[51] nasty, or unpleasant[50,51] things are being said or done to them. The surveys also indicate that bullying occurs when a student is teased a lot[51] or repeatedly[50] in a way that is unpleasant[51] or is disliked,[50] and/or when a youth is excluded or left out of things deliberately[50] or purposely.[51] The surveys do not recognize as bullying such circumstances as when two students of about the same strength or power argue or fight[50,51] or when teasing is friendly,[50,51] playful,[50] and fun.[51]

The HBSC[52] and GSHS[53] are two World Health Organization cross-national youth health surveys, administered in almost 150 countries and territories around the world, through a large array of languages. Forty percent of these languages use words to describe bullying that, when translated[54] to English, signify concepts like assault, flouting, harassment, imposition, insult, intimidation, maltreatment, mistreatment, mobbing, mocking, provocation, suffering, terrorism, tormenting, or tyranny (Table 1.1).

Table 1.1. Meaning of Words Utilized in HBSC and GSHS in Languages Other Than English to Indicate the Concept of Bullying

Language/Country	Word	English Translation
Albanian (Albania)	Nëpërkëmbja	Maltreatment
Arabic (Egypt, Iraq, Libya)	المضايقات (almdayqat)	Harassment
Armenian	Ահաբեկման (Ahabekman)	Terrorism
Bulgarian	Тормоза (tormoza)	Harassment
Chinese (Mandarin)	欺负的 (Qīfù de)	Bullied
Croatian	Zlostavljanjem	By abuse
Czech	Šikanování	Bullying
Danish	Mobning	Bullying
Dutch	Pesten	Bullying
Estonian	Kiusamisest	From bullying
Finnish	Kiusaamista	Bullying
French (Canada)	Intimidation Taxage	Intimidation Imposition
French (France, Djibouti)	Brimades	Bullying
Gaelic	Bhulaíocht	Bullying
German	Schikanieren	Harass
Hebrew	הטרדות (hat'radah) הצקות (hatz'kot)	Harassment Bullying
Hungarian	Bántalmazás	Abuse
Italian	Bullismo	Bullying
Kiswahili (Swahili)	Kunyanyaswa	Harassment
Latvian	Nirgāšanās	Mockery
Lithuanian	Tyčiojamasi	Bullied
Maltese	Ibbulijar	Bullying
Norwegian	Mobbing	Bullying
Polish	Dręczenia	Tormenting
Portuguese (Mozambique)	Intimidação	Bullying
Portuguese (Portugal)	Provocação	Provocation
Romanian	Intimidare	Intimidation

Table 1.1. Continued

Language/Country	Word	English Translation
Romanian	Batjocorire Agresare	Flouting Assault
Russian (Russia)	Оскорблении (Oskorblenii)	Insulted
Russian (Tajikistan)	Буллингом Bullingom	Bullying
Slovakian	Šikanovania	Bullying
Slovenian	Trpinčenju	Suffering
Spanish (Spain)	Maltrato	Mistreatment
Spanish) (Latin America)	Intimidación	Intimidation
Swedish	Mobbning	Bullying
Tagalog	Pananakot	Intimidation
Turkish	Zorbalik	Tyranny
Ukrainian	Образа (Obraza)	Insult
Vietnamese	Bắt nạt	Bullying
Welsh	Bwlio	Bullying

The Notion of Bullying across Social Settings

The wide-ranging concept of bullying, which encompasses elements of physical aggression, verbal harassment, and/or indirect maltreatment, as applied to the notion of school peer victimization, can also be used in a core definition of bullying occurring in other social settings. Furthermore, the notion of bullying can also include other elements based on unique ecological and cultural aspects of different milieus. In this context, bullying in the workplace can be typified by being "compelled to do tasks that are harmful to one's health" or being "exposed to [an] unmanageable workload" (see Chapter 12, Table 12.1). Furthermore, bullying among prisoners may be characterized by being "forced to buy … goods for another prisoner" or "forced to send one's private cash to another prisoner's family" (see Chapter 19).

Medical Concept of Bullying

Health practitioners are faced with a public health need to determine whether their patients are being bullied and/or bullying others, as well as whether they are suffering from associated health risks. Therefore, the medical concept of bullying is evolving.

Physicians need to recognize bullying as a multifaceted form of maltreatment that encompasses physical aggression (hitting, pushing, punching, or kicking), verbal harassment (threatening, teasing, name-calling, or making faces or dirty gestures), and indirect or relational mistreatment (ignoring someone or excluding someone on purpose). Daring a person to perform a dangerous, illegal, or inappropriate action under the threat of losing approval, or of not being liked or loved, should also be considered a form of bullying.[55] In a medical context, it may be difficult to include elements of intentionality, recurrence, and imbalance of power in the notion of bullying, although these elements are included in its original research definition.[45] Some people may bully others without planning or intending to do so, because their behavior could be the result of faulty regulation of impulse control, as in individuals with Tourette disorder or impulse control disorder.[55] Yet, the bullying victim may be affected regardless of the intentionality of the perpetrator, an imbalance of power, and or the frequency of bullying.[55]

In determining whether an incident of bullying indeed occurred, it is necessary to bear in mind that the experience of being bullied is in the "eye of the beholder,"[55] because "a person who was previously bullied may be sensitized to future occurrences and perceive an act of mistreatment when other people may not consider it as such."[55] Furthermore, the personal awareness of having been bullied often incurs the feeling of having been physically or emotionally "hurt." Conversely, some people may report and describe, within a clinical anamnesis, that they have been exposed to behaviors that clearly meet the definition of bullying, but the individuals fail to recognize that behavior as mistreatment because they do not feel that they have been "hurt." Furthermore, they may indicate that in the past a similar incident harmed them, but by now they have become used to it and "don't care."

Spectrum of Maltreatment

A central tenet of this book is to consider bullying within a spectrum of maltreatment, where at its core bullying is identified as harassment or intimidation, and with one end of the spectrum being abuse, aggression, or violence, and the opposite end being neglect, rejection, or exclusion.

Furthermore, bullying can be associated with other forms of maltreatment (polyvictimization; see Chapter 3), and it can be understood as diverse types of victimization or crime (Table 1.2).

Table 1.2. Types of Maltreatment

Assault	Bullying	Corporal punishment	Dating violence
Domestic violence	Extortion	Fraud	Hazing
Human trafficking	Kidnapping	Physical abuse	Psychological abuse
Random shootings	Rape	Road rage	Robbery
Sexual abuse	Sexual assault	Sexual harassment	Stalking
Terrorism	Theft	Threats	Vandalism

Traditionally, the study of different forms of victimization has been compartmentalized because of research and/or legal requirements. Now, the study of bullying requires us to explore the spectrum of maltreatment, and in this context, important psychosocial issues emerge at a level not seen in the last five decades, since the lethal aspects of child abuse came to public awareness.[56]

Notes

1. Review of newspapers utilizing the term *bullying* in the headline or lead paragraph, through Access World News from News Bank, Factiva from Dow Jones, Google News, Historical Newspapers from Pro Quest, Nexis Uni® from LexisNexis, and Times Digital Archive.
2. Gómez L. Muerte de un niño africano en la jungla del gueto londinense. *El País*. December 3, 2000.
3. Bullying debe ser prevenido pelas escolas. *Correio da Manha* (Portugal). April 16, 2015:Quinta feira.
4. A 14 ans, victime de bullying d'un collégien. *L'Express* (Port Louis). July 9, 2020.
5. Van Dyke JE. The "bullying" of Cuba. *New York Times*. March 1, 1902:8.
6. Davis OK. China prompts Japs to change bullying ways: moves Nippon to switch from indemnity demands. *Chicago Daily Tribune*. August 4, 1915:7.
7. Wireless to *The New York Times*. Nazi bullying fails, *London Times* says: Hitlerite methods likened to the policy of 'deliberate ruthlessness of 1914.' *New York Times*. July 30, 1934:2.
8. Axis bullying in the Balkans sneers at Greece, Duce visits Yugoslav. *The Times Friday*. October 22, 1940:4.
9. Tokyo police ordered to quit bullying people. *Chicago Daily Tribune*. October 26, 1946:11.
10. Bullying alleged at Guards' depot. *The Times Tuesday*. July 2, 1963:10.
11. Bullying of Army cadets alleged. *The Times Tuesday*. September 16, 1969:6.
12. Parents say girl died after school bullying. *The Times Tuesday*. December 11, 1973:2.
13. Devlin T. Schoolmasters call for bullying inquiry. *The Times Friday*. March 22, 1974:4.
14. David Watts suicide highlights bullying in Japan. *The Times Thursday*. October 24, 1985:10.
15. Makihara K. Bullying in Japan's public schools is major social issue. The Associated Press. December 3, 1985.
16. The Associated Press. In Japan, children's bullying can lead to murder and suicide. *The Record*. December 15, 1985.
17. Researcher suggests bullying on the rise. *St. Petersburg Times*. April 11, 1987.
18. Bullying problem is a serious one. *The State* (Columbia, SC). June 4, 1988.
19. Researcher touts program to clamp down on schoolyard bullying. *Evening Tribune*. February 15, 1988.
20. Dakin Andone. CNN, Finland found a proven way to combat bullying. Here's what it'll take to make it work in the U.S. Fri August 11, 2017, CNN Health, https://www.cnn.com/2017/08/11/health/finland-us-bullying-prevention-trnd/index.html. Accessed October 10, 2023.
21. Jeffrey Pierre and Cory Turner. Experts say we can prevent school shootings. Here's what the research say. National Public Radio, NPR, WAMU 88.5, American University Radio, https://www.npr.org/2022/05/26/1101571302/what-schools-can-do-to-prevent-school-shootings. Accessed October 10, 2023.
22. Srabstein J. Deaths linked to bullying and hazing. *Int J Adolesc Med Health*. 2008;20(2):235–239.

23. Boy's suicide is tragic reminder of schoolyard bullying problem in Japan. *The Dallas Morning News*. December 2, 1995.
24. Boy aged 14 'hanged himself after campaign of bullying.' *The Independent* (London, England). September 3, 2005.
25. Bullying at school likely had role in teen girl's suicide, coroner says. *Houston Chronicle*. May 14, 2010.
26. Taunting Facebook posts prompt arrests in Fla. bullying-suicide case. *The Star-Ledger* (Newark, NJ). October 16, 2013.
27. Putting a face on school bullying. *Daily Telegraph* (Sydney, Australia). October 31, 2000.
28. 52% say bullying is a big problem—children worried about violence in their schools. *The Daily Mirror* (London, England). November 16, 2005.
29. Taiwan's school bullying menace—cases spark outcry as acts get more violent; leaders vow to get tough. *The Straits Times* (Singapore). January 3, 2011.
30. Bullying at school single biggest problem for pupils. *The Witness* (South Africa). December 5, 2012.
31. Top Swedish school closed over bullying. *The Daily Telegraph* (London, England). September 4, 2013.
32. Holly Rosenkrantz, Bullying Prevention for Teachers and Parents. US News, September 22, 2021. https://www.usnews.com/education/k12/articles/bullying-prevention-for-teachers-and-parents. Accessed October 10, 2023.
33. Bullying reaches to cyberspace—cyberbullying increasing in prominence. *The Tribune-Star* (Terre Haute, IN). April 28, 2009.
34. Cyberbullying a growing problem for one in 10 kids. *Sunday Territorian* (Darwin, Australia). April 18, 2010.
35. Cyberbullying 'as difficult to stop as abuse in playground.' *The Herald and the Sunday Herald* (Glasgow, Scotland). November 22, 2013.
36. Bullying at work increases. *The Times*. July 10, 1995.
37. Bullying on the rise at work. *The Daily Record* (Glasgow, Scotland). February 15, 2000.
38. Bullying is rampant in workplace, expert says. *Tulsa World* (OK). October 18, 2008.
39. Workplace bullying 'out of control.' *The Examiner* (Launceston, Australia). July 12, 2012.
40. Search of articles with the term *bullying*, either in the title or in the abstract, through National Center for Biotechnology Information, US National Library of Medicine, PubMed. https://www.ncbi.nlm.nih.gov/pubmed. Accessed July 8, 2022.
41. Olweus D. *Mobbning i Skolan: Vad Vi Vet Och Vad Vi Kan Göra*. Cited in Olweus D. *Bullying at School: What We Know and What We Can Do*. Oxford, England: Blackwell Publishers; 1993:9.
42. Olweus D. *Bullying at School: What We Know and What We Can Do*. Oxford, England: Blackwell Publishers; 1993:9.
43. Bullying. https://www.merriam-webster.com/dictionary/bullying. Accessed July 8, 2022.
44. Bullying. https://dictionary.cambridge.org/us/dictionary/english/bullying. Accessed July 8, 2022.
45. Olweus D. Sweden. In: *The nature of school bullying: a cross-national perspective*. Smith PK, Morita Y, Junger-Tas J, Olweus D, Catalano R, Slee P, eds. London, England: Routledge; 1969:11.
46. Smith PK, Levan S. Perceptions and experiences of bullying in younger pupils. *Br J Educ Psychol.* 1995;65:489–500.

47. Review of: Ala. Code—Title 16: Education—§16-28B-3; Alaska Stat.—§14.33.250; Education Act, SA 2012, c E-0.3; Ark. Code Ann. §6-18-514; Colo. Rev. Stat. 22-32-109.1; Conn. Gen. Stat. §10-222d (2012); Del. Code—§4112D; D.C. L19-0167; Fla. Stat.—§1006.147; Ga. Code—Educ.—Title 20, §20-2-751.4; Guam 17 GCA §3112.1.; Haw. Admin. R. §8-19-2; Idaho Stat. 18-917A; Ill. Comp. Stat. 105 ILCS 5/27-23.7; Ind. Code IC 20-8.1-5.1-0.2; Iowa Code 280.28; Kan. Stat. 72-8256; Ky. Rev. Stat. KRS 525.070; La. Rev. Stat. §17:416.13; Me. Rev. Stat. Title 20-A §6554; Manitoba, The Public Schools Act, C.C.S.M. c. P250, 1.2(1)(2); Md. Code §7-424.; Mass. Gen. Laws, Part I, Title XII, ch 71, §370; Mich. Comp. Laws, §380.1310b; Miss. Code §37-11-67; Mo. Rev. Stat. 160.775; N.Y. Educ. Law §11; N.C. Gen. Stat. §115C-407.15; N.D. Cent. Code 15.1-19-17; Ohio Rev. Code 3313.666; Okla. Stat. §70-24-100.3; Ontario Bill 13, Accepting Schools Act, 2012; Or. Rev. Stat. §339.351; Puerto Rico, Laws of Puerto Rico Annotated 3 L.P.R.A. §144g-1; R.I. Gen. Laws §16-21-33; S.C. Code §59-63-120; S.D. Codified Laws §13-32-15; Tenn. Code Ann. §49-6-4502; Tex. Educ. Code §37.0832; Utah Code 53A-11a-102; Vt. Stat. §1.16 V.S.A. §11(a)(32); Va. Code §22.1-276.01; W. Va. Code §18-2C-2; Wisc. Stat. 118.127 (2).
48. Craig W, Edge HM. Bullying and fighting. In: *The Health of Canada's Young People: A Mental Health Focus*. Public Health Agency of Canada. http://www.phac-aspc.gc.ca/hp-ps/dca-dea/publications/hbsc-mental-mentale/bullying-intimidation-eng.php. Accessed July 8, 2022.
49. Gladden RM, Vivolo-Kantor AM, Hamburger ME, Lumpkin CD. *Bullying Surveillance among Youths: Uniform Definitions for Public Health and Recommended Data Elements, Section 2, The Uniform Definition, Version 1.0*. Atlanta, GA; National Center for Injury Prevention and Control and US Department of Education; 2014. http://www.cdc.gov/violenceprevention/pdf/bullying-definitions-final-a.pdf. Accessed July 8, 2022.
50. Health Behavior in School-Aged Children (HBSC) 2005/06 Survey. International Standard Version of the Mandatory Questionnaire, Being Bullied, page 22, based on Olweus D. The revised Olweus Bully/Victim Questionnaire. Mimeo; 1996. HEMIL, University of Bergen, N-5015 Bergen, Norway; HBSC 2002. http://filer.uib.no/psyfa/HEMIL-senteret/HBSC/2006_Mandatory_Questionnaire.pdf. Accessed July 8, 2022.
51. Global School-based Student Health Survey (GSHS). Core Questionnaire Violence and Unintentional Injury Module, Questions about Bullying. GSHS Core Questionnaire Modules, Final. https://www3.paho.org/hq/dmdocuments/2010/cuestionario2009eng.pdf. Accessed July 8, 2022.
52. Health Behavior in School-Aged Children (HBSC). *World Health Organization Collaborative Cross-National Survey*. http://www.hbsc.org. Accessed July 8, 2022.
53. Global School-based Student Health Survey (GSHS). The GSHS was developed by the World Health Organization (WHO) in collaboration with United Nations' UNICEF, UNESCO, and UNAIDS, and with technical assistance from CDC. GSHS is a school-based survey conducted primarily among students 13 to 17 years old. http://www.cdc.gov/GSHS/. Accessed July 8, 2022.
54. By use of Google Translate, https://translate.google.com/.
55. Srabstein JC. The prevention of bullying: a whole school and community model. In: Shute RH, Slee PT, Murray-Harvey R, Dix KL, eds. *Mental Health and Wellbeing: Educational Perspectives*. Adelaide, Australia: Shannon Research Press; 2011:297–305.
56. Kempe CH, Silverman FN, Steele BF, Droegemueller W, Silver HK. The battered-child syndrome. *JAMA*. 1962;181:17–24. Cited in Srabstein JC. Be aware of bullying: a critical public health responsibility. *Virtual Mentor*. 2009;11(2):173–177.

2
The Prevalence of Bullying

Bullying Happens Everywhere

There is an evolving understanding that bullying occurs across the life span[1-7] and around the world.[8] Furthermore, "it can be simultaneously present in different social settings both in and beyond the school mileu."[9] A more comprehensive understanding of the distinctive aspects of bullying in various environments is explored in Chapters 11 through 20. This chapter reviews the global prevalence of bullying and examines some sociodemographic factors associated with this form of maltreatment.

Global Prevalence of Bullying and Regional Differences

School Bullying

The worldwide occurrence of school bullying has been examined by Due and Holstein[8] via a second analysis of the 2001–2002 Health Behavior in School-aged Children (HBSC) survey[10] and the Global School-based Student Health Survey (GSHS)[11] as administered from 2003 to 2007. The Due and Holstein study,[8] which drew its data from more than 200,000 adolescents (age 13 to 15) in 66 countries and regions, documented that, on average, 32.1% of students in HBSC countries were bullied at least once in the preceding two months, and 37.4% in GSHS countries were victimized by peers in the previous 30 days.

More than 15 years later, a 2017–2018 HBSC[12] survey of national representative samples of students 11 to 15 years old in Canada and 41 European countries and territories showed that an average of 9.0% of the students reported having been bullied, at least twice, in the previous two months, with the prevalence ranging from 2.5% to 26.0% (Table 2.1).

Based on available data from the GSHS[13] implemented between 2010 and 2019 in 36 countries and regions, an average of 48.55% of adolescents 13 to 15 years old reported having been bullied in school once or more frequently in the previous 30 days, with the prevalence ranging from 13.3% to 74.0% (Table 2.2).

Data from the 2009–2010 US HBSC[50] indicate that 16.7% of students 10 to 17 years old were bullied in school once or twice in the preceding couple of months. Female students (17.7%) were slightly more frequently bullied than male students (15.5%), while the frequency of being bullied decreased from 19% in the sixth and seventh grade to 12% in tenth grade.

According to the 2019 Youth Risk Behavior Surveillance System (YRBSS),[51] 19.5% of US adolescents in grades 9 to 12 reported having been bullied, on school property, during the 12 months preceding the survey.[52] Female students (23.6%) were more frequently bullied than male students (15.4%), while the prevalence of bullying victimization among

Table 2.1. Frequency of Being Bullied at School at Least Twice in the Previous Two Months among 13- to 15-year-old Students, by Country or Region, Based on HBSC Data from 2017–2018[12]

Albania	6.0%	France	5.0%	North Macedonia	7.0%
Austria	8.0%	Germany	9.5%	Norway	2.5%
Armenia	4.5%	Greece	6.5%	Poland	6.5%
Azerbaijan	10.0%	Greenland	14.5%	Portugal	6.0%
Belgium (Flemish)	7.5%	Hungary	12.0%	Romania	9.0%
Belgium (French)	7.0%	Iceland	2.5%	Russia	14.5%
Bulgaria	16.5%	Ireland	10.5%	Scotland	14.0%
Canada	15.5%	Italy	5.0%	Slovakia	9.0%
Croatia	9.0%	Latvia	19.0%	Slovenia	8.5%
Czechia	6.0%	Lithuania	26.0%	Spain	3.5%
Denmark	5.5%	Luxembourg	9.5%	Sweden	8.5%
England	14.0%	Malta	8.5%	Switzerland	6.5%
Estonia	15.0%	Moldova	15.0%	Ukraine	16.5%
Finland	8.0%	Netherlands	4.5%	Wales	12.0%

Table 2.2. Frequency of Bullying at Least Once in the Previous Month among 13- to 15-year-old Students, by Country or Region, Based on GSHS Data from 2010–2019[13]

Afghanistan 2014[14]	44.2%	Fiji Islands 2016[26]	29.9%	Oman 2015[38]	42.3%
Argelia 2011[15]	51.7%	French Polynesia 2015[27]	25.1%	Philippines 2019[39]	41.8%
Argentina 2012[16]	24.5%	Guatemala 2015[28]	22.8%	Samoa 2011[40]	74.0%
Bahamas 2013[17]	23.6%	Lebanon 2017[29]	24.5%	Swaziland 2013[41]	32.1%
Bangladesh 2014[18]	23.6%	Malaysia 2012[30]	20.9%	Tanzania 2014[42]	26.9%
Barbados 2011[19]	13.3%	Maldives 2014[31]	30.1%	Tokelau 2014[43]	40.5%
Belize 2011[20]	30.7%	Mauritania 2010[32]	47.2%	Tonga 2010[44]	50.3%
Bhutan Urban 2016[21]	29.9%	Mauritius 2017[33]	25.3%	Trinidad and Tobago 2017[45]	15.4%
Brunei 2014[22]	23.4%	Mongolia 2013[34]	30.5%	United Arab Emirates 2016[46]	27.1%
Cambodia 2013[23]	22.4%	Morocco 2016[35]	38.2%	Vanuatu 2011[47]	67.3%
Cook Islands 2015[24]	30.9%	Mozambique 2015[36]	45.0%	Vietnam 2013[48]	26.1%
Egypt 2011[25]	70.0%	Niue 2010[37]	35.5%	West Bank 2010[49]	52.9%

lesbian, gay, or bisexual students was higher (32%) than among heterosexual students (17.1%).[52]

The significantly higher risk of bullying among lesbian, gay, bisexual, and transgender (LGBT) youth has been highlighted in numerous studies.[53-63]

Gender Nonconformity and School Bullying

Children who do not follow the expectations of behavior for their biological sex are described as gender noncomforming.[64]

Analysis of data from a US population-based longitudinal study of a large national cohort (N = 10,655)[64] documented that the frequency of bullying victimization (9.7%) in the previous year among boys in the upper decile of gender nonconformity was significantly higher than the prevalence of peer victimization (5.2%) experienced by conforming boys. There was no statistically significant difference in bullying experienced by gender-conforming girls compared to their nonconforming peer females.

Semenya et al[65] conducted a study in Samoa that compared 100 heterosexual adult men to 103 gay transgender adult men (known as *fa'afafine*) to ascertain the degree of association between childhood gender atypicality and recalled early years of bullying victimization. The research did not document a significant difference between the two groups in the rates of childhood bullying victimization, despite a significantly higher frequency of earlier gender nonconformity reported by the *fa'afafine* as compared to the heterosexual men (21.18% vs. 8.28%).[65] The study was limited in its power to demonstrate causality, due to its cross-sectional design and reliance on recalled information, yet the authors suggested that Samoans' relative tolerance and acceptance of gender-atypical behavior may explain why the prevalence of bullying does not seem to be significantly augmented by gender nonconformity when there is a cultural open-mindedness.[65]

School Bullying by Race, Ethnicity, or Being Foreign-Born

According to a second analysis[50] of the 2009–2010 US HBSC data, being bullied once or twice in the preceding two months occurred at a higher frequency (18.4%) among white adolescents than among African Americans (13.0%) or Hispanics (15.0%).[50]

There are some reports documenting higher frequency of bullying among the indigenous segment of a population as compared to their non-aboriginal neighbors.[66–71]

A cross-sectional survey of more than 12,000 men and women 36 to 79 years old residing in Central and Northern Norway has documented a very significantly high frequency (36%) of reported discrimination and bullying against Sami-speaking indigenous people, as compared to a low prevalence of this type of mistreatment (3.5%) among non-Sami-speaking or "ethnic Norwegians."[66] Another report[67] of the same study indicated that "Sami women were more likely to report emotional, physical, and sexual violence than non-Sami women."

An examination[68] of bullying prevalence among 204 First Nation young people (age 10 to 16) living in a reserve within the Saskatoon Tribal Council has shown that the youth experienced, in the previous month, rates of physical, verbal, social, and electronic bullying that were significantly higher than the frequencies of the same types of victimization among Canadian youth of the same age living in the city of Saskatoon.[69]

It has been reported that Māori (New Zealand indigenous) high school students have a moderate risk of being ethnically bullied as compared to their New Zealand European (Pākehā) peers [adjusted odds ratio (AOR) = 1.61],[70] yet the risk was much higher among students of Asian descent than among Pākehā pupils (AOR = 5.36).[70]

A cross-sectional analysis of data from almost 4,000 children 12 to 13 years old in the nationally representative Longitudinal Study of Australian Children showed that indigenous Australian children reported the highest risk of bullying victimization and racial discrimination.[71]

Maynard et al[72] conducted a very comprehensive study to ascertain the prevalence of bullying victimization among foreign-born[73] youth in the United States, based on a secondary analysis of the 2009–2010 HBSC data.[50] This research documented that, as compared to their US-born peers, first-generation immigrant US adolescents are at a significant risk of suffering from one or more types of bullying, and they have a high probability of being bullied with comments about their race or color (AOR = 2.14).

School Bullying by Area of Residence (Urban, Suburban, or Rural)

Based on second analysis[50] of the 2009–2010 US HBSC data, being bullied once or twice in the previous two months occurred at a statistically significant higher frequency (18%) among students living in rural areas[74] than among students from urban[75] or suburban areas (16%).

A cross-sectional study[76] of Icelandic children age 11 to 15 (based on HBSC data) showed that being bullied was significantly associated with living in a rural area (OR = 1.50).

School Bullying by Parental Occupation/Socioeconomic Status (SES)

A secondary analysis[50] of the 2009–2010 US HBSC data showed that there was a statistically significant higher frequency (20%–21%) of being bullied once or twice in the previous two months among students whose fathers were restaurant, factory, or transportation workers as well as technical, office, or sales employees, as compared to the 15% bullying frequency reported by students whose fathers were professionals, business owners, or managers. No statistically significant difference in prevalence of bullying was found among students based on their mother's occupation.

Låftman et al[77] analyzed data from the Swedish Living Conditions Survey of 2008 to 2011, which was based on a sample of almost 4,000 adolescents, and found that youngsters were significantly more at risk of being bullied (AOR = 1.45) if they lived in a household with "no cash margin, defined as the ability to pay an unexpected bill of 8,000 Swedish Kronor or about 800 euros." Also, adolescents living with one custodial parent were significantly more at risk (AOR = 1.51) of being subject to at least one type of harassment, at least weekly, than adolescents who lived with both custodial parents.[77]

Physical or Developmental Aspects Associated with Bullying

Physical Characteristics Linked to Bullying

Using the 2015 YRBSS, Johns et al[78] analyzed data from a sample of more than 7,700 female students to ascertain whether their BMI might compound sexual minority girls' risk for harassment. The findings[78] indicated that the risk of being bullied on school property was higher for students who were both heterosexual and overweight (AOR = 1.34) than for heterosexual peers who had normal BMI. Furthermore, the risk was even higher among peers who were from a sexual minority and were overweight (AOR = 2.73).[78]

De Oliveira et al[79] investigated the reasons for school bullying reported by Brazilian students. Their findings, which were based on cross-sectional data from a 2012 epidemiologic survey of more than 109,000 ninth grade students from public and private schools, indicated that almost 35% of the students reported body or facial appearance as being causes of bullying.

In an effort to ascertain the contribution of general physical and dentofacial features to bullying, Al-Bitar et al[80] conducted a cross-sectional study of a representative sample of 920 Jordanian students age 11 to 12 living in Amman. Their study[80] showed that dentofacial features were the most frequent (50%) physical aspect reported by victims of bullying, followed by an average of one third of the victims who were bullied because of visible characteristics like their strength, weight, hair, height, or clothes. Furthermore, an average of 15% of the victims were targeted due to the characteristics of their eyes, nose, ears, and lips, their wearing glasses, or their having freckles. Among the most frequent (76%) dentofacial features identified as targets for bullying in this study[80] were spacing between teeth or missing teeth, shape or color of the teeth, or prominent anterior teeth.

Developmental Conditions Associated with Peer Victimization

Mayes et al[81] studied the frequency of bullying behavior, based on maternal reports, among a sample of 1,707 children and adolescents. The researchers compared peer victimization among youth with clinically diagnosed psychiatric disorders and controls. Their findings showed that the highest rates of "often" or "very often" peer victimization were found among young people who were diagnosed with autism (43.5%) or intellectual disability (35.2%), while the rates were much lower among controls (1.6%).

An investigation led by Pfeffer[82] assessed prevalence rates of interpersonal violence in a national sample of 262 US children and adolescents with a diagnosis of autism spectrum disorder, and the study documented that 74% of the youth had been assaulted or bullied in the previous 12 months and 84% had been subjected to those types of maltreatment in their lifetime.

Cyberbullying

A review of the 2017–2018 HBSC[83] survey indicated that an average of 13.25% of adolescents (13 to 15 years old) in 41 European and North American countries and regions reported that

Table 2.3. Frequency of Being Cyberbullied at School at Least Once in the Previous Two Months among 13- to 15-year-old Students, by Country or Region, Based on HBSC Data from 2017–2018[12]

Albania	12.0%	France	6.0%	North Macedonia	8.0%
Austria	8.0%	Germany	8.5%	Norway	7.5%
Armenia	9.5%	Greece	4.0%	Poland	18.5%
Azerbaijan	8.0%	Greenland	17.5%	Portugal	7.0%
Belgium (Flemish)	7.0%	Hungary	19.0%	Romania	16.5%
Belgium (French)	8.0%	Iceland	10.0%	Russia	21.0%
Bulgaria	17.5%	Ireland	14.5%	Scotland	17.5%
Canada	12.5%	Italy	10.0%	Slovakia	11.0%
Croatia	12.5%	Latvia	19.0%	Slovenia	12.0%
Czechia	9.5%	Lithuania	23.5%	Spain	4.0%
Denmark	9.0%	Luxembourg	10.0%	Sweden	15.5%
England	19.5%	Malta	14.0%	Switzerland	7.5%
Estonia	16.0%	Moldova	14.5%	Ukraine	22.0%
Finland	14.5%	Netherlands	6.5%	Wales	14.5%

they had been cyberbullied at least once in the preceding two months,[83] with the prevalence ranging from 4.0% to 23.5% (Table 2.3).

Data from the 2009–2010 US HBSC[50] indicated that 4.0% of US students age 10 to 17 were cyberbullied outside school, once or twice, in the preceding couple of months. Female students were slightly more frequently (4.7%) bullied than male students (3.2%), while the frequency of being cyberbullied did not differ significantly between sixth and tenth grade.

According to the 2019 YRBSS,[51] 15.7% of US adolescents in grades 9 to 12 reported having been electronically bullied, through texting, Instagram, Facebook, or other social media, during the 12 months preceding the survey. Female adolescents were significantly more frequently cyberbullied (20.4%) than were males (10.9%).[51] Gay, lesbian, and bisexual adolescents were significantly more frequently cyberbullied (26.6%) than were heterosexual teenagers (14.1%). Also, white adolescents were significantly more frequently cyberbullied (18.6%) than were African American adolescents (8.6%) and Hispanic youths (12.7%).[51]

Based on second analysis[50] of the 2009–2010 US HBSC data, there are not significant differences in prevalence of being cyberbullied once or twice in the preceding two months according to place of residence (urban, suburban, or rural). Yet, students whose fathers were low-service laborer (restaurant, factory, or transportation workers) were more frequently cyberbullied (4.8%) than were students whose fathers were in other occupations, whose average frequency of being cyberbullied was 3.55%.[50]

Workplace Bullying

The 2010 European Working Conditions Survey,[84] encompassing interviews of 44,000 workers in 34 European countries, has shown that an average of 3% of workers have experienced harassment or bullying at work in the previous year, with prevalence ranging from 1% to 10% (Table 2.4).

An online survey[85] to establish the prevalence of workplace bullying, based on a sample of 1,215 adult Americans, was conducted in 2021 by Zogby Analytics[86] at the request of the Workplace Bullying Institute.[87] The study[85] showed that 13% of the respondents had experienced, at the time of survey and/or through the previous year, repeated mistreatment at work, in the form of abusive conduct that was threatening, intimidating, and humiliating, being verbally abused, or having their work sabotaged.[85] Seventeen percent of the respondents experienced workplace mistreatment sometime in the year preceding the survey. These results show an increase in the prevalence of workplace bullying as documented by a similar survey conducted in 2007[88] that showed 9% of the respondents reported being mistreated at work at the time of the survey or during the previous year, and only 10% had experienced this form of victimization before but not in the previous year.[88]

Table 2.4. Frequency of Workplace Bullying in the Previous Year, by European Countries, Based on Data from the 2010 European Working Conditions Survey[84]

Albania	2.0%	Latvia	5.0%
Austria	7.0%	Lithuania	5.0%
Belgium	9.0%	Luxembourg	7.0%
Bulgaria	1.0%	Malta	3.0%
Croatia	3.0%	Montenegro	3.0%
Cyprus	2.0%	Netherlands	8.0%
Czechia	2.0%	North Macedonia	4.0%
Denmark	3.0%	Norway	4.0%
Estonia	2.0%	Poland	1.0%
Finland	6.0%	Portugal	2.0%
France	10.0%	Romania	2.0%
Germany	5.0%	Slovakia	1.0%
Greece	3.0%	Slovenia	5.0%
Hungary	2.0%	Spain	2.0%
Ireland	5.0%	Sweden	3.0%
Italy	1.0%	Turkey	1.0%
Kosovo	1.0%	United Kingdom	5.0%

Workplace Bullying and Cultural Distance

The role of cultural distance from a host culture as a moderator variable in the risk for workplace bullying was examined[89] in a cross-sectional study of 363 bus drivers and mechanics employed in a Finnish transport company. The concept of cultural distance was defined in this study as the gap between the country of origin and the native language of that country and the Finnish language and its way of life. Cultural distance was represented by three groups: the "culturally closest group," which included workers from Estonia and Sweden; an "intermediate" group, encompassing workers from Russia, the former Yugoslavia, and Russian-speaking Estonians: and a "distant" group composed of immigrants from sub-Saharan and North Africa. The immigrants of close cultural proximity had the same rates of workplace bullying as their native Finnish colleagues. The risk of being bullied was almost three times higher among immigrants in the intermediate cultural distance group and nearly eight times higher in the most distant group. Social exclusion was the most prominent form of bullying experienced by the immigrant workers.

Future Directions

Worldwide, there is a public health need to conduct periodic surveys of national and regional occurrence of youth exposure to, and participation in, bullying and other forms of maltreatment, across social settings. The enhancement of current items included in periodic assessments like the HBSC survey[10] and the GSHS[11] is a first step toward this objective. The availability of suitable national representative samples of youth populations should offer a better understanding of regional sociocultural risks linked to the occurrence bullying and other forms of maltreatment, as well as the effectiveness of policies implemented to ensure their prevention. Similarly, national differences in the prevalence of workplace bullying should be regularly investigated by governmental entities dealing with occupational health, through periodic and systematic surveys to determine the frequency and characteristics of victimization in the workplace.

Beyond epidemiologic data from surveys of nonclinical populations, research should aim to ascertain the prevalence of bullying among individuals of all ages who are being evaluated in medical settings.

Notes

1. Ilola AM, Lempinen L, Huttunen J, Ristkari T, Sourander A. Bullying and victimisation are common in four-year-old children and are associated with somatic symptoms and conduct and peer problems. *Acta Paediatr.* 2016;105(5):522–528.
2. Rose CA, Richman DM, Fettig K, Hayner A, Slavin C, Preast JL. Peer reactions to early childhood aggression in a preschool setting: defenders, encouragers, or neutral bystander. *Dev Neurorehabil.* 2016;19(4):246–254.
3. Camodeca M, Caravita SC, Coppola G. Bullying in preschool: the associations between participant roles, social competence, and social preference. *Aggress Behav.* 2015;41(4):310–321.

4. Perren S, Alsaker FD. Social behavior and peer relationships of victims, bully-victims, and bullies in kindergarten. *J Child Psychol Psychiatry*. 2006;47(1):45–57.
5. Craig W, Harel-Fisch Y, Fogel-Grinvald H, et al. A cross-national profile of bullying and victimization among adolescents in 40 countries. *Int J Public Health*. 2009;54(suppl 2):216–224.
6. Chadaga AR, Villines D, Krikorian A. Bullying in the American graduate medical education system: a national cross-sectional survey. *PLOS One*. 2016;11(3):1–14.
7. Burnes D, Pillemer K, Caccamise PL, Mason A, Henderson CR Jr, Berman J. Prevalence of and risk factors for elder abuse and neglect in the community: a population-based study. *J Am Geriatr Soc*. 2015;63(9):1906–1912.
8. Due P, Holstein BE, Soc MS. Bullying victimization among 13 to 15-year-old school children: results from two comparative studies in 66 countries and regions. *Int J Adolesc Med Health*. 2008;20(2):209–221.
9. Srabstein, JC. (2011). The prevention of bullying: a whole school and community model. In: Slute RH, Slee PT, Murray-Harvey R, Dix KL, eds. *Mental Health and Wellbeing: Educational Perspective*. Adelaide, Australia: Shannon Research Press; 2011:300.
10. The Health Behavior in School-aged Children (HBSC) survey http://hbsc.org/about/ is a research collaboration with the World Health Organization (WHO) Regional Office for Europe. The survey has been performed every four years for the past three decades, in countries and regions across Europe and North America. This cross-sectional study obtains insight into young people's well-being, their health behaviors, and their social context. Its questionnaire covers multiple public health areas, including bullying and fighting, health complaints, substance use, injuries, and eating behaviors, among many others.
11. The Global School-based Student Health Survey (GSHS) was developed by the World Health Organization (WHO) and the Centers for Disease Control and Prevention (CDC). GSHS (www.cdc.gov/GSHS/) is conducted primarily among students 13 to 17 years old. Its 10 core questionnaire modules address the leading causes of morbidity and mortality among adolescents worldwide. It includes, among others, questions about bullying, fighting, unintentional injury, and alcohol/substance use.
12. Based on the findings of the HBSC survey conducted in 2017–2018 among 227,441 students (age 11–15) living in 45 countries and regions. Among the 20 areas of health behaviors surveyed, the students were asked about having been bullied at least twice in the previous two months. An average country prevalence of bullying was calculated based on data for girls and boys age 11, 13, and 15, and results can be found in
Inchley J, Currie D, Budisavljevic S, et al., eds. *Spotlight on Adolescent Health and Well-being. Findings from the 2017/2018 Health Behavior in School-aged Children (HBSC) Survey in Europe and Canada. International Report.* Vol 2. *Key Data*. Copenhagen: WHO Regional Office for Europe; 2020:98–99. License: CC BY-NC-SA 3.0 IGO, Bullying. https://apps.who.int/iris/bitstream/handle/10665/332104/9789289055017-eng.pdf.
13. Data from the GSHS, which has assessed students age 13 to 15 living in 36 countries or regions, at a specific year between 2010 and 2019. Among the many sectors of health behaviors surveyed, the students were asked about having been bullied at least once or more in the preceding 30 days. The frequency of responses of being bullied by the students was obtained from the respective countries' or territories' most recent fact sheets or codebooks (see Notes 14 to 49).
14. Global School-based Student Health Survey, Afghanistan, 2014, Fact Sheet. https://cdn.who.int/media/docs/default-source/ncds/ncd-surveillance/data-reporting/afghanistan/gshs/

2014-gshs-afghanistan-fact-sheet.pdf?sfvrsn=39a13746_3&download=true. Accessed July 15, 2022.

15. Global School-based Student Health Survey, Argelia, 2011, Fact Sheet. https://cdn.who.int/media/docs/default-source/ncds/ncd-surveillance/data-reporting/algeria/2011-gshs-fs-algeria.pdf?sfvrsn=dbcd449d_2&download=true. Accessed July 15, 2022.
16. Global School-based Student Health Survey, Argentina, 2012, Fact Sheet. https://cdn.who.int/media/docs/default-source/ncds/ncd-surveillance/data-reporting/argentina/gshs/argentina_gshs_fs_2012_national.pdf?sfvrsn=5f99eb0f_5&download=true. Accessed July 15, 2022.
17. Global School-based Student Health Survey, Bahamas, 2013, Fact Sheet. https://cdn.who.int/media/docs/default-source/ncds/ncd-surveillance/data-reporting/bahamas/gshs/2013_bahamas_fact_sheet.pdf?sfvrsn=8ffa7e96_7&download=true. Accessed July 15, 2022.
18. Global School-based Student Health Survey, Bangladesh, 2014, Fact Sheet. https://cdn.who.int/media/docs/default-source/ncds/ncd-surveillance/data-reporting/bangladesh/gshs/2014-gshs-bangladesh-fact-sheet.pdf?sfvrsn=d685bf4b_2&download=true. Accessed July 15, 2022
19. Global School-based Student Health Survey, Barbados, 2011, Fact Sheet. https://www.paho.org/hq/dmdocuments/2011/GSHS-barbados-factsheet-2011.pdf. Accessed July 15, 2022.
20. Global School-based Student Health Survey, Belize, 2011, Fact Sheet. https://cdn.who.int/media/docs/default-source/ncds/ncd-surveillance/data-reporting/belize/gshs/2011_gshs_fs_belize.pdf?sfvrsn=c27c81c4_5&download=true. Accessed July 15, 2022.
21. Global School-based Student Health Survey, Bhutan Urban, 2016, Fact Sheet. https://cdn.who.int/media/docs/default-source/ncds/ncd-surveillance/data-reporting/bhutan/gshs/bhutan-gshs-fs-urban-2016.pdf?sfvrsn=5e3d69ad_2&download=true. Accessed July 15, 2022.
22. Global School-based Student Health Survey, Brunei Darussalam, 2014, Fact Sheet. http://www.ppkk.gov.bn/Shared%20Documents/DOCUMENT%2015%20(2014BUH%20Fact%20Sheet%20GSHS%20Global%20School%20Health%20Survey).pdf. Accessed July 15, 2022.
23. Global School-based Student Health Survey, Cambodia, 2013, Fact Sheet. https://cdn.who.int/media/docs/default-source/ncds/ncd-surveillance/data-reporting/cambodia/gshs/2013_cambodia_gshs_fact_sheet.pdf?sfvrsn=3fde50db_3&download=true. Accessed July 15, 2022.
24. Global School-based Student Health Survey, Cook Islands, 2015, Fact Sheet. https://cdn.who.int/media/docs/default-source/ncds/ncd-surveillance/data-reporting/cook-islands/gshs/gshs-fs-cook-islands-2015.pdf?sfvrsn=b6b57041_3&download=true. Accessed July 15, 2022.
25. Global School-based Student Health Survey, Egypt, 2011, Fact Sheet. https://cdn.who.int/media/docs/default-source/ncds/ncd-surveillance/data-reporting/egpyt/gshs/egypt-gshs-fs-2011.pdf?sfvrsn=faf83394_2&download=true. Accessed July 15, 2022.
26. Global School-based Student Health Survey, Fiji Islands, 2016, Fact Sheet. https://cdn.who.int/media/docs/default-source/ncds/ncd-surveillance/data-reporting/fiji/gshs/gshs-fs-fiji-2016.pdf?sfvrsn=943e4d7a_3&download=true. Accessed July 15, 2022.
27. Global School-based Student Health Survey, French Polynesia, 2015, Fact Sheet. https://cdn.who.int/media/docs/default-source/ncds/ncd-surveillance/data-reporting/french-polynesia/gshs/gshs-fs-french-polynesia-2015.pdf?sfvrsn=db458dd8_3&download=true. Accessed July 15, 2022.

28. Global School-based Student Health Survey, Guatemala, 2015, Fact Sheet. https://cdn.who.int/media/docs/default-source/ncds/ncd-surveillance/data-reporting/guatemala/gshs/gshs_fs_guatemala_2015.pdf?sfvrsn=6ddea764_5&download=true. Accessed July 15, 2022.
29. Global School-based Student Health Survey, Lebanon, 2017, Report. https://www.moph.gov.lb/userfiles/files/GSHS_Report_2017.pdf. Accessed July 15, 2022.
30. Global School-based Student Health Survey, Malaysia, 2012, Fact Sheet. https://cdn.who.int/media/docs/default-source/ncds/ncd-surveillance/data-reporting/malaysia/gshs/malaysia-2012-gshs-fs-national.pdf?sfvrsn=56e59de7_3&download=true. Accessed July 15, 2022.
31. Global School-based Student Health Survey, Maldives, 2014, Fact Sheet. https://cdn.who.int/media/docs/default-source/ncds/ncd-surveillance/data-reporting/maldives/gshs/2014-maldives-gshs-fs.pdf?sfvrsn=392d9a2e_2&download=true. Accessed July 15, 2022.
32. Global School-based Student Health Survey, Mauritania, 2010, Fact Sheet. https://cdn.who.int/media/docs/default-source/ncds/ncd-surveillance/data-reporting/mauritania/gshs/mauritania-2010-gshs-fs.pdf?sfvrsn=21337d1a_2&download=true. Accessed July 15, 2022.
33. Global School-based Student Health Survey, Mauritius, 2017, Fact Sheet. https://cdn.who.int/media/docs/default-source/ncds/ncd-surveillance/data-reporting/mauritius/gshs/mauritius-2017-gshs-fs.pdf?sfvrsn=9cff0522_2&download=true. Accessed July 15, 2022.
34. Global School-based Student Health Survey, Mongolia, 2013, Fact Sheet. file:///C:/Users/jsrab/Downloads/2013_Mongolia_GSHS_Fact_Sheet.pdf. Accessed July 15, 2022.
35. Global School-based Student Health Survey, Morocco, 2016, Fact Sheet. https://cdn.who.int/media/docs/default-source/ncds/ncd-surveillance/data-reporting/morocco/gshs/morocco-2016-gshs-fs.pdf?sfvrsn=737818ae_3&download=true. Accessed July 15, 2022.
36. Global School-based Student Health Survey, Mozambique, 2015, Fact Sheet. https://cdn.who.int/media/docs/default-source/ncds/ncd-surveillance/data-reporting/mozambique/gshs/gshs-fs-mozambique-2015.pdf?sfvrsn=8f6d1733_2&download=true. Accessed July 15, 2022.
37. Global School-based Student Health Survey, Niue, 2010, Fact Sheet. https://cdn.who.int/media/docs/default-source/ncds/ncd-surveillance/data-reporting/niue/gshs/niue-gshs-fs-2010.pdf?sfvrsn=6103a6a5_2&download=true. Accessed July 15, 2022.
38. Global School-based Student Health Survey, Oman, 2015, Fact Sheet. https://cdn.who.int/media/docs/default-source/ncds/ncd-surveillance/data-reporting/oman/gshs/2015-oman-gshs-fact-sheet.pdf?sfvrsn=f8f56471_2&download=true. Accessed July 15, 2022.
39. Global School-based Student Health Survey, Philippines, 2019, Fact Sheet. https://cdn.who.int/media/docs/default-source/ncds/ncd-surveillance/data-reporting/philippines/2019-philippines-fact-sheet.pdf?sfvrsn=7e3888af_1&download=true. Accessed July 17, 2022.
40. Global School-based Student Health Survey, Samoa, 2011, Fact Sheet. https://cdn.who.int/media/docs/default-source/ncds/ncd-surveillance/data-reporting/samoa/gshs/samoa-2011-gshs-fs.pdf?sfvrsn=92caa54b_2&download=true. Accessed July 17, 2022.
41. Global School-based Student Health Survey, Swaziland, 2013, Fact Sheet. https://cdn.who.int/media/docs/default-source/ncds/ncd-surveillance/data-reporting/eswatini/gshs/2013-swaziland-gshs-fs.pdf?sfvrsn=a3557f63_2&download=true. Accessed July 17, 2022.
42. Global School-based Student Health Survey, Tanzania, 2014, Fact Sheet. https://cdn.who.int/media/docs/default-source/ncds/ncd-surveillance/data-reporting/united-republic-of-tanzania/gshs/2014_tanzania_gshs_fact_sheet.pdf?sfvrsn=a66324b7_3&download=true. Accessed July 17, 2022.

43. Global School-based Student Health Survey, Tokelau, 2014, Fact Sheet. https://cdn.who.int/media/docs/default-source/ncds/ncd-surveillance/data-reporting/tokelau/gshs/2014-gshs-tokelau-fact-sheet.pdf?sfvrsn=700e47af_2&download=true. Accessed July 17, 2022.
44. Global School-based Student Health Survey, Tonga, 2010, Fact Sheet. https://cdn.who.int/media/docs/default-source/ncds/ncd-surveillance/data-reporting/tonga/gshs/2010-gshs-fs-tonga.pdf?sfvrsn=f4b5a57f_2&download=true. Accessed July 17, 2022.
45. Global School-based Student Health Survey, Trinidad and Tobago, 2017, Fact Sheet. https://cdn.who.int/media/docs/default-source/ncds/ncd-surveillance/data-reporting/trinidad-and-tobago/gshs/trinidad_and_tobago__trinidad_2017_gshs_fs.pdf?sfvrsn=5e5f4895_5&download=true. Accessed July 17, 2022.
46. Global School-based Student Health Survey, United Arab Emirates, 2016, Fact Sheet. https://cdn.who.int/media/docs/default-source/ncds/ncd-surveillance/data-reporting/united-arab-emirates/gshs/uae-2016-gshs-fact-sheet.pdf?sfvrsn=7ac30a41_3. Accessed July 17, 2022.
47. Global School-based Student Health Survey, Vanuatu, 2011, Fact Sheet. https://cdn.who.int/media/docs/default-source/ncds/ncd-surveillance/data-reporting/vanuatu/gshs/vanuatu-2011-gshs-fs.pdf?sfvrsn=cfc090da_4&download=true. Accessed July 17, 2022.
48. Global School-based Student Health Survey, Vietnam, 2013, Fact Sheet. https://cdn.who.int/media/docs/default-source/ncds/ncd-surveillance/data-reporting/viet-nam/gshs/2013-gshs-viet-nam-fact-sheet.pdf?sfvrsn=dd133dd1_2&download=true. Accessed July 17, 2022.
49. Global School-based Student Health Survey, West Bank, 2010, Fact Sheet. https://cdn.who.int/media/docs/default-source/ncds/ncd-surveillance/palestine/opt_west_bank_gshs_fs_2010.pdf?sfvrsn=8696fe1f_1&download=true. Accessed July 17, 2022.
50. Second online frequency analysis of data from Iannotti RJ. *Health Behavior in School-Aged Children (HBSC), 2009–2010. ICPSR34792-v1*. Ann Arbor, MI: Inter-university Consortium for Political and Social Research [distributor], November 20, 2013. https://www.icpsr.umich.edu/icpsrweb/NAHDAP/studies/34792. Accessed July 22, 2022.
51. Data from the 2019 Youth Risk Behavior Surveillance System (YRBSS), which includes national, state, territorial, tribal government, and local school-based surveys of representative samples of students in the ninth through twelfth grades in the United States. The surveys, conducted by departments of health and education, provide data representative of mostly public high school students in each jurisdiction. Among the several health risk behaviors surveyed, the students were asked about having been bullied in the previous 12 months on school property, having been bullied electronically (being bullied through e-mail, chat rooms, instant messaging, websites, or texting), or having been subjected to physical or sexual violence in a dating relationship. Overview of the YRBSS can be found at https://www.cdc.gov/healthyyouth/data/yrbs/overview.htm. Accessed October 13, 2023. Access to respective online analyses of the questions of being bullied on school property, being electronically bullied, and/or suffering from physical or sexual dating violence at all locations in 2019 can be found at the Centers for Disease Control, High School YRBS, Unintentional Injuries and Violence, Behaviors that Contribute to Violence, https://nccd.cdc.gov/youthonline/App/QuestionsOrLocations.aspx?CategoryId=C01.
52. Centers for Disease Control and Prevention (CDC). 1991–2019 High School Youth Risk Behavior Survey Data. http://yrbs-explorer.services.cdc.gov/. Accessed July 22, 2022.
53. Earnshaw VA, Bogart LM, Poteat VP, Reisner SL, Schuster MA. Bullying among lesbian, gay, bisexual, and transgender youth. *Pediatr Clin North Am*. 2016;63(6):999–1010.

54. Coulter RW, Herrick AL, Friedman MR, Stall RD. Sexual-orientation differences in positive youth development: the mediational role of bullying victimization. *Am J Public Health.* 2016;106(4):691–697.
55. Bouris A, Everett BG, Heath RD, Elsaesser CE, Neilands TB. Effects of victimization and violence on suicidal ideation and behaviors among sexual minority and heterosexual adolescents. *LGBT Health.* 2016;3(2):153–161.
56. Schuster MA, Bogart LM, Elliott MN, et al. A longitudinal study of bullying of sexual-minority youth. *N Engl J Med.* 2015;372(19):1872–1874.
57. Andersen JP, Zou C, Blosnich J. Multiple early victimization experiences as a pathway to explain physical health disparities among sexual minority and heterosexual individuals. *Soc Sci Med.* 2015;133:111–119.
58. Mueller AS, James W, Abrutyn S, Levin ML. Suicide ideation and bullying among US adolescents: examining the intersections of sexual orientation, gender, and race/ethnicity. *Am J Public Health.* 2015;105(5):980–985.
59. O'Malley Olsen E, Kann L, Vivolo-Kantor A, Kinchen S, McManus T. School violence and bullying among sexual minority high school students, 2009–2011. *J Adolesc Health.* 2014;55(3):432–438.
60. Patrick DL, Bell JF, Huang JY, Lazarakis NC, Edwards TC. Bullying and quality of life in youths perceived as gay, lesbian, or bisexual in Washington State, 2010. *Am J Public Health.* 2013;103(7):1255–1261.
61. Wensley K, Campbell M. Heterosexual and non-heterosexual young university students' involvement in traditional and cyber forms of bullying. *Cyberpsychol Behav Soc Netw.* 2012;15(12):649–654.
62. Russell ST, Ryan C, Toomey RB, Diaz RM, Sanchez J. Lesbian, gay, bisexual, and transgender adolescent school victimization: implications for young adult health and adjustment. *J Sch Health.* 2011;81(5):223–230.
63. Berlan ED, Corliss HL, Field AE, Goodman E, Austin SB. Sexual orientation and bullying among adolescents in the Growing Up Today Study. *J Adolesc Health.* 2010;46(4):366–371.
64. Roberts AL, Rosario M, Slopen N, Calzo JP, Austin SB. Childhood gender nonconformity, bullying victimization, and depressive symptoms across adolescence and early adulthood: an 11-year longitudinal study. *J Am Acad Child Adolesc Psychiatry.* 2013;52(2):143–152.
65. Semenyna SW, Vasey PL. Bullying, physical aggression, gender-atypicality, and sexual orientation in Samoan males. *Arch Sex Behav.* 2017;46:1375–1381.
66. Hansen KL, Melhus M, Høgmo A, Lund E. Ethnic discrimination and bullying in the Sami and non-Sami populations in Norway: the SAMINOR study. *Int J Circumpolar Health.* 2008;67(1):97–113.
67. Eriksen AM, Hansen KL, Javo C, Schei B. Emotional, physical and sexual violence among Sami and non-Sami populations in Norway: The SAMINOR 2 questionnaire study. *Scand J Public Health.* 2015;43(6):588–596.
68. Lemstra M, Rogers M, Redgate L, Garner M, Moraros J. Prevalence, risk indicators and outcomes of bullying among on-reserve First Nations youth. *Can J Public Health.* 2011;102(6):462–466.
69. Lemstra ME, Nielsen G, Rogers MR, Thompson AT, Moraros JS. Risk indicators and outcomes associated with bullying in youth aged 9–15 years. *Can J Public Health.* 2012;103(1):9–13. Cited in Lemstra et al.[35]

70. Crengle S, Robinson E, Ameratunga S, Clark T, Raphael D. Ethnic discrimination prevalence and associations with health outcomes: data from a nationally representative cross-sectional survey of secondary school students in New Zealand. *BMC Public Health.* 2012;12:45.
71. Priest N, King T, Bécares L, Kavanagh AM. Bullying victimization and racial discrimination among Australian children. *Am J Public Health.* 2016;106(10):1882–1884.
72. Maynard BR, Vaughn MG, Salas-Wright CP, Vaughn S. Bullying victimization among school-aged immigrant youth in the United States. *J Adolesc Health.* 2016;58(3):337–344.
73. For the purpose of this section, the terms *foreign born* and *immigrant* are used interchangeably. Yet, we need to recognize that the notion of "foreign born" is established and reflects a system of citizenship. Consequently, in a country like the United States, where citizenship is attained by birth (i.e., birthright citizenship—*jus soli*), the term *foreign persons* refers to all foreign-born residents in the population and includes both naturalized citizens and noncitizens. Conversely, in countries like Germany, where citizenship is acquired by ancestry or "blood" (*jus sanguinis*), a foreign person is either a foreign-born or native-born person who is not of German descent (see Note 40). See Grieco, E. *Defining 'foreign born' and 'foreigner' in international migration statistics.* Migration Information Source, July 1, 2002. Washington, DC: Migration Policy Institute. https://www.migrationpolicy.org/article/defining-foreign-born-and-foreigner-international-migration-statistics/. Accessed July 24, 2022.
74. "The distinction between urban and rural population is not amenable to a single definition applicable to all countries." Population Density and Urbanization, United Nations Statistics Division. https://unstats.un.org/unsd/demographic/sconcerns/densurb/densurbmethods.htm. Accessed July 24, 2022.
75. What is defined by the term *urban* varies between counties. In the United States, an urban area is an "agglomeration of 2,500 or more inhabitants, generally having population densities of 1,000 persons per square mile or more." In Canada, an urban area is a place of "1,000 or more inhabitants, having a population density of 400 or more per square kilometer." For details about each country, see United Nations, *2015 Demographic Yearbook*, definition of Urban, pages 118–122. https://unstats.un.org/unsd/demographic-social/products/dyb/dybsets/2015.pdf. Accessed July 24, 2022.
76. Garmy P, Vilhjalmsson R, Kristjánsdóttir G. Bullying in school-aged children in Iceland: a cross-sectional study. *J Pediatr Nurs.* 2018;38:e30–e34.
77. Låftman SB, Fransson E, Modin B, Östberg V. National data study showed that adolescents living in poorer households and with one parent were more likely to be bullied. *Acta Paediatr.* 2017;106(12):2048–2054.
78. Johns MM, Lowry R, Demissie Z, Robin L. Harassment and mental distress among adolescent female students by sexual identity and BMI or perceived weight status. *Obesity.* 2017;25(8):1421–1427.
79. Oliveira WA, Silva MA, Mello FC, Porto DL, Yoshinaga AC, Malta DC. The causes of bullying: results from the National Survey of School Health (PeNSE). *Rev Lat Am Enfermagem.* 2015;23(2):275–282.
80. Al-Bitar ZB, Al-Omari IK, Sonbol HN, Al-Ahmad HT, Cunningham SJ. Bullying among Jordanian schoolchildren, its effects on school performance, and the contribution of general physical and dentofacial features. *Am J Orthod Dentofacial Orthop.* 2013;144(6):872–878.

81. Mayes SD, Calhoun SL, Baweja R, Mahr F. Maternal ratings of bullying and victimization: differences in frequencies between psychiatric diagnoses in a large sample of children. *Psychol Rep*. 2015;116(3):710–722.
82. Pfeffer RD. Childhood victimization in a national sample of youth with autism spectrum disorders. *J Policy Pract Intellect Disabil*. 2016;13(4):311–319.
83. Based on the findings of the HBSC survey conducted in 2017–2018 among 227,441 students (age 11–15) living in 45 countries and regions. Among the 20 areas of health behaviors surveyed, the students were asked about having been cyberbullied at least once in the previous two months. An average for country prevalence of bullying was calculated based on data for girls and boys age 11, 13, and 15 found at: Inchley J, Currie D, Budisavljevic S, et al., eds. *Spotlight on Adolescent Health and Well-being. Findings from the 2017/2018 Health Behavior in School-aged Children (HBSC) Survey in Europe and Canada. International Report*. Vol 2. *Key Data*. Copenhagen, Denmark: WHO Regional Office for Europe; 2020:102–103. License: CC BY-NC-SA 3.0 IGO, Bullying. https://apps.who.int/iris/bitstream/handle/10665/332091/9789289055000-eng.pdf. Accessed July 22, 2022.
84. European Foundation for the Improvement of Living and Working Conditions (Eurofound). *European Working Conditions Survey 2010*. https://www.researchgate.net/publication/281645178_5th_EWCS_overview_report. Accessed October 13, 2023.
85. Namie G. *WBI U.S. Workplace Bullying Survey*. The Fifth National Scientific WBI Study, Zogby Analytics, Pollster, Workplace Bullying Institute. 2021. https://workplacebullying.org/wp-content/uploads/2021/04/2021-Full-Report.pdf. Accessed July 25, 2022.
86. Zogby Analytics. About the Zogby Poll®. https://zogbyanalytics.com/about-us. Accessed July 25, 2022.
87. Workplace Bullying Institute. https://workplacebullying.org/. Accessed July 25, 2022.
88. Namie G, Christensen D, Phillips D. *WBI U.S. Workplace Bullying Survey*. Workplace Bullying Institute; 2014. http://workplacebullying.org/multi/pdf/WBI-2014-US-Survey.pdf. Accessed July 25, 2022.
89. Bergbom B, Vartia-Vaananen M, Kinnunen U. Immigrants and natives at work: exposure to workplace bullying. *Employee Relat*. 2015;37(2):158–175.

3
Polyvictimization and Revictimization

What Is Known?

A key epidemiologic aspect of evaluating patients who have been victimized[1] is the finding that they are likely to have been repeatedly exposed in their lifetime to the same and/or different types of maltreatment. This means we need to examine both revictimization and polyvictimization, as well as to review what is known about their epidemiology and health consequences.

The following composite[2] vignette provides a clinical framework for the discussion.

Composite Clinical Vignette

A psychiatric consultation was requested by a primary care physician on behalf of a young adult female patient who was recently suffering frequent tension headaches, possibly associated with significant stress at her workplace.

Present Medical and Psychiatric History

For the previous three months, the patient had been experiencing daily frontal headaches without any proven organic etiology, as well as intermittent depression with vague suicidal ideation, significant irritability, marked anxiety, occasional episodes of panic attacks, initial and middle insomnia, nightmares, flashbacks, auditory hallucinations of derogatory comments, hyper-alertness, and progressive inattention to detail. The symptoms were associated with episodic alcohol abuse, smoking 20 cigarettes per day, frequent absenteeism, and a decline in her work performance.

Past Medical and Psychiatric History

Episodes of Acute and Frequent Symptoms

At age 7, the patient required five months of individual therapy to treat significant daily anxiety, irritability, nightmares, and abdominal pain without organic etiology.

When the patient was 12 years old, she experienced daily depression with suicidal ideation, marked irritability, difficulties in falling and staying asleep, frequent headaches, and a decline in academic performance, requiring six months of individual therapy.

At age 15, the patient was hospitalized for five days after a suicide attempt. She also experienced mood swings, marked irritability linked to self-injuries, significant middle insomnia, nightmares, flashbacks, panic attacks, daily smoking, episodic alcohol abuse, significant weight gain, episodes of running away, and academic decline.

At age 18, the patient experienced three months of daily depression, vague suicidal ideation, irritability, anxiety, initial insomnia, decline in academic performance, and dropping out of her first year of tertiary education.

Occurrence of Chronic and Occasional Symptoms

The patient had a long history of intermittent, brief, mild irritability, sadness, and/or anxiety, at least once a week, occurring before and after the past four episodes of acute and frequent symptoms.

Exposure to Victimization

Present Experience with Victimization

For the three months preceding this evaluation, the patient had been subjected to workplace bullying by her immediate supervisor. This maltreatment was characterized by being given tasks above her skill level with unreasonable deadlines, having her opinions and contributions ignored, being subjected to negative comments about her skills and performance, being treated with sarcasm, being reprimanded in front of others, and being given hints to quit her job.

A colleague recently subjected the patient to mocking and disrespectful gestures, spread rumors about her, intimidated her, and threatened her with harm. The patient's complaints to her employer's personnel department remained unresolved.

Past Exposure to Different Types of Victimization

At age 5, the patient escaped, with her mother and older brother, from criminal violence in her native country and sought refuge in the United States. During the perilous journey to the United States, they were subjected to threats, intimidation, and neglect by the people smuggling them across the border.

The patient's father had sought refuge in the United States two years earlier, escaping kidnapping and torture.

Throughout her childhood, the patient was exposed to frequent loud arguments between her parents, with mutual name-calling and constant criticism. Her parents resorted to "reasonable corporal punishment" by moderate spanking on the buttocks to deal with their children's behavioral problems. For many years, the patient was poked, teased, and frightened with scary stories by her older brother.

In second grade (age 7), the patient experienced frequent school bullying: she was excluded by her peers, who often subjected her to racial slurs. She was involved in some physical fights with classmates and some verbal arguments with teachers, leading to in-school suspension and corporal punishment.

In seventh grade (age 12), she was frequently teased in school about her shyness, being thin, being short, wearing glasses, and having crooked teeth. Once she was told by a classmate that she was a loser and she should kill herself. While running away from peers who were threatening her, she fell and hurt her head.

At age 15 (tenth grade), while she was dating a classmate, she experienced intimate partner violence (IPV), characterized by feeling controlled by her boyfriend: he told her what to wear, he didn't let her hang out with her friends, he had to be with her all the time, and he was very jealous. During arguments, the pair called each other names and occasionally threatened to hurt themselves and/or each other.

At age 18, while in college, the patient was sexually assaulted during a date. The assault was reported, but the investigation could not sustain the allegation. A month later, messages were placed on Facebook calling the patient a "fat slut." During that period, she was subjected to frequent teasing and harassment by her college roommate.

This clinical vignette not only illustrates the frequent symptoms and psychosocial risks associated with exposure to bullying and other forms of maltreatment (discussed further in Chapters 4 and 5), but also, above all, highlights how polyvictimization and revictimization can occur in the life of a patient (Table 3.1).

Definition and Epidemiology of Polyvictimization

The notion that children and adults are prone to be exposed to multiple types of victimization was advanced by several studies[3-7] published in the 1990s and reviewed by Saunders[8] in 2003. The concept of polyvictimization and its prevalence in youth were outlined and highlighted by Finkelhor et al[9] in a pivotal longitudinal study conducted during 2002–2004. The research[9] was conducted using a nationally representative sample of 2,030 children and adolescents (2 to 17 years old) living in the United States, and was based on a survey via the Juvenile Victimization Questionnaire (JVQ),[10] which covers 34 forms of offenses against youth.[11] The study documented that 22% of the participants were polyvictims, defined "as children who experienced four or more types of victimization in one year."[9] Among the whole sample, 15% were categorized as "low polyvictims" (exposed to four to six victimizations in one year), while 7% of the participants were labeled "high polyvictims" (subjected to seven or more victimizations in one year).[9] Compared to nonvictimized participants, low polyvictims had a higher percentage of males (65% vs. 45%), were older (mean age 11 years vs. 9 years old), and were more likely to live in larger cities (22% vs. 13%). The high polyvictims, in contrast to children who were not victimized, were more likely to be black (22% vs. 15%), to come from a lower economic status (36% vs. 19%), and to reside in a one-parent household (36% vs. 18%).[9] Polyvictimization occurred very frequently (90% or more) among children who experienced a sexual assault by a peer, an attempted or completed rape, or a sexual exposure, while polyvictimization occurred less frequently (< 50%) among those suffering from bullying or assault by peers or siblings.[9]

Table 3.1. Exposure to Similar or Different Types of Victimization, by Age of Occurrence

Age of Occurrence	Domestic Violence	Corporal Punishment	Sibling Bullying	School Bullying	Cyberbullying	Intimate Partner Violence	Workplace Bullying	Community Violence
5 years old or younger	✓	✓	✓					✓
7 years old	✓	✓	✓	✓				
12 years old	✓	✓	✓	✓				
15 years old	✓		✓			✓		
18 years old	✓		✓	✓	✓	✓		
24 years old							✓	

Table 3.2. Lifetime Prevalence of Polyvictimization: Comparison among Countries

Country	Study	Sample (N) Age	Lifetime Prevalence of Polyvictimization
United States	Finkelhor et al[12]	N = 1,467	10.66%*
Canada	Cyr et al[13]	N = 2,801 2–17 years old	9.0%*
Chile	Pinto-Cortez et al[14]	N = 718 17–28 years old	14.7%*
China	Chan[15]	N = 18,341 15–17 years old	14.0%**
Spain	Pereda et al[16]	N = 1,107 12–17 years old	7.9%*
Vietnam	Le et al[17]	N = 1,606 Mean age, 16.5 years	14.6 %***

*Percentage of participants with number of victimizations in the top 10th percentile.

** Percentage of participants with four types of victimization or more.

***Percentage of participants with the highest number of victimizations (15 or more).

A subsequent study by Finkelhor et al[12] ascertained the lifetime prevalence of polyvictimization in a national sample of 1,467 children (2 to 17 years old), by analyzing data from the second wave of their two-year longitudinal research,[9] which combined information about both past-year and lifetime victimization, yielding a total lifetime measurement. The investigators found that close to 80% of the participants reported at least one victimization in their lifetime, with 3.7 being the mean number of episodes of victimization reported by the participants.[12] In the context of this study,[12] polyvictims were defined as the 10% of the children and adolescents with the highest victimization score, while different thresholds were calculated by age group. The research[12] documented that an average of 10.66% of the children and adolescents participating in the study met the threshold score of polyvictimization, which ranged from nine or more episodes of maltreatment for children 6 years old or younger to a tally of 15 or more reported incidents of victimization for adolescents age 15 or older.

Following Finkelhor's research,[12] several other studies in different countries[13-17] have used the JVQ and have found lifetime prevalence of polyvictimization ranging from ~ 8.0% in Spain[16] to nearly 15.0% in Chile[14] and Vietnam[17] (Table 3.2).

Definition and Epidemiology of Revictimization

A report[18] derived from Finkelhor's two-year longitudinal study[9] underscored the notion of revictimization by showing a substantial persistence of victimization over two years: 66% of youth experiencing peer or sibling victimization in the first year were revictimized in the following year. In fact, young people who were exposed to a single type of victimization in the first year of the study had a significant possibility of suffering the same kind of maltreatment during the second year, with relative risk ratios fluctuating from 2.2 for peer or sibling victimization to 6.9 for sexual victimization.[18] Furthermore, the research[18] also demonstrated that one kind of victimization occurring in the first year of the study was associated with increased risk of another type of victimization happening in the second year, as exemplified by peer or sibling victimization occurring in the first year being associated with a 3.2 relative risk of sexual victimization in the following year.[18] Moreover, polyvictimization reported in the first year of the survey was shown to be significantly associated (risk ratio = 5.1) with recurrence in the second year, and it was 6.8 times as likely to be linked with sexual victimization in the subsequent year.[13] In the first year of the study, the most significant variables found to be associated with repeated polyvictimization in the second year were: witnessing nonfamily victimization, the experience of anger/aggression, moving to a worse neighborhood, and experiencing physical assault or property crime.[18]

The epidemiology of women's revictimization was examined by Kimerling et al[19] in a population-based sample of 11,056 adult women who participated in the 2002–2004 California Women's Health Survey. The research[19] documented that, among women who were subjected to any type of childhood violence, the frequency of adult victimization was 50.2%, compared to only 14% among women who did not report childhood violence. More specifically, the study[19] showed that women who experienced any childhood violence (physical or sexual) were 5.5 times more likely to experience physical assault as an adult and 4.7 times more likely to be subjected to adult sexual assault, even after adjusting for age, ethnicity, education, and poverty.

Further support for the finding that childhood victimization is significantly associated with lifetime revictimization was provided by Widom et al[20] through a prospective cohort study. Individuals with exposure to childhood physical and sexual abuse and neglect during the years 1967 to 1971, along with a matched control group, were interviewed in person in 2000–2002 and were assessed using the Lifetime Trauma and Victimization History.[21] The Widom study[20] showed that individuals who experienced childhood victimization were at a significantly higher risk than controls of being subsequently physically harmed (OR = 2.14) or kidnapped (OR = 2.10), witnessing somebody else being sexually attacked (OR = 3.22), being coerced into unwanted sex (OR = 2.64), or being assaulted with a weapon (OR = 2.01).[20]

The prevalence of revictimization in a clinical population was brought to light by Faergemann et al[22] in a population study at the Odense Municipality in Denmark. The study included all victims of violence treated at the open-access Emergency Department at Odense University Hospital or subjected to medicolegal autopsy at the Institute of Forensic Medicine, University of Southern Denmark, during 1991 to 2001. During the 12 years, there were a total of 14,307 incidents involving 10,216 different people, of whom 22% were repeat victims, who accounted for 44% of all contacts with the Emergency Department and/or the Institute of Forensic Medicine during that period, with a median number of two clinical contacts.

Health Impact of Polyvictimization

Turner et al[23] studied the association between lifetime polyvictimization and trauma symptoms, such as anger, depression, anxiety, and dissociation, through a survey of a nationally representative sample of 4,053 children and adolescents 2 to 17 years old and their caregivers. The participants were assessed using the JVQ[10] and the Trauma Symptom Checklist for

Children (age 10–17 years; TSCC)[24] or Trauma Symptom Checklist for Young Children (age 2–9 years; TSCYC).[25] The study[23] documented an almost linear increment in symptoms with each additional exposure to different victimization types. At the level of 11 victimizations, which delineated the lower margin of the "serious polyvictim group,"[23] the intensity of symptomatology became markedly high, ranging from 1.25 to 2 SDs above the sample mean.[23]

An investigation conducted by Chan[15] to ascertain the association between victimization and health outcomes among a sample of 18,341 Chinese adolescents (age 15 to 17) showed that polyvictims, defined as youth having been subjected to four or more victimizations during their lifetime, were significantly more likely to report posttraumatic stress disorder (PTSD), depression, deliberate self-harm, suicidal ideation, and poorer health quality of life than nonvictims as well as victims of one to three types of violence.[15]

The association of polyvictimization with psychiatric symptoms, diagnoses, and impairment in a clinical population was investigated by Ford et al[26] through a chart review of 295 child psychiatric outpatient admissions at the University of Connecticut Health Center from 2007 to 2009, with the cases closed by 2010. Polyvictimization was found to be significantly associated with a diagnosis of PTSD (OR = 11.77); severe delinquent and aggressive behaviors (OR = 5.93), as established by the Child Behavior Checklist[27]; and a marked to severe psychiatric impairment (OR = 4.57), as determined by the Clinical Global Impressions Severity Score.[28]

Baldwin et al[29] conducted a genetically sensitive cohort study of 2,232 children followed from birth to 18 years of age, as part of the Environmental Risk Longitudinal Twin Study,[30] to further understand the role of childhood victimization as a risk factor for elevated inflammation biomarkers in young adulthood. Their research[29] demonstrated that, at age 18, females who were polyvictimized in childhood (exposed to two or more victimizations) had significantly higher serum levels (1.19) of C-reactive protein (CRP) than nonvictimized females (0.75), while no significant association was found in male polyvictims. The significant link between polyvictimization during childhood among females and elevated adult CRP levels was found to be independent of latent genetic influence, childhood socioeconomic status, waist–hip ratio, and body temperature at the time of CRP evaluation.[29]

Health Impact of Revictimization

The significant link between psychological distress and women's revictimization has been highlighted by Kimerling et al,[31] who analyzed data from the 2002–2004 California Women's Health Survey and documented that, compared to women who were never victimized, women who reported revictimization (exposure to violence in both childhood and adulthood) were more likely to experience anxiety [adjusted OR (AOR) = 3.1], depression (AOR = 3.4), and, above all, PTSD (AOR = 12.4).[31] This study supported the previous body of research evidence showing the cumulative psychological effect of revictimization.[32-37]

Future Directions

There is a need for further research on global and regional differences in the lifetime prevalence of polyvictimization and revictimization and their impact on physical and mental health. In this context, future studies should continue the research trajectory established by

Finkelhor et al[3,9,18] by surveying nonclinical national or regional population-based samples of children, adolescents, and adults, as well as clinical populations being evaluated at emergency departments and inpatient or outpatient psychiatric units. The experience of polyvictimization or revictimization and its associated cumulative effect should be taken into consideration and included in the assessment and anamnesis of any person seeking psychiatric treatment.

Notes

1. Since 2000, the author has clinically evaluated and treated more than 1,500 children, adolescents, and adults exposed to bullying and other forms of victimization. This clinical service was respectively provided at a pediatric hospital-based child and adolescent outpatient psychiatric clinic as well as at a local government clinic for victims of crimes.
2. Based on a composite of many clinical evaluations (see Note 1).
3. Finkelhor D, Dziuba-Leatherman J. Children as victims of violence: A national survey. *Pediatrics*. 1994;94(4):413–420. Cited by Saunders (see Note 8).
4. Kilpatrick DG, Saunders BE. Prevalence and consequences of child victimization: results from the National Survey of Adolescents. Final report (NIJ Grant 93-IG-CX-0023). Charleston, SC: Author; 1999. Cited by Saunders (see Note 8).
5. Green BL, Goodman LA, Krupnick JL, et al. Outcomes of single versus multiple trauma exposure in a screening sample. *J Trauma Stress*. 2000;13(2):271–286. Cited by Saunders (see Note 8).
6. Kessler RC, Sonnega A, Bromet E, Hughes M, Nelson CB. Posttraumatic stress disorder in the National Comorbidity Survey. *Arch Gen Psychiatry*. 1995;52(12):1048–1060. Cited by Saunders (see Note 8).
7. Resnick HS, Kilpatrick DG, Dansky BS, Saunders BE, Best CL. Prevalence of civilian trauma and posttraumatic stress disorder in a representative national sample of women. *J Consult Clin Psychol*. 1993;61(6):984–991. Cited by Saunders (see Note 8).
8. Saunders BE. Understanding children exposed to violence: toward an integration of overlapping fields. *J Interpers Violence*. 2003;18(4):356–376.
9. Finkelhor D, Ormrod RK, Turner HA. Polyvictimization and trauma in a national longitudinal cohort. *Dev Psychopathol*. 2007;19(1):149–166.
10. Hamby SL, Finkelhor D, Ormrod R, Turner H. *The Juvenile Victimization Questionnaire (JVQ): Administration and Scoring Manual*. Durham, NH: Crimes Against Children Research Center; 2005. https://www.unh.edu/ccrc/sites/default/files/media/2022-02/the-juvenile-victimization-questionnaire-jvq-administration-scoring-manual.pdf. Accessed February 13, 2022.
11. "The JVQ obtains reports on 34 forms of offenses against youth that cover five general areas of concern: Conventional Crime, Child Maltreatment, Peer and Sibling Victimization, Sexual Assault, and Witnessing and Indirect Victimization."[10]
12. Finkelhor D, Ormrod RK, Turner HA. Lifetime assessment of poly-victimization in a national sample of children and youth. *Child Abuse Negl*. 2009;33(7):403–411.
13. Cyr K, Chamberland C, Clément MÈ, et al. Polyvictimization and victimization of children and youth: results from a population survey. *Child Abuse Negl*. 2013;37(10):814–820.
14. Pinto-Cortez C, Gutiérrez-Echegoyen P, Henríquez D. Child victimization and polyvictimization among young adults in northern Chile. *J Interpers Violence*. 2018:0886260518759058.

15. Chan KL. Victimization and poly-victimization among school-aged Chinese adolescents: prevalence and associations with health. *Prev Med.* 2013;56(3-4):207–210.
16. Pereda N, Guilera G, Abad J. Victimization and polyvictimization of Spanish children and youth: results from a community sample. *Child Abuse Negl.* 2014;38(4):640–649.
17. Le MT, Holton S, Nguyen HT, Wolfe R, Fisher J. Poly-victimization among Vietnamese high school students: prevalence and demographic correlates. *PLOS One.* 2015;10(5):e0125189.
18. Finkelhor D, Ormrod RK, Turner HA. Re-victimization patterns in a national longitudinal sample of children and youth. *Child Abuse Negl.* 2007;31(5):479–502.
19. Kimerling R, Alvarez J, Pavao J, Kaminski A, Baumrind N. Epidemiology and consequences of women's revictimization. *Womens Health Issues.* 2007;17(2):101–106.
20. Widom CS, Czaja SJ, Dutton MA. Childhood victimization and lifetime revictimization. *Child Abuse Negl.* 2008;32(8):785–796.
21. Widom CS, Dutton MA, Czaja SJ, DuMont KA. The development and validation of a new instrument to assess lifetime trauma and victimization history. *J Trauma Stress.* 2005;18(5):519–532. Cited by Widom et al.[20]
22. Faergemann C, Lauritsen JM, Brink O, Stovring H. The epidemiology of repeat contacts with an emergency department or an institute of forensic medicine due to violent victimization in a Danish urban population. *J Forensic Leg Med.* 2007;14(6):333–339.
23. Turner HA, Finkelhor D, Ormrod R. Poly-victimization in a national sample of children and youth. *Am J Prev Med.* 2010;38(3):323–330.
24. Briere J. *Trauma Symptom Checklist for Children.* Odessa, FL: Psychological Assessment Resources; 1996:00253–8.
25. Briere J, Johnson K, Bissada A, et al. The Trauma Symptom Checklist for Young Children (TSCYC): reliability and association with abuse exposure in a multi-site study. *Child Abuse Negl.* 2001;25(8):1001–1014.
26. Ford JD, Wasser T, Connor DF. Identifying and determining the symptom severity associated with polyvictimization among psychiatrically impaired children in the outpatient setting. *Child Maltreat.* 2011;16(3):216–226.
27. Achenbach TM. *Manual for the Child Behavior Checklist/4-18.* Burlington, VT: University Associates in Psychiatry; 1991. Cited by Ford et al.[26]
28. Guy W. *Assessment Manual for Psychopharmacology.* Washington, DC: US Department of Health, Education and Welfare; 1976. Cited by Ford et al.[26]
29. Baldwin JR, Arseneault L, Caspi A, et al. Childhood victimization and inflammation in young adulthood: a genetically sensitive cohort study. *Brain Behav Immun.* 2018;67:211–217.
30. Trouton A, Spinath FM, Plomin R. Twins Early Development Study (TEDS): a multivariate, longitudinal genetic investigation of language, cognition, and behavior problems in childhood. *Twin Res Hum Genet.* 2002;5(5):444–448. Cited Baldwin et al.[29]
31. Kimerling R, Alvarez J, Pavao J, Kaminski A, Baumrind N. Epidemiology and consequences of women's revictimization. *Womens Health Issues.* 2007;17(2):101–106.
32. Messman-Moore TL, Long PJ, Siegfried NJ. The revictimization of child sexual abuse survivors: an examination of the adjustment of college women with child sexual abuse, adult sexual assault, and adult physical abuse. *Child Maltreat.* 2000;5(1):18–27.
33. Hanson RK. The psychological impact of sexual assault on women and children: a review. *Ann Sex Res.* 1990;3(2):187–232. Cited by Messman-Moore et al.[32]

34. Follette VM, Polusny MA, Bechtle AE, Naugle AE. Cumulative trauma: the impact of child sexual abuse, adult sexual assault, and spouse abuse. *J Trauma Stress*. 1996;9(1):25–35. Cited by Messman-Moore et al.[32]
35. Murphy SM, Kilpatrick DG, Amick-McMullan A, et al. Current psychological functioning of child sexual assault survivors: a community study. *J Interpers Violence*. 1988;3(1):55–79. Cited by Messman-Moore et al.[32]
36. Gidycz CA, Coble CN, Latham L, Layman MJ. Sexual assault experience in adulthood and prior victimization experiences: a prospective analysis. *Psychol Women Q*. 1993;17(2):151–168. Cited by Messman-Moore et al.[32]
37. Sappington AA, Pharr R, Tunstall A, Rickert E. Relationships among child abuse, date abuse, and psychological problems. *J Clin Psychol*. 1997;53(4):319–329. Cited by Messman-Moore et al.[32]

4

Morbidity Associated with Bullying and Other Forms of Victimization

The main clinical lesson derived from the evaluation and treatment of patients[1] who have been exposed to, and/or participated in, bullying and other forms of victimization is that they are likely to suffer from a pattern of frequently occurring physical and emotional symptoms, as illustrated in the following clinical vignette, which is based on a composite of the author's many patients.[1]

Clinical Vignette

A psychiatric consultation was requested by a pediatrician on behalf of a young adolescent female patient who has recently been suffering of frequent tension headaches possibly associated with stress in school.

History of Presenting Problem

For the previous three months, the patient had been experiencing daily frontal headaches without any proven organic etiology, as ascertained by a recent neurological evaluation.

Furthermore, she has been suffering from recent intermittent depression with vague suicidal ideation, significant irritability, marked anxiety with occasional episodes of panic attack, initial and middle insomnia, nightmares, flashbacks, dissociation, auditory hallucinations with derogatory comments, and hyper-alertness. These symptoms have been associated with frequent school absenteeism and a decline in her academic performance.

For the previous six months, as she started sixth grade, the patient has been frequently bullied in school by being teased because of her shyness, being thin, being short, wearing glasses, and having crooked teeth. Once she was told by a classmate that she was a loser and she should kill herself. While running away from peers who were threatening her, she fell and hurt her head.

Past History

In second grade, the patient experienced frequent school bullying in the form of being excluded by her peers, who often subjected her to racial slurs. During that time, she experienced intermittent abdominal pain, headaches, nausea, sadness, anxiety, and sleep difficulties.

While there is a lack of published clinical reports supporting a significant link between exposure to bullying and health problems, there is an extensive body of available studies, mostly based on surveys of nonclinical populations, documenting a significant level of physical and emotional morbidity among individuals who are victims and or perpetrators of bullying and other forms of maltreatment. This literature is cited throughout this chapter in the relevant discussions of physical and emotional problems.

What Is Known?

Based on a second analysis of data from the Health Behavior in School-aged Children (HBSC) survey,[2] studies[3–5] have documented a significant association between participation in bullying and frequent physical and emotional symptoms. In 2005, Srabstein and Piazza[5] conducted a second review of the 1996 United States HBSC[6] and showed that 9.5% of adolescents reported a cluster of symptoms, occurring almost daily, including irritability, depression, anxiety, and insomnia, as well as one or more physical symptoms (headaches, stomachaches, backaches, and dizziness), associated with their experience as a victim and/or as a perpetrator of bullying.

This chapter reviews each of these symptoms as well as other expressions of morbidity associated with bullying and other forms of victimization or maltreatment.

Headaches

School Bullying and Headaches

Gini et al.[7] have validated the significant association between school bullying victimization and headaches through a meta-analysis of three longitudinal and 17 cross-sectional studies that included a total of 173,775 children and adolescents. Their meta-analysis showed that young people who are bullied are at a significantly higher risk of suffering from headaches than are their nonbullied peers.

A study by Ilola et al.[8] focused on a population-based sample of 931 4-year-old children attending their check-up at a health clinic, and the study documented that victims of bullying have a high risk of suffering headaches [adjusted OR (AOR) = 8.10].

Cyberbullying and Headaches

A study by Li et al,[9] which was based on a survey of 3,378 middle school students in eastern, western, and central China, showed that students who were cyberbullying victims were at higher risk (AOR = 2.0 to 2.1) of suffering often to always from headaches, as compared to peers who were not exposed to, or involved in, cyberbullying, even after adjustment for spending three or more hours per day online.

Workplace Bullying and Headaches

A three-year longitudinal survey[10] of a random cohort from the Norwegian general population (16 to 66 years old) showed that, among work-related psychosocial and organizational hazards, workplace bullying/harassment was the highest risk factor (AOR = 3.94) for headaches, exceeding the risk with high role conflict (AOR = 2.86), low social climate (AOR = 2.21), and downsizing (AOR = 2.38).[10]

Adverse Childhood Experiences and Headaches

Several studies[11-21] have documented that adolescents and adults who suffered from migraine headaches are very likely to have experienced childhood maltreatment.

Anda et al.[17] analyzed data related to adverse childhood experiences used in a survey of more than 17,000 adult Kaiser Health Plan members who were undertaking a complete preventive medical evaluation. The analysis showed an increased prevalence of frequent headaches associated with childhood experience of physical, emotional, or sexual abuse; witnessing domestic violence; parental separation or divorce; or growing up with mentally ill, substance-abusing, or criminal household members.[17] Furthermore, Anda et al documented a dose–response relationship between the number of adverse childhood experiences and the prevalence of frequent headaches.[17]

A study conducted by Brennenstuhl et al,[14] based on a sample of almost 23,000 men and women assessed through the 2012 Canadian Community Health Survey–Mental Health, validated that exposure to either childhood physical or sexual abuse or witnessing parental domestic violence was associated with migraine headaches in both men and women, even after adjustment for lifetime depression and anxiety, health behaviors, and sociodemographic variables. The study also showed that men and women suffering from three adverse childhood events have twice the risk of migraine compared to those who did not experience any adverse event.[14]

Intimate Partner Violence and Headaches

Cripe et al.[22] interviewed more than 2,000 Peruvian women during their postpartum hospital stay, querying them about their lifetime experience with headaches and migraine and with physical and sexual violence. Their study demonstrated that women with experiences of lifetime physical and/or sexual violence have increased risks of migraine in comparison to women without a history of violence, and this link was maintained after adjustment for maternal age, parity, and access to basic foods. This association was more robust among women with a history of sexual violence only (AOR = 2.51) and among women with any lifetime physical or sexual violence and depressive symptoms (AOR = 2.72).[22]

Suggested Common Pathophysiology for Childhood Maltreatment and Headaches

Tietjen et al have suggested in several reports[11,12,15,19-21] that a common pathophysiology explains the significant association between childhood maltreatment and headaches. They have highlighted dysregulation of the HPA axis and the autonomic, immune, and metabolic systems as being a common consequence of both maltreatment and migraine.[11]

Furthermore, they underscored that the same brain areas are affected structurally and functionally by childhood abuse and by headache, including the limbic system, which is connected to pain regions in the brainstem.[11] Additionally, they suggested that early life stresses may increase the possibility of migraine through gene and environment interaction as well as epigenetic modifications via DNA methylation.[11]

The Psychosocial Impact of Headaches

Several studies[23-30] have examined and highlighted the serious effect of headaches on the lives of young[23-25] and adult[26-30] populations in terms of quality of life,[24-25] absenteeism,[23,30] utilization of medical services,[30] work productivy,[26,28] performance,[22] and economic losses.[29]

Irritability

Recently, a number of reports have highlighted the clinical, developmental, and epidemiologic relevance of irritability[31-52] and its bearing within the diagnostic concept of disruptive mood dysregulation.[31,46] Yet, there are fewer studies focusing on irritability or anger than studies concentrating on depression or anxiety.[53] This may explain in part the lack of understanding among the public, and perhaps health professionals, of the significance of irritability as a symptom of dysregulation of mood and emotional distress, and its potential risk to others, because it may mediate physical or verbal aggression. So far, few studies have underscored the link between irritability or anger and participation in school bullying.[4,54-60]

Irritability Linked to School Bullying

A study by Srabstein et al,[4] using a second review of the 1997–1998 US HBSC, aimed at ascertaining the link between exposure to, and/or participation in, school bullying and morbidities. The study showed a very significant association between suffering from irritability several times a week and being bullied and/or bullying others at least once a week (AOR = 3.07). The association was significant among students who were only victims (AOR = 2.62) as well as among those who only bullied others (AOR = 2.97).[4]

A similar link between bullying and irritability was found by Arslan et al.[55] through a survey of more than 1,300 Turkish students in grades 5 to 9. The survey documented a high risk of irritability among victimizers (OR = 2.82) and among students who were both victims and perpetrators (OR = 2.78) as compared to peers not involved in bullying.[55]

Depression

Many studies[61-116] have underscored the significant link between feeling depressed, sad, or low with exposure to bullying and other forms of maltreatment occurring across social settings and along the life span.

Depression Linked to Victimization among Peers

Of reports about depression and bullying published since 1999,[85] 75% were related to victimization among school peers.[61-85] Most of the studies used cross-sectional data, which have shown a significant link between school bullying and depression, but the methodology precluded the determination of causality. Yet, some longitudinal studies[66,67,73,75,80,82] have underscored the impact of school bullying on adulthood depression. These findings are in line with the results of reports showing the important effect of many types of childhood maltreatment and adversity on the development of depression in adulthood.[109-116]

A recent study by Connolly and Beaver,[68] based on sibling data from the National Longitudinal Survey of Youth 1997, showed that the combination of genetic and nonshared environmental effects accounts for peer victimization and maladaptive development, including symptoms of depression and anxiety.

It should be noted that there is published evidence showing the significant mediator effect of depression between bullying and suicide or substance abuse.[62,63]

Cyberbullying and Depression

The significant link between cyberbullying and depression has been supported in a cross-sectional study by Selkie et al,[93] based on a sample of 265 female students from four colleges. This investigation demonstrated that students who had experienced cyberbullying as a victim or as a bully had three to four times higher risk for depression than students with no cyberbullying experience. Among those who experienced cyberbullying as a victim, there were no significant associations with depression when compared to peers not involved in this type of victimization.

It is worth citing the longitudinal study by Gámez-Guadix et al.[94] of 845 adolescents who were assessed on two occasions, six months apart. The study showed that exposure to cyberbullying, as evident in the first assessment, predicted depressive symptoms six months later, and that more depressive symptoms documented in the first assessment predicted more cyberbullying at the subsequent evaluation.

A prospective study by Feinstein et al.[92] used 565 college-age young adults who completed online surveys at two time points three weeks apart. The study found that cybervictimization was associated with increases in both depressive symptoms and rumination over time, with rumination being the moderator, at least for women.

Workplace Bullying and Depression

A few Scandinavian longitudinal studies[86-88] have demonstrated the significant association between workplace bullying and depression.

In 2003, Kivimäki et al.[86] examined data from a prospective study based on two surveys in a cohort of 5,432 hospital employees in Finland, showing that the link between prolonged workplace bullying and depression was significant, even after adjustment for age, income, and gender (OR = 4.2).

A two-year study of Danish workers conducted by Gullander et al.[87] investigated a prospective association between self-labeled and witness-reported workplace bullying and the risk of new-onset of depression. The study demonstrated that the odds ratio for new-onset depression among participants reporting bullying occasionally was 2.17, and among the frequently bullied, it was 9.63. Yet, there was no association between witnessing bullying (bystanders) and new-onset depression. Conversely, the notion that bystanding (witnessing) workplace bullying is related to future depressive symptoms, primarily among women, was supported by a Swedish longitudinal study by Emdad et al,[88] who studied 2,563 employees with more than one year at the workplace in four large enterprises.

Takaki et al.[89] sought to ascertain whether workplace bullying mediates between job strains and symptoms of depression and sleep disturbance, through a cross-sectional study of approximately 2,000 employees from 50 Japanese organizations. The research revealed that the total effects of job strain on depression or sleep disturbance were all positive and significant ($P < .05$) in both genders. The mediation effects of workplace bullying were also all positive and significant ($P < .05$) in both genders. After adjustment for workplace social support, the mediation effects were decreased, especially in women, but they remained significant ($P < .05$).[89]

Bullying among Siblings and Depression

A longitudinal study conducted by Arsenault[90] showed that children who reported being bullied by siblings several times a week at age 12 were twice as likely to suffer from depression at age 18, in comparison to children who were not bullied by siblings.

A prospective cohort study led by Bowes et al.[91] has documented a strong causality relationship between sibling bullying and young adulthood depression, even after adjustment for individual and family confounders, such as earlier depression and/or peer victimization, physical or sexual abuse, foster care, or domestic violence.

Intimate Partner Violence and Depression

There is a significant body of research documenting the association of intimate partner violence (IPV) and depression.[95-108]

Gao et al.[95] first reported a significant link between IPV and postnatal depression. Their study showed that women who were victims of physical violence were more than twice as likely to report postnatal depressive symptoms than those who were not.

Research by Ludemir et al.[96] concluded that IPV during pregnancy is strongly associated with postnatal depression, independently of physical or sexual violence.

In 2016, Shamu et al.[97] reported very strong associations between postnatal depression and severe (three or more events) emotional IPV or severe combined forms of IPV. Furthermore, suicidal ideation was significantly associated with severe emotional IPV.

Gilchrist et al.[105] investigated the link between depressive symptoms, ever being afraid of a partner, and hazardous drinking by using cross-sectional screening data from 7,667 randomly selected patients from a large primary care cohort study of 30 metropolitan and rural general practices in Victoria, Australia. Their study[105] showed that men and women who had ever been afraid of a partner or who were hazardous drinkers had on average higher depressive symptom scores than those who had never been afraid or who were not hazardous drinkers.[105] Yet, there was a stronger association between depressive symptoms and ever being afraid of a partner compared to hazardous drinking for both males and females, even after adjustment for age group, income, employment status, marital status, living alone, and education level.[105]

Dougé et al.[106] studied the moderating effect of employment status and social support on the severity of depression associated with IPV. Their report showed that exposure to IPV was associated with more severe depressive symptoms among women with low social support and unemployment, although the effect of recent (vs. lifetime) IPV was most pronounced among women with high social support or employed women.

Childhood Maltreatment and Depression

A meta-analysis of published literature conducted by Mandelli et al.[104] to assess childhood trauma as a risk factor for depressive disorders showed that emotional abuse had the strongest association with adult depression (OR = 2.78), trailed by neglect (OR = 2.75) and sexual abuse (OR = 2.42).

The effect of the timing of childhood trauma on adulthood depression was explored by Dunn et al.[111] in a study involving 2,892 African American adults. This investigation demonstrated that those participants who were exposed to early childhood maltreatment (birth to 5 years of age) had depressive symptoms scores that were 1.5 times as high as those who were fist exposed during middle childhood and almost twice as high as those affected during adolescence.[111]

Research by Russell et al.[116] investigated the association between witnessing domestic abuse in childhood and depression in young adulthood. This study was based on a sample of 1,175 young adults from Miami, Florida, who were first surveyed in 1998–2000 about having witnessed domestic violence and were further assessed in 2000–2002 for depressive symptoms. The results provided evidence that recollection of frequent (10 or more times) experiences of having witnessed their mother or close female relative being physically abused was significantly (AOR = 1.71) associated with experiencing depressive symptoms during young adulthood, even after adjustment for demographic variables, family structure, adverse family experiences, and target of abuse.[116]

Anxiety

A wide range of published reports have demonstrated the significant association between different forms of maltreatment and anxiety.[55,117,90,91,107-128]

Peer Victimization and Anxiety

The first studies showing a signification linkage between being bullied and anxiety were based on data from cross-sectional surveys that also ascertained the association of school bullying with depression and other symptoms.[55,117,118]

Salmon et al.[118] confirmed previous observations made by Olweus[119] that "bullied children are more anxious and bullies equally or less anxious than their peers."[119]

Due et al.[3] analyzed data from the 1997–1998 HBSC, based on a national representative sample of more than 123,000 adolescent students in 28 European countries, and documented that males and females who were bullied weekly had twice the risk of "feeling nervous" in comparison to their peers who were not bullied or were bullied less frequently.

A second analysis of the US data of the 1997–1998 HBSC[4] showed that adolescents who were victims of bullying and those who were both victims and perpetrators were at 2.6 times higher risk of feeling nervous once a week or more frequently than those who had no bullying experience. The risk was lower among those who were perpetrators only (AOR = 1.47).[4]

The cross-sectional nature of the last three studies[3,4,118] precludes any inference of causality, which was ascertained by Pabian and Vandebosch,[120] who examined short-term longitudinal associations between feelings of social anxiety and involvement in bullying among more than 2,100 adolescents. Their results indicated that having a higher level of social anxiety seems to be a risk factor for later bullying victimization, but victimization did not predict later levels of social anxiety. Furthermore, perpetrators of bullying experienced higher levels of anxiety six months later, but anxiety did not foretell later bullying perpetration.[120]

McCabe et al.[121] reported that, among adults with anxiety disorders, a significantly greater percentage (92%) of individuals with a diagnosis of social anxiety were bullied or severely teased in childhood, in comparison to adults with a diagnosis of obsessive-compulsive disorder (50%) or panic disorder (32%).

A cross-sectional study to ascertain the link between school bullying and anxiety among more than 1,900 children and adolescents in an ethnic autonomous county of Gansu, China, was conducted by Gong et al.[129] in December 2019. This research showed that increased symptoms of generalized anxiety were significantly linked to being a victim of either verbal (OR = 3.08), physical (OR = 3.24), or relational bullying (OR = 3.72). Symptoms of generalized anxiety were significantly associated with being a perpetrator of verbal (OR = 2.12), physical (OR = 1.85), or relational peer victimization (OR = 1.78). It is of interest that both victims and perpetrators had higher levels of anxiety associated with a greater number of types of bullying that they were exposed to or involved in, "suggesting a dose–response relation between school bullying involvement and anxiety."[129]

Cyberbullying and Anxiety

The previously cited investigation by Gong et al.[129] indicated that anxiety symptoms were significantly linked to being cyberbullied (OR = 3.47) or to cyberbullying others (OR = 1.59).

A longitudinal study of almost 2,500 adolescents (age 12 to 13), conducted by Fahy et al,[122] documented that youngsters who were cybervictims or cyberbully victims were at significantly higher risk (OR = 1.52 and 1.44, respectively) of reporting symptoms of social anxiety at one-year follow-up, in comparison to their peers who were not involved in cyberbullying, after adjustment for confounding factors, including baseline mental health.

Bullying among Siblings and Anxiety

Bowes et al.[91] showed that children who reported being bullied by a sibling several times a week had a significant risk of anxiety at age 18, even after adjustment for individual and family characteristics (AOR = 1.51).

Workplace Bullying and Anxiety

Rodriguez-Muñoz et al.[123] conducted a two-wave longitudinal study of almost 350 Spanish workers to examine the relationship between workplace bulling and psychological health. Cross-lagged structural equation modeling analyses showed that workplace bullying occurring at the beginning of the study was significantly related to anxiety experienced six months later. Conversely, anxiety suffered at the first wave of the study was significantly linked to workplace bullying half a year later.

A one-year longitudinal study[124] of more than 2,000 Norwegian nurses also showed that high exposure to workplace bullying has an adverse impact on later levels of anxiety regardless of coping style.

IPV and Anxiety

A descriptive cross-sectional study conducted by Mapayi et al.[125] among 373 Nigerian women demonstrated that there was a 21-fold increase in the risk of IPV among women with anxiety, after controlling for significant sociodemographic variables.

Fonseca-Machado et al.[126] documented that women who were victims of IPV during pregnancy had higher symptom scores of trait and state anxiety than nonvictims.

Childhood Exposure to Maltreatment and Anxiety

An investigation by Rehan et al,[127] based on the assessment of more than 14,000 Finnish adult twins of both sexes and their siblings, determined that for both genders, major early years experiences of abuse and neglect increased the likelihood of suffering from clinical anxiety or depression, compared to less severe incidents of childhood maltreatment. Among men, the link between childhood maltreatment and anxiety in adulthood was only evident with incidents of severe emotional and physical abuse and physical neglect, but no significant association was observed for severe sexual abuse and severe emotional neglect. On the other hand, women were more likely to suffer from adult anxiety in association with all types of severe childhood maltreatment as compared to other less severe experiences of maltreatment.[127]

Bruce et al.[128] ascertained which types of childhood maltreatment were associated with severity of social anxiety disorder (SAD). Their study, which was based on 156 treatment-seeking adult outpatients with a primary diagnosis of generalized SAD who completed the Childhood Trauma Questionnaire–Short Form, showed that all types of maltreatment except for sexual and physical abuse were related to greater severity of social anxiety.[128]

Insomnia

Peer Victimization and Sleep Difficulties/Nightmares

A few studies, based on health surveys of nationally representative sample of adolescents, have established that there is a significant link between participating in peer victimization as a victim and/or as a perpetrator and suffering from sleep difficulties.[3-5] A report by van Geel et al,[130] based on a meta-analysis of 21 studies with a total of 363,539 children and adolescents, underscored the "significant effect between peer victimization and sleep problems, with victimized children reporting more sleep problems than children who did not report victimization [OR = 2.14 (95% = 2.01–2.44), I^2 = 93.07]."[130]

Kubiszewski et al.[131] investigated the subjective sleep disorders and sleep/wake patterns associated with participation in bullying among 1,422 French preadolescent and adolescent students. The study showed that victims of bullying showed significantly more subjective sleep disturbances than perpetrators or students not involved in bullying. Perpetrators had sleep schedules that were significantly more irregular, and their sleep duration was shorter than that of their schoolmates.[131]

Adolescents with sleep bruxism, characterized by clenching or grinding of the teeth and or by bracing or thrusting the mandible, have been found more likely to be exposed to episodes of verbal bullying (OR = 6.20).[132]

Wolke and Lereya conducted a longitudinal study[133] of almost 6,800 British children age 8 through 13; the study showed that victims of bullying are at significant risk of having nightmares or night terrors. In contrast, perpetrators were not shown to have an increased risk for parasomnias.

Cyberbullying and Sleep Difficulties

A cross-sectional survey 19,436 Japanese students, conducted by Tochigi et al,[134] examined the relationship between school bullying and sleep pattern or nocturnal cellular phone usage. The results showed that "bullying status was significantly associated with irregular bedtime (OR = 1.23 and 1.41 for pure bullies and bully-victims, respectively) and e-mail exchange or calling after lights-out (OR = 1.53 and 1.31 for pure bullies and bully-victims, respectively), after controlling for domestic violence and substance usage."[134]

Research by Li et al.[9] found that Chinese students who were cyberbullied were at a significant risk (AOR = 2.2) of suffering, often or always, from sleep problems.

Workplace Bullying and Sleep Difficulties

A study conducted by Yoo et al,[135] based on data from the 4th Korean Working Conditions Survey (KWCS) of 2014, which assessed a total of 25,138 wage workers, established that workplace violence was a risk factor for sleep disturbance in the preceding 12 months (OR = 3.77). Complaints of sleep disturbance symptoms were increased when the perpetrator was a colleague or boss (OR = 5.70) rather than a client (OR = 2.9).[135] For the purpose of this study,[135] the definition of workplace violence included verbal abuse, unwanted sexual attention, threatening or humiliating behavior, physical violence, bullying/harassment, and sexual harassment.

A cross-sectional survey of almost 7,700 men and women in the working population of the southeast of France conducted by Niedhammer et al.[136] showed that, beyond a significant association of workplace bullying and sleep disturbances, past exposure to bullying increased the risk of sleep instability among females, and the more frequent the exposure to bullying, the higher the risk. Furthermore, women who were both bullied and witnessed others being bullied had a higher risk of sleep difficulties.[136]

A cause-and-effect relationship between workplace bullying and sleep difficulties was supported by a longitudinal study published by Hansen et al.[137] The study, which used a two-year follow-up of almost 3,400 Danish workers, showed that employees who were frequently bullied at baseline had a significant risk (AOR = 1.61) at two-year follow-up of experiencing disturbed sleep and unsatisfactory awakening, as well as having poor quality of sleep, even after adjustment for age, gender, body mass index (BMI), alcohol, and smoking.[137]

In a longitudinal study that used a two-year follow-up of more than 7,600 public and private Danish employees, Nabe-Nielsen et al.[138] documented that disturbed sleep and difficulty awakening were involved in a small way (12.8%) in mediating the significant association between workplace bullying and long-term sickness or absence.

IPV and Sleep Difficulties/Nightmares

In a cross-sectional study of 634 Peruvian women, Sanchez et al.[139] examined the association between IPV and stress-related sleep disturbance, as well as poor sleep quality, during early pregnancy. For this investigation, sleep disturbance was assessed with the Ford Insomnia Response to Stress Test,[140] a standardized self-rating questionnaire that measures the likelihood of the occurrence of sleep disturbance in response to commonly experienced stressors, while sleep quality was evaluated using the Pittsburgh Sleep Quality Index[141] to assess sleep duration, disturbance, latency, habitual sleep efficiency, use of sleep medicine, daytime dysfunction due to sleepiness, and overall quality of sleep. The study[139] determined that, compared to women who did not experience IPV, women who experienced IPV were more likely to have stress-related sleep disturbance (AOR = 1.54) and poor sleep quality (AOR = 1.93).

An investigation conducted by Rauer and El-Sheikh,[142] which examined cross-sectional and longitudinal relations between IPV and sleep problems in men and women, showed cross-sectional links between IPV and sleep that were evident in both partners, in particular between psychological IPV and sleep.[142] This study also demonstrated that sleep problems predicted increased perpetration of psychological IPV over time for both men and women.[142] Furthermore, cross-partner effects emerged only for men, revealing that men's sleep problems were strongly affected by their partner's earlier perpetration of IPV and sleep difficulties.[142]

A 2015 study by Romito et al.[143] evaluated the association of psychological health symptoms and partner violence among 178 adult women attending five anti-violence centers in Italy. The findings documented that 60% of participants reported nightmares. After adjustment for confounders (women's age, having children, living vs. not living with the perpetrator, education, employment, nationality, and the Anti-Violence Center), the results indicated that participants who were exposed to a high level of IPV were at high risk of suffering nightmares (AOR = 4.41).

Childhood Exposure to Maltreatment and Sleep Difficulties/ Nightmares

Several reports have underscored the significant link between childhood exposure to maltreatment and sleep difficulties.[144-150]

Sadeh et al.[144] conducted a study of 39 children age 7 to 14 hospitalized in a psychiatric inpatient unit, and the results showed that "physically abused children spent less of their bedtime in sleep than did sexually abused and non-abused children ($F = 2.91$, $P < .05$)."[144] Also, "physically abused children (with or without history of sexual abuse) spend proportionally less time in quiet-motionless sleep ($F = 3.54$, $P < .05$)."[144] No other group differences were found for sleep onset time,; total sleep period, true sleep time, or longest sleep period.[144]

Research by Lind et al.[145] involving more than 8,000 adult twins documented that reported childhood sexual abuse significantly predicted insomnia among females (OR = 1.67).[145]

Sleep paralysis, which manifests as a feeling of paralysis of the skeletal muscles during during transitions between sleep and awake states, has been found to be more frequently reported by adults with a history of confirmed or unconfirmed childhood sexual abuse than by individuals without a history of such abuse.[146]

A survey of more than 800 US adults (60 years old and older)[147] found that early parental emotional abuse was significantly associated with more sleep complaints (difficulties falling asleep or staying asleep, waking up too early in the morning, and/or feeling fatigued during the day). This association was only partially explained by current unsupportive interactions with family, friends, or significant others and emotional distress.[147]

Gelaye et al.[148] conducted a cross-sectional study of more than 600 Peruvian women and established that women who experienced any childhood abuse had 1.65-fold increased odds of stress-related sleep disturbance and 2.11-fold increased odds of poor sleep quality during early pregnancy as compared with women who reported no abuse.

Sleep disturbance in the third trimester of pregnancy related to childhood emotional abuse has been found to be a mediator of reduced fetal heart rate variability, an indicator of parasympathetic nervous system performance.[149] This finding indicates an intergenerational transmission of health risk.[149]

Petrov et al.[150] studied 589 community-dwelling adults and showed the mediator role of sleep disturbance, as well as inflammation, in the indirect association between childhood abuse and hypertension in adulthood.[150]

A meta-analysis of five studies[151-155] conducted by Schønning et al.[156] showed that, compared to nonmaltreated peers, young people subjected to maltreatment are at a higher risk (OR = 3.15) of experiencing nightmares.

Backache

School Bullying and Backache

There are few reports[3-5] documenting a significant association between peer victimization and backache. The large international cross-sectional study led by Due et al.[3] examined the association between bullying and physical symptoms, and it showed that there was a significant risk of back pain among both male (OR = 1.97) and female students (OR = 1.88) who were bullied weekly.

Workplace Bullying and Backache

A study by Min et al,[157] based on the First KWCS[158] of more than 10,000 employees, documented a significant association between the experience of workplace injustice, defined as discrimination, violence, and harassment at work in the previous year, and increased risk of backache [prevalence ratio (PR)[159] = 1.6] and musculoskeletal pain (PR = 1.5), after adjustment for personal,[160] occupational,[161] and job-related[162] characteristics.

The role of gender as a moderator in the prospective relationship between exposure to workplace bullying and ensuing back and neck pain was investigated by Glambek et al.[163] in a two wave (six time lag) survey of 5,000 Norwegian workers. The investigation showed that workplace bullying significantly contributed to subsequent back and neck pain, with low baseline levels of pain among men increasing with exposure to bullying, while in females the baseline high levels of pain remained steady even after being subjected to bullying.[163]

IPV and Back Pain

Gilkey et al.[164] conducted a cross-sectional survey of 963 students at Colorado State University to ascertain risk factors associated with back pain, and they found that being in an emotionally abusive relationship was significantly associated with backache (AOR = 2.78).

Similar findings were documented by Vives-Cases et al.[165] through a National Health Survey of more than 13,000 Spanish women who were more likely to suffer from back pain (AOR = 2.34) if they had experienced IPV, as compared to women who had not experienced that form of victimization.

Childhood Maltreatment and Back Pain

A study by Leisner et al.[166] of 103 adult patients with established chronic low back pain (CLBP) and who reported a history of childhood abuse found that the patients exhibited "higher spatial extent of pain, higher affective and sensory pain sensation and more pain disability compared to CLBP patients who had not experienced abuse."[166] Multivariate analysis documented that only spatial extent of pain was directly linked to childhood abuse, while the link between childhood maltreatment and sensory pain sensation was mediated by anxiety and dissociation.[166]

Tesarz et al.[167] investigated whether maltreatment during childhood was linked to specific alterations in pain perception. Their study used 176 adult patients with established nonspecific CLBP being assessed at a tertiary care pain center at the Heidelberg University Hospital and 27 pain-free controls. The study showed that, in comparison to those without a history of childhood victimization, all patients who suffered nonspecific CLBP and who were subjected to any type of childhood maltreatment had a significantly reduced pressure pain threshold.[167]

Stomachache or Abdominal Pain

School Bullying and Stomachache

Several reports have highlighted the association between school bullying and frequent stomachaches.[3-5,168-172] The causal relationship between bullying and abdominal pain was documented by Fekkes et al.[170] in a prospective cohort study of 1,118 Dutch children (9 to 11 years old), which showed that being bullied had a strong relation to the development of abdominal pain in girls (OR = 4.98), although there was no such relationship in boys (OR = 0.34).[170]

Cyberbullying and Stomachache

Sourander et al.[171] conducted a population-based cross-sectional study of 2,215 Finnish adolescents (age 13 to 16) that showed that recurrent abdominal pain (occurring once a week or more frequently) was very significantly associated with being both a victim and a perpetrator of cyberbullying (AOR = 2.7), as well as being a victim only (AOR = 2.6) and, to a slightly lesser degree, being a cyberbully only (AOR = 1.8).[171]

IPV and Abdominal Pain

Bonomi et al.[172] investigated the wide range of morbidity associated with a history of IPV experienced after age 18 by conducting a telephone survey of more than 3,500 women randomly sampled from a large US health plan. The study documented that, compared to women who were never abused, those women who were exposed to IPV in the previous year were at a significant risk (AOR = 1.47) of suffering from abdominal pain.[172]

Childhood Maltreatment and Abdominal Pain

A longitudinal study of 845 children from age 4 through 12 years, conducted by van Tilburg et al.[173] to investigate the link between childhood maltreatment and gastrointestinal symptoms, demonstrated a significant association between youth recall of ever having been psychologically, physically, or sexually abused and suffering, at age 12, from abdominal pain and nausea/vomiting (OR = 1.5 to 2.1). The effects became insignificant when adjusted for anxiety and depression, except for the link between physical abuse and nausea/vomiting (OR = 1.5).[173]

Musculoskeletal Pain/Fibromyalgia

School Bullying and Musculoskeletal Pain/Fibromyalgia

The association between perceived social support in school and musculoskeletal complaints was studied by Bru et al.[174] among 1,071 eighth grade students randomly selected from 24

Norwegian municipalities. The research showed that exposure to peer harassment and perceived lack of academic support was significantly associated with musculoskeletal as well as emotional complaints, especially in students reporting learning difficulties.

Kashikar-Zuck et al.[175] studied 55 adolescents (12 to 18 years old) with juvenile primary fibromyalgia syndrome (JPFS) who were compared to 55 adolescents without chronic illness to ascertain the quality of peer relations. The researchers found that students with JPFS were less well liked and were less often selected as a best friend, showing an association between possible peer rejection and musculoskeletal pain.

Workplace Bullying and Musculoskeletal Pain/Fibromyalgia

The link between the exposure to workplace bullying and development of fibromyalgia, which is characterized by widespread muscle pain, tenderness, fatigue, and sleep disturbances,[176] was investigated by Kivimäki et al.[177] through a prospective study of more than 4,700 Finnish hospital employees who completed a survey in 1998 and 2000. The study found a significant association (AOR = 4.36) between workplace bullying and suffering from fibromyalgia, after adjustment for age, sex, income, obesity, and smoking.

Cross-sectional research by Vignoli et al.[178] involving 512 Italian retail workers showed that job-related strain (i.e., feeling emotionally drained from work) was the mediator in the link between workplace bullying and musculoskeletal disorders.

The association between workplace bullying and pain has been shown to be dependent on a gene–environment interaction. In a study based on a nationally representative sample of 987 Norwegian employees, Jacobsen et al.[179] documented that the relationship between bullying and pain intensity was significantly stronger for workers with a genetic variation of the *SLC6A4* genotype; specifically, it was greater among employees with $L_A L_A$ genotype than among workers with the $SL_A/L_AL_G/SL_G$ genotype.

Inflammation

School Bullying and Inflammation

The link between school bullying and low-grade inflammation persisting into adulthood, as measured by C-reactive protein (CRP) levels, was investigated by Copeland et al.[180] in a prospective population based Great Smoky Mountains study involving 1,420 children, with up to nine waves of data per subject covering childhood and adolescence (ages 9 to 16) and young adulthood (ages 19 and 21). The research showed that "being bullied predicted greater increases in CRP levels, whereas bullying others predicted lower increases in CRP compared with those uninvolved in bullying." These results were strong even after adjustment for BMI, substance use, physical and mental health status, and exposure to other childhood adversities.[180]

The significant association between exposure to bullying in childhood and inflammation as well as adiposity at midlife was ascertained by Takizawa et al.[181] in a 50-year prospective birth cohort study of all births in Britain in one week of 1958. The investigation found that participants who were frequently bullied in childhood had higher levels of inflammation as indicated by CRP readings than nonbullied participants. Furthermore, women who had been occasionally or frequently bullied as children presented with greater midlife adiposity than women who had not been bullied.[181]

IPV and Inflammation

Newton et al.[182]conducted a cross-sectional study of 68 midlife divorced women to ascertain a link between history of IPV and circulating biological markers of inflammation. Their research established that CRP levels were positively correlated with a history of having been stalked, even after adjustment for current depression and PTSD symptoms, yet this association was diminished with adjustment for BMI.

Childhood Maltreatment and Inflammation

The life-course association between childhood maltreatment and adult inflammation was ascertained by Danese et al.[183] in a birth cohort of almost 1,000 individuals born between April 1972 and March 1973 in Dunedin, New Zealand. The study followed the individuals to age 32 years as part of the Dunedin Multidisciplinary Health and Development Study.[184-186] Danese et al.[183] found that children who were maltreated (defined as exposure to maternal rejection, harsh discipline, disruptive caregiver changes, and physical or sexual abuse) presented with significant and graded increase in the risk (risk ratio = 1.80) for clinically relevant CRP levels in adulthood. This significant association was independent of the influence of co-occurring early life risks (risk ratio = 1.58), stress in adulthood (risk ratio = 1.58), and adult health and behavior (risk ratio = 1.76).[183]

Abnormal Weight Gain

School Bullying and Weight Gain

The association between bullying in the first year of school and greater weight gain in early adolescence was investigated by Sutin et al.[187] based on data drawn from the Longitudinal Study of Australian Children. More than 3,900 children participated in the study, with their BMI and waist circumference being measured every two years from ages 4 to 15, bullying being reported by parents at age 6 and participants reporting depressive symptoms from age 12 to 13.The study documented that children with obesity at age 4 had more than 50% increased risk of being bullied at age 6, but then, and of note, suffering bullying at age 6 was significantly associated with excess weight gain (BMI and waist circumference) between 6 and 15 years of age, with this association being partially mediated by depression reported at age 12.

IPV and Weight Gain

The link between exposure to IPV in late adolescence and five-year weight gain in young women was investigated by Mason et al.[188] in a longitudinal study of 619 females from the Minneapolis-St. Paul area. The research showed that IPV in late adolescence was significantly linked to an increment in BMI of 1.8 kg/m^2 among young adult women who were suffering from depression as compared to those without depression, even after adjustment for socioeconomic variables and baseline BMI. Yet, there was no difference in BMI changes associated with depression among women without exposure to IPV.[188]

The effects of IPV during the perinatal period on inadequate and excessive gestational weight gain was studied by Alhusen et al.[189] with data from more than 251,000 US mothers who gave birth from 2004 through 2011. The investigation reported that women who suffered physical IPV during the year before pregnancy had a mildly significant risk (AOR = 1.14) of excessive gestational weight gain as compared to those who did not suffer IPV in the last year prior to pregnancy, after adjustment for age, race, education, income level, marital status, smoking, adequacy of prenatal care, and pre-pregnancy BMI.[189]

Childhood Maltreatment and Weight Gain

By studying 472 pregnant women in Pittsburgh, Pennsylvania, Diesel et al.[190] investigated whether maternal pre-pregnancy obesity or excessive gestational weight gain was linked to a maternal history of childhood maltreatment. The results showed a significant link between moderate to severe physical abuse in childhood and obesity in pre-pregnancy, after adjustment for race, tobacco use, alcohol consumption, and marijuana use. The risk of prenatal obesity was higher among women with a history of childhood maltreatment and elevated prenatal anxiety or depression, as compared to women with childhood maltreatment and less anxiety or depression.[190]

Diabetes

Workplace Bullying and Diabetes

The link between workplace bullying and violence with increased risk of type 2 diabetes was investigated by Xu et al.[191] in a prospective multicohort study that included 4,505 men and women from Sweden, Denmark, and Finland. The investigators determined that both men and women who were bullied at work had, after adjustment for BMI, 1.37 times higher risk of developing diabetes than workers who were not bullied.

IPV and Diabetes

The association between IPV and the incidence of type 2 diabetes was assessed by Mason et al.[192] in a study involving 64,732 female registered nurses. This investigation showed a small association [adjusted hazard ratio (HR) = 1.18] between physical IPV and type 2 diabetes, but a stronger risk for type 2 diabetes (adjusted HR = 1.61) was found among participants subjected to severe psychological violence.[192]

Childhood Maltreatment and Diabetes

The risk of developing diabetes in adulthood among individuals with a history of childhood physical abuse, sexual abuse, or exposure to IPV was investigated by Shields et al,[193] who used a sample of 21,878 men and women from the 2012 Canadian Community Health Survey–Mental Health (CCHS-MH).[194] Their results showed that self-reported diabetes was significantly linked, after adjustment for sociodemographic factors, with a history of severe and frequent (more than 10 times) childhood physical abuse (AOR = 1.8), severe and frequent (more than three times) childhood sexual abuse (AOR = 2.2), and the co-occurrence of both childhood physical and sexual abuse, either severe and frequent or both severe (AOR = 2.6).[193] There was some attenuation in the risks for diabetes when controlling for mediating factors, such as smoking status, obesity, physical activity level, high blood pressure, and lifetime depression, resulting in a 41% reduction in the risk of diabetes with a history of severe and frequent childhood physical abuse (AOR = 1.4).[193] The effects of mediating variables were not pronounced in the association between severe and frequent childhood sexual abuse and diabetes (AOR = 2.0). Finally, there was no significant association found in this study between childhood exposure to IPV and diabetes.[193]

Li et al.[195] studied 121 adults (19 to 60 years old) recruited in Birmingham, Alabama, to examine whether a history of childhood maltreatment, including physical or emotional neglect and emotional, physical, or sexual abuse, is an independent risk factor for prediabetes. Their results indicated that participants with a history of childhood maltreatment, in contrast to those without exposure to this form of victimization, showed a significantly higher level of 1-hour glucose during the oral glucose tolerance test. Furthermore, 20% of individuals with a history of childhood maltreatment show evidence of prediabetes as manifested by impaired fasting glucose and/or impaired glucose tolerance, in contrast to only 10% of individuals with no history of childhood maltreatment.[195]

Cardiovascular Disease

Workplace Bullying and Cardiovascular Disease

The study by Kivimäki et al.[86] that showed a significant link between workplace bullying and depression also investigated the effect of workplace bullying on cardiovascular disease (CVD). Using two consecutive surveys completed in 1998 and 2000, the investigators showed a significant risk (AOR = 2.31) for CVD, identified as reported myocardial infarction, angina pectoris, cerebrovascular disease, or hypertension, among employees subjected to workplace bullying. Adjustment for being overweight lessened the risk (AOR = 1.62) between exposure to workplace victimization and CVD.[86]

The prospective association of workplace bullying and workplace violence with new-onset CVD was examined by Xu et al.[196] in a multicohort study involving 79,201 adult participants from the Swedish and Danish labor force. Participants were linked to the national registries in each country and had no prior CVD. Information on workplace bullying or violence within 12 months prior to baseline was available. The research documented that, after adjustment for demographic and educational variables, workplace bullying was associated with a significant risk (adjusted HR = 1.59) of CVD onset, defined as a first hospitalization with coronary or cerebrovascular disease.[196] Furthermore, experiencing workplace violence was associated with a HR of 1.25 for CVD onset.

IPV and CVD

Clark et al.[197] investigated the effect of being exposed to, or participating in, IPV in adolescence or young adulthood (ages 16 and 22) and blood pressure outcomes as well as hypertension onset during adulthood (average age 29). The data were from 9,699 participants in waves 3 (2001–2002) and 4 (2008–2009) of the National Longitudinal Study of Adolescent Health,[198] which used a nationally representative sample of US adolescents in grades 7 to 12 during the 1994–95 school year. The study found that, after adjustment for confounders, men experiencing severe victimization and involved in severe perpetration had systolic blood pressure 2.6 mm Hg higher than the systolic pressure in men without IPV.[197] Furthermore, in contrast to men not experiencing IPV, men involved in both severe victimization and perpetration had a higher risk (AOR = 1.59) of hypertension in adulthood, defined as a systolic blood pressure ≥ 140 mm Hg, a diastolic blood pressure ≥ 90 mm Hg, or taking hypertensive medication.[197] The other categories of IPV were not associated with blood pressure or onset of hypertension in men, and IPV was not found to be linked to onset of hypertension in women.[197]

Childhood Maltreatment and CVD

Ho et al.[199] conducted a retrospective cohort study to establish and quantify the underlying pathways linking child maltreatment and CVD. The study was based on data from more than 152,000 adult participants in the UK Biobank.[200] The research showed a significant association between child maltreatment and an incident of CVD, defined, according to the ICD 10,[201] as "death or hospital admission for ischemic heart disease (including myocardial infarction), atrial fibrillation, heart failure, or stroke." Furthermore, the study[199] indicated that there was "evidence of a of a dose–response relationship between the number of maltreatment types and incident CVD." Moreover, the link between childhood maltreatment and CVD was mainly mediated by depressive symptoms (56%), "followed by smoking (14.7%), high-density lipoprotein cholesterol (8.7%), and sleep duration (2.4%)."[199]

Disruption in Cognitive Processes

School Bullying and Inattention

An indication of the concurrent and longitudinal contribution of exposure to bullying, at age 11 and 14 years, to inattention, as measured by Conners Parent Rating,[202] can be found in a longitudinal study by Singham et al,[203] who studied 11,108 twins to determine the extent that exposure to bullying causes mental health problems, including inattention. The study found that, in a concurrent analysis at age 11, past-year exposure to bullying was significantly associated with "parent-rated inattention,"[202] and this link remained significant even after controlling for all shared environmental and genetic influences in monozygotic analysis. The contribution of exposure to bullying at age 14 to inattention at age 16 continues to be significant, even after adjustment for dizygotic differences.[203]

School Bullying and Dissociation

Evidence of a significant association between bullying in childhood and adolescence and dissociation in young adulthood can be found in a study by Sesar et al.[204] involving 249 students from Mostar University in Bosnia and Herzegovina, who completed the Retrospective Bullying Questionnaire developed by Schäfer et al.[205] and the Trauma Symptom Checklist 40 (TSC-40),[206] which includes a Dissociation Subscale.[207] The research[204] showed that participants who were exposed to bullying had significantly higher levels of dissociation than those who were not exposed to bullying. Furthermore, participants who were exposed to bullying in all periods of school (first to fourth grade, fifth to eighth grade, and high school) reported significantly higher scores on dissociation symptoms than those who suffered bullying in only two or one period of school.[204]

Childhood Maltreatment and Dissociation

Levels of dissociation in relation to early maltreatment were examined by Hulette et al.[208] in a study of 67 foster children (average age 9 years) who had been maltreated in early childhood. The foster children were compared to 51 nonmaltreated community children of similar age. The investigation[208] documented that almost 21% of foster children presented with a possible clinically significant dissociation, as evidenced by a Child Dissociative Checklist[209] score of 12 or above, as compared to 2% in the community comparison group. Higher levels of dissociation were evident among females as well as among those children who had higher number of foster placement transitions.[208]

Intrusive Memories

The experience of recurrent, involuntary, and intrusive traumatic memories is a "unique symptom of posttraumatic stress disorder"[210] recognized in ICD-11[211] and in DSM-V[212] diagnostic criteria. So far, there is a lack of published research specifically addressing the prevalence of intrusive memories or flashbacks among individuals who were exposed to bullying or other forms of victimization, but a number of reports[213-220] document the significant association of bullying and other types of ill-treatment with all core symptoms[211,212] in posttraumatic stress disorder.[221-224]

Psychotic Symptoms

Peer Victimization and Psychotic Symptoms

The link between peer victimization and psychotic symptoms was examined in a nonclinical prospective birth cohort study by Schreier et al.[225] The study included 6,437 children born in

Southwest England between 1991 and 1992. The children were part of the Avon Longitudinal Study of Parents and Children and participated in annual psychological and physical assessments from 7 to 12 years of age. The results[225] documented a significant risk (AOR = 1.94) for psychotic symptoms (hallucinations and delusions) among 12-year-old children who were exposed to bullying at age 8 and/or 10 years, after adjustment for other prior psychopathology, family adversity, and child's IQ.[225]

Catone et al.[226] conducted a cross-sectional study to assess the association of specific bullying victimization with psychotic experiences,[227] such as paranoia, hallucinations, cognitive disorganization, grandiosity, and anhedonia, as well as negative symptoms, such as affective flattening or blunting, poverty of speech, and lack of motivation. The research[226] was based on the assessment of 50 adolescent patients, ages 12 to 18 years, who were found to have psychotic experiences, within the screening of a total of 324 patients being seen at the Complex Unit of Child and Adolescent Neuropsychiatry at the University of Campania Luigi Vanvitelli in Naples, Italy. Catone et al.[226] showed that patients who were verbally bullied had a significantly high risk of experiencing paranoia (AOR = 3.45), after adjustment for sociodemographics, anxiety, depression, physical bullying, social manipulation, and attack on property. Similarly, paranoia was found to be significantly linked (AOR = 2.34) with the experience of being socially manipulated as a form of peer victimization, even after adjustment for similar confounders.[226]

The association between peer victimization and hallucinatory experiences among early adolescents was found to be mediated by dissociation in a study by Yamasaki et al.[228] involving a population-based cross-sectional survey of 4,277 10-year-old children born in the metropolitan area of Tokyo, Japan.

Stanyon et al.[229] conducted research to determine the role of bullying in the association between autistic traits and psychotic experiences in adolescence, based on longitudinal data from the Tokyo Teen Cohort study.[230] The investigation identified a significant ($P < .001$) indirect effect between autistic traits and psychotic experiences via bullying victimization, even after controlling for known confounders.

IPV and Psychotic Experiences

Sha et al.[231] investigated the link between IPV and psychotic experiences among 1,615 participants from four cities in the United States (New York City, Philadelphia, Baltimore, and Washington DC). The study documented that being exposed to any form of IPV (threat, physical, or sexual) was significantly associated with either paranoia, thought insertion, hallucination, or a "strange experience," defined as a "feeling something strange and unexplainable was going on that other people would find hard to believe."[231] In an analysis mutually adjusted for each type of IPV, as well as age, education, race/ethnicity, sexual orientation, household income, city of residence, and prior mental health diagnosis, it was found that physical IPV was not significantly associated with any psychotic experiences, while threat IPV had the highest level of significant association ($P < .001$) with hallucinations (AOR = 9.58), paranoia (AOR = 5.27), and strange experiences (AOR = 4.56). A lower degree of significant association ($P < .05$) was found between sexual IPV and strange experiences (AOR = 2.31), paranoia (AOR = 2.59), and hallucinations (AOR = 2.86).[231]

Childhood Maltreatment and Psychotic Symptoms

A study by Holshausen et al.[232] evaluated the relation between history of sexual, physical, and emotional abuse or neglect and psychotic symptoms among 129 adolescents and young adults (age 12 to 21) from a midsize city in Ontario, Canada, who met the diagnostic criteria for a current episode of major depressive disorder.[233] The investigation demonstrated that participants with psychotic symptoms, such as hallucinations, delusions, or incoherence/loosening of associations, were significantly more likely (OR = 3.86) to report a history of severe sexual maltreatment as compared to those without psychotic symptoms, even after considering the overall role of depression severity as a significant predictor.[232]

Injuries

School Bullying and Injuries

Peyton et al.[234] examined the association between peer victimization and injuries, in a study based on the analysis of responses provided by 1,606 students who participated in Oman's 2010 Global School-based Student Health Survey.[235] This survey documented a significant association among boys (OR = 4.5) who had been bullied one or more days during the previous 30 days and having a serious injury in the previous year. Among girls, this association was significant (OR = 2.4) but less significant than among boys.

Data derived from the 2012–2013 Global School-based Student Health Survey were analyzed by Beck et al.[236] to identify risk behaviors and other exposures associated with injuries among more than 35,000 students (13 to 15 years old), from Argentina, Bolivia, Chile, and Uruguay. The results showed that males and females had three times the risk of sustaining an injury in the previous year if they were bullied one or more times in the previous month.

IPV and Injuries

An assessment of injuries resulting from IPV was conducted by Fanslow and Robinson,[237] who used a cross-sectional survey of a New Zealand random population-based sample of 2,885 women age 18 to 64. The study showed that 33% of participants (n = 956) had experienced physical and/or sexual IPV in their lifetime, and 16% (n = 482) reported being injured at least once because of the violence. Abrasions and bruises were the most common form of injury (reported by 14% of the women surveyed), followed by cuts, punctures, bites, ear or eye injuries, fractures, head injuries, and sprains or dislocations, which were suffered by almost 3% to 5% of the participants, while 1% to 2% were affected by burns, deep cuts, broken teeth, and other injuries.[237]

Childhood Maltreatment and Injuries

Vaithianathan et al.[238] published a study aimed at determining whether children who have been classified as at a "high risk" of maltreatment are also at elevated risk of injury in early childhood. This population-based study, which used two New Zealand birth cohorts born in 2010 and 2011, helped in developing a model to predict the risk that a child would have a substantiated allegation of maltreatment (physical or emotional abuse or neglect) by 2 years of age. The children who were at the top 10% of scores of the predictive risk model of maltreatment had a very significant relative risk (OR = 9.6) of hospitalization for maltreatment-related injury by the time they were 2 years old.[238]

A retrospective, one-year population-based study of child maltreatment-related injuries was conducted by Forjuoh[239] based on all 1995 hospital child maltreatment discharges in Pennsylvania. The investigation documented a total of 348 maltreated–injured children (from birth to age 19 years), representing an incidence of 10.8 per 100,000 persons. Hospitalized maltreated–injured children, as compared to children hospitalized for injuries not related to maltreatment, were significantly more likely to be urgently referred by a physician, to be transferred from other facilities, to be less than 5 years old, to have a longer hospital stay, and to be three times as likely to die.[239]

Future Directions

There is a need for future studies, based on clinical populations, to further assess the scope and prevalence of symptoms and other expressions of morbidity associated with exposure to bullying and other forms of victimization. These studies should carefully consider the potential causal and summative effect of polyvictimization and/or revictimization throughout the life span (see Chapter 3). Furthermore, it is important to medical and public health that clinical research ascertain the prevalence of diagnostic entities that may precede, or may be the outcome of, victimization, either by contributing as a moderating factor or by being the expression of its toxicity. In particular, emphasis should be given to the prevalence of adjustment disorder, acute stress reaction,[240] posttraumatic stress disorder,[211] and complex posttraumatic stress disorder[241] associated with exposure to bullying and other forms of victimization.

Notes

1. For the past two decades, the author has clinically evaluated and treated more than 1,500 children, adolescents, and adults exposed to bullying and other forms of victimization. This clinical service was provided at a pediatric hospital-based child and adolescent outpatient psychiatric clinic as well as at a local government clinic for victims of trauma.
2. Health Behavior in School-Aged Children (HBSC) is a cross-national, school-based research study conducted in collaboration with the World Health Organization (WHO) Regional Office in Europe. The HBSC started in 1982 to collect information on health-related attitudes and behaviors of young people, and the HBSC survey is conducted every four years in many countries and regions across Europe and North America. https://hbsc.org/about/. Accessed October 3, 2022.

3. Due P, Holstein BE, Lynch J, et al. Bullying and symptoms among school-aged children: international comparative cross sectional study in 28 countries. *Eur J Public Health.* 2005;15(2):128–132.

4. Srabstein JC, McCarter RJ, Shao C, Huang ZJ. Morbidities associated with bullying behaviors in adolescents. School based study of American adolescents. *Int J Adolesc Med Health.* 2006;18(4):587–596.
5. Srabstein J, Piazza T. Is there a syndrome of bullying? *Int J Adolesc Med Health.* 2012;24(1):91–96.
6. World Health Organization. *Health Behavior in School-Aged Children, 1995-1996: [United States].* Ann Arbor, MI: Inter-university Consortium for Political and Social Research [distributor]; 2008. https://www.icpsr.umich.edu/web/NAHDAP/studies/3154/versions/V3. Accessed October 3, 2022.
7. Gini G, Pozzoli T, Lenzi M, Vieno A. Bullying victimization at school and headache: a meta-analysis of observational studies. *Headache.* 2014;54(6):976–986.
8. Ilola AM, Lempinen L, Huttunen J, Ristkari T, Sourander A. Bullying and victimisation are common in four-year-old children and are associated with somatic symptoms and conduct and peer problems. *Acta Paediatr.* 2016;105(5):522–528.
9. Li J, Wu Y, Hesketh T. Internet use and cyberbullying: impacts on psychosocial and psychosomatic wellbeing among Chinese adolescents. *Comput Hum Behav.* 2023;138:107461.
10. Tynes T, Johannessen HA, Sterud T. Work-related psychosocial and organizational risk factors for headache: a 3-year follow-up study of the general working population in Norway. *J Occup Environ Med.* 2013;55(12):1436–1442.
11. Tietjen GE, Buse DC, Collins SA. Childhood maltreatment in the migraine patient. *Curr Treat Options Neurol.* 2016;18(7):31.
12. Tietjen GE. Childhood maltreatment and headache disorders. *Curr Pain Headache Rep.* 2016;20(4):26.
13. Altintaş E, Karakurum Göksel B, Saritürk Ç, Taşkintuna N. Evaluation of relationship between childhood maltreatment and medication overuse headache. *Noro Psikiyatr Ars.* 2015;52(3):267–271.
14. Brennenstuhl S, Fuller-Thomson E. The painful legacy of childhood violence: migraine headaches among adult survivors of adverse childhood experiences. *Headache.* 2015;55(7):973–983.
15. Tietjen GE, Buse DC, Fanning KM, Serrano D, Reed ML, Lipton RB. Recalled maltreatment, migraine, and tension-type headache: results of the AMPP study. *Neurology.* 2015;84(2):132–140.
16. Tietjen GE, Peterlin BL. Childhood abuse and migraine: epidemiology, sex differences, and potential mechanisms. *Headache.* 2011;51(6):869–879.
17. Anda R, Tietjen G, Schulman E, Felitti V, Croft J. Adverse childhood experiences and frequent headaches in adults. *Headache.* 2010;50(9):1473–1481.
18. Fuh JL, Wang SJ, Juang KD, Lu SR, Liao YC, Chen SP. Relationship between childhood physical maltreatment and migraine in adolescents. *Headache.* 2010;50(5):761–768.
19. Tietjen GE, Brandes JL, Peterlin BL, et al. Childhood maltreatment and migraine (part I). Prevalence and adult revictimization: a multicenter headache clinic survey. *Headache.* 2010;50(1):20–31.
20. Tietjen GE, Brandes JL, Peterlin BL, et al. Childhood maltreatment and migraine (part II). Emotional abuse as a risk factor for headache chronification. *Headache.* 2010;50(1):32–41.
21. Tietjen GE, Brandes JL, Digre KB, et al. History of childhood maltreatment is associated with comorbid depression in women with migraine. *Neurology.* 2007;69(10):959–968.

22. Cripe SM, Sanchez SE, Gelaye B, Sanchez E, Williams MA. Association between intimate partner violence, migraine and probable migraine. *Headache*. 2011;51(2):208–219.
23. Rousseau-Salvador C, Amouroux R, Annequin D, Salvador A, Tourniaire B, Rusinek S. Anxiety, depression and school absenteeism in youth with chronic or episodic headache. *Pain Res Manag*. 2014;19(5):235–240.
24. Lima AS, de Araújo RC, Gomes MR, et al. Prevalence of headache and its interference in the activities of daily living in female adolescent students. *Rev Paul Pediatr*. 2014;32(2):256–261.
25. Kernick D, Reinhold D, Campbell JL. Impact of headache on young people in a school population. *Br J Gen Pract*. 2009;59(566):678–681.
26. Selekler HM, Gökmen G, Alvur TM, Steiner TJ. Productivity losses attributable to headache, and their attempted recovery, in a heavy-manufacturing workforce in Turkey: implications for employers and politicians. *J Headache Pain*. 2015;16(1):96.
27. Linde M, Gustavsson A, Stovner LJ, et al. The cost of headache disorders in Europe: the Eurolight project. *Eur J Neurol*. 2012;19(5):703–711.
28. Selekler MH, Gökmen G, Steiner TJ. Productivity impact of headache on a heavy-manufacturing workforce in Turkey. *J Headache Pain*. 2013;14:88.
29. Kessler RC, Shahly V, Stang PE, Lane MC. The associations of migraines and other headaches with work performance: results from the National Comorbidity Survey Replication (NCS-R). *Cephalalgia*. 2010;30(6):722–734.
30. Rasmussen BK, Jensen R, Olesen J. Impact of headache on sickness absence and utilisation of medical services: a Danish population study. *J Epidemiol Community Health*. 1992;46(4):443–446.
31. Roy AK, Lopes V, Klein RG. Disruptive mood dysregulation disorder: a new diagnostic approach to chronic irritability in youth. *Am J Psychiatry*. 2014;171(9):918–924.
32. Mulraney M, Melvin G, Tonge B. Brief report: can irritability act as a marker of psychopathology? *J Adolesc*. 2014;37(4):419–423.
33. Leibenluft E, Stoddard J. The developmental psychopathology of irritability. *Dev Psychopathol*. 2013;25(4 Pt 2):1473–1487.
34. Pedrelli P, Nyer M, Holt D, et al. Correlates of irritability in college students with depressive symptoms. *J Nerv Ment Dis*. 2013;201(11):953–958.
35. Krieger FV, Leibenluft E, Stringaris A, Polanczyk GV. Irritability in children and adolescents: past concepts, current debates, and future opportunities. *Rev Bras Psiquiatr*. 2013;35(suppl 1):S32–S39.
36. Judd LL, Schettler PJ, Coryell W, Akiskal HS, Fiedorowicz JG. Overt irritability/anger in unipolar major depressive episodes: past and current characteristics and implications for long-term course. *JAMA Psychiatry*. 2013;70(11):1171–1180.
37. Stringaris A, Maughan B, Copeland WS, Costello EJ, Angold A. Irritable mood as a symptom of depression in youth: prevalence, developmental, and clinical correlates in the Great Smoky Mountains Study. *J Am Acad Child Adolesc Psychiatry*. 2013;52(8):831–840.
38. Deveney CM, Connolly ME, Haring CT, Bones BL, Reynolds RC, Kim P. Neural mechanisms of frustration in chronically irritable children. *Am J Psychiatry*. 2013;170(10):1186–1194.
39. Birmaher B, Goldstein BI, Axelson DA, et al. Mood lability among offspring of parents with bipolar disorder and community controls. *Bipolar Disord*. 2013;15(3):253–263.
40. Hunt JI, Case BG, Birmaher B, et al. Irritability and elation in a large bipolar youth sample: relative symptom severity and clinical outcomes over 4 years. *J Clin Psychiatry*. 2013;74(1):e110–e117. https://doi.org/10.4088/JCP.12m07874

41. Kovess-Masfety V, Alonso J, Angermeyer M, et al. Irritable mood in adult major depressive disorder: results from the world mental health surveys. *Depress Anxiety.* 2013;30(4):395–406.
42. Leigh E, Smith P, Milavic G, Stringaris A. Mood regulation in youth: research findings and clinical approaches to irritability and short-lived episodes of mania-like symptoms. *Curr Opin Psychiatry.* 2012;25(4):271–276.
43. Drabick DA, Gadow KD. Deconstructing oppositional defiant disorder: clinic-based evidence for an anger/irritability phenotype. *J Am Acad Child Adolesc Psychiatry.* 2012;51(4):384–393.
44. Stringaris A, Zavos H, Leibenluft E, Maughan B, Eley TC. Adolescent irritability: phenotypic associations and genetic links with depressed mood. *Am J Psychiatry.* 2012;169(1):47–54.
45. Stringaris A. Irritability in children and adolescents: a challenge for DSM-5. *Eur Child Adolesc Psychiatry.* 2011;20(2):61–66.
46. Leibenluft E. Severe mood dysregulation, irritability, and the diagnostic boundaries of bipolar disorder in youths. *Am J Psychiatry.* 2011;168(2):129–142.
47. Stringaris A, Cohen P, Pine DS, Leibenluft E. Adult outcomes of youth irritability: a 20-year prospective community-based study. *Am J Psychiatry.* 2009;166(9):1048–1054.
48. Hunt J, Birmaher B, Leonard H, et al. Irritability without elation in a large bipolar youth sample: frequency and clinical description. *J Am Acad Child Adolesc Psychiatry.* 2009;48(7):730–739.
49. Fava M, Hwang I, Rush AJ, Sampson N, Walters EE, Kessler RC. The importance of irritability as a symptom of major depressive disorder: results from the National Comorbidity Survey Replication. *Mol Psychiatry.* 2010;15(8):856–867.
50. Perlis RH, Fava M, Trivedi MH, et al. Irritability is associated with anxiety and greater severity, but not bipolar spectrum features, in major depressive disorder. *Acta Psychiatr Scand.* 2009;119(4):282–289.
51. Farchione TR, Birmaher B, Axelson D, Kalas C, Monk K, Ehmann M. Aggression, hostility, and irritability in children at risk for bipolar disorder. *Bipolar Disord.* 2007;9(5):496–503.
52. Leibenluft E, Cohen P, Gorrindo T, Brook JS, Pine DS. Chronic versus episodic irritability in youth: a community-based, longitudinal study of clinical and diagnostic associations. *J Child Adolesc Psychopharmacol.* 2006;16(4):456–466.
53. Based on a PubMed search of *irritability*, *anger*, *depression*, and *anxiety* as MESH terms appearing in the title, we found fewer studies focusing on irritability (< 900) or anger (< 3,900) than those concentrating on depression (> 172,000) or anxiety (> 52,000). https://pubmed.ncbi.nlm.nih.gov/. Accessed October 4, 2022.
54. Barker ED, Salekin RT. Irritable oppositional defiance and callous unemotional traits: is the association partially explained by peer victimization? *J Child Psychol Psychiatry.* 2012;53(11):1167–1175.
55. Arslan S, Hallett V, Akkas E, Akkas OA. Bullying and victimization among Turkish children and adolescents: examining prevalence and associated health symptoms. *Eur J Pediatr.* 2012;171(10):1549–1557.
56. Chen HW, Gardner ES, Clarkson T, et al. Bullying perpetration and victimization in youth: associations with irritability and anxiety. *Child Psychiatry Hum Dev.* 2022;53(5):1075–1082.
57. Rieffe C, Camodeca M, Pouw LB, Lange AM, Stockmann L. Don't anger me! Bullying, victimization, and emotion dysregulation in young adolescents with ASD. *Eur J Dev Psychol.* 2012;9(3):351–370.
58. Natvig GK, Albrektsen G, Qvarnstrøm U. Psychosomatic symptoms among victims of school bullying. *J Health Psychol.* 2001;6(4):365–377.

59. Gobina I, Zaborskis A, Pudule I, Kalnins I, Villerusa A. Bullying and subjective health among adolescents at schools in Latvia and Lithuania. *Int J Public Health*. 2008;53(5):272–276.

60. Santric-Milicevic M, Stevanovic A, Popovac N, et al. Participation in bullying and associated health characteristics, risk factors and leisure activities: a profile of school-age children in Serbia. *Int J Environ Res Public Health*. 2022;19(15):9159.

61. Cardoso JB, Szlyk HS, Goldbach J, Swank P, Zvolensky MJ. General and ethnic-biased bullying among Latino students: exploring risks of depression, suicidal ideation, and substance use. *J Immigr Minor Health*. 2018;20:816–822.

62. Kodish T, Herres J, Shearer A, Atte T, Fein J, Diamond G. Bullying, depression, and suicide risk in a pediatric primary care sample. *Crisis*. 2016;37:241–244.

63. Hong L, Guo L, Wu H, et al. Bullying, depression, and suicidal ideation among adolescents in the Fujian Province of China: a cross-sectional study. *Medicine*. 2016;95(5):e2530. https://www.ncbi.nlm.nih.gov/pmc/articles/PMC4748877/pdf/medi-95-e2530.pdf. Accessed October 13, 2023.

64. Guo L, Hong L, Gao X, Zhou J, Lu C, Zhang WH. Associations between depression risk, bullying and current smoking among Chinese adolescents: modulated by gender. *Psychiatry Res*. 2016;237:282–289.

65. Undheim AM, Wallander J, Sund AM. Coping strategies and associations with depression among 12- to 15-year-old Norwegian adolescents involved in bullying. *J Nerv Ment Dis*. 2016;204(4):274–279.

66. Bland P. Bullying in adolescence linked to depression in young adults. *Practitioner*. 2015;259(1784):5.

67. Bowes L, Joinson C, Wolke D, Lewis G. Peer victimisation during adolescence and its impact on depression in early adulthood: prospective cohort study in the United Kingdom. *Br J Sports Med*. 2016;50(3):176–183.

68. Connolly EJ, Beaver KM. Considering the genetic and environmental overlap between bullying victimization, delinquency, and symptoms of depression/anxiety. *J Interpers Violence*. 2016;31(7):1230–1256.

69. Boyes ME, Cluver LD. Relationships between familial HIV/AIDS and symptoms of anxiety and depression: the mediating effect of bullying victimization in a prospective sample of South African children and adolescents. *J Youth Adolesc*. 2015;44(4):847–859.

70. Yen CF, Lin IM, Liu TL, Hu HF, Cheng CP. Mediating effects of depression and anxiety on the relationship between bullying involvement and pain problems among adolescents in Taiwan. *Compr Psychiatry*. 2014;55(6):1415–1421.

71. Klomek AB, Kleinman M, Altschuler E, Marrocco F, Amakawa L, Gould MS. Suicidal adolescents' experiences with bullying perpetration and victimization during high school as risk factors for later depression and suicidality. *J Adolesc Health*. 2013;53(1):S37–S42.

72. Hamilton JL, Shapero BG, Stange JP, Hamlat EJ, Abramson LY, Alloy LB. Emotional maltreatment, peer victimization, and depressive versus anxiety symptoms during adolescence: hopelessness as a mediator. *J Clin Child Adolesc Psychol*. 2013;42(3):332–347.

73. Roberts AL, Rosario M, Slopen N, Calzo JP, Austin SB. Childhood gender nonconformity, bullying victimization, and depressive symptoms across adolescence and early adulthood: an 11-year longitudinal study. *J Am Acad Child Adolesc Psychiatry*. 2013;52(2):143–152.

74. Madowitz J, Knatz S, Maginot T, Crow SJ, Boutelle KN. Teasing, depression and unhealthy weight control behaviour in obese children. *Pediatr Obes*. 2012;7(6):446–452.

75. Klomek AB, Kleinman M, Altschuler E, Marrocco F, Amakawa L, Gould MS. High school bullying as a risk for later depression and suicidality. *Suicide Life Threat Behav*. 2011;41(5):501–516.
76. Kindrick K, Castro J, Messias E. Sadness, suicide, and bullying in Arkansas: results from the Youth Risk Behavior Survey–2011. *J Ark Med Soc*. 2013;110(5):90–91.
77. Kaltiala-Heino R, Fröjd S. Correlation between bullying and clinical depression in adolescent patients. *Adolesc Health Med Ther*. 2011;2:37–44.
78. Luk JW, Wang J, Simons-Morton BG. Bullying victimization and substance use among US adolescents: mediation by depression. *Prev Sci*. 2010;11(4):355–359.
79. Kaltiala-Heino R, Fröjd S, Marttunen M. Involvement in bullying and depression in a 2-year follow-up in middle adolescence. *Eur Child Adolesc Psychiatry*. 2010;19(1):45.
80. Due P, Damsgaard MT, Lund R, Holstein BE. Is bullying equally harmful for rich and poor children? A study of bullying and depression from age 15 to 27. *Eur J Public Health*. 2009;19(5):464–469.
81. Fleming LC, Jacobsen KH. Bullying and symptoms of depression in Chilean middle school students. *J Sch Health*. 2009;79(3):130–137.
82. Lund R, Nielsen KK, Hansen DH, et al. Exposure to bullying at school and depression in adulthood: a study of Danish men born in 1953. *Eur J Public Health*. 2009;19(1):111–116.
83. Klomek AB, Sourander A, Kumpulainen K, et al. Childhood bullying as a risk for later depression and suicidal ideation among Finnish males. *J Affective Disord*. 2008;109(1):47–55.
84. Klomek AB, Marrocco F, Kleinman M, Schonfeld IS, Gould MS. Bullying, depression, and suicidality in adolescents. *J Am Acad Child Adolesc Psychiatry*. 2007;46(1):40–49.
85. Kaltiala-Heino R, Rimpelä M, Marttunen M, Rimpelä A, Rantanen P. Bullying, depression, and suicidal ideation in Finnish adolescents: school survey. *BMJ*. 1999;319(7206):348–351.
86. Kivimäki M, Virtanen M, Vartia M, Elovainio M, Vahtera J, Keltikangas-Järvinen L. Workplace bullying and the risk of cardiovascular disease and depression. *Occup Environ Med*. 2003;60(10):779.
87. Gullander M, Hogh A, Hansen ÅM, et al. Exposure to workplace bullying and risk of depression. *J Occup Environ Med*. 2014;56(12):1258–1265.
88. Emdad R, Alipour A, Hagberg J, Jensen IB. The impact of bystanding to workplace bullying on symptoms of depression among women and men in industry in Sweden: an empirical and theoretical longitudinal study. *Int Arch Occup Environ Health*. 2013;86(6):709–716.
89. Takaki J, Taniguchi T, Fukuoka E, et al. Workplace bullying could play important roles in the relationships between job strain and symptoms of depression and sleep disturbance. *J Occup Health*. 2010;52(6):367–374.
90. Arseneault L. Sibling bullying is associated with anxiety, depression and self-harm. *Evid Based Ment Health*. 2015;18(3):83.
91. Bowes L, Wolke D, Joinson C, Lereya ST, Lewis G. Sibling bullying and risk of depression, anxiety, and self-harm: a prospective cohort study. *Pediatrics*. 2014;134(4):e1032–e1039.
92. Feinstein BA, Bhatia V, Davila J. Rumination mediates the association between cyber-victimization and depressive symptoms. *J Interpers Violence*. 2014;29(9):1732–1746.
93. Selkie EM, Kota R, Chan YF, Moreno M. Cyberbullying, depression, and problem alcohol use in female college students: a multisite study. *Cyberpsychol Behav Soc Netw*. 2015;18(2):79–86.
94. Gámez-Guadix M, Orue I, Smith PK, Calvete E. Longitudinal and reciprocal relations of cyberbullying with depression, substance use, and problematic internet use among adolescents. *J Adolesc Health*. 2013;53(4):446–452.

95. Gao W, Paterson J, Abbott M, Carter S, Iusitini L. Pacific Islands Families Study: intimate partner violence and postnatal depression. *J Immigr Minor Health.* 2010;12(2):242–248.
96. Ludermir AB, Lewis G, Valongueiro SA, de Araújo TV, Araya R. Violence against women by their intimate partner during pregnancy and postnatal depression: a prospective cohort study. *Lancet.* 2010;376(9744):903–910.
97. Shamu S, Zarowsky C, Roelens K, Temmerman M, Abrahams N. High-frequency intimate partner violence during pregnancy, postnatal depression and suicidal tendencies in Harare, Zimbabwe. *Gen Hosp Psychiatry.* 2016;38:109–114.
98. Dienemann J, Boyle E, Baker D, Resnick W, Wiederhorn N, Campbell J. Intimate partner abuse among women diagnosed with depression. *Issues Ment Health Nurs.* 2000;21(5):499–513.
99. Caetano R, Cunradi C. Intimate partner violence and depression among Whites, Blacks, and Hispanics. *Ann Epidemiol.* 2003;13(10):661–665.
100. Nixon RD, Resick PA, Nishith P. An exploration of comorbid depression among female victims of intimate partner violence with posttraumatic stress disorder. *J Affective Disord.* 2004;82(2):315–320.
101. Martin SL, Li Y, Casanueva C, Harris-Britt A, Kupper LL, Cloutier S. Intimate partner violence and women's depression before and during pregnancy. *Violence Against Women.* 2006;12(3):221–239.
102. Koopman C, Ismailji T, Palesh O, et al. Relationships of depression to child and adult abuse and bodily pain among women who have experienced intimate partner violence. *J Interpers Violence.* 2007;22(4):438–455.
103. Deyessa N, Berhane Y, Alem A, et al. Intimate partner violence and depression among women in rural Ethiopia: a cross-sectional study. *Clin Pract Epidemiol Ment Health.* 2009;5(1):8.
104. Mburia-Mwalili A, Clements-Nolle K, Lee W, Shadley M, Yang W. Intimate partner violence and depression in a population-based sample of women: Can social support help? *J Interpers Violence.* 2010;25(12):2258–2278.
105. Gilchrist G, Hegarty K, Chondros P, Herrman H, Gunn J. The association between intimate partner violence, alcohol and depression in family practice. *BMC Fam Pract.* 2010;11(1):72.
106. Dougé N, Lehman EB, McCall-Hosenfeld JS. Social support and employment status modify the effect of intimate partner violence on depression symptom severity in women: results from the 2006 Behavioral Risk Factor Surveillance System Survey. *Womens Health Issues.* 2014 Aug 31;24(4): e425–e434.
107. Breet E, Seedat S, Kagee A. Posttraumatic stress disorder and depression in men and women who perpetrate intimate partner violence. *J Interpers Violence.* 2016:0886260516660297.
108. Kamimura A, Nourian MM, Assasnik N, Franchek-Roa K. Depression and intimate partner violence among college students in Iran. *Asian J Psychiatry.* 2016;23:51–55.
109. Steine IM, Winje D, Krystal JH, et al. Cumulative childhood maltreatment and its dose–response relation with adult symptomatology: findings in a sample of adult survivors of sexual abuse. *Child Abuse Negl.* 2017;65:99–111.
110. Nelson J, Klumparendt A, Doebler P, Ehring T. Childhood maltreatment and characteristics of adult depression: meta-analysis. *Br J Psychiatry.* 2017;210(2):96–104.
111. Dunn EC, Nishimi K, Powers A, Bradley B. Is developmental timing of trauma exposure associated with depressive and post-traumatic stress disorder symptoms in adulthood? *J Psychiatr Res.* 2017;84:119–127.

112. Schalinski I, Teicher MH, Nischk D, Hinderer E, Müller O, Rockstroh B. Type and timing of adverse childhood experiences differentially affect severity of PTSD, dissociative and depressive symptoms in adult inpatients. *BMC Psychiatry*. 2016;16(1):295.
113. Marackova M, Prasko J, Matousek S, et al. The impact of childhood adversities on anxiety and depressive disorders in adulthood. *Neuroendocrinol Lett*. 2016;37(7):478–484.
114. Mandelli L, Petrelli C, Serretti A. The role of specific early trauma in adult depression: a meta-analysis of published literature. Childhood trauma and adult depression. *Eur Psychiatry*. 2015;30(6):665–680.
115. Dunn EC, McLaughlin KA, Slopen N, Rosand J, Smoller JW. Developmental timing of child maltreatment and symptoms of depression and suicidal ideation in young adulthood: results from the National Longitudinal Study of Adolescent Health. *Depress Anxiety*. 2013;30(10):955–964.
116. Russell D, Springer KW, Greenfield EA. Witnessing domestic abuse in childhood as an independent risk factor for depressive symptoms in young adulthood. *Child Abuse Negl*. 2010;34(6):448–453.
117. Srabstein J, Piazza T. Public health, safety and educational risks associated with bullying behaviors in American adolescents. *Int J Adolesc Med Health*. 2008;20(2):223–233.
118. Salmon G, James A, Smith DM. Bullying in schools: self-reported anxiety, depression, and self-esteem in secondary school children. *BMJ*. 1998;317(7163):924–925.
119. Olweus D. Bullying at school: basic facts and effects of a school based intervention program. *J Child Psychol Psychiatry*. 1994;35:1171–1190.
120. Pabian S, Vandebosch H. An investigation of short-term longitudinal associations between social anxiety and victimization and perpetration of traditional bullying and cyberbullying. *J Youth Adolesc*. 2016;45(2):328.
121. McCabe RE, Antony MM, Summerfeldt LJ, Liss A, Swinson RP. Preliminary examination of the relationship between anxiety disorders in adults and self-reported history of teasing or bullying experiences. *Cognitive Behav Ther*. 2003;32(4):187–193.
122. Fahy AE, Stansfeld SA, Smuk M, Smith NR, Cummins S, Clark C. Longitudinal associations between cyberbullying involvement and adolescent mental health. *J Adolesc Health*. 2016;59(5):502–509.
123. Rodríguez-Muñoz A, Moreno-Jiménez B, Sanz-Vergel AI. Reciprocal relations between workplace bullying, anxiety, and vigor: a two-wave longitudinal study. *Anxiety Stress Coping*. 2015;28(5):514–530.
124. Reknes I, Einarsen S, Pallesen S, Bjorvatn B, Moen BE, Magerøy N. Exposure to bullying behaviors at work and subsequent symptoms of anxiety: the moderating role of individual coping style. *Ind Health*. 2016;54(5):421–432.
125. Mapayi B, Makanjuola RO, Mosaku SK, et al. Impact of intimate partner violence on anxiety and depression amongst women in Ile-Ife, Nigeria. *Arch Womens Ment Health*. 2013;16:11–18.
126. Fonseca-Machado MD, Monteiro JC, Haas VJ, Abrão AC, Gomes-Sponholz F. Intimate partner violence and anxiety disorders in pregnancy: the importance of vocational training of the nursing staff in facing them. *Rev Lat Am Enfermagem*. 2015;23(5):855–864.
127. Rehan W, Antfolk J, Johansson A, Jern P, Santtila P. Experiences of severe childhood maltreatment, depression, anxiety and alcohol abuse among adults in Finland. *PLOS One*. 2017;12(5):e0177252.

128. Bruce LC, Heimberg RG, Blanco C, Schneier FR, Liebowitz MR. Childhood maltreatment and social anxiety disorder: implications for symptom severity and response to pharmacotherapy. *Depress Anxiety*. 2012;29(2):132–139.
129. Gong Z, Reinhardt JD, Han Z, Ba Z, Lei S. Associations between school bullying and anxiety in children and adolescents from an ethnic autonomous county in China. *Psychiatry Res*. 2022:114649.
130. van Geel M, Goemans A, Vedder PH. The relation between peer victimization and sleeping problems: a meta-analysis. *Sleep Med Rev*. 2016;27:89–95.
131. Kubiszewski V, Fontaine R, Potard C, Gimenes G. Bullying, sleep/wake patterns and subjective sleep disorders: findings from a cross-sectional survey. *Chronobiol Int*. 2014;31(4):542–553.
132. Tochigi M, Nishida A, Shimodera S, et al. Irregular bedtime and nocturnal cellular phone usage as risk factors for being involved in bullying: a cross-sectional survey of Japanese adolescents. *PLOS One*. 2012;7(9):e45736.
133. Serra-Negra JM, Pordeus IA, Corrêa-Faria P, Fulgêncio LB, Paiva SM, Manfredini D. Is there an association between verbal school bullying and possible sleep bruxism in adolescents? *J Oral Rehab*. 2017;44(5):347–353.
134. Wolke D, Lereya ST. Bullying and parasomnias: a longitudinal cohort study. *Pediatrics*. 2014;134(4):e1040–e1048.
135. Yoo T, Ye B, Kim JI, Park S. Relationship of workplace violence and perpetrators on sleep disturbance—data from the 4th Korean Working Conditions Survey. *Ann Occup Environ Med*. 2016;28(1):59.
136. Niedhammer I, David S, Degioanni S, Drummond A, Philip P; 143 occupational physicians. Workplace bullying and sleep disturbances: findings from a large scale cross-sectional survey in the French working population. *Sleep*. 2009;32(9):1211–1219.
137. Hansen ÅM, Hogh A, Garde AH, Persson R. Workplace bullying and sleep difficulties: a 2-year follow-up study. *Int Arch Occup Environ Health*. 2014;87(3):285–294.
138. Nabe-Nielsen K, Grynderup MB, Lange T, et al. The role of poor sleep in the relation between workplace bullying/unwanted sexual attention and long-term sickness absence. *Int Arch Occup Environ Health*. 2016;89(6):967–979.
139. Sanchez SE, Islam S, Zhong QY, Gelaye B, Williams MA. Intimate partner violence is associated with stress-related sleep disturbance and poor sleep quality during early pregnancy. *PLOS One*. 2016;11(3):e0152199.
140. Drake C, Richardson G, Roehrs T, Scofield H, Roth T. Vulnerability to stress-related sleep disturbance and hyperarousal. *Sleep*. 2004;27(2):285–291. Cited by Sanchez et al.[139]
141. Buysse DJ, Reynolds CF III, Monk TH, Berman SR, Kupfer DJ. The Pittsburgh Sleep Quality Index: a new instrument for psychiatric practice and research. *Psychiatry Res*. 1989;28(2):193–213. Cited by Sanchez et al.[139]
142. Rauer AJ, El-Sheikh M. Reciprocal pathways between intimate partner violence and sleep in men and women. *J Fam Psychol*. 2012;26(3):470.
143. Romito P, Feresin MC, Bastiani F, Saurel-Cubizolles MJ. Psychological symptoms and intensity of partner violence: A study of women attending an anti-violence center in Italy. *Health Care Women Int*. 2022;43(7-8):931–945.
144. Sadeh A, McGuire JP, Sachs H, Seifer R, Tremblay A, Civita R, Hayden RM. Sleep and psychological characteristics of children on a psychiatric inpatient unit. *J Am Acad Child Adolesc Psychiatry*. 1995;34(6):813–819.

145. Lind MJ, Aggen SH, Kendler KS, York TP, Amstadter AB. An epidemiologic study of childhood sexual abuse and adult sleep disturbances. *Psychol Trauma*. 2016;8(2):198.
146. Abrams MP, Mulligan AD, Carleton RN, Asmundson GJ. Prevalence and correlates of sleep paralysis in adults reporting childhood sexual abuse. *J Anxiety Disord*. 2008;22(8):1535–1541.
147. Poon CY, Knight BG. Impact of childhood parental abuse and neglect on sleep problems in old age. *J Gerontol B Psychol Sci Soc Sci*. 2011;66(3):307–310.
148. Gelaye B, Kajeepeta S, Zhong QY, et al. Childhood abuse is associated with stress-related sleep disturbance and poor sleep quality in pregnancy. *Sleep Med*. 2015;16(10):1274–1280.
149. Gustafsson H, Doyle C, Gilchrist M, Werner E, Monk C. Maternal abuse history and reduced fetal heart rate variability: abuse-related sleep disturbance is a mediator. *Dev Psychopathol*. 2017;29(3):1023–1034.
150. Petrov ME, Davis MC, Belyea MJ, Zautra AJ. Linking childhood abuse and hypertension: sleep disturbance and inflammation as mediators. *J Behav Med*. 2016;39(4):716–726.
151. April-Sanders A, Duarte CS, Wang S, et al. Childhood adversity and sleep disturbances: longitudinal results in Puerto Rican children. *Int J Behav Med*. 2021;28(1):107–115. Cited by Schønning et al (see Note 156).
152. Choquet M, Darves-Bornoz JM, Ledoux S, Manfredi R, Hassler C. Self-reported health and behavioral problems among adolescent victims of rape in France: results of a cross-sectional survey. *Child Abuse Negl*. 1997;21(9):823–832. Cited by Schønning et al (see Note 156).
153. Langevin R, Hébert M, Guidi E, Bernard-Bonnin AC, Allard-Dansereau C. Sleep problems over a year in sexually abused preschoolers. *Paediatr Child Health*. 2017;22(5):273–276. Cited by Schønning et al (see Note 156).
154. Mignot S, Fritel X, Loreal M, et al. Identifying teenage sexual abuse victims by questions on their daily lives. *Child Abuse Negl*. 2018;85:127–136. Cited by Schønning et al (see Note 156).
155. Wells RD, McCann J, Adams J, Voris J, Ensign J. Emotional, behavioral, and physical symptoms reported by parents of sexually abused, nonabused, and allegedly abused prepubescent females. *Child Abuse Negl*. 1995;19(2):155–163. Cited by Schønning et al (see Note 156).
156. Schønning V, Sivertsen B, Hysing M, Dovran A, Askeland KG. Childhood maltreatment and sleep in children and adolescents: a systematic review and meta-analysis. *Sleep Med Rev*. 2022:101617.
157. Min JY, Park SG, Kim SS, Min KB. Workplace injustice and self-reported disease and absenteeism in South Korea. *Am J Ind Med*. 2014;57(1):87–96.
158. Park J, Lee N. First Korean Working Conditions Survey: a comparison between South Korea and EU countries. *Ind Health*. 2009;47(1):50–54. Cited by Min et al.157
159. Prevalence ratio (PR). For details, see Zocchetti C, Consonni D, Bertazzi PA. Relationship between prevalence rate ratios and odds ratios in cross-sectional studies. *Int J Epidemiol*. 1997;26(1):220–223. Cited by Min et al.[157]
160. Adjusted for personal characteristics (age, sex, education, income, smoking, alcohol consumption, and income). See Min et al.[157]
161. Adjusted for occupational characteristics (occupational status, employment status, working time, working day, and shift work). See Min et al.[157]
162. Adjusted for job-related characteristics (job insecurity, job satisfaction, being well informed about health and safety risks, and exposure to occupational hazards). See Min et al.[157]
163. Glambek M, Nielsen MB, Gjerstad J, Einarsen S. Gender differences in the relationship between workplace bullying and subjective back and neck pain: a two-wave study in a Norwegian probability sample. *J Psychosomat Res*. 2018;106:73–75.

164. Gilkey DP, Keefe TJ, Peel JL, Kassab OM, Kennedy CA. Risk factors associated with back pain: a cross-sectional study of 963 college students. *J Manipulative Physiol Ther*. 2010;33(2):88–95.
165. Vives-Cases C, Ruiz-Cantero MT, Escribà-Agüir V, Miralles JJ. The effect of intimate partner violence and other forms of violence against women on health. *J Public Health*. 2010;33(1):15–21.
166. Leisner S, Gerhardt A, Tesarz J, Janke S, Seidler GH, Eich W. Childhood abuse experiences and chronic low back pain: direct and mediated effects of childhood abuse in different pain dimensions of nonspecific chronic low back pain [in German]. *Schmerz*. 2014;28(6):600–606. Abstract in English at https://www.ncbi.nlm.nih.gov/pubmed/25179418. Accessed October 4, 2022. Cited by Tesarz et al (see Note 167).
167. Tesarz J, Eich W, Treede RD, Gerhardt A. Altered pressure pain thresholds and increased wind-up in adult patients with chronic back pain with a history of childhood maltreatment: a quantitative sensory testing study. *Pain*. 2016;157(8):1799–1809.
168. Boey CC, Goh KL. The significance of life-events as contributing factors in childhood recurrent abdominal pain in an urban community in Malaysia. *J Psychosomat Res*. 2001;51(4):559–562.
169. Fekkes M, Pijpers FI, Verloove-Vanhorick SP. Bullying behavior and associations with psychosomatic complaints and depression in victims. *J Pediatr*. 2004;144(1):17–22.
170. Fekkes M, Pijpers FI, Fredriks AM, Vogels T, Verloove-Vanhorick SP. Do bullied children get ill, or do ill children get bullied? A prospective cohort study on the relationship between bullying and health-related symptoms. *Pediatrics*. 2006;117(5):1568–1574.
171. Sourander A, Klomek AB, Ikonen M, et al. Psychosocial risk factors associated with cyberbullying among adolescents: a population-based study. *Arch Gen Psychiatry*. 2010;67(7):720–728.
172. Bonomi AE, Anderson ML, Reid RJ, Rivara FP, Carrell D, Thompson RS. Medical and psychosocial diagnoses in women with a history of intimate partner violence. *Arch Intern Med*. 2009;169(18):1692–1697.
173. van Tilburg MA, Runyan DK, Zolotor AJ, et al. Unexplained gastrointestinal symptoms after abuse in a prospective study of children at risk for abuse and neglect. *Ann Fam Med*. 2010;8(2):134–140.
174. Bru E, Boyesen M, Munthe E, Roland E. Perceived social support at school and emotional and musculoskeletal complaints among Norwegian 8th grade students. *Scand J Educ Res*. 1998;42(4):339–356.
175. Kashikar-Zuck S, Lynch AM, Graham TB, Swain NF, Mullen SM, Noll RB. Social functioning and peer relationships of adolescents with juvenile fibromyalgia syndrome. *Arthritis Care Res*. 2007;57(3):474–480.
176. Wallace DJ. The fibromyalgia syndrome. *Ann Med*. 1997;29(1):9–21. Cited by >Kivimäki> et al (see Note 177).
177. Kivimäki M, Leino-Arjas P, Virtanen M, et al. Work stress and incidence of newly diagnosed fibromyalgia: prospective cohort study. *J Psychosomat Res*. 2004;57(5):417–422.
178. Vignoli M, Guglielmi D, Balducci C, Bonfiglioli R. Workplace bullying as a risk factor for musculoskeletal disorders: the mediating role of job-related psychological strain. *Biomed Res Int*. 2015;2015:712642.
179. Jacobsen DP, Nielsen MB, Einarsen S, Gjerstad J. Negative social acts and pain: evidence of a workplace bullying and 5-HTT genotype interaction. *Scand J Work Environ Health*. 2018;44(3):283–290.

180. Copeland WE, Wolke D, Lereya ST, Shanahan L, Worthman C, Costello EJ. Childhood bullying involvement predicts low-grade systemic inflammation into adulthood. *Proc Natl Acad Sci*. 2014:201323641.
181. Takizawa R, Danese A, Maughan B, Arseneault L. Bullying victimization in childhood predicts inflammation and obesity at mid-life: a five-decade birth cohort study. *Psychol Med*. 2015;45(13):2705–2715.
182. Newton TL, Fernandez-Botran R, Miller JJ, Lorenz DJ, Burns VE, Fleming KN. Markers of inflammation in midlife women with intimate partner violence histories. *J Womens Health*. 2011;20(12):1871–1880.
183. Danese A, Pariante CM, Caspi A, Taylor A, Poulton R. Childhood maltreatment predicts adult inflammation in a life-course study. *Proc Natl Acad Sci*. 2007;104(4):1319–1324.
184. Stanton WR, ed. *From Child to Adult: The Dunedin Multidisciplinary Health and Development Study*. New York, NY: Oxford University Press; 1996.
185. Silva PA. The Dunedin Multidisciplinary Health and Development Study: a 15 year longitudinal study. *Paediatr Perinat Epidemiol*. 1990;4(1):76–107.
186. The Dunedin Study. https://dunedinstudy.otago.ac.nz/. Accessed October 4, 2022.
187. Sutin AR, Robinson E, Daly M, Terracciano A. Parent-reported bullying and child weight gain between ages 6 and 15. *Child Obes*. 2016;12(6):482–487.
188. Mason SM, Ayour N, Canney S, Eisenberg ME, Neumark-Sztainer D. Intimate partner violence and 5-year weight change in young women: a longitudinal study. *J Womens Health*. 2017;26(6):677–682.
189. Alhusen JL, Geller R, Dreisbach C, Constantoulakis L, Siega-Riz AM. Intimate partner violence and gestational weight gain in a population-based sample of perinatal women. *J Obstet, Gynecol Neonatal Nurs*. 2017;46(3):390–402.
190. Diesel JC, Bodnar LM, Day NL, Larkby CA. Childhood maltreatment and the risk of pre-pregnancy obesity and excessive gestational weight gain. *Matern Child Nutr*. 2016;12(3):558–568.
191. Xu T, Hanson LL, Lange T, et al. Workplace bullying and violence as risk factors for type 2 diabetes: a multicohort study and meta-analysis. *Diabetologia*. 2018;61(1):75–83.
192. >Mason> SM, >Wright> RJ, >Hibert> EN, >et al>. Intimate partner violence and incidence of type 2 diabetes in women. *Diabetes Care*. 2013;36(5):1159–1165.
193. Shields ME, Hovdestad WE, Pelletier C, Dykxhoorn JL, O'Donnell SC, Tonmyr L. Childhood maltreatment as a risk factor for diabetes: findings from a population-based survey of Canadian adults. *BMC Public Health*. 2016;16(1):879.
194. Canada Statistics. Canadian Community Health Survey—Mental Health, Detailed Information for 2012. http://www23.statcan.gc.ca/imdb/p2SV.pl?Function=getSurvey&SDDS=5015. Accessed October 4, 2022.
195. Li L, Garvey WT, Gower BA. Childhood maltreatment is an independent risk factor for prediabetic disturbances in glucose regulation. *Front Endocrinol*. 2017;8:151.
196. Xu T, Magnusson Hanson LL, Lange T, et al. Workplace bullying and workplace violence as risk factors for cardiovascular disease: a multi-cohort study. *Eur Heart J*. 2019;40(14):1124–1134.
197. >Clark> CJ, >Everson-Rose> SA, >Alonso> A, >et al>. Effect of partner violence in adolescence and young adulthood on blood pressure and incident hypertension. *PLOS One*. 2014;9(3):e92204.

198. >Harris> KM, >Halpern> CT, >Whitsel> E, >et al>. The National Longitudinal Study of Adolescent to Adult Health: research design. 2009. http://www.cpc.unc.edu/projects/addhealth/design. Accessed October 4, 2022.
199. Ho FK, Celis-Morales C, Gray SR, et al. Child maltreatment and cardiovascular disease: quantifying mediation pathways using UK Biobank. *BMC Med.* 2020;18(1):1–10. https://www.ukbiobank.ac.uk/learn-more-about-uk-biobank/about-us. Accessed September 20, 2023.
200. Biobank, About Us, Background. "UK Biobank is a large-scale biomedical database and research resource, containing in-depth genetic and health information from half a million UK participants." https://www.ukbiobank.ac.uk/learn-more-about-uk-biobank/about-us. Accessed October 13, 2023.
201. ICD-10 (*International Classification of Diseases*, 10th revision) codes I20, I21, I25, I48, I50, I60, I61, I63, I64. Cited by Ho et al.[199]
202. Conners CK. *Conners' Rating Scales–Revised: Technical Manual.* New York, NY: Multi-Health System Inc; 2003. Cited by Singham et al (see Note 203).
203. Singham T, Viding E, Schoeler T, et al. Concurrent and longitudinal contribution of exposure to bullying in childhood to mental health: the role of vulnerability and resilience. *JAMA Psychiatry.* 2017;74(11):1112–1119.
204. Sesar K, Barišić M, Pandža M, Dodaj A. The relationship between difficulties in psychological adjustment in young adulthood and exposure to bullying behaviour in childhood and adolescence. *Acta Med Acad.* 2012;41(2):131–144. doi:10.5644/ama2006-124.46
205. >Schäfer> M, >Korn> S, >Smith> PK, >et al>. Lonely in the crowd: recollections of bullying. *Br J Dev Psychol.* 2004;22(3):379–394. Cited by Sesar et al.[204]
206. Briere J, Runtz M. The Trauma Symptom Checklist (TSC-33) early data on a new scale. *J Interpers Violence.* 1989;4(2):151–163. Cited by Sesar et al.[204]
207. This subscale includes the following items: flashbacks ("sudden vivid distracting memories"), spacing out ("going away in your mind"), dizziness, memory problems, feeling that things are "unreal," and feelings that you are not always in your body. http://s1097954.instanturl.net/trauma-symptom-checklist-40-tsi-40/. Accessed October 4, 2022.
208. Hulette AC, Freyd JJ, Fisher PA. Dissociation in middle childhood among foster children with early maltreatment experiences. *Child Abuse Negl.* 2011;35(2):123.
209. Putnam FW, Helmers K, Trickett PK. Development, reliability, and validity of a child dissociation scale. *Child Abuse Negl.* 1993;17(6):731–741. Cited by Hulette et al.[208]
210. Brewin CR. Re-experiencing traumatic events in PTSD: new avenues in research on intrusive memories and flashbacks. *Eur J Psychotraumatol.* 2015;6(1):27180.
211. World Health Organization. ICD-11 for Mortality and Morbidity Statistics (2018), 6B40 Post traumatic stress disorder, Description. https://icd.who.int/browse11/l-m/en#/http://id.who.int/icd/entity/2070699808. Accessed October 4, 2022.
212. Recurrent, involuntary, and distressing memories; recurrent distressing dreams; dissociative reactions; intense or prolonged psychological distress; marked physiological reactions; avoidance of stimuli associated with the traumatic event; negative alterations in cognitions and mood associated with the trauma; marked alterations in arousal and reactivity, as listed in American Psychiatric Association. *Diagnostic and Statistical Manual of Mental Disorders.* 5th ed. Arlington, VA: American Psychiatric Association; 2013.
213. Hébert M, Langevin R, Daigneault I. The association between peer victimization, PTSD, and dissociation in child victims of sexual abuse. *J Affective Disord.* 2016;193:227–232.

214. Andersen LP, Hogh A, Elklit A, Andersen JH, Biering K. Work-related threats and violence and post-traumatic symptoms in four high-risk occupations: short-and long-term symptoms. *Int Arch Occup Environ Health.* 2018:1–4.
215. Idsoe T, Dyregrov A, Idsoe EC. Bullying and PTSD symptoms. *J Abnorm Child Psychol.* 2012;40(6):901–911.
216. Malinauskiene V, Einarsen S. Workplace bullying and post-traumatic stress symptoms among family physicians in Lithuania: an occupation and region specific approach. *Int J Occup Med Environ Health.* 2014;27(6):919–932.
217. >Ranney> ML, >Patena> JV, >Nugent> N, >et al>. PTSD, cyberbullying and peer violence: prevalence and correlates among adolescent emergency department patients. *Gen Hosp Psychiatry.* 2016;39:32–38.
218. Litman L, Costantino G, Waxman R, et al. Relationship between peer victimization and posttraumatic stress among primary school children. *J Trauma Stress.* 2015;28(4):348–354.
219. Shorey RC, Fite PJ, Menon SV, Cohen JR, Stuart GL, Temple JR. The association between PTSD symptoms and IPV perpetration across 6 years. *J Interpers Violence.* 2018:0886260518800310.
220. Castro M, Alcántara-López M, Martínez A, Fernández V, Sánchez-Meca J, López-Soler C. Mother's IPV, child maltreatment type and the presence of PTSD in children and adolescents. *Int J Environ Res Public Health.* 2017;14(9):1077.
221. Wolfe VV. The Children's Impact of Traumatic Events Scale II (CITES-II). In: Wolfe VV,ed. Unpublished Assessment Instrument. Child and Adolescent Centre, London Health Sciences Centre, Canada; 2002. Cited by Hébert et al.[213]
222. Weiss DS, Marmar CR. *The Impact of Event Scale—Revised.* New York, NY: Guilford Press; 1997:399–411. Cited by Andersen et al.[214]
223. Foa EB, Johnson KM, Feeny NC, Treadwell KR. The Child PTSD Symptom Scale: A preliminary examination of its psychometric properties. *J Clin Child Psychol.* 2001;30(3):376–384. Cited by Ranney et al.[217]
224. Steinberg AM, Brymer MJ, Decker KB, Pynoos RS. The University of California at Los Angeles Post-traumatic Stress Disorder Reaction Index. *Curr Psychiatry Rep.* 2004;6(2):96–100. Cited by Litman et al.[218]
225. Schreier A, Wolke D, Thomas K, et al. Prospective study of peer victimization in childhood and psychotic symptoms in a nonclinical population at age 12 years. *Arch Gen Psychiatry.* 2009;66(5):527–536.
226. Catone G, Marotta R, Pisano S, et al. Psychotic-like experiences in help-seeking adolescents: dimensional exploration and association with different forms of bullying victimization–a developmental social psychiatry perspective. *Int J Social Psychiatry.* 2017;63(8):752–762.
227. Ronald A, Sieradzka D, Cardno AG, Haworth CM, McGuire P, Freeman D. Characterization of psychotic experiences in adolescence using the Specific Psychotic Experiences Questionnaire: findings from a study of 5000 16-year-old twins. *Schizophr Bull.* 2013;40(4):868–877. Cited by Catone et al.[226]
228. >Yamasaki> S, >Ando> S, >Koike> S, >et al>. Dissociation mediates the relationship between peer victimization and hallucinatory experiences among early adolescents. *Schizophr Res Cognition.* 2016;4:18–23.
229. Stanyon D, Yamasaki S, Ando S, et al. The role of bullying victimization in the pathway between autistic traits and psychotic experiences in adolescence: data from the Tokyo Teen Cohort study. *Schizophr Res.* 2022;239:111–115.

230. The Tokyo Teen Cohort study "is a large population-based longitudinal survey assessing the health and development in a general sample of adolescents living in three municipalities in the Tokyo metropolitan area born between September 2002 and August 2004."[229]
231. Shah R, Von Mach T, Fedina L, Link B, DeVylder J. Intimate partner violence and psychotic experiences in four US cities. *Schizophr Res.* 2018;195:506–512.
232. Holshausen K, Bowie CR, Harkness KL. The relation of childhood maltreatment to psychotic symptoms in adolescents and young adults with depression. *J Clin Child Adolesc Psychol.* 2016;45(3):241–247.
233. American Psychiatric Association. *Diagnostic and Statistical Manual of Mental Disorders.* 4th ed. Washington, DC: American Psychiatric Association; 1994.
234. Peyton RP, Ranasinghe S, Jacobsen KH. Injuries, violence, and bullying among middle school students in Oman. *Oman Med J.* 2017;32(2):98.
235. Abdou SA, Al-Murzahmi SN. *Oman Global School-based Student Health Survey 2010.* Muscat, Oman: Ministry of Health; 2012. Cited by Peyton et al.[234]
236. Beck NI, Arif I, Paumier MF, Jacobsen KH. Adolescent injuries in Argentina, Bolivia, Chile, and Uruguay: results from the 2012–2013 Global School-based Student Health Survey (GSHS). *Injury.* 2016;47(12):2642–2649.
237. Fanslow JL, Robinson EM. Physical injuries resulting from intimate partner violence and disclosure to healthcare providers: results from a New Zealand population-based study. *Inj Prev.* 2011;17(1):37–42.
238. Vaithianathan R, Rouland B, Putnam-Hornstein E. Injury and mortality among children identified as at high risk of maltreatment. *Pediatrics.* 2018;141(2):e20172882.
239. Forjuoh SN. Child maltreatment related injuries: incidence, hospital charges, and correlates of hospitalization. *Child Abuse Negl.* 2000;24(8):1019–1025.
240. World Health Organization. ICD-11 for Mortality and Morbidity Statistics, QE84 Acute stress reaction. https://icd.who.int/browse11/l-m/en#/http://id.who.int/icd/entity/505909942. Accessed October 4, 2022.
241. World Health Organization. ICD-11 for Mortality and Morbidity Statistics, 6B41 Complex post-traumatic stress disorder. https://icd.who.int/browse11/l-m/en#/http%253a%252f%252fid.who.int%252ficd%252fentity%252f585833559. Accessed October 4, 2022.

5
Psychosocial Problems and Risk Behaviors Linked to Bullying and Other Forms of Victimization

What Is Known?

Bullying and other forms of victimization have been associated with an array of psychosocial problems and risk behaviors, including poor health-related quality of life, absenteeism, poor academic performance, school dropout, physical fights, carrying a weapon, adolescent pregnancy, self-injurious behavior, suicide attempt, substance abuse, and criminality.

Poor Health-Related Quality of Life

Quality of Life

The World Health Organization (WHO) has defined quality of life (QoL) as "an individual's perception of their position in life in the context of culture and value systems in which they live, and in relation to their goals, expectations, standards and concerns."[1] WHO has developed an international assessment of this subjective construct, known as WHOQAR, which is organized into six broad areas, including the physical and psychological domains, level of independence, social relationships, environment, and spirituality/religion/personal beliefs.[2]

Health-Related Quality of Life

> Health-related quality of life (HRQoL) is a multidimensional concept that includes domains related to physical, mental, emotional, and social functioning. It goes beyond direct measures of population health, life expectancy, and causes of death, and focuses on the impact health status has on quality of life. A related concept of HRQoL is well-being, which assesses the positive aspects of a person's life, such as positive emotions and life satisfaction.[3]

Peer Victimization and HRQoL

Wilkins-Shumer et al.[4] initially documented that adolescents who were bullied more than once a week experienced a significantly higher negative impact on their psychosocial well-being, as manifested by a lower HRQoL rating, when compared to their peers who were victimized less frequently or not at all.[4]

A subsequent study by Frisén and Bjarnelind[5] further confirmed that being bullied was associated with poorer ratings of HRQoL. Furthermore, their study showed that adolescents who bullied others had poorer ratings on some aspects of HRQoL.[5] Moreover, students who reported being bullied during the last high school years experienced more difficulties with their general health and estimated their mental health as poorer in comparison to adolescents who reported being bullied sometime during first through sixth grade.[5]

It should be noted that there is documented evidence indicating that the magnitude of the link between victimization and lower ratings of QoL varies according to the causes of peer bullying. This notion was supported by a study conducted by Patrick et al.[6] that showed that students who were bullied because they were perceived as being gay, lesbian, or bisexual had significantly lower QoL scores that those who were mistreated for other reasons.[6]

A study conducted by Chen and Huang[7] indicated that college students who experienced verbal and relational bullying, both before and during college, reported lower HRQoL.

Workplace Bullying and HRQoL

Fattori et al.[8] assessed the HRQoL associated with workplace bullying among patients with different chronic medical conditions. Their research, with data from more than 1,700 participants, showed that workplace bullying was associated with worse HRQoL scores, above and beyond the detrimental effect of other concurrent medical conditions.[8]

Intimate Partner Violence and HRQoL

The effect of intimate partner violence (IPV) on HRQoL was explored by Costa et al.[9] in a randomized sample of almost 3,500 adult men and women from six European cities. The study documented that physical HRQoL was significantly lower in women who in the previous 12 months had been involved in physical IPV as both victims or perpetrators than in non-abused women.[9] Furthermore, women who were victims-only of sexual coercion in the previous year, as well as those who were victims-only or both victims and perpetrators in concomitant physical and sexual IPV, had significantly lower scores of mental HRQoL than women not involved in IPV.[9]

Moreover, significantly lower mental HRQoL was found among men who, in the previous year, were involved in physical IPV, both as victims and as perpetrators, as well as those who were concurrently participating in physical and sexual IPV, as victims and perpetrators, as compared with men not involved in IPV.[9]

Cyberbullying and HRQoL

An analysis of how HRQoL varies depending on the role played in cyberbullying was conducted by González-Cabrera et al.[10] through a four-month longitudinal study (December 2015–April 2016) based on the participation of 920 Spanish students (11 to 18 years old) who were assessed with the use of the Cyberbullying Test,[11] a self-report questionnaire about participation in cyberbullying as a victim, perpetrator, or bystander, and the KIDSCREEN-52,[12] an instrument to measure different dimensions of HRQoL. This investigation documented that cyber victims and cyberbully victims report inferior QoL in all the dimensions ($P < .001$), as compared to those participants who were not involved in cyberbullying or were bystanders.

Absenteeism

School Bullying and Cyberbullying and the Risk of Absenteeism

A significant association between bullying and school absenteeism due to safety concerns was highlighted by Steiner and Rasberry[13] in a study based on a large national sample of US high school students who were part of the 2013 Youth Risk Behavior Survey. Steiner and Rasberry[13] documented that adolescents who were bullied either in school or in cyberspace had a significantly higher risk of school absenteeism, due to fears of endangerment, as compared to young people who were not bullied. Furthermore, female and male students who were exposed to both types of bullying "had more than five and six times the odds, respectively, of missing school because of safety concerns."[13]

Workplace Bullying and Absenteeism

The link between workplace mistreatment and absenteeism was examined in a study by Asfaw et al.[14] through an analysis of 2010 National Health Interview Survey data from more than 13,000 employed adults. The research showed that "being mistreated was associated with a 42% increase in the number of missed workdays, controlling for covariates."[14] Additionally, the study indicated that absent days of work differed by 2.45 days between mistreated and nonmistreated workers, incurring $4.1 billion in sickness absenteeism costs in 2010.[14]

Poor Academic Performance

Peer Victimization and Poor Academic Performance

Mundy et al.[15] quantified the association between peer victimization and academic performance in a large sample of Australian children 8 to 9 years old. Their analysis demonstrated that girls and boys who were exposed to both physical and verbal victimization exhibited significantly lower performance on reading than their peers who were not mistreated, even after controlling for emotional symptoms. Furthermore, female students who were both physically and verbally bullied performed at a lower level in spelling, grammar, and writing. Poor performance in numeracy was exhibited by students of both genders who were physically victimized. A causal relationship could not be established, given the cross-sectional nature of the study.

The risk to academic performance linked to peer victimization was also highlighted in a study by Wang et al.,[16] which documented a significant relation between peer victimization and grade point average (GPA), even after taking into consideration school climate scores, individual variability in school climate scores, ethnicity, absenteeism, household income, parental education, percentage of minority students, type of school, and bullying perpetration.

IPV and Poor Academic Performance

Brewer et al.[17] investigated the association between IPV and academic performance in a study based on a national sample of more than 85,000 US undergraduate students from 128 tertiary education institutions. The study documented that students who reported IPV were likely to have a lower cumulative grade average and increased academic difficulties, with the association being mediated through psychological distress.

Childhood Maltreatment and Poor Academic Performance

The relationship between childhood maltreatment and school performance was investigated by Zolotor et al.,[18] in a longitudinal study of a cohort of children at risk of maltreatment who were followed from birth through 8 years of age. The investigation showed that a confirmed maltreatment report was significantly associated with poorer academic performance, even after controlling for gestational age, caregiver's age and employment status, and caregiver report of child's anxiety and depression.

Carrying a Weapon

Bullying and Carrying a Weapon

The link between participation in school bullying, as a victim or as a perpetrator, and carrying weapons to school was first highlighted by Nansel et al.,[19] in cross-sectional study of a US representative sample of more than 15,000 students in grades 6 to 10 who participated in the 1998 Health Behavior in School-aged Children (HBSC) survey. Nansel et al.[19] documented that the risk of carrying a weapon was higher among those who bullied others in school [adjusted OR (AOR) = 2.6] as compared to those who were bullied in school (AOR = 1.5), as well as among those students who bullied others outside school (AOR = 5.9) as compared to those who were bullied outside the school (AOR = 4.1).

The association between bullying participation and carrying weapons was further underscored by Van Geel et al.[20] in research based on meta-analysis of 22 studies involving more than 257,000 youths, ranging in age from 11 to 21 years, which showed that, in comparison to noninvolved peers, victims of bullying were at risk of carrying weapons (OR = 1.97), while this risk was higher among perpetrators (OR = 3.25) and bully-victims (OR = 4.95). Furthermore, studies done in the United States found stronger relations between being a bully-victim and weapon-carrying (OR = 7.84) than were found in studies from other countries (OR = 3.62).[20]

A study by Esselmont,[21] based on a second analysis of data available from the 2001–2002 US HBSC survey, demonstrated that the effects of school bullying victimization on weapon-carrying are mediated by the students' perception of school safety.[21]

Physical Fights

Bullying and Physical Fights

The study by Nansel et al.,[19] which examined the link between bullying and carrying weapons, also documented that students who have been bullied in school weekly were at risk of being involved in frequent fighting (AOR = 1.7), and that the risk was higher among those who bullied others in school (AOR = 3.1) or away from school (AOR = 3.5). Furthermore, there was a significant risk of being injured in a fight among those who, away from school, were bullied weekly (AOR = 3.5) or bullied others weekly (AOR = 3.3).

School Dropout

Bullying and School Dropout

A "harassing/bullying school environment" was found to be a factor significantly linked (AOR = 1.70) to school dropout in a study conducted by Prakash et al.,[22] based on a cross-sectional survey of 2,275 female adolescent students in Karnataka, India. This significant association was evident even after adjustment for individual, family, and village/school characteristics. Yet, at the individual level, no significant link was found between having been teased or sexually harassed in the previous 12 months and school dropout (OR = 1.04).

IPV and School Dropout

Currently, there is no published evidence of school dropout being significantly associated with being exposed to IPV, at the individual level. Yet, as in the case of school bullying,[22] the prevalence of physical and or sexual IPV in an area has been found to be associated with the prevalence of school dropout in the area. In a study by Sanz-Barbero et al.,[23] based on the analysis of a cross-sectional sample of 5,976 European ever-partnered women age 18 to 29, it was shown that "living in a country with a medium/high level of school dropout increases the probability of experiencing physical and/or sexual IPV (PR = 1.4) as well as psychological IPV (PR = 1.2)."[23]

Childhood Maltreatment and School Dropout

Barker et al.[24] assessed the impact of childhood maltreatment on high school completion in a cross-sectional study involving 974 young adults in Vancouver, Canada. The investigation[24] documented that, after a thorough adjustment for a range of confounding variables, four types of childhood maltreatment were significantly and independently linked with incompletion of high school education, including physical abuse (AOR = 1.63), emotional abuse (AOR = 2.20), physical neglect (AOR = 1.55), and emotional neglect (AOR = 1.69).

Adolescent Pregnancy

School Bullying and Adolescent Pregnancy

Lehti et al.[25] conducted a birth cohort study of more than 2,500 Finnish girls to examine the association between participation in bullying behavior at age 8 and becoming a mother before the age of 20. The investigation[25] showed that the highest risk for becoming an adolescent mother was found among the participants who, during childhood, bullied others (AOR = 2.2), followed by those who were both victims and perpetrators (AOR = 1.8), after adjustment for family-related risk factors and childhood psychopathology. Yet, no significant association was found for those who were pure victims.

A similar study by Lehti et al.[26] involving a birth cohort of more than 2,700 Finnish boys showed that the participants who at age 8 were involved in bullying as both victims and perpetrators were significantly at risk (AOR = 2.6) of becoming fathers before age 22, after adjustment for parental education and childhood psychopathology.

Self-injurious Behavior

Bullying Victimization and Self-injurious Behavior

The association between victimization by bullying and direct self-injurious behavior (D-SIB) was investigated by Brunstein-Klomek et al.,[27] with D-SIB being defined as "intentional self-inflicted damage of the surface of an individual's body by self-cutting, burning, hitting, biting and skin damage by other methods."[28] The research,[27] based on cross-sectional study of more than 11,000 students in 10 European countries, documented a significant relationship between any type of peer victimization (physical, verbal, or relational) with any lifetime, occasional, or repetitive D-SIB, even after adjustment for risk[29] and protective[30] covariables. The highest risk (AOR = 2.22) for repetitive D-SIB (five or more times in lifetime) was found among participants who were exposed to physical victimization.[27]

Victimization and Exposure to Pro-Self-Harm Web Sites

Minkkinen et al.[31] studied the association between victimization and exposure to Web sites showing ways of physical self-harm and/or committing suicide. Their research,[31] based on a cross-sectional survey of 3,567 individuals 15 to 30 years old from the United States, United Kingdom, Germany, and Finland, documented that offline victimization was significantly associated (AOR = 2.97) with exposure to pro-self-harm Web sites only among British respondents, after adjustment for covariables, including female sex, age, education, main occupation, living alone, social media activity, belongingness to primary groups (family or friends), and being an online victim.

Childhood Maltreatment and Nonsuicidal Self-injury

An investigation to determine a link between direct and indirect forms of childhood maltreatment and nonsuicidal self-injury (NSSI) was conducted by Armiento et al.[32] in a cross-sectional study of 747 children and adolescents (8 to 18 years old) through 10 community mental health clinics in Ontario, Canada. The research found that, after controlling for age and sex, only witnessing domestic violence was significantly associated (AOR = 1.6) with NSSI, while a nonsignificant link was found for physical or sexual abuse.

Suicide Attempts

Peer Victimization and Suicide Attempts

Brunstein-Klomek et al.[33] examined the bidirectional effect and the chronicity versus infrequent impact of physical, verbal, and relational bullying victimization on suicide attempts as well as suicidal ideation and depression. The study, based on a longitudinal assessment of 2,933 adolescents from 10 European countries, showed that participants who suffered from physical victimization at baseline were 2.18 times more prone to attempt suicide at three months than those who were not exposed to physical victimization. Furthermore, those who suffered physical victimization at three months were 4.72 times more likely to try to commit suicide at 12 months than those who did not suffer from physical victimization. Moreover, the students who attempted suicide between baseline and three-month follow-up were 2.49 times more at risk of experiencing physical victimization at 12 months when compared to participants who did not attempt suicide during that period. All these findings remained significant even after controlling for the impact of depression and socioeconomic variables.[33]

Cyberbullying and Suicide Attempts

The association between cyberbullying and suicidal behaviors among 15-year-old adolescents in Israel, Lithuania, and Luxembourg was studied by Zaborskis et al.[34] with analysis of data derived from the 2013–2014 HBSC[35] carried out in those three countries. The analysis showed that adolescents who were cyberbullied, when compared to those who were not, were very significantly at risk (AOR = 4.30) of attempting suicide, after adjustment for bullying others or being bullied at school, gender, family affluence, family structure, and child–parent communication.[34]

IPV and Suicide Attempt

Peltzer and Pengpid[36] analyzed the link between IPV and suicidal threats or attempts in a cross-sectional study involving 14,288 women attending antenatal care or general outpatient clinics in nine Thai hospitals. The research documented a significant association (AOR = 7.11) between being exposed to threats of mild violence and suicidal threats or attempts. The investigators also found that "danger," as manifested by "risk factors that have been associated with homicide in situations involving abuse,"[37] was very significantly (AOR = 63.17) linked to suicidal behaviors.[36]

Childhood Maltreatment and Suicide Attempts

An examination of the relationship between childhood maltreatment and suicide attempts in adolescence was done by Ammerman et al.[38] through the analysis of data derived from the US National Longitudinal Study of Adolescent Health,[39] which involved 4,834 adolescents who completed three waves of the longitudinal study (1995 through 2001–2002).[39] The findings indicated a significant association between childhood maltreatment and suicide attempts in adolescence only among females.[38] The primary mediator of this association was found to be a history of having received counseling in the previous 12 months, followed by having a friend who had attempted suicide in the previous year.[38]

Substance Abuse

School Bullying and Substance Abuse

Luukkonen et al.[40] examined the putative link between substance use and bullying behavior in a study of 508 Finnish adolescents (age 12 to 17) admitted to a psychiatric adolescent unit at Oulo University Hospital in Northern Finland. The research showed that, after adjustment for age, family type, parental employment, family's psychiatric and substance abuse history, and patient's psychiatric disorders, the male patients who reported having threatened or intimidated others three or four times were significantly more at risk, as compared to those who had not participated in bullying as victims and/or perpetrators, to be involved in regular daily smoking (AOR = 3.02), drinking alcohol at least once a week (AOR = 2.34), using hard drugs (AOR = 3.47), and having a diagnosed substance-related disorder (AOR = 2.32).[40] Furthermore, the female patients who had bullied others three or four times were significantly more at risk, as compared to those who had not participated in bullying, in being involved in regular daily smoking (AOR = 14.83), having high nicotine dependence (AOR = 31.50), using alcohol at least once a week (AOR = 2.20), using cannabis (AOR = 8.28), using any hard drugs (AOR = 6.43), and having a substance-related disorder (AOR = 5.24).[40]

Childhood Sexual Abuse and Substance Abuse

The association between childhood abuse and substance abuse was examined by Tonmyr and Shields[41] through the analysis of data from the survey of 14,063 Canadian adults who participated in the 2004–2005 Canadian Gender, Alcohol and Culture International Study.[42] The analysis[41] documented that, after controlling for socioeconomic factors and depression, the male participants who were exposed to sexual abuse, in contrast to those who were not abused, were at significantly higher risk (AOR = 1.5) of being a heavy drinker (consuming 15 or more drinks per week in the last year) or using marijuana in the previous 12 months (AOR = 2.2). Female participants who were victims of sexual abuse, when compared to those who were not abused, were at a significantly higher risk (AOR = 2.6) of being a "hazardous drinker," as defined by the Alcohol Use Disorders Identification Test (AUDIT).[43] Furthermore, females who were victims of sexual abuse were found to be more at risk (AOR = 2.1) of using marijuana in the previous 12 months than those who were not sexually abused.[41]

Criminality

School Bullying and Criminality

Several studies have explored the link between bullying at school and later criminality.[44-47] Sourander et al.[44] investigated the effect of school bullying behavior on delinquency during young adulthood, in a birth cohort study involving 5,351 Finnish children born in 1981. The study linked surveys of the children at age 8 with information from the National Police Registry when the birth cohort were 23 to 26 years old. The research[44] documented that, after controlling for psychopathology score and parental educational level, in comparison to those who did not bully others, male participants who self-reported and/or were reported by their parents and/or teachers to have bullied others almost every day were at significantly high risk during young adulthood to be involved in four or five crimes (AOR = 6.6), violent offenses (AOR = 3.9), and traffic offenses (AOR = 2.8). No significant association was found among males between being victimized in childhood and adult delinquency. Similarly, among females, no significant link was found between being a victim at age 8 and adult criminality.[44]

Sibling Bullying and Antisocial Behavior or Criminality

Dantchev and Wolke[48] explored the association between sibling bullying in early adolescence and high-risk behavior, including antisocial behavior and criminal involvement, in a study involving almost 7,000 individuals from the Avon Longitudinal Study of Parents and Children.[49] This research documented that, after adjustment for confounders,[50] the participants who bullied their siblings were at a significantly higher risk (AOR = 1.66) of antisocial behavior at age 18 to 20 years, as compared to participants not involved in sibling bullying. The risk for adult antisocial behavior was found to be higher (AOR = 2.75) if the participant was involved in bullying both siblings and peers. The types of antisocial behavior examined in this study included being rowdy/rude in public, shoplifting, buying something knowing that it was stolen, breaking into a vehicle or a house to steal something, vandalism, hurting animals on purpose, and physical aggression with the intention of hurting somebody. No significant association was found, after adjustment for confounders,[50] between bullying siblings during adolescence and adult criminal involvement as manifested by being arrested, being given a summons, or appearing in court, or by spending time in prison, a young offenders' institution, or a security unit.[48]

Future Directions

In future, it will be of significant public health value for research to determine the prevalence of behavioral risks and psychosocial problems affecting individuals who report being exposed to, or involved in, different forms of victimization, while ascertaining the mediator role of any physical or emotional symptoms known to be significantly associated with bullying and other forms of victimization, as reviewed in Chapter 4.

Notes

1. WHOQOL Group. Development of the WHOQOL: Rationale and current status. *Int J Mental Health*. 1994;23:24–56. Cited by Skevington et al. (see Note 2).
2. Skevington SM, Lotfy M, O'Connell KA; WHOQOL Group. The World Health Organization's WHOQOL-BREF quality of life assessment: psychometric properties and results of the international field trial. A report from the WHOQOL group. *Qual Life Res*. 2004;13(2):299–310.
3. People H. 2020 Foundation Health Measure Report: Health-Related Quality of Life and Well-Being. https://wayback.archive-it.org/5774/20220415162323/https://www.healthypeople.gov/sites/default/files/HRQoLWBFullReport.pdf. Accessed September 21, 2023.
4. Wilkins-Shurmer A, O'Callaghan MJ, Najman JM, Bor W, Williams GM, Anderson MJ. Association of bullying with adolescent health-related quality of life. *J Paediatr Child Health*. 2003;39(6):436–441.
5. Frisén A, Bjarnelind S. Health-related quality of life and bullying in adolescence. *Acta Paediatr*. 2010;99(4):597–603.
6. Patrick DL, Bell JF, Huang JY, Lazarakis NC, Edwards TC. Bullying and quality of life in youths perceived as gay, lesbian, or bisexual in Washington State, 2010. *Am J Public Health*. 2013;103(7):1255–1261.
7. Chen YY, Huang JH. Precollege and in-college bullying experiences and health-related quality of life among college students. *Pediatrics*. 2015;135(1):18–25.;
8. Fattori A, Neri L, Aguglia E, et al. Estimating the impact of workplace bullying: humanistic and economic burden among workers with chronic medical conditions. *Biomed Res Int*. 2015;2015:708908. doi:10.1155/2015/708908
9. Costa D, Hatzidimitriadou E, Ioannidi-Kapolou E, et al. Intimate partner violence and health-related quality of life in European men and women: findings from the DOVE study. *Qual Life Res*. 2015;24(2):463–471.
10. González-Cabrera J, León-Mejía A, Beranuy M, Gutiérrez-Ortega M, Álvarez-Bardón A, Machimbarrena JM. Relationship between cyberbullying and health-related quality of life in a sample of children and adolescents. *Qual Life Res*. 2018;27(10):2609–2618.
11. Garaigordobil M. Psychometric properties of the Cyberbullying Test, a screening instrument to measure cybervictimization, cyberaggression, and cyberobservation. *J Interpers Violence*. 2017;32(23):3556–3576. Cited by González-Cabrera et al.[10]
12. The KIDSCREEN Group Europe. *The KIDSCREEN Questionnaires: Quality of Life Questionnaires for Children and Adolescents*. Lengerich, Germany: Pabst Science Publishers; 2006. Cited by González-Cabrera et al.[10]

13. Steiner RJ, Rasberry CN. Brief report: associations between in-person and electronic bullying victimization and missing school because of safety concerns among US high school students. *J Adolescence*. 2015;43:1–4.
14. Asfaw AG, Chang CC, Ray TK. Workplace mistreatment and sickness absenteeism from work: results from the 2010 National Health Interview survey. *Am J Ind Med*. 2014;57(2):202–213.
15. Mundy LK, Canterford L, Kosola S, Degenhardt L, Allen NB, Patton GC. Peer victimization and academic performance in primary school children. *Academic Pediatr*. 2017;17(8):830–836.
16. Wang W, Vaillancourt T, Brittain HL, et al. School climate, peer victimization, and academic achievement: results from a multi-informant study. *Sch Psychol Q*. 2014;29(3):360.
17. Brewer N, Thomas KA, Higdon J. Intimate partner violence, health, sexuality, and academic performance among a national sample of undergraduates. *J Am Coll Health*. 2018;66(7):683–692.
18. Zolotor A, Kotch J, Dufort V, Winsor J, Catellier D, Bou-Saada I. School performance in a longitudinal cohort of children at risk of maltreatment. *Matern Child Health J*. 1999;3(1):19–27.
19. Nansel TR, Overpeck MD, Haynie DL, Ruan WJ, Scheidt PC. Relationships between bullying and violence among US youth. *Arch Pediatr Adolesc Med*. 2003;157(4):348–353.
20. Van Geel M, Vedder P, Tanilon J. Bullying and weapon carrying: a meta-analysis. *JAMA Pediatrics*. 2014;168(8):714–720.
21. Esselmont C. Carrying a weapon to school: the roles of bullying victimization and perceived safety. *Deviant Behav*. 2014;35(3):215–232.
22. Prakash R, Beattie T, Javalkar P, et al. Correlates of school dropout and absenteeism among adolescent girls from marginalized community in north Karnataka, South India. *J Adolescence*. 2017;61:64–76.
23. Sanz-Barbero B, Pereira PL, Barrio G, Vives-Cases C. Intimate partner violence against young women: prevalence and associated factors in Europe. *J Epidemiol Community Health*. 2018;72(7):611–616.
24. Barker B, Kerr T, Dong H, Wood E, Debeck K. High school incompletion and childhood maltreatment among street-involved young people in Vancouver, Canada. *Health Soc Care Community*. 2017;25(2):378–384.
25. Lehti V, Sourander A, Klomek A, et al. Childhood bullying as a predictor for becoming a teenage mother in Finland. *Eur Child Adolesc Psychiatry*. 2011;20(1):49–55.
26. Lehti V, Klomek AB, Tamminen T, et al. Childhood bullying and becoming a young father in a national cohort of Finnish boys. *Scand J Psychol*. 2012;53(6):461–466.
27. Klomek AB, Snip A, Apter A, et al. Association between victimization by bullying and direct self-injurious behavior among adolescents in Europe: a ten-country study. *Eur Child Adolesc Psychiatry*. 2016;25(11):1183–1193.
28. Brunner R, Kaess M, Parzer P, et al. Life-time prevalence and psychosocial correlates of adolescent direct self-injurious behavior: a comparative study of findings in 11 European countries. *J Child Psychol Psychiatry*. 2014;55(4):337–348. Cited by Klomek et al.[27]
29. Risk covariables include depression, anxiety, suicide attempts, suicidal ideation, loneliness, alcohol consumption, drug consumption, and gender.
30. Protective covariables include parent support, peer support, and prosocial behavior.
31. Minkkinen J, Oksanen A, Kaakinen M, Keipi T, Räsänen P. Victimization and exposure to pro-self-harm and pro-suicide websites: a cross-national study. *Suicide Life Threat Behav*. 2017;47(1):14–26.

32. Armiento J, Hamza CA, Stewart SL, Leschied A. Direct and indirect forms of childhood maltreatment and nonsuicidal self-injury among clinically referred children and youth. *J Affective Disord.* 2016;200:212–217.
33. Brunstein Klomek A, Barzilay S, Apter A, et al. Bi-directional longitudinal associations between different types of bullying victimization, suicide ideation/attempts, and depression among a large sample of European adolescents. *J Child Psychol Psychiatry.* 2019;60(2):209–215.
34. Zaborskis A, Ilionsky G, Tesler R, Heinz A. The association between cyberbullying, school bullying, and suicidality among adolescents: findings from the cross-national study HBSC in Israel, Lithuania, and Luxembourg. *Crisis.* 2019;40(2):100–114.
35. Inchley J, Currie D, Young T, et al. Growing up unequal: gender and socioeconomic differences in young people's health and well-being. In: *Health Behaviour in School-aged Children (HBSC) Study: International Report from the 2013–2014 Survey.* Copenhagen, Denmark: WHO Regional Office for Europe; 2016. Cited by Zaborskis et al.[34]
36. Peltzer K, Pengpid S. Associations between intimate partner violence, depression, and suicidal behavior among women attending antenatal and general outpatient hospital services in Thailand. *Nigerian J Clin Pract.* 2017;20(7):892–899.
37. Campbell JC. Nursing assessment for risk of homicide with battered women. *Adv Nurs Sci.* 1986;8(4):36–51. Cited by Peltzer and Pengpid.[36]
38. Ammerman BA, Serang S, Jacobucci R, Burke TA, Alloy LB, McCloskey MS. Exploratory analysis of mediators of the relationship between childhood maltreatment and suicidal behavior. *J Adolescence.* 2018;69:103–112.
39. Harris KM, Halpern CT, Whitsel E, et al. National Longitudinal Study of Adolescent Health: research design. https://addhealth.cpc.unc.edu/documentation/study-design/. Accessed September 21, 2023. Cited by Ammerman et al.[38]
40. Luukkonen AH, Riala K, Hakko H, Räsänen P. Bullying behaviour and substance abuse among underage psychiatric inpatient adolescents. *Eur Psychiatry.* 2010;25(7):382–389.
41. Tonmyr L, Shields M. Childhood sexual abuse and substance abuse: A gender paradox? *Child Abuse Negl.* 2017;63:284–294.
42. Bloomfield K, Allamani A, Beck F, et al. *Gender, Culture and Alcohol Problems: A Multinational Study—Project Final Report.* Berlin, Germany: Institute for Medical Informatics, Biometrics and Epidemiology; 2005. Cited by Tonmyr and Shields.[41]
43. Babor TF, Higgins-Biddle JC, Saunders JB, Monteiro MG. *The Alcohol Use Disorders Identification Test (AUDIT): Guidelines for Use in Primary Care.* World Health Organization, Department of Mental Health and Substance Abuse; 2001. https://iris.who.int/bitstream/handle/10665/67205/W?sequence=1. Accessed September 21, 2023. Cited by Tonmyr and Shields.[41]
44. Sourander A, Klomek AB, Kumpulainen K, et al. Bullying at age eight and criminality in adulthood: findings from the Finnish Nationwide 1981 Birth Cohort Study. *Soc Psychiatry Psychiatr Epidemiol.* 2011;46(12):1211–1219.
45. Olweus D. Bullying at school and later criminality: findings from three Swedish community samples of males. *Crim Behav Ment Health.* 2011;21(2):151–156.
46. Jiang D, Walsh M, Augimeri LK. The linkage between childhood bullying behaviour and future offending. *Crim Behav Ment Health.* 2011;21(2):128–135.
47. Howell KH, Cater ÅK, Miller-Graff LE, Schwartz LE, Graham-Bermann SA. The relationship between types of childhood victimisation and young adulthood criminality. *Crim Behav Ment Health.* 2017;27(4):341–353.

48. Dantchev S, Wolke D. Sibling bullying at 12 years and high-risk behavior in early adulthood: a prospective cohort study. *Aggress Behav.* 2018;45(1):18–32.

49. Boyd A, Golding J, Macleod J, et al. Cohort profile: the 'children of the 90s'—the index offspring of the Avon Longitudinal Study of Parents and Children. *Int J Epidemiol.* 2013;42(1):111–127. Cited by Dantchev and Wolke.[48]

50. Confounders considered in the adjusted model analysis include gender, maternal education, marital status, maternal depression, domestic violence, maltreatment, peer bullying, child psychiatric problems, internalizing and externalizing problems, and IQ.[49]

6
Mortality Linked to Bullying and Other Forms of Maltreatment

More than three decades ago, a flow of Japanese news reports[1-6] about deaths associated with school bullying led to worldwide awareness of the nature and risks associated with this form of maltreatment. In fact, the initial research on prevention of school bullying led by Olweus was prompted by the suicides of three Norwegian students who were bullied.[7]

Yet, after all these years, we do not have data estimating the magnitude of the mortality rate linked to bullying.

What Is Known?

Information Derived from News Reports

The extent of lethality associated with bullying is, so far, known only through deaths that were made public through the media.

A study[8] based on a survey of English-language newspapers from around the world documented 250 deaths associated with a history of bullying, hazing,[9] or ragging[10] reported from 1950 to 2007, with 67% of the deaths occurring between 1997 and 2007. Most of the reports (62%) originated from Europe, primarily from the United Kingdom. This is in no way an indication of geographical differences in the prevalence of bullying-related deaths, but perhaps it is a reflection of global diversities in the methodology or guidelines for coroners' inquests to ascertain the possible association between bullying and unnatural or unexpected deaths.

A survey[11] by country or dependent territory in the Americas of nonduplicated news reports of fatal injurious events related to bullying or violence affecting children and adolescents, published in the local language from July 2011 through June 2012, documented 17 cases of bullying-related suicides occurring in six countries[12] and at least 18 homicides of adolescents in nine nations.[13]

A review[14] of nonduplicated news reports about cases of death linked to bullying covered in English language newspapers from January 1, 2016, through December 31, 2016, documented at least 74 cases[15-89] of unnatural or unexpected death associated with bullying or other forms of maltreatment, occurring in 25 countries, with most of the deaths (75%) occurring among people 18 years old and younger. The reported deaths were mainly associated with school bullying (41%), urban terrorism (30%), cyberbullying (13%), and workplace bullying (7%), while 9% were linked to other forms of victimization, such as rape,[70] family violence,[52] and witchcraft killings.[69]

This review[14] and previous similar studies[8,11] provide a glimpse of the tip of the iceberg that is mortality related to bullying and other forms of victimization, while the real dimensions remain unknown. The findings would have been larger if the search had been conducted in languages other than English[79-84] or had included terms for other forms of victimization, such as intimate partner or domestic violence,[85] child maltreatment,[88-89] or elder abuse.[90]

Suicide Related to Bullying and Other Forms of Maltreatment

There are no available published studies documenting the national or regional prevalence of completed suicide events related to bullying and other forms of maltreatment. Yet, there are many reports supporting the significant association of different types of victimization, including bullying, and suicide attempts[91-99] or completed suicides.[94]

Bullying and Risk of Suicide Attempts

Bang and Park[91] conducted a cross-sectional study of almost 1,200 Korean students (in grades 7 and 8) showing that bullying victimization was significantly associated with suicide attempts after controlling for socioenvironmental characteristics, depression, and psychosis [adjusted odds ratio (AOR) = 2.49].

Barzilay et al.[92] conducted a cross-sectional analysis, based on data from more than 11,000 students in 10 European countries, aimed at examining the risk and protective factors moderating the association of physical, verbal, and relational bullying with suicidal ideation and attempts. Their findings established that physical bullying was linked with a 39% increase in the probability for suicidal ideation, that relational bullying was associated with a 28% rise in the chances for suicide attempt, and that verbal bullying was associated with suicide attempts among adolescents with anxiety who perceived low parental support.

Research undertaken by Luukkonen et al.,[93] based on a sample of 508 Finnish adolescents admitted to a psychiatric inpatient unit, demonstrated that there was a greater risk of suicide attempts in girls who were victims of bullying (AOR = 2.07) or who bullied others (AOR = 3.27), after adjustment for age, school factors, family factors, and psychiatric disorders. Yet the study did not show any similar significant association among boys.

A longitudinal study, published in 2009 by Klomek et al.,[94] based on more than 5,300 Finish children, explored the link between childhood bullying behaviors occurring at 8 years of age and suicide attempts and completed suicides up to age 25. Their analysis documented that boys who frequently bully others or are being bullied are at high risk for later suicides and completed suicides, but this association is not significant after adjustment for symptoms of depression and conduct disorder. Conversely, frequent bullying victimization of girls is significantly linked to later suicide attempts and completed suicides, even after controlling clinical indications of depression and conduct disorder.

Sinyor et al.[95] conducted a review of coroner records of 94 suicide deaths of young people 10 to 19 years old that occurred in the city of Toronto from 1998 to 2011, to determine the frequency of bullying as a contributing factor to youth suicide. The study showed that bullying was present in 6.4% of the deaths and that there were no cases where cyberbullying was detected. Furthermore, depression was detected in 40.4% of cases, while the most common stressors found were problems with parents (21.3%), romantic partner conflicts (17.0%), academic difficulties (10.6%), and criminal and/or legal troubles (10.6%).[95]

A two-year study conducted by Geoffroy et al.[96] with the participation of almost 1,200 adolescents from Quebec demonstrated that those who were victimized by peers at age 13 experienced significantly higher risk of suicide attempt two years later (OR = 3.05), even after adjustment for baseline suicidality, mental health problems, socioeconomic status, intelligence, family functioning and structure, hostile-reactive parenting, and maternal lifetime suicidal ideation/suicide attempt.

It is of note that a significant link between participating in bullying as a bully, victim, or bully victim, and subsequent suicidal/self-injurious behavior, after adjustment for multiple confounders, has been shown in preadolescent children in the United Kingdom, through a prospective birth cohort study of more than 6,000 children carried out by Winsper et al..[97] Above all, this study gave evidence that "bully/victims" and "chronic victims" were at high risk for suicidal/self-injurious behavior at age 8 and 10 years, as reported by themselves, mothers, and teachers, while the risk for lethal behaviors was only significant among "pure bullies" at age 8 according to teachers and self-reports.[97]

Cyberbullying and Suicide Attempts

Messias et al.[98] analyzed data of the 2011 CDC Youth Risk Behavior Survey, a nationally representative sample of more than 15,000 adolescents living in the United States, to ascertain association between victimization in school, cyberbullying, or both and suicide attempts. Their findings, adjusted for age, gender, and race, showed that students who reported being cyberbullied were at a higher risk (AOR = 3.7) of experiencing suicide attempts requiring treatment than those who were only bullied in school (AOR = 1.6), but they were at less risk than those who were bullied both in school and cyberspace (AOR = 4.2). These findings are limited by the cross-sectional aspects of the study as well as by the lack of adjustment for the experience of sadness or depression.

A similar study led by Sampasa-Kanyinga et al.,[99] which analyzed data from the 2011 Eastern Ontario Youth Risk Behavior Survey (based on a population of almost 3,000 Canadian adolescent students attending schools in Eastern Ontario), reported that victims of cyberbullying were at risk (OR = 1.40) of attempting suicide as compared to their peers who were not exposed to school bullying or cyberbullying, after adjustment for grade, gender, sedentary activities, smoking, alcohol use, marijuana use, and computer abuse. Yet, the risk was reduced (OR = 1.09) in an adjusted model that included depression, clearly indicating the significant moderating role of this covariable in the link between cyberbullying and suicide attempts.

Intimate Partner Violence and Suicidal Behaviors

Cavanaugh et al.[100] examined the prevalence and correlates of suicidal threats and attempts among more than 600 racially and ethnically diverse adult female victims of intimate partner violence (IPV). Their analysis documented that almost 23% of the women reported having threatened suicide during their lifetime. The likelihood of suicidal threats or attempts was highest among IPV victims at extreme danger of lethal assaults (AOR = 3.7) as measured by the Danger Assessment[101] and among those who reported chronic or disabling illness (AOR = 2.4).

Childhood Maltreatment and Suicide Attempts

The effects of different types of childhood maltreatment, including emotional or physical neglect, as well as physical, emotional, or sexual abuse, on the risk of attempting suicide were examined by Hoertel et al.,[102] who analyzed data drawn from a nationally representative sample of more than 34,600 US residents older than 18. The research showed that, "after adjusting for socioeconomic characteristics and psychopathology, all types of childhood maltreatment were significantly associated with a lifetime history of suicide attempt in the general population and with a younger age at first suicide attempt among attempters."[102]

Homicide Related to Bullying and Other Forms of Maltreatment

Deaths due homicide or aggravated assault may be associated with previous exposure to bullying or other forms of victimization. Furthermore, because any form of maltreatment may include physical aggression, then it can be construed that every death due to homicide or aggravated assault is, by itself, an extreme expression or consequence of victimization.[11]

In this context, we can find published reports addressing the frequency of homicide among victims of school, Internet, or workplace bullying, IPV, and childhood maltreatment.

School Violence and Homicide

A population-based surveillance investigation based on data from multiple sources, led by Anderson et al.[103] and aimed at studying school-violent deaths in the United States, showed that 183 homicides (6% of which were homicide/suicides) occurred from 1994 to 1999. The study also found a significant increase in the homicide rates for students killed in "multiple-victim events." Furthermore, the study revealed that students who were homicide victimizers were more significantly at risk than their peers who were homicide victims to have communicated some form of suicidal behavior prior to the incident (OR = 9.00), to be gang member (OR = 3.77), to have received psychological counselling (OR = 3.20), to have been treated for depression (OR = 3.48), and to have been bullied by their peers (OR = 2.57).[103] Anderson et al. recognized the limitation of their study, which used data based on a small number of deaths and which was the product of secondary sources that could have been subject to "error and bias."[103]

Using the US Digest of Education Statistics,[104] we can calculate that, between 1995 and 2015, 434 US students (K–12) were killed in school, representing 1.25% of homicide deaths for children ages 5 to 18 during those 25 years (Table 6.1).

According to Kahn et al.,[105] almost 3% of US students in grades 9 to 12 were injured in a physical fight one or more times during the year 2015 and had to be treated by a physician or

Table 6.1. Deaths at School and Homicides Among Youth Age 5 to 18, 1995–2015

Years	Number of School Deaths	Number of Homicides	School Deaths as Percent of Homicides
1995–2000	141	11,069	1.27%
2000–2005	93	8,227	1.13%
2005–2010	111	8,894	1.24%
2010–2015	89	6,539	1.36%
1995–2015	434	34,729	1.25%

Source: Data from National Center of Education Statistics.[104]

nurse. During the same year, 0.7% of US adolescents age 14 to 17 were victims of physical assault requiring them to be seen in a hospital emergency department.[106]

Cyberviolence and Homicide or Seriously Violent Behavior

In 2006, Ybarra et al.[107] conducted an online survey of almost 1,600 youths age 10 to 15 to examine the link between violence on the Internet and other media and self-reported seriously violent behavior, including shooting or stabbing someone, aggravated assault resulting in the need for medical care, robbery using a weapon, or sexual assault. The degree of risk of the adolescents reporting one or more seriously violent behaviors in the previous year was contingent on the context of violence depicted on different websites visited in the previous 12 months.

The study found that youngsters who looked at Internet pages showing pictures of war, death, or terrorism had a lower level of recounting participation in one or more incidents of seriously violent behavior (AOR = 1.2) than those who visited "hate sites" (AOR = 4.7) or websites showing satanic rituals (AOR = 5.1). The cross-sectional aspects of the study[107] allow only identification of a significant association and preclude determining a cause–effect relationship, which could be ascertained only through longitudinal studies.

Workplace Violence and Homicide

Data from the US Bureau of Labor Statistics Census and the US Bureau of Labor Statistics Census of Fatal Occupational Injuries (CFOI)[108,109] have been used in published studies[110-113] about occupational homicides in the United States. Menéndez et al.[110] showed that taxi and limousine drivers who are male, Hispanic, non-Hispanic black, or work in the South and Midwest experience the highest homicide rates, after adjustment for all other demographic variables examined.

Konda et al.[111] documented that 28% of homicides that occurred in the retail industry from 2003 to 2008 were non-robbery-related: 34% were perpetrated by customers, 31% by someone in a personal relationship with an employee, and 24% by coworker violence.[111] Fifty of the workplace homicides were due to arguments.[111]

A study by Tiesman et al.[112] analyzed workplace injury deaths among law enforcement officers between 1992 and 2002 and established that, during this 11-year period, 2,280 workers died from an occupational injury, with almost half of the fatalities due to homicide.

Tiesman et al.[113] also analyzed the CFOI to investigate aspects of US workplace homicides among women between 2003 and 2008. The research demonstrated that, during those five years, 648 women were feloniously killed on the job, with robbery of a store being the leading criminal intent (39%), followed by homicides perpetrated by intimate partners (22%).

A *Morbidity and Mortality Weekly Report* on fatal occupational injuries in the United States during 2005[114] documented that 10% (n = 564) of the total fatal injuries (N = 5,702) were due to homicides. Almost 80% of these deaths occurred among employees in the services industry (46%) and workers employed in the transportation, warehousing, and utilities sector (33%).

According to the US Bureau of Labor Statistics,[115] during 2019 there were 454 workplace homicides, representing 9% of all fatal work injuries for that year, with nearly 20% of all workplace deaths occurring among women (88 of 437) due to homicide, compared to 7.5% of all workplace deaths among men (366 of 4,896).

Intimate Partner Homicide

Stöckl et al.[116] conducted a systematic review to estimate global and regional prevalence of intimate partner homicide, based on data from 66 countries. Their study documented that 13.5% of homicides were carried out by an intimate partner, and this percentage was six times higher for female homicides (38.6%) than for male homicides (6.3%). The median percentage of intimate partner homicides among slain females was greatest in southeast Asia (58.8%), high-income countries (41.2%), the Americas (40.5%), and Africa (40.5%).[116] The occurrence was smaller in the Western Pacific (19.1%), the low- and middle-income European region (20.0%), and the Eastern Mediterranean area (14.4%). Intimate partner homicides among male victims were found to be highest in high-income countries (6.3%), the African region (4.1%), and middle-income European area (3.6%).[116] Overall, this research highlighted the lack of data about intimate partner homicide in many countries, as well as the lack of information about the victim–offender relationship.

Maltreatment and Homicide

A UNICEF report[117] on child maltreatment deaths in 30 rich nations,[118] members of the Organization for Economic Co-operation and Development (OECD),[119] indicated that "almost 3,500 children under the age of 15 die from maltreatment (physical abuse and neglect) every year in the industrialized world," with an average rate of death from maltreatment and undetermined causes of 1.05/100,000. The lowest incidence (0.1–0.3/100,000) was recorded in Spain, Greece, Italy, Ireland, and Norway, while the highest rates (2.4–3.7/100,000) were found in the United States, Mexico, and Portugal.[118] Furthermore, the UNICEF report showed that "infants under 1 year are in greatest danger of death from maltreatment, with a risk level approximately three times higher than for those age 1 to 4 (who themselves face almost double the risk of 5- to 14-year-olds)."[118]

A US Department of Health and Human Services report on child maltreatment in the United States,[120] based on data from 2008, documented that more than 1,700 children died due to child abuse or neglect, representing an overall rate of child fatalities of 2.33 deaths per 100,000. Almost 40% of the deaths were caused by different forms of maltreatment; neglect alone accounted for almost 32% of the fatalities, while physical abuse was associated with 23% of the deaths.[120]

Accidental or Other Unnatural Deaths Related to Victimization

As discussed in Chapter 4, bullying is significantly associated with injuries.[121-126]

Engström et al.[127] documented that the risk of being injured is 5.5 times higher among children exposed to an episode of victimization within 15 minutes before the injury than during periods of no victimization. This research supported the notion that peer victimization is an injury trigger, possibly through disturbance of the concentration and attention processes of the victim.[127]

Accidental deaths have been reported as being associated with incidents of bullying or victimization characterized by daring somebody "to perform a dangerous, illegal, or inappropriate action under the threat of losing approval or of not being liked or loved,"[128] as has happened in hazing-related deaths, "where alcohol intoxication was frequently the cause or a significant factor of the fatality."[8]

Future Directions

As a first step in estimating the global prevalence of mortality associated with bullying and other forms of maltreatment, every coroner or medical examiner report should systematically include information about bullying or any other form of victimization or maltreatment experienced by a victim of suicide within the previous 1 or 2 months. Information concerning exposure to victimization should be gathered as part of the investigation to ascertain possible factors related to suicide in the same context as depression, alcohol and drug abuse, and major life stresses. Thus, while we recognize the multiple correlates of suicide, we should start highlighting the role of bullying or other forms of victimization and eventually estimate their contribution to the relative risk of this type of unnatural death.

In the case of homicides, it should be considered that an intentional homicide is an extreme form of victimization or maltreatment, for which global mortality statistics are already available.[129]

Notes

1. Review of news on "bullying" and "death" (from 1980 to 1986) through Factiva, a global news database, owned by Dow Jones and Company.
2. Watts D. Suicide highlights bullying in Japan: Takashi Kabasawa kills himself. *New York Times*. Boston Globe, Washington Post, The Toronto Star. October 24, 1985.

3. The Associated Press. "Bullying" "suicide" prompts inquiry in Japan. November 23, 1985.
4. Walkom T. Bullies bring death to Japanese classes. *The Globe and Mail*. December 9, 1985.
5. The Associated Press. In Japan, children's bullying can lead to murder and suicide. *The Record*. December 15, 1985.
6. Reuters. Children's suicide rate up sharply in Japan. *The Toronto Star*. May 30, 1986.
7. Olweus D. *Bullying at School: What We Know and What We Can Do*. Oxford, UK: Blackwell Publishers; 1993:2.
8. Srabstein J. Deaths linked to bullying and hazing. *Int J Adolesc Med Health*. 2008;20(2):235–239.
9. "Hazing is any activity expected of someone joining or participating in a group that humiliates, degrades, abuses, or endangers them, regardless of a person's willingness to participate. There are three components that define hazing:
   1. It occurs in a group context
   2. Humiliating, degrading, or endangering behavior
   3. Happens regardless of an individual's willingness to participate"

   Stop Hazing, What is Hazing https://stophazing.org/issue/#:~:text=Hazing%20is%20any%20activity%20expected,Humiliating%2C%20degrading%2C%20or%20endangering%20behavior. Accessed September 21, 2023.
10. "Ragging is a set of undisciplined activities undertaken by the seniors to break the ice with the juniors, who have been suddenly thrown into a totally new environment. The contention of seniors behind all such activities is simply to bring the freshers down to earth, because in their opinion the freshers do not respect the seniors and by doing all such inhuman activities under the garb of 'introduction,' the seniors rag the freshers so that the freshers may respect them and be under their control. Over the years in all over the world and especially in South Asia, the practice of 'ragging' has come to be meant as an extreme 'harassment,' 'terror' and even 'physical and mental torture' of freshers." Supreme Court of India. *University of Kerala vs Council, Principals', Colleges, Kerala ... on 11 February, 2009, Judgment, section 10.* https://indiankanoon.org/doc/1460097/. Accessed September 21, 2023.
11. Srabstein JC. News reports of bullying-related fatal and nonfatal injuries in the Americas. *Rev Panam Salud Publica*. 2013;33(5):378–382.
12. Supplementary material to Srabstein JC. News reports of bullying-related fatal and nonfatal injuries in the Americas. *Rev Panam Salud Publica*. 2013;33(5):378–382. Annex 2, pages 7–8. https://www.scielosp.org/media/assets/rpsp/v33n5/a10v33n5_ms01.pdf. Accessed November 10, 2022.
13. Supplementary material to Srabstein JC. News reports of bullying-related fatal and nonfatal injuries in the Americas. *Rev Panam Salud Publica*. 2013;33(5):378–382. Annex 3, pages 9–10. https://www.scielosp.org/media/assets/rpsp/v33n5/a10v33n5_ms01.pdf. Accessed November 10, 2022.
14. Srabstein J. Unpublished review of English unduplicated news, by country, of deaths associated with bullying. This survey was conducted using LexisNexis® Academic and Google News by country, with search on the terms *bullying* AND *death* from January 1 through December 31, 2016.
15. Smith B, Kitching C. Thousands of mourners turn out for funeral of "bullied" 11-year-old boy found dead in his bedroom. *Mirror*. October 4, 2016. https://www.mirror.co.uk/news/uk-news/thousands-mourners-turn-out-funeral-8973098. Accessed November 10, 2022.
16. Family says 11-year-old committed suicide because of bullying. Toledo, OH: WTVG Action News. http://www.13abc.com/content/news/Family-says-11-year-old-committed-suicide-because-of-bullying-390526152.html. Accessed 10/11/2022.

17. Houston S. Man, 21, found dead after claims he was subjected to cyber bullying. *Daily Record*. September 8, 2016. https://www.dailyrecord.co.uk/news/local-news/man-21-found-dead-after-8795941. Accessed November 10, 2022.
18. Ellingham J. Girl remembered as "wonderful student." NZHerald.co.nz. March 15, 2016. http://www.nzherald.co.nz/nz/news/article.cfm?c_id=1&objectid=11605578. Accessed November 10, 2022.
19. Brisbane Year 7 student takes own life after being bullied for sexuality. News.com.au. November 25, 2016. http://www.news.com.au/lifestyle/parenting/school-life/brisbane-year-7-student-takes-own-life-after-being-bullied-for-sexuality/news-story/b98bcb64168eb9ead21f435001981119. Accessed November 10, 2022.
20. Salinger T. Suicide of 12-year-old Pennsylvania boy Evan Ziemniak "was his response to stop the pain" of bullying. *New York Daily News*. April 4, 2016. http://www.nydailynews.com/news/national/suicide-12-year-old-boy-bullying-article-1.2588304. Accessed November 10, 2022.
21. Cotter SP. Father: Bullying cut daughter's life short. *York Dispatch*. May 27, 2016. http://www.yorkdispatch.com/story/news/2016/05/27/father-bullying-cut-daughters-life-short/85055224/. Accessed November 10, 2022.
22. Sharman J. Polish teenager who took her own life was "victim of bullying," coroner told. *Independent*. February, 22, 2017. http://www.independent.co.uk/news/uk/home-news/dagmara-przybysz-polish-bullied-racism-pool-academy-cornwall-inquest-coroner-a7593381.html. Accessed November 10, 2022.
23. Warrenton parents say bullying caused daughter to take her life. St. Louis, MO: Fox 2NOW. http://fox2now.com/2016/04/26/warrenton-parents-say-bullying-caused-daughter-to-take-her-life/. Accessed November 10, 2022.
24. Tributes flood in for 14-year-old schoolboy Jack Scott. *Evening Times*. June 16, 2016. http://www.eveningtimes.co.uk/news/14560619.Tributes_flood_in_for_14_year_old_schoolboy_Jack_Scott/. Accessed November 10, 2022.
25. McLeod K, Hyland J. Teenager takes her own life after suffering torrent of bullying on social media. *Daily Record*. July 9, 2016. http://www.dailyrecord.co.uk/news/scottish-news/teenager-takes-life-after-suffering-8382697. Accessed November 10, 2022.
26. Stefanovich O. People should know: Sisters open up about 13-year-old brother's suicide in Fort Albany. *CBC News*. October 20, 2016. http://www.cbc.ca/news/canada/sudbury/fort-albany-young-boy-suicide-1.3812627. Accessed November 10, 2022.
27. Del Valle L. Ohio child cancer survivor kills herself over bullying. CNN. November 1, 2016. https://www.cnn.com/2016/10/31/health/cancer-survivor-bully-trnd/index.html. Accessed November 10, 2022.
28. Murray R. Grandma in support call after heartbreak of grandson's suicide. *Wiltshire Times*. May 19, 2016. http://www.wiltshiretimes.co.uk/news/14504318.display/. Accessed November 10, 2022.
29. Worley W. Mother of cyber bullying victim pens heartbreaking open letter in response to his suicide. *Independent*. October 6, 2016. http://www.independent.co.uk/news/uk/home-news/mother-open-letter-cyber-bullying-victim-suicide-online-social-media-a7347531.html. Accessed November 10, 2022.
30. Thomson B. Families hope suicide outreach service at Wangaratta will save lives. *The Border Mail*. July 28, 2016 https://www.bordermail.com.au/story/4060769/a-lifeline/. Accessed November 10, 2022.

31. Matthew Wooby, 12, found dead after being bullied. BBC News. August 25, 2016. http://www.bbc.com/news/uk-england-suffolk-37186184. Accessed November 10, 2022.
32. Santosh Kumar RB. Bengaluru boy's suicide note names "bully," cops tread with caution. *The Indian Express.* July 2016. http://indianexpress.com/article/india/india-news-india/bengaluru-boy-suicide-note-bully-ragging-raunak-banerjee-baldwin-school-2898200/. Accessed August 31, 2017.
33. Oliphant V. Schoolgirl found hanged posted "death is near" message on social media. *Express.* June 3, 2016. http://www.express.co.uk/news/uk/676661/Bullied-Bolton-schoolgirl-death-is-near-online-social-media-post-found-hanged-bedroom. Accessed November 10, 2022.
34. Holley P. A boy who killed himself wrote a letter about bullying. His struggles may have started at home. *Washington Post.* August 16, 2016. https://www.washingtonpost.com/news/morning-mix/wp/2016/08/16/a-boy-who-killed-himself-wrote-a-letter-about-bullying-his-struggles-may-have-started-at-home/?utm_term=.7f293d353a63. Accessed November 10, 2022.
35. Oduor B. Kendu Bay boy's death investigated after bullying claims. *Daily Nation.* October 17, 2016. http://www.nation.co.ke/counties/homa-bay/Kendu-Bay-boy-s-death-investigated-after-bullying-claims-/3444904-3420072-jq8l7p/index.html. Accessed November 10, 2022.
36. Lack B. Bullying not severe enough to cause teenager's suicide. *The Times.* July 21, 2016. https://www.thetimes.co.uk/article/bullying-not-severe-enough-to-cause-teenager-s-suicide-pq0xf26zm. Accessed November 10, 2022.
37. Mum of former Guildford College student found dead at home dedicates life to campaign against bullying. *Surrey.* January 4, 2017. http://www.getsurrey.co.uk/news/surrey-news/mum-former-guildford-college-student-12406717. Accessed November 10, 2022.
38. Richter N. Family mourns after bullying takes the life of a 9-year-old. WTRF.com. September 13, 2016. https://www.wtrf.com/archives/family-mourns-after-bullying-takes-the-life-of-a-9-year-old/. Accessed November 10, 2022.
39. Egan L. Parents, school board clash after son's suicide. KSL.com. September 29, 2016. https://www.ksl.com/?sid=41662195&nid=148&title=parents-school-board-clash-after-sons-suicide. Accessed November 10, 2022.
40. McCowan C. Girl, 15, commits suicide after friends share nude Snapchat video taken without permission. News Channel 8 WFLA. https://www.wfla.com/news/girl-15-commits-suicide-after-friends-share-nude-snapchat-video-taken-without-permission/. Accessed November 10, 2022.
41. Jouvenal J. Female firefighter's suicide is a 'fire bell in the night.' *Washington Post.* August 22, 2016. https://www.washingtonpost.com/local/public-safety/female-reghters-suicide-is-a-re-bell-in-the-night/2016/08/22/11c73a16-3956-11e6-a254-2b336e293a3c_story.html?utm_term=.7e486269d618. Accessed November 10, 2022.
42. Pells R. Mother of teacher who died blames stress and anxiety piled on by 'extreme' workload. *Independent.* November 11, 2016. https://www.independent.co.uk/news/education/education-news/laurian-bold-gabrielle-hollingworth-academy-rochdale-mother-teacher-who-died-blames-stress-anxiety-piled-extreme-workload-a7412471.html. Accessed November 10, 2022.
43. Murió el chico que se disparó en la cabeza porque le decían "Obama." *Infobae.* November 2, 2016. https://www.infobae.com/sociedad/2016/11/02/murio-el-chico-que-se-disparo-en-la-cabeza-porque-le-decian-obama/. Accessed November 10, 2022.

44. Jones S. Schoolboy, 13, 'bullied into hanging himself after teammates blame him for losing online game League of Legends.' *Mirror News*. October 18, 2016. http://www.mirror.co.uk/news/uk-news/schoolboy-13-bullied-hanging-himself-9071265. Accessed November 10, 2022.
45. McNeill S. Teenage girl stabbed to death in bedroom by Palestinian attacker in occupied West Bank. June30, 2016. ABC.net.au. http://www.abc.net.au/news/2016-07-01/teenage-girl-stabbed-to-death-in-bedroom-by-palestinian-attacker/7559630. Accessed November 10, 2022.
46. Liebermann O, Almasy S, Tal A. American fatally stabbed in Israel terror attack that wounds 10 others. CNN. March 9, 2016. http://www.cnn.com/2016/03/08/middleeast/israel-violence/index.html. Accessed November 10, 2022.
47. Carma H. Teen who was relentlessly bullied kills herself in front of her family. CNN. December 1, 2016. https://www.cnn.com/2016/12/01/health/teen-suicide-cyberbullying-trnd. Accessed November 10, 2022.
48. Shichijo R. Aomori officials investigate bullying in boy's suicide. August 27, 2016. *Tokyo Daily News*. http://www.tokyoreporter.com/2016/08/27/aomori-officials-investigate-bullying-in-boys-suicide/. Accessed November 10, 2022.
49. Intern commits suicide after suffering from workplace bullying at Korean company. Nextshark. February 29, 2016. https://nextshark.com/won-so-yeon-lf-corp-suicide/. Accessed November 10, 2022.
50. Ying TP.Victim snaps, stabs bully to death. *The Strait Times*. May 9, 2016. https://www.nst.com.my/news/2016/05/144618/victim-snaps-stabs-bully-death. Accessed November 10, 2022.
51. Fan of JJ Lin dead, cyber-bullying suspected. *The Strait Times*. October 31, 2016. http://www.straitstimes.com/lifestyle/fan-of-jj-lin-dead-cyber-bullying-suspected. Accessed November 11, 2022.
52. Davies G. Pregnant Afghan 14-year-old is tortured and burned to death by her in-laws in revenge for her father eloping with their niece. *Daily Mail*. July 18, 2016.http://www.dailymail.co.uk/news/article-3695881/Pregnant-14-year-old-tortured-burned-death-Afghanistan-laws-revenge-father-eloping-niece.html. Accessed November 10, 2022.
53. Burrows T. Bangladeshi boy, 10, is murdered by co-workers in a textiles factory after they inserted a high-pressure nozzle into his rectum. MailonLine. July 25, 2016. http://www.dailymail.co.uk/news/article-3706589/Bangladeshi-boy-10-murdered-workers-textiles-factory-inserted-high-pressure-nozzle-rectum.html. Accessed November 10, 2022.
54. 20 killed in Bangladesh hostage bloodbath. *Daily Mail*. July 2, 2016. http://www.dailymail.co.uk/wires/afp/article-3671027/Bangladesh-commandos-end-hostage-siege-kill-six-gunmen.html. Accessed November 10, 2022.
55. Samuelson K. University English professor hacked to death with machetes in Bangladesh in brutal ISIS attack. *Daily Mail*. April 23, 2016. http://www.dailymail.co.uk/news/article-3555000/University-professor-hacked-death-Bangladesh.html. Accessed November 10, 2022.
56. Tomlison S. US embassy worker who ran Bangladesh's only LGBT magazine is hacked to death by 'Islamist militants.' *Daily Mail*. April 25, 2016. http://www.dailymail.co.uk/news/article-3557877/Editor-Bangladesh-s-LGBT-magazine-hacked-death-Islamist-militants-person-receiving-threats-online.html. Accessed November 10, 2022.
57. Elderly Buddhist monk hacked to death in Bangladesh temple. *The Telegraph*. May 14, 2016. http://www.telegraph.co.uk/news/2016/05/14/elderly-buddhist-monk-hacked-to-death-in-bangladesh-temple/. Accessed November 10, 2022.
58. Hawken A. Hindu man hacked to death on the streets of Bangladesh by two men on motorcycles after he 'criticised the prophet Mohammed.' *Daily Mail*. April 30, 2016. http://

www.dailymail.co.uk/news/article-3567027/Hindu-man-hacked-death-streets-Bangladesh-two-men-motorcycles-criticised-prophet-Mohammed.html. Accessed November 10, 2022.

59. Manik Julfikar A, Najar N. Militant Islamists are suspected in slaying of Hindu priest in Bangladesh. *New York Times*. June 7, 2016. https://www.nytimes.com/2016/06/08/world/asia/bangladesh-hindu-priest-killed.html. Accessed November 10, 2022.
60. Boyle D. Islamic militants hack Christian convert to death in Bangladesh: killers slash victim's throat in busy street attack. March 22, 2016. http://www.dailymail.co.uk/news/article-3504096/Islamic-militants-hack-Christian-convert-death-Bangladesh-Killers-slash-victim-s-throat-busy-street-attack.html. Accessed November 10, 2022.
61. No changes mooted following Thai Army bastardisation death. April 7, 2016. https://aecnewstoday.com/2016/no-changes-mooted-following-thai-army-bastardisation-death/#axzz4qysd6tzU. Accessed November 10, 2022.
62. Two 5th grade school girls drown after school bully pushes them into Bangkok canal. *Chiangrai Times*. March 25, 2016. https://www.chiangraitimes.com/news-asia-thailand/two-5th-grade-school-girls-drown-after-school-bully-pushes-them-into-bangkok-canal/. Accessed November 10, 2022.
63. Rook E. Turkish LGBTQ activists protest gruesome murder of transgender woman. *LGBQT Nation*. August 21, 2016. https://www.lgbtqnation.com/2016/08/turkish-lgbtq-activists-protest-gruesome-murder-transgender-woman/. Accessed November 10, 2022.
64. Fraňková R. Death of bullied teacher puts spotlight on poor training. Radio Praha. February 17, 2016. http://www.radio.cz/en/section/curraffrs/death-of-bullied-teacher-puts-spotlight-on-poor-training. Accessed November 10, 2022.
65. Williamson L. French school bullying deaths stir intense debate. BBC News. September 30, 2016. http://www.bbc.com/news/world-europe-37505349. Accessed November 10, 2022.
66. Masters J, Borghese L. Tiziana Cantone's family calls for justice after suicide over sex tape. September 16, 2016. http://www.cnn.com/2016/09/16/europe/tiziana-cantone-sex-tape-suicide/index.html. Accessed November 10, 2022.
67. Bullying in focus after Norway teen's death. *The Local*. January 6, 2016. https://www.thelocal.no/20160106/bullying-in-focus-after-norway-teens-death. Accessed November 10, 2022.
68. Stabbing death of 15yo schoolboy by 'Arab migrant' classmate in Sweden sparks outrage. RT.com. January 17, 2016. https://www.rt.com/news/329243-sweden-migrant-stabbed-teenager/. Accessed November 10, 2022.
69. Ligomeka B. 17 albinos killed in Malawi. News 24. http://www.news24.com/Africa/News/17-albinos-killed-in-malawi-20160509-2. Accessed November 10, 2022.
70. Shefars N. Moroccan rape victim commits suicide after release of her 8 rapists. *Morocco World News*. August 8, 2016. https://www.moroccoworldnews.com/2016/08/193475/moroccan-rape-victim-commit-suicide-release-8-rapists/. Accessed November 10, 2022.
71. Smith J. High school senior, 18, shoots herself in front of her horrified parents after being tormented by anonymous bullies who used encrypted messaging apps to tease her. *Daily Mail*. December 1, 2016. http://www.dailymail.co.uk/news/article-3992188/High-school-senior-18-shoots-terror-stricken-parents-tormented-anonymous-bullies-used-encrypted-messaging-apps-tease-her.html. Accessed November 10, 2022.
72. Hawkesbury student who took her own life was target of bullying, friends say. CBC News. September 9, 2016. http://www.cbc.ca/news/canada/ottawa/eastern-ontario-teen-suicide-blamed-bullying-1.3756124. Accessed November 10, 2022.

73. Suspect in Saskatchewan shooting teased, called himself 'black sheep:' Friends. *MacLean's*. January 25, 2016. http://www.macleans.ca/news/canada/la-loche-teen-appears-in-court-on-murder-charges-in-mass-shooting/. Accessed November 10, 2022.
74. Parry H. Heartbroken brother of high school student, 16, who committed suicide after being tormented online for months writes moving message calling for end to cyber bullying. January 9, 2016. https://www.dailymail.co.uk/news/article-3391659/Heartbroken-brother-high-school-student-16-committed-suicide-tormented-online-months-writes-moving-message-calling-end-cyber-bullying.html. Accessed November 10, 2022.
75. Harper P. Superhero send-off: mourners dress as superheroes for funeral of 18-year-old comic book fan who took his life after years of bullying. *The Sun*. December 9, 2016. https://www.thesun.co.uk/news/2368017/mourners-dress-as-superheroes-for-funeral-of-comic-book-fan/. Accessed November 10, 2022.
76. Niedermeier J. Student commits suicide while suit pending against school. *Great Falls Tribune*. February 25, 2016. http://www.greatfallstribune.com/story/news/2016/02/25/student-commits-suicide-suit-pending-school/80931212/. Accessed November 10, 2022.
77. Robson S. Teenage girl 'beaten to death by gang of bullies in school toilets following row over boy.' *The Mirror*. April 22, 2016. http://www.irishmirror.ie/news/world-news/teenage-girl-beaten-death-gang-7808672. Accessed November 10, 2022.
78. Man faces murder, kidnapping charges in death of 11-year-old girl. NBC 4. May 4, 2016. http://nbc4i.com/2016/05/04/man-faces-murder-kidnapping-charges-in-death-of-11-year-old-girl/. Accessed November 10, 2022.
79. Garcia M. The tragic goodbye of Oriana, a victim of school bullying. CNN. May 2, 2017. http://cnnespanol.cnn.com/2017/05/02/el-tragico-adios-de-oriana-una-victima-del-acoso-escolar/. Accessed November 10, 2022.
80. Joven de 15 años se suicidó de un disparo a causa del bullying. *El Litoral*. September 29, 2016. http://www.ellitoral.com/index.php/id_um/136379-joven-de-15-anos-se-suicido-de-un-disparo-a-causa-del-bullying-en-una-escuela-de-venado-tuerto. Accessed November 10, 2022.
81. Investigarán si la muerte de un joven fue por causa de hostigamiento escolar. *El Litoral*. June 22, 2016. http://www.ellitoral.com/index.php/diarios/2016/06/22/educacion/EDUC-01.html. Accessed November 10, 2022.
82. Estudante que sofria bullying é espancado até a morte no Pará. *O Dia*. September 1, 2016. http://odia.ig.com.br/brasil/2016-09-01/estudante-que-sofria-bullying-e-espancado-ate-a-morte-no-para.html. Accessed November 10, 2022.
83. CNDH investiga muerte de niño en Michoacán por acoso escolar. *La Razon*. April 29, 2016. https://www.razon.com.mx/mexico/cndh-investiga-muerte-de-nino-en-michoacan-por-acoso-escolar/. Accessed November 10, 2022.
84. Van Malderen S. Pesters die Madison (14) tot zelfmoord dreven nu zelf opgejaagd wild. "Ze deden hetzelfde bij andere meisjes." HLN. February 6, 2016. https://www.hln.be/binnenland/pesters-die-madison-14-tot-zelfmoord-dreven-nu-zelf-opgejaagd-wild-ze-deden-hetzelfde-bij-andere-meisjes~a13b6f06/#:~:text=apf8Y7Uo1Y-,Pesters%20die%20Madison%20(14)%20tot%20zelfmoord%20dreven%20nu%20zelf%20opgejaagd,heel%20wat%20heftige%20reacties%20losgeweekt. Accessed November 10, 2022.
85. Jeltsen M. Man charged with murder for allegedly driving his partner to suicide. Huffpost. June 23, 2016. http://www.huffingtonpost.com/entry/jessica-haban-domestic-violence-suicide_us_576ab898e4b09926ce5d4a53. Accessed November 10, 2022.

86. Sawyer L, Chanen D, Jany L. Man, two teens dead after south Minneapolis domestic shooting. *Star Tribune*. September 30, 2016. http://www.startribune.com/police-investigate-homicide-in-wenonah-neighborhood/395409531/. Accessed November 10, 2022.
87. Rosella L. Court documents show murdered City of Brampton employee beaten with brick, strangled. *Brampton Guardian*. December 27, 2016. https://www.bramptonguardian.com/news-story/7038388-court-documents-show-murdered-city-of-brampton-employee-beaten-with-brick-strangled/. Accessed November 10, 2022.
88. Cohen S, Moore T, Schram J. Boy beaten to death with broomstick was abused for months. *New York Post*. September 28, 2016. http://nypost.com/2016/09/28/boy-beaten-to-death-was-abused-for-months-with-broom-stick/. Accessed November 10, 2022.
89. McDermott MM. Brook's grandfather seeks Trump's attention on abuse. *Democrat and Chronicle*. December 30, 2016. http://www.democratandchronicle.com/story/news/2016/12/30/brooks-grandfather-seeks-trumps-attention-abuse/95995056/. Accessed November 10, 2022.
90. Stickney R, Summers D. Caregiver arrested after elderly Oceanside woman dies. NBC 7 San Diego. July 12, 2016. http://www.nbcsandiego.com/news/local/Caregiver-Arrested-After-Elderly-Oceanside-Woman-Dies-386352971.html. Accessed November 10, 2022.
91. Bang YR, Park JH. Psychiatric disorders and suicide attempts among adolescents victimized by school bullying. *Australasian Psychiatry*. 2017; 25(4):376–380.
92. Barzilay S, Klomek AB, Apter A, et al. Bullying victimization and suicide ideation and behavior among adolescents in Europe: a 10-country study. *J Adolesc Health*. 2017;61(2):179–186..
93. Luukkonen AH, Räsänen P, Hakko H, Riala K. Bullying behavior is related to suicide attempts but not to self-mutilation among psychiatric inpatient adolescents. *Psychopathology*. 2009;42(2):131–138.
94. Klomek AB, Sourander A, Niemelä S, et al. Childhood bullying behaviors as a risk for suicide attempts and completed suicides: a population-based birth cohort study. *J Am Acad Child Adolesc Psychiatry*. 2009;48(3):254–261.
95. Sinyor M, Schaffer A, Cheung AH. An observational study of bullying as a contributing factor in youth suicide in Toronto. *Can J Psychiatry*. 2014;59(12):632–638.
96. Geoffroy MC, Boivin M, Arseneault L, et al. Associations between peer victimization and suicidal ideation and suicide attempt during adolescence: results from a prospective population-based birth cohort. *J Am Acad Child Adolesc Psychiatry*. 2016;55(2):99–105.
97. Winsper C, Lereya T, Zanarini M, Wolke D. Involvement in bullying and suicide-related behavior at 11 years: a prospective birth cohort study. *J Am Acad Child Adolesc Psychiatry*. 2012;51(3):271–282.
98. Messias E, Kindrick K, Castro J. School bullying, cyberbullying, or both: correlates of teen suicidality in the 2011 CDC Youth Risk Behavior Survey. *Compr Psychiatry*. 2014;55(5):1063–1068.
99. Sampasa-Kanyinga H, Roumeliotis P, Xu H. Associations between cyberbullying and school bullying victimization and suicidal ideation, plans and attempts among Canadian schoolchildren. *PLOS One*. 2014;9(7):e102145.
100. Cavanaugh CE, Messing JT, Del-Colle M, O'Sullivan C, Campbell JC. Prevalence and correlates of suicidal behavior among adult female victims of intimate partner violence. *Suicide Life Threat Behav*. 2011;41(4):372–383..
101. Campbell JC. Danger assessment. 2003 Cited in Cavanaugh et al.[100] https://www.dangerassessment.org/uploads/pdf/DAEnglish2010.pdf. Accessed November 10, 2022.

102. Hoertel N, Franco S, Wall MM, et al. Childhood maltreatment and risk of suicide attempt: a nationally representative study. *J Clin Psychiatry*. 2015;76(7):916–923.
103. Anderson M, Kaufman J, Simon TR, et al.; School-Associated Violent Deaths Study Group. School-associated violent deaths in the United States, 1994–1999. *JAMA*. 2001;286(21):2695–2702.
104. National Center of Education Statistics. *2021 Digest of Education Statistics*. Table 228.10, School-associated violent deaths of all persons, homicides and suicides of youth ages 5–18 at school, and total homicides and suicides of youth ages 5–18, by type of violent death: 1992–93 through 2018–19. https://nces.ed.gov/programs/digest/d21/tables/dt21_228.10.asp. Accessed November 10, 2022.
105. Kann L, McManus T, Harris WA, et al. Youth risk behavior surveillance—United States, 2015. *MMWR Surveillance Summaries*. 2016;65(6):1–74.
106. Centers for Control Disease and Prevention, National Center for Injury Prevention and Control. *WISQARS™ Fatal Injury Reports, National, Regional and State, 1981–2015, Homicides*. Atlanta, GA: Centers for Control Disease and Prevention. https://webappa.cdc.gov/sasweb/ncipc/mortrate.html. Accessed November 10, 2022.
107. Ybarra ML, Diener-West M, Markow D, Leaf PJ, Hamburger M, Boxer P. Linkages between Internet and other media violence with seriously violent behavior by youth. *Pediatrics*. 2008;122(5):929–937.
108. US Department of Labor, Bureau of Labor Statistics. *Census of Fatal Occupational Injuries (CFOI)—Current and Revised Data*. Washington DC: US Department of Labor, Bureau of Labor Statistics. https://www.bls.gov/iif/oshcfoi1.htm. Accessed November 23, 2022.
109. US Department of Labor, Bureau of Labor Statistics. *Data Tools, Census of Fatal Occupational Injuries (2001 Forward). Top Picks*. Washington DC: US Department of Labor, Bureau of Labor Statistics. https://data.bls.gov/cgi-bin/surveymost?fw. Accessed November 10, 2022. or *Create Customized Tables*. https://data.bls.gov/cgi-bin/dsrv?fw. Accessed November 10, 2022.
110. Menéndez CK, Socias-Morales C, Daus MM. Work-related violent deaths in the US taxi and limousine industry 2003 to 2013: disparities within a high-risk working population. *J Occup Environ Med*. 2017;59(8):768..
111. Konda S, Tiesman HM, Hendricks S, Gurka KK. Non-robbery-related occupational homicides in the retail industry, 2003–2008. *Am J Ind Med*. 2014;57(2):245–253.
112. Tiesman HM, Hendricks SA, Bell JL, Amandus HE. Eleven years of occupational mortality in law enforcement: the census of fatal occupational injuries, 1992–2002. *Am J Ind Med*. 2010;53(9):940–949.
113. Tiesman HM, Gurka KK, Konda S, Coben JH, Amandus HE. Workplace homicides among US women: The role of intimate partner violence. *Ann Epidemiol*. 2012;22(4):277–284.
114. Centers for Disease Control and Prevention (CDC). Fatal occupational injuries—United States, 2005. *MMWR*. 2007;56(13):297..
115. US Department of Labor, Bureau of Labor Statistics. *Homicides and Other Workplace Assaults by Gender in 2019*. Washington DC: US Department of Labor, Bureau of Labor Statistics. https://www.bls.gov/opub/ted/2021/homicides-and-other-workplace-assaults-by-gender-in-2019.htm. Accessed November 20, 2022.
116. Stöckl H, Devries K, Rotstein A, et al. The global prevalence of intimate partner homicide: a systematic review. *Lancet*. 2013;382(9895):859–865.

117. UNICEF. *A League Table of Child Maltreatment Deaths in Rich Nations*. Innocenti Report Card No.5, September 2003. Florence, Italy: UNICEF Innocenti Research Centre. https://www.unicef-irc.org/publications/pdf/repcard5e.pdf. Accessed November 10, 2022.

118. Rich nations are "The group of countries that produce two-thirds of the world's goods and services."[120]

119. The OECD member countries are Australia, Austria, Belgium, Canada, the Czech Republic, Denmark, Finland, France, Germany, Greece, Hungary, Iceland, Ireland, Italy, Japan, the Republic of Korea, Luxembourg, Mexico, the Netherlands, New Zealand, Norway, Poland, Portugal, the Slovak Republic, Spain, Sweden, Switzerland, Turkey, the United Kingdom of Great Britain and Northern Ireland, and the United States of America.[120]

120. US Department of Health and Human Services, Administration on Children, Youth and Families. *Child Maltreatment 2008*. Washington, DC: US Government Printing Office; 2008. https://www.acf.hhs.gov/sites/default/files/documents/cm08_0.pdf. Accessed November 20, 2022.

121. Peltzer K, Pengpid S. Unintentional injuries and psychosocial correlates among in-school adolescents in Malaysia. *Int J Environ Res Public Health*. 2015;12(11):14936–14947.

122. Peltzer K, Pengpid S. Nonfatal injuries and psychosocial correlates among middle school students in Cambodia and Vietnam. *Int J Environ Res Public Health*. 2017;14(3):280.

123. Denny VC, Cassese JS, Jacobsen KH. Nonfatal injury incidence and risk factors among middle school students from four Polynesian countries: the Cook Islands, Niue, Samoa, and Tonga. *Injury*. 2016;47(5):1135–1142.

124. Beck NI, Arif I, Paumier MF, Jacobsen KH. Adolescent injuries in Argentina, Bolivia, Chile, and Uruguay: results from the 2012–2013 Global School-based Student Health Survey (GSHS). *Injury*. 2016;47(12):2642–2649.

125. Peyton RP, Ranasinghe S, Jacobsen KH. Injuries, violence, and bullying among middle school students in Oman. *Oman Med J*. 2017;32(2):98.

126. Wahdan MM, Sayed AM, Elaziz KM, El-Hoseiny MM, Al-Gwaily MM. Prevalence of injuries among high school students in eastern and western parts of Cairo, Egypt. *Injury*. 2016;47(12):2650–2654.

127. Engström K, Hallqvist J, Möller J, Laflamme L. Do episodes of peer victimization trigger physical injury? A case-crossover study of Swedish school children. *Scand J Soc Med*. 2005;33(1):19–25.

128. Srabstein JC. The prevention of bullying: a whole school and community model. In: Shute RH, Slee PT, Murray-Harvey R, Dix KL, eds. *Mental Health and Wellbeing: Educational Perspectives*. Adelaide, Australia: Shannon Research Press; 2011:297–305.

129. UNODC, Global Study on Homicide 2019 (Vienna, 2019). https://www.unodc.org/documents/data-and-analysis/gsh/Booklet1.pdf. Accessed September 21, 2023.

7
Prevention of Bullying and Other Forms of Victimization

The seminal work of Olweus[1] on the prevention of bullying has been followed in the last three decades by many research-based strategies to prevent this form of victimization, primarily in school,[2-20] and by a few approaches to prevent it from taking place in cyberspace,[21-27] the workplace,[28-31] and dating relations,[32-54] as well as to prevent childhood maltreatment.[55-60]

What Is Known?

Prevention Programs for School Bullying

Several existing systematic reviews[61-72] provide summaries and in-depth examinations of the available school-based prevention and intervention programs.[73-124]

In 2002, Rigby[61] presented one of the first comprehensive meta-evaluations of methods and approaches to reduce bullying in preschool and early elementary school by assessing the effectiveness of 13 studies implemented in nine countries. Only the Norwegian study, conducted by Olweus[74,75] from May 1983 to May 1985 and evaluated in the Bergen sample, showed "substantial reductions in self-reported bullying (up to 50%) and reduction in other antisocial behaviors,"[61] and this level of improvement was not achieved by the other reviewed studies.

In 2007, Vreeman and Carol[64] published a frequently cited[76] systematic review of comprehensively assessed school-based strategies to reduce bullying. Their initial extensive search led to the selection of 26 studies for evaluation, including ten curriculum programs,[77-86] ten multidisciplinary or whole-school strategies,[1,6,87-94] four social skills groups,[95-98] one mentoring program,[99] and one social worker support study.[100] The antibullying strategies examined in the review offered mixed outcomes. Only one program[84] of the ten curriculum studies[77-86] showed definite improvement, which was only evident in an indirect outcome, an "increased generation of responses to a simulated bullying situation by the intervention group."[84] Furthermore, the program by King et al.[99] showed that mentored students were significantly less likely at posttest to have bullied a peer during the previous 30 days, as compared to pretest, yet the results were not compared with the control group. Moreover, the study by Bagley and Pritchard[100] examining the effects of an increase in the number of school social workers focusing on problem behaviors, including bullying, demonstrated a significant decrease in self-reported bullying, as compared to matched controls, but this was evident only in elementary school, while worsening of bullying was found in secondary school. In contrast, seven of the ten whole-school approach programs examined in the study showed decreased bullying, although with less definite outcome among younger children. The Olweus multidisciplinary whole-school intervention approach,[102] as implemented in Bergen, Norway,

Table 7.1. Bullying Prevention and/or Intervention Programs with Reported Levels of Significant Effectiveness

Study	Type of Program	Outcome	Study	Type of Program	Outcome
Finland study in Turku and Helsinki[101]	Whole-school approach	Significant reduction in reports of being bullied, especially among youngest students[101]	Prevention of bullying in German schools, 1994–1996[105] (Olweus program)	Whole-school approach	Significant reduction only in low-level bullying and in young students[105]
Olweus Program Norwegian Project, 1983–1985, Bergen Sample[102]	Whole-school approach	Substantial reduction in self-reported bullying (up to 50%)[102]	Antibullying interventions in Kempele, Finland (1990–1998)[106]	Whole-school approach	Significant reductions in bullying after one year and sustained over seven years[106]
Seville Study[103]	Whole-school approach	Significant reductions in students involved in bullying[103]	Promoting positive bystander behavior (1999–2000)[107]	Curriculum for bystanders to discourage bullying	Significant reduction in self-reported victimization[107]
Olweus Program Southeastern United States[104]	Whole-school approach	In some schools, significant reduction in reports of being bullied only among boys and after one year[104]	Support group method (1996–1997)[108]	Intervention to tackle cases of bullying	Some 80% of cases of bullying reported as immediately stopped; 14% after a delay[108]

Source: Based on Rigby and Slee.[65]

emerged in this review,[64] as well as in others,[61,65] as perhaps the most effective antibullying strategy, with reductions in victimization after eight months of 48% for boys and 58% for girls. Yet, its replication by Roland[2] in Rogaland, Norway, showed the opposite result: an increase by 44% of victimization among boys.

In 2008, Rigby and Slee[65] published an excellent summary of 32 school initiatives to reduce bullying, providing a concise description of the nature of the programs, the characteristics of the participants, an explanation of the assessment methods and design, and an account of the main outcomes. Of the reviewed programs, eight (25%) showed some level of significant reduction in bullying behaviors[65] (Table 7.1).

The Most Widely Recognized School Bullying Prevention Programs

After multiple international efforts to develop and implement bullying intervention strategies, the Olweus[1,109-118] and KiVa[119] programs rank as the most recognized and globally implemented programs so far.

Olweus Program

Olweus and Limber[109] published a comprehensive article that provided a succinct description of the Olweus Bullying Prevention Program (OBPP), its development, the subsequent evaluations of its effectiveness, and its dissemination in Norway and the United States.

The OBPP engages in a "restructuring of the school environment"[109] by having adults present sincere, kind, and constructive attention to the students; by providing resolved constraints on unwelcome conduct; by using nonphysical and nonhostile penalties when rules are transgressed; and by providing role models. The OBPP uses four large categories of modules at the school, classroom, individual, and community levels. The approach includes training for all school staff, involving parents, holding weekly class meetings, ensuring immediate intervention when bullying is observed, meeting with perpetrators and victims separately, and developing school–community partnerships.[109] Following its implementation and replication in Norway, the OBPP has been evaluated in different areas of the United States, including South Carolina,[116] Pennsylvania,[117] Washington,[110] and California.[118]

KiVa Antibullying Program

The KiVa Antibullying Program (KiVa is the Finnish acronym for *Kiusaamista Vastaan*, which means "against bullying", is a Finnish national antibullying strategy developed at the University of Turku, Finland, and implemented in grades 4 through 6 during the 2007–2008 academic year.[119] KiVa prevents the occurrence of bullying and intervenes in single instances through general and specified measures that are applied at three different developmental levels (in grades 1 to 3, 4 to 6, and 7 to 9).[119] Kärnä et al.[119] described the components of the version for grades 4 to 6, which include lessons to raise students' awareness of the responsibility that the group has in preserving bullying or not, ways to foster empathy and support for bullying victims, and general guidance for parents.[119] For elementary school students, a computer game is included that offers new information and helps students to learn new skills and to apply their newly acquired knowledge and expertise in real-life situations.[119] Intervention for each case of bullying is addressed by a team of three teachers or school staff, through individual and group meetings with the perpetrators and the victims, as well as by providing support to the victim from "prosocial and high-status classmates."[119] The KiVa program incorporates many elements of the Olweus whole-school approach while underscoring and promoting the role of bystanders.[119]

A study to ascertain the effectiveness of the KiVa program during the first nine months of its nationwide implementation in Finland was conducted by Kärnä et al.[120] with 150,000 students (8 to 16 years old) in 888 Finish schools. The study showed that the KiVa program reduced both victimization and bullying, with control/intervention odds ratios of 1.22 for victimization and 1.18 for bullying.[120]

Beyond Finland, the efficacy of the KiVa program has been, or is being, evaluated in Chile,[121] Italy,[122] Wales,[123] and the Netherlands.[124]

Prevention Strategies beyond School Bullying

Cyberbullying Prevention

Wölfer et al.[23] reported details of the German cyberbullying prevention strategy called Media Heroes and evaluated its effectiveness. This program,[23] first implemented in five German schools, was included in the regular school curriculum and was aimed at reducing cyberbullying by providing psychoeducational and social skills training. The goals were to raise students' awareness of the nature and consequences of cyberbullying, to foster social responsibility, and to enhance the class climate, while also helping students gain experience in self-protection.[23] The long-term effects of the program were assessed via a longitudinal nine-month study conducted with 593 middle school students; multilevel analysis demonstrated the effectiveness of Media Heroes in reducing cyberbullying in intervention classes in comparison to the control group.[23]

Cross et al.[24] described the Australian cyberbullying prevention approach known as Cyber Friendly Schools (CFS), a whole-school approach based on a "social-ecological conceptual framework."[24] The CFS program used a teaching and learning strategy to reduce cyberbullying by way of focusing on the online environments where students spent time, addressing the students' social competence in making positive cyber relationships, adopting Internet privacy and protection, promoting conduct and online skills as well social responsibility, and raising awareness of legal issues, while fostering reporting online.[24] The CFS program's efficacy was investigated through a prospective randomized trial conducted by Cross et al.[24] in Western Australia, using 3,382 grade 8 students. The program[24] was implemented from grade 8 through grade 9 and the students were surveyed for participation in, or exposure to, cyberbullying at the beginning of grade 8 (baseline), at the end of grade 9, and at the end of grade 10.[24] The study showed that the CFS program "was associated with steeper declines in the odds of cyber victimization and cyber perpetration" from baseline to the end of the first year, but not for the subsequent period.[24]

Del Rey et al.[25] highlighted the effectiveness of the ConRed Program, a Spanish cyberbullying intervention initiative also known as "The Knowing, Building and Living Together on the Internet Program" (Conocer, Construir and Convivir en la Red, ConRed).[125] This program utilizes a whole-school approach based on a curriculum geared to foster empathy and sessions to raise awareness on Internet safety and to promote bullying prevention.[25] Its effectiveness was ascertained through a longitudinal study[25] of a sample of 875 secondary school students in the city of Cordoba, Spain. The study included pre- and posttest measurements applied to the experimental and control groups one week before and after the intervention, which lasted three months.[25] The control group was exposed to only the curriculum focused on social competencies in living together (in Spanish, *convivencia*) and empathy, without lessons on cyberbehavior.[25] The research documented that there was a reduction in cyberbullying participation among experimental cybervictims, cyberaggressors, and cyber/bully victims in comparison to the controls.[25]

The effectiveness of the KiVa program[119] in addressing cyberbullying and cybervictimization was assessed by Williford et al.[126] in a study involving 18,412 Finnish students in grades 4 to 9. The investigation showed that KiVa students reported fewer occurrences of cybervictimization at posttest than control students reported.[126]

A meta-analysis by Van Cleemput et al.[127] of several school-based cyberbullying prevention strategies indicated a small but significant level of reduction in cyberbullying by the KiVa program (Hedges' $g = .23$), by the Media Heroes (Hedges' $g = .19$), and by the ConRed program (Hedges' $g = .15$).[127]

Dating Violence Prevention

Since the late 1990s, a number of evidence-based dating violence prevention programs have emerged. De La Rue et al.[128] evaluated the efficacy of 17 school-based programs[32-48] (Table 7.2)

Table 7.2. School-Based Programs for the Prevention of Dating Violence

Program	Target Age	Program Characteristics
Love U2: Increasing your relationship smarts[32]	High school students	Didactic materials, experiential activities
Pilot study of a dating violence prevention program[33]	Eleventh and twelfth grade students	Psychoeducation, focusing on multidimensional aspects of "courtship" aggression
Acquaintance rape education program[34]	Ninth grade students	Role-playing, reflection, discussion, video media
Safe Dates Project[35]	Eighth and ninth grade students	Lecture, poster contest, and a theater production performed by peers
Connections: Relationships and Marriage[36]	High school students	Lecture only
Men as Allies[37]	High school students	Lecture and participatory discussion
Ending Violence[38]	Ninth grade students	Lecture and discussion of laws and legal issues surrounding dating violence
The Power to Choose[39]	Middle school students	Video presentations, multimedia lectures, school posters
Skills for Violence-Free Relationships[40]	Seventh grade students	Participatory discussion devoted to challenging stereotypes and conflict resolution
Dating violence prevention program[41]	Sixth to eighth grade students	Group discussions, experiential exercises
Dating and Sexual Responsibility[42]	Tenth grade students	Video media, role play, discussion, lecture
Rape-awareness program[43]	High school students	Lecture
The Youth Project[44]	Ninth grade students	Role-playing, conflict resolution strategies; two-hour workshop
Rhode Island Teen Dating Violence Prevention Program[45]	Six and seventh grade students	Workshop presentations
Shifting Boundaries[46]	Six and seventh grade students	Lecture and discussion focusing on setting boundaries and deterrence of unwanted behavior
Reaching and Teaching Teens to Stop Violence[47]	Six and seventh grade students	Didactic materials, modeling, role-playing, experiential exercises
Fourth R: Skills for Youth Relationships[48]	Ninth grade students	Video resources, role-playing exercises, rubrics, handouts

Source: Studies reviewed by De La Rue et al.[128]

aimed at decreasing or preventing teen dating violence or sexual violence in intimate relationships. The investigators concluded that the prevention strategies may influence "knowledge and attitudes," but that "the results for dating violence perpetration and victimization were less encouraging."[128]

The Safe Dates Project,[35] a widely cited[49] evidence-based strategy for the prevention of adolescent dating violence, consists of a curriculum with nine 50-minute sessions, one 45-minute play to be performed by students, and a poster contest.[50] Safe Dates focuses on explaining care relationships, defining dating abuse, describing the causes and consequences of abuse, discussing how to help friends, learning how to overcome gender stereotypes, acquiring skills for effective communication, learning to recognize and manage anger, and learning how to prevent sexual assault.[50] It also provides parents and teachers with information about resources.

Forshee et al.[51] assessed the effects of the Safe Dates program in a study involving 1,700 eighth and ninth grade students in a rural area of North Carolina. The intervention-group students were given school and community activities (crisis lines, support groups, materials for parents), while the controls were provided with community resources only. The study showed that the adolescents who were given both school and community activities reported significantly less psychological abuse perpetration and less perpetration of violence against a current dating partner than those who were controls.

In a subsequent study, Forshee et al.[52] evaluated the effects of Safe Dates over four years of follow-up. The results showed that, in comparison to controls, adolescents who were exposed to the Safe Dates program reported perpetrating significantly less psychological, moderate physical, and sexual dating violence through the four years of follow-up.

Foshee et al.[53] assessed the effects of the Family for Safe Dates (FSD), a family-based teen dating abuse prevention program, in a study involving 324 families, recruited nationwide, of whom 140 were randomly assigned to the program, which included six mailed activity booklets, while the rest of participating families were designated controls. At three-month follow-up, the program was shown to be significantly ($P = .04$) associated with less physical victimization.

Finally, the Safe Dates program has been shown to be effective in the prevention of other forms of youth violence, including peer victimization and carrying weapons to school.[54]

Workplace Bullying Prevention

Gillen et al.[129] evaluated the effectiveness of workplace bullying prevention strategies. The researchers reviewed five[28-31,130] randomized and cluster-randomized controlled trials of employee-directed interventions, with controls before and after study. The review determined that there was very low-quality evidence that the programs prevented workplace bullying.

Child Maltreatment Prevention

In 2016, Constantino[55] published a review of available strategies for the prevention of child maltreatment, summarizing the experience with home visitation programs and evidence-based interventions. The review[55] cited a comprehensive analysis of home visitations for infants and toddlers ("Home Visiting Evidence of Effectiveness Review"[56]) and underscored the nurse– family partnership model as "having achieved the strongest evidence base, with one order of magnitude reductions in the incidence of child maltreatment among at-risk groups,"[55] albeit clarifying that, until 2016, the studies "have largely been restricted to families with first-born infants."[55,57] Among available evidence-based parenting education programs, Constantino[55] drew attention to Triple P[58] and The Incredible Years[59] as the programs that "have shown more promise for child maltreatment prevention,"[55] while emphasizing the merits of the preventive intervention for maltreated infants and toddlers in foster care described by Zeanah et al.[60] In this program,[60] child psychiatrists with expertise in infancy provide regularly updated intervention recommendations to the court; the recommendations relate to safety of visitation, delivery of mental healthcare to the birth parents, regular evaluation of the parent–child relationship, and ultimately advice regarding reunification.[55] Evaluation[60] of this prevention approach showed that, in comparison to controls, children who benefited from the intervention had a 53% to 68% relative risk reduction for returning with a subsequent incident of maltreatment. Also, mothers who were exposed to intervention had a 63% to 75% relative risk reduction for maltreating another child subsequently.[60]

Future Directions

The development of the next generation of programs for the prevention of bullying and other forms of victimization should be guided by the evolving evidence that bullying is a form of maltreatment that occurs across social settings, at times simultaneously, and along the life span, and that it is associated with other forms of victimization as well as morbidity and mortality. Furthermore, it should be noted that there is no available evidence-based strategy yet published for the prevention of bullying in social settings like home or prisons, although some programs, such as KiVa[126] and Safe Dates,[54] have been applied to more than one setting. Moreover, there are no published data documenting any significant reduction in morbidity or mortality associated with bullying by any of the available prevention strategies, while the most widely recognized primary prevention programs have been able to reduce the frequency of bullying incidents no more than 50% to 60%.[61,65] In this context, future programs for the prevention of bullying and other forms of victimization should aim to:

- Prevent the occurrence of victimization across social settings and along the life span
- Reduce the morbidity and mortality associated with victimization

These goals could be achieved by providing all members of the community, from preschool through old age, with periodic and developmentally appropriate exposure to three levels of bullying/victimization prevention:

- Primary prevention, to raise awareness of bullying and other forms of maltreatment and to develop knowledge of the health problems related to victimization, while fostering mutual respect and sensitivity to others
- Secondary prevention, to detect exposure to bullying and other forms of victimization, along with appropriate intervention to preclude further occurrences
- Tertiary prevention, to provide treatment of the morbidity related to victimization and to prevent mortality

Notes

1. Olweus D. Bullying at school: basic facts and effects of a school-based intervention program. *J Child Psychol Psychiatry*. 1994;35(7):1171–1190. Cited by Vreeman and Carroll (see Note 64).

2. Roland E. Bullying in school: three national innovations in Norwegian schools in 15 years. *Aggress Behav.* 2000;26:135–143. http://www.std-support.net/ext/asset/upload/Erling%20article%20(1).pdf. Accessed October 4, 2022.
3. Stevens V, De Bourdeaudhuij I, Van Oost P. Anti-bullying interventions at school: aspects of programme adaptation and critical issues for further programme development. *Health Promot Int.* 2001;16(2):155–167.
4. Bosworth K, Espelage D, DuBay T, Dahlberg LL, Daytner G. Using multimedia to teach conflict-resolution skills to young adolescents. *Am J Prev Med.* 1996;12(suppl 5):65–74.
5. Salmivalli C. Participant role approach to school bullying: implications for interventions. *J Adolescence.* 1999;22(4):453–459.
6. Twemlow SW, Fonagy P, Sacco FC, Gies ML, Evans R, Ewbank R. Creating a peaceful school learning environment: a controlled study of an elementary school intervention to reduce violence. *Am J Psychiatry.* 2001;158(5):808–810. Cited by Vreeman and Carroll (see Note 64).
7. Rahey L, Craig WM. Evaluation of an ecological program to reduce bullying in schools. *Can J Couns.* 2002;36(4):281.
8. Meraviglia MG, Becker H, Rosenbluth B, Sanchez E, Robertson T. The Expect Respect Project: creating a positive elementary school climate. *J Interpers Violence.* 2003;18(11):1347–1360.
9. Frey KS, Hirschstein MK, Snell JL, Edstrom LV, MacKenzie EP, Broderick CJ. Reducing playground bullying and supporting beliefs: an experimental trial of the Steps to Respect program. *Dev Psychol.* 2005;41(3):479.
10. Li KK, Washburn I, DuBois DL, et al. Effects of the Positive Action programme on problem behaviours in elementary school students: a matched-pair randomised control trial in Chicago. *Psychol Health.* 2011;26(2):187–204.
11. Shek DT, Ma HK, Sun RC. Development of a new curriculum in a positive youth development program: the Project PATHS in Hong Kong. *Sci World J.* 2011;11:2207–2218.
12. Sapouna M, Wolke D, Vannini N, et al. Virtual learning intervention to reduce bullying victimization in primary school: a controlled trial. *J Child Psychol Psychiatry.* 2010;51(1):104–112.
13. Salmivalli C, Poskiparta E. Making bullying prevention a priority in Finnish schools: the KiVa Antibullying Program. *New Dir Stud Leadersh.* 2012;133:41–53.
14. Alsaker FD, Valkanover S. The Bernese program against victimization in kindergarten and elementary school. *New Dir Stud Leadersh.* 2012;133:15–28.
15. Bonell C, Allen E, Christie D, et al. Initiating change locally in bullying and aggression through the school environment (INCLUSIVE): study protocol for a cluster randomised controlled trial. *Trials.* 2014;15(1):381.
16. Palladino BE, Nocentini A, Menesini E. Evidence-based intervention against bullying and cyberbullying: evaluation of the NoTrap! program in two independent trials. *Aggress Behav.* 2016;42(2):194–206.
17. Trip S, Bora C, Sipos-Gug S, et al. Bullying prevention in schools by targeting cognitions, emotions, and behavior: evaluating the effectiveness of the REBE-ViSC program. *J Couns Psychol.* 2015;62(4):732.
18. Gusmões JD, Sanudo A, Valente JY, Sanchez ZM. Violence in Brazilian schools: analysis of the effect of the Tamojunto prevention program for bullying and physical violence. *J Adolescence.* 2018;63:107–117.
19. Chaux E, Barrera M, Molano A, et al. Classrooms in peace within violent contexts: field evaluation of Aulas en Paz in Colombia. *Prev Sci.* 2017;18(7):828–838.

20. da Silva JL, de Oliveira WA, Braga IF, et al. The effects of a skill-based intervention for victims of bullying in Brazil. *Int J Environ Res Public Health.* 2016;13(11):1042.
21. Roberto AJ, Eden J, Savage MW, Ramos-Salazar L, Deiss DM. Outcome evaluation results of school-based cyber safety promotion and cyberbullying prevention intervention for middle school students. *Health Commun.* 2014;29(10):1029–1042.
22. Lee MS, Zi-Pei W, Svanström L, Dalal K. Cyber bullying prevention: intervention in Taiwan. *PLOS One.* 2013;8(5):e64031.
23. Wölfer R, Schultze-Krumbholz A, Zagorscak P, Jäkel A, Göbel K, Scheithauer H. Prevention 2.0: targeting cyberbullying @ school. *Prev Sci.* 2014;15(6):879–887.
24. Cross D, Shaw T, Hadwen K, et al. Longitudinal impact of the Cyber Friendly Schools program on adolescents' cyberbullying behavior. *Aggress Behav.* 2016;42(2):166–180.
25. Del Rey R, Casas JA, Ortega R. Impact of the ConRed program on different cyberbullying roles. *Aggress Behav.* 2016;42(2):123–135.
26. Schultze-Krumbholz A, Schultze M, Zagorscak P, Wölfer R, Scheithauer H. Feeling cybervictims' pain—the effect of empathy training on cyberbullying. *Aggress Behav.* 2016;42(2):147–156.
27. Doane AN, Kelley ML, Pearson MR. Reducing cyberbullying: a theory of reasoned action-based video prevention program for college students. *Aggress Behav.* 2016;42(2):136–146.
28. Kirk BA, Schutte NS, Hine DW. The effect of an expressive-writing intervention for employees on emotional self-efficacy, emotional intelligence, affect, and workplace incivility. *J Appl Soc Psychol.* 2011;41(1):179–195., Cited by Gillen et al. (see Note 129).
29. Leiter MP, Day A, Oore DG, Spence Laschinger HK. Getting better and staying better: assessing civility, incivility, distress, and job attitudes one year after a civility intervention. *J Occup Health Psychology.* 2012;17(4):425. Cited by Gillen et al. (see Note 129).
30. McGrath L, Jones RS, Hastings RP. Outcomes of anti-bullying intervention for adults with intellectual disabilities. *Res Dev Disabil.* 2010;31(2):376–380. Cited by Gillen et al. (see Note 129).
31. Osatuke K, Moore SC, Ward C, Dyrenforth SR, Belton L. Civility, respect, engagement in the workforce (CREW) nationwide organization development intervention at Veterans Health Administration. *J Appl Behav Sci.* 2009;45(3):384–410. Cited by Gillen et al. (see Note 129).
32. Adler Baeder F, Kerpelman JL, Schramm DG, Higginbotham B, Paulk A. The impact of relationship education on adolescents of diverse backgrounds. *Fam Relat.* 2007;56(3):291–303.
33. Avery-Leaf S, Cascardi M, O'Leary KD, Cano A. Efficacy of a dating violence prevention program on attitudes justifying aggression. *J Adolesc Health.* 1997;21(1):11–17.
34. Fay KE, Medway FJ. An acquaintance rape education program for students transitioning to high school. *Sex Educ.* 2006;6(3):223–236.
35. Foshee VA, Linder GF, Bauman KE, et al. The Safe Dates Project: theoretical basis, evaluation design, and selected baseline findings. *Am J Prev Med.* 1996;12(5):39–47.
36. Gardner SP, Giese K, Parrott SM. Evaluation of the Connections: Relationships and Marriage curriculum. *Fam Relat.* 2004;53(5):521–527.
37. Hillenbrand-Gunn TL, Heppner MJ, Mauch PA, Park HJ. Men as allies: the efficacy of a high school rape prevention intervention. *J Couns Dev.* 2010;88(1):43–51.
38. Jaycox LH, McCaffrey D, Eiseman B, et al. Impact of a school-based dating violence prevention program among Latino teens: randomized controlled effectiveness trial. *J Adolesc Health.* 2006;39(5):694–704.

39. Jones LE. The Minnesota School Curriculum Project: a statewide domestic violence prevention project in secondary schools. In: B. Levy (Ed.), *Dating Violence: Young Women in Danger.* Seattle, WA: Seal Press; 1991:258–266.
40. Krajewski SS, Rybarik MF, Dosch MF, Gilmore GD. Results of a curriculum intervention with seventh graders regarding violence in relationships. *J Fam Violence.* 1996;11(2):93–112.
41. Macgowan MJ. An evaluation of a dating violence prevention program for middle school students. *Violence Vict.* 1997;12(3):223.
42. Pacifici C, Stoolmiller M, Nelson C. Evaluating a prevention program for teenagers on sexual coercion: a differential effectiveness approach. *J Consult Clin Psychol.* 2001;69(3):552.
43. Proto-Campise L, Belknap J, Wooldredge J. High school students' adherence to rape myths and the effectiveness of high school rape-awareness programs. *Violence Against Women.* 1998;4(3):308–328.
44. Sanchez-Cesareo, M. *Outcome Evaluation of the Youth Project: A School Based Teen Dating Violence Prevention Program* [dissertation]. DePaul University; 2002. ProQuest Dissertations and Theses (305508868).
45. Silverman AB. *Evaluating the efficacy of the Rhode Island Teen Dating Violence Prevention Program (TDVPP): A Process and Outcome Approach to Determining the Success of Both Primary and Secondary Prevention Projects.* University of Rhode Island; 2000.
46. Taylor BG, Stein ND, Mumford EA, Woods D. Shifting Boundaries: an experimental evaluation of a dating violence prevention program in middle schools. *Prev Sci.* 2013;14(1):64–76.
47. Weisz AN, Black BM. Evaluating a sexual assault and dating violence prevention program for urban youths. *Soc Work Res.* 2001;25(2):89–100.
48. Wolfe DA, Crooks C, Jaffe P, et al. A school-based program to prevent adolescent dating violence: a cluster randomized trial. *Arch Pediatr Adolesc Med.* 2009;163(8):692–699.
49. According to Google Scholar, Foshee et al., The Safe Dates Project,[35] has been cited by 683 publications. https://scholar.google.com/scholar?hl=en&as_sdt=0%2C21&q=The+Safe+Dates+Project%3A+Theoretical+basis%2C+evaluation+design%2C+and+selected+baseline+findings.+&btnG=. Updated September 9, 2022.
50. US Department of Justice, National Institute of Justice, Office of Justice Programs. *Program Profile, Safe Dates.* https://www.crimesolutions.gov/ProgramDetails.aspx?ID=142. Accessed October 4, 2022.
51. Foshee VA, Bauman KE, Arriaga XB, Helms RW, Koch GG, Linder GF. An evaluation of Safe Dates, an adolescent dating violence prevention program. *Am J Public Health.* 1998;88(1):45–50.
52. Foshee VA, Bauman KE, Ennett ST, Suchindran C, Benefield T, Linder GF. Assessing the effects of the dating violence prevention program "Safe Dates" using random coefficient regression modeling. *Prev Sci.* 2005;6(3):245.
53. Foshee VA, Reyes HL, Ennett ST, Cance JD, Bauman KE, Bowling JM. Assessing the effects of Families for Safe Dates, a family-based teen dating abuse prevention program. *J Adolesc Health.* 2012;51(4):349–356..
54. Foshee VA, Reyes LM, Agnew-Brune CB, et al. The effects of the evidence-based Safe Dates dating abuse prevention program on other youth violence outcomes. *Prev Sci.* 2014;15(6):907–916.
55. Constantino JN. Child maltreatment prevention and the scope of child and adolescent psychiatry. *Child Adolesc Psychiatr Clin.* 2016;25(2):157–165.

56. Avellar S, Paulsell D, Sama-Miller E, Grosso PD, Akers L, Kleinman R. Home visiting evidence of effectiveness review: executive summary. *Math Policy Res.* 2015. https://www.mathematica.org/publications/september-2019-home-visiting-evidence-of-effectiveness-review-executive-summary. Accessed October 4, 2022. Cited by Constantino.[55]
57. Lanier P, Jonson-Reid M. Comparing primiparous and multiparous mothers in a nurse home visiting prevention program. *Birth.* 2014;41(4):344–352. Cited by Constantino.[55]
58. Prinz RJ, Sanders MR, Shapiro CJ, Whitaker DJ, Lutzker JR. Population-based prevention of child maltreatment: the US Triple P system population trial. *Prev Sci.* 2009;10(1):1–2. Cited by Constantino.[55]
59. Hurlburt MS, Nguyen K, Reid J, Webster-Stratton C, Zhang J. Efficacy of the Incredible Years group parent program with families in Head Start who self-reported a history of child maltreatment. *Child Abuse Negl.* 2013;37(8):531–543. Cited by Constantino.[55]
60. Zeanah CH, Larrieu JA, Heller SS, et al. Evaluation of a preventive intervention for maltreated infants and toddlers in foster care. *J Am Acad Child Adolesc Psychiatry.* 2001;40(2):214–221. Cited by Constantino.[55]
61. Rigby K. Meta evaluation of methods and approaches to reducing bullying in pre-schools and early primary school in Australia. Canberra: Commonwealth Attorney-General's Department, Canberra, 2002; 2008. https://pdfs.semanticscholar.org/9309/e8b289e1cb761d84c6e9a03b2ae02632cb0f.pdf?_ga=2.36089120.1410045772.1549207442-1791718516.1549207442. Accessed October 4, 2022.
62. Smith PK, Ananiadou K, Cowie H. Interventions to reduce school bullying. *Can J Psychiatry.* 2003;48(9):591–599..
63. Smith PK, Pepler D, Rigby K, eds. *Bullying in Schools: How Successful Can Interventions Be?* Cambridge, England: Cambridge University Press; 2004..
64. Vreeman RC, Carroll AE. A systematic review of school-based interventions to prevent bullying. *Arch Pediatr Adolesc Med.* 2007;161(1):78–88.
65. Rigby K, Slee P. Interventions to reduce bullying. *Int J Adolesc Med Health.* 2008;20(2):165–184.
66. Cantone E, Piras AP, Vellante M, et al. Interventions on bullying and cyberbullying in schools: a systematic review. *Clin Pract Epidemiol Ment Health.* 2015;11(suppl 1 M4):58.
67. Lee S, Kim CJ, Kim DH. A meta-analysis of the effect of school-based anti-bullying programs. *J Child Health Care.* 2015;19(2):136–153.
68. National Research Council. *Building Capacity to Reduce Bullying: Workshop Summary.* Washington, DC: National Academies Press; 2014..
69. Silva JL, Oliveira WA, Mello FC, Andrade LS, Bazon MR, Silva MA. Anti-bullying interventions in schools: a systematic literature review. *Ciênc. Saúde Colet.* 2017;22(7):2329–2340.
70. Voight A, Nation M. Practices for improving secondary school climate: a systematic review of the research literature. *Am J Commun Psychol.* 2016;58(1-2):174–191.
71. Bradshaw CP. Translating research to practice in bullying prevention. *Am Psychol.* 2015;70(4):322.
72. Fox KA, Shjarback JA. What works to reduce victimization? Synthesizing what we know and where to go from here. *Violence Vict.* 2016;31(2):285.
73. The Bernese Study, Switzerland; The Chicago Study, United States; The Toronto Study, Canada; The Sheffield Cooperative Learning Study, Sheffield, England; The Finland Study, Turku and Helsinki; The Texas Study, United States; The Norwegian Project, as evaluated in the Bergen sample; The Norwegian Project, as evaluated in the Rogaland sample; The Sheffield Study,

England; The Home Office Study, Liverpool and London, England; The Seville Study, Spain; The Flanders Study, Belgium; The New South Wales Study, Australia.

74. Olweus D. Bully/victim problems among school children: basic facts and effects of a school-based intervention program. In: Pepler DJ, Rubin KH, eds. *The Development and Treatment of Childhood Aggression*. Hillsdale, NJ: Erlbaum; 1991:411–448. Cited by Rigby.[61]
75. Olweus D. *Bullying at School*. Oxford, England: Blackwell Publishers; 1993. Cited by Rigby.[61]
76. Vreeman and Carroll[64] has been cited by 1,131 publications, according to Google Scholar. https://scholar.google.com/scholar?hl=en&as_sdt=0%2C21&q=A+systematic+review+of+school-based+interventions+to+prevent+bullying.+&btnG=. Accessed September 23, 2023.
77. Baldry AC, Farrington DP. Evaluation of an intervention program for the reduction of bullying and victimization in schools. *Aggress Behav*. 2004;30(1):1–5. Cited by Vreeman and Carroll.[64]
78. Boulton MJ, Flemington I. The effects of a short video intervention on secondary school pupils' involvement in definitions of and attitudes towards bullying. *Sch Psychol Int*. 1996;17(4):331–345. Cited by Vreeman and Carroll.[64]
79. Cowie HS, Smith PK, Boulton M, Laver R. *Cooperation in the Multi-Ethnic Classroom*. London, England: David Fulton; 1994. Cited by Vreeman and Carroll.[64]
80. Elliot H, Faupel A. Children's solutions to bullying incidents. *Educ Psychol Pract*. 1997;13:21–28. Cited by Vreeman and Carroll.[64]
81. Englert D. *Investigating the Effectiveness of Violence Intervention in a Primary Education Setting: A Comparison of Programs* [dissertation]. University of Mississippi; 1999. Cited by Vreeman and Carroll.[64]
82. Kaiser-Ulrey C. *Bullying in Middle School: A Study of B.E.S.T.—Bullying Eliminated from Schools Together—An Anti-Bullying Program for Seventh Grade Students*. Tallahassee Florida State University College of Education; 2003. Cited by Vreeman and Carroll.[64]
83. ŘíČan PA, Ondrová K, Svatoš J. The effect of a short, intensive intervention upon bullying in four classes in a Czech town. *Ann NY Acad Sci*. 1996;794(1):399–400. Cited by Vreeman and Carroll.[64]
84. Stevens V, Bourdeaudhuij I, Oost P. Bullying in Flemish schools: an evaluation of anti-bullying intervention in primary and secondary, schools. *Br J Educ Psychol*. 2000;70(2):195–210. Cited by Vreeman and Carroll.[64]
85. Teglasi H, Rothman L. STORIES: a classroom-based program to reduce aggressive behavior. *J Sch Psychol*. 2001;39(1):71–94. Cited by Vreeman and Carroll.[64]
86. Warden D, Moran E, Gillies J, Mayes G, Macleod L. An evaluation of a children's safety training programme. *Educ Psychol*. 1997;17(4):433–448. Cited by Vreeman and Carroll.[64]
87. Alsaker FD, Valkanover S. Early diagnosis and prevention of victimization in kindergarten. In: Juvonen J, Graham S, eds. *Peer Harassment in School*. New York, NY: Guilford Press; 2001:175–195. Cited by Vreeman and Carroll.[64]
88. Melton GB, Limber SP, Cunningham P, et al. *Violence Among Rural Youth*. Washington, DC: Office of Juvenile Justice and Delinquency Prevention; 1998. Cited by Vreeman and Carroll.[64]
89. Menesini E, Codecasa E, Benelli B, Cowie H. Enhancing children's responsibility to take action against bullying: evaluation of a befriending intervention in Italian middle schools. *Aggress Behav*. 2003;29(1):1–4. Cited by Vreeman and Carroll.[64]
90. Metzler CW, Biglan A, Rusby JC, Sprague JR. Evaluation of a comprehensive behavior management program to improve school-wide positive behavior support. *Educ Treat Child*. 2001:448–479. Cited by Vreeman and Carroll.[64]

91. Mitchell J, Palmer S, Booth M, Powell Davies G. A randomised trial of an intervention to develop health promoting schools in Australia: the Southwestern Sydney Study. *Aust NZ J Public Health*. 2000;24242–22446. Cited by Vreeman and Carroll.[64]
92. Rahey L, Criag W. Evaluation of an ecological program to reduce bullying in schools. *Can J Couns*. 2002;36281–36296. Cited by Vreeman and Carroll.[64]
93. Roland E. Bullying in school: three national innovations in Norwegian schools in 15 years. *Aggress Behav*. 2000;135–143. Cited by Vreeman and Carroll.[64]
94. Sanchez E, Robertson T, Lewis C, Rosenbluth B, Bohman T, Casey D. Preventing bullying and sexual harassment in elementary schools: the Expect Respect model. In: Geffner R, Loring M, Young C, eds. *Bullying Behavior: Current Issues, Research, and Interventions*. Vol 2. New York, NY: Haworth Maltreatment & Trauma Press; 2001:157–180. Cited by Vreeman and Carroll.[64]
95. DeRosier ME. Building relationships and combating bullying: effectiveness of a school-based social skills group intervention. *J Clin Child Adolesc Psychol*. 2004;33(1):196–201. Cited by Vreeman and Carroll.[64]
96. Fast J, Fanelli F, Salen L. How becoming mediators affects aggressive students. *Child Sch*. 2003;25(3):161–171. Cited by Vreeman and Carroll.[64]
97. Meyer N, Lesch E. An analysis of the limitations of a behavioural programme for bullying boys from a subeconomic environment. *S Afr J Child Adolesc Ment Health*. 2000;12(1):59–69. Cited by Vreeman and Carroll.[64]
98. Tierney T, Dowd R. The use of social skills groups to support girls with emotional difficulties in secondary schools. *Support Learn*. 2000;15(2):82–85. Cited by Vreeman and Carroll.[64]
99. King KA, Vidourek RA, Davis B, McClellan W. Increasing self-esteem and school connectedness through a multidimensional mentoring program. *J Sch Health*. 2002;72(7):294–299. Cited by Vreeman and Carroll.[64]
100. Bagley C, Pritchard C. The reduction of problem behaviours and school exclusion in at-risk youth: an experimental study of school social work with cost–benefit analyses. *Child Fam Soc Work*. 1998. Cited by Vreeman and Carroll.[64]
101. Salmivalli C, Kaukiainen A, Voeten M. Anti-bullying intervention: implementation and outcome. *Br J Educ Psychol*. 2005;75(3):465–487. Cited by Rigby and Slee.[65]
102. Olweus D. The Olweus Bullying Prevention Programme: design and implementation issues and a new national initiative in Norway. In: Smith PK, Pepler D, Rigby K, eds. *Bullying in Schools: How Successful Can Interventions Be?* Cambridge, England: Cambridge University Press; 2004:13–36. Cited by Rigby and Slee.[65]
103. Onega R, Del Rey R, Mora-Merchan JA. SAVE model: an anti-bullying intervention in Spain. In: Smith PK, Pepler D, Rigby K, eds. *Bullying in Schools: How Successful Can Interventions Be?* Cambridge, England: Cambridge University Press; 2004:167–185. Cited by Rigby and Slee.[65]
104. Limber SP, Nation M, Tracy AJ, Melton GB, Flerx V. Implementation of the Olweus Bullying Prevention Programme in the southeastern United States. In: Smith PK, Pepler D, Rigby K, eds. *Bullying in Schools: How Successful Can Interventions Be?* Cambridge, England: Cambridge University Press; 2004:55–79. Cited by Rigby and Slee.[65]
105. Hanewinkel R. Prevention of bullying in German schools: an evaluation of an anti-bullying approach. In: Smith PK, Pepler D, Rigby K, eds. *Bullying in Schools: How Successful Can Interventions Be?* Cambridge, England: Cambridge University Press; 2004:81–97. Cited by Rigby and Slee.[65]

106. Koivisto M. A follow-up survey of antibullying interventions in the comprehensive schools of Kempele in 1990–98. In: Smith PK, Pepler D, Rigby K, eds. *Bullying in Schools: How Successful Can Interventions Be?* Cambridge, England: Cambridge University Press; 2004:275–288. Cited by Rigby and Slee.[65]
107. Salmivalli C, Kaukiainen A, Voeten M. Anti-bullying intervention: implementation and outcome. *Br J Educ Psychol.* 2005;75(3):465–487. Cited by Rigby and Slee.[65]
108. Smith PK, Howard S, Thompson F. Use of the support group method to tackle bullying, and evaluation from schools and local authorities in England. *Pastoral Care Educ.* 2007;25(2):4–13. Cited by Rigby and Slee.[65]
109. Olweus D, Limber SP. Bullying in school: evaluation and dissemination of the Olweus Bullying Prevention Program. *Am J Orthopsychiatry.* 2010;80(1):124–134.
110. Bauer NS, Lozano P, Rivara FP. The effectiveness of the Olweus Bullying Prevention Program in public middle schools: a controlled trial. *J Adolesc Health.* 2007;40(3):266–274.
111. Black S, Washington E, Trent V, Harner P, Pollock E. Translating the Olweus Bullying Prevention Program into real-world practice. *Health Promot Pract.* 2010;11(5):733–740.
112. Bowllan NM. Implementation and evaluation of a comprehensive, school-wide bullying prevention program in an urban/suburban middle school. *J Sch Health.* 2011;81(4):167–173.
113. Schroeder BA, Messina A, Schroeder D, et al. The implementation of a statewide bullying prevention program: preliminary findings from the field and the importance of coalitions. *Health Promot Pract.* 2012;13(4):489–495.
114. Beckman L, Svensson M. The cost-effectiveness of the Olweus Bullying Prevention Program: results from a modelling study. *J Adolescence.* 2015;45:127–137..
115. Olweus D, Limber SP. *Olweus bullying prevention program teacher guide.* Center City, MN: Hazelden; 2007.
116. Melton GB, Limber SP, Cunningham P, et al. *Violence among Rural Youth. Final Report.* Washington, DC: US Department of Justice Programs, Office of Juvenile Justice and Delinquency Prevention. Unpublished report. Cited by Olweus and Limber.[109]
117. Black SA, Jackson E. Using bullying incident density to evaluate the Olweus Bullying Prevention Programme. *Sch Psychol Int.* 2007;28(5):623–638. Cited by Olweus and Limber.[109]
118. Pagliocca PM, Limber SP, Hashima P. Evaluation report for the Chula Vista Olweus Bullying Prevention Program. Unpublished report prepared for the Chula Vista (CA) Police Department. 2007. Cited by Olweus and Limber.[109]
119. Kärnä A, Voeten M, Little TD, Poskiparta E, Kaljonen A, Salmivalli C. A large-scale evaluation of the KiVa antibullying program: Grades 4–6. *Child Dev.* 2011;82(1):311–330.
120. Kärnä A, Voeten M, Little TD, Poskiparta E, Alanen E, Salmivalli C. Going to scale: A non-randomized nationwide trial of the KiVa antibullying program for grades 1–9. *J Consult Clin Psychol.* 2011;79(6):796.
121. Gaete J, Valenzuela D, Rojas-Barahona C, Valenzuela E, Araya R, Salmivalli C. The KiVa antibullying program in primary schools in Chile, with and without the digital game component: study protocol for a randomized controlled trial. *Trials.* 2017;18(1):75.
122. Nocentini A, Menesini E. KiVa anti-bullying program in Italy: evidence of effectiveness in a randomized control trial. *Prev Sci.* 2016;17(8):1012–1023.
123. Clarkson S, Axford N, Berry V, et al. Effectiveness and micro-costing of the KiVa school-based bullying prevention programme in Wales: study protocol for a pragmatic definitive parallel group cluster randomised controlled trial. *BMC Public Health.* 2015;16(1):104.

124. The KiVa Anti-Bullying Program in the Netherlands, Waves 1–5. https://b2find.eudat.eu/dataset/ac46da44-00f4-5f12-ae19-d9584c37f9f3. Accessed September 23, 2023.
125. Del Rey Alamillo R, Casas JA, Ortega R. The ConRed Program, an evidence-based practice [in Spanish]. *Comunicar*. 2012;20(39):129.
126. Williford A, Elledge LC, Boulton AJ, DePaolis KJ, Little TD, Salmivalli C. Effects of the KiVa antibullying program on cyberbullying and cybervictimization frequency among Finnish youth. *J Clin Child Adolesc Psychol*. 2013;42(6):820–833.
127. Van Cleemput K, DeSmet A, Vandebosch H, et al. A systematic review of studies evaluating anti-cyberbullying programs. Paper presented at Etmaal van Communicatiewetenschap; February 3–4, 2014; Wageningen, Netherlands. Cited by Espelage DL, Hong JS. Cyberbullying prevention and intervention efforts: current knowledge and future directions. *Can J Psychiatry*. 2017;62(6):374–380.
128. De La Rue L, Polanin JR, Espelage DL, Piggot TD, De La Rue L. School-based interventions to reduce dating and sexual violence: a systematic review. *Campbell Syst Rev*. 2014;7. https://onlinelibrary.wiley.com/doi/full/10.4073/csr.2014.7.
129. Gillen PA, Sinclair M, Kernohan WG, Begley CM, Luyben AG. Interventions for prevention of bullying in the workplace. *Cochrane Database Syst Rev*. 2012;4.
130. Hoel H, Giga SI, with contributions from Brian Faragher. Destructive interpersonal conflict in the workplace: the effectiveness of management interventions. *Br Occup Health Res Found*. 2006:1–85. Cited by Gillen et al.[129]

8
Detection of Bullying and Other Forms of Victimization

What Is Known?

The growing recognition that bullying and other forms of victimization are associated with an array of health and safety risks constitutes a challenge to health practitioners to detect bullying and victimization. In this context, detection is an essential tool in the secondary prevention of victimization and related toxicity and opens the opportunity for appropriate intervention to stop ongoing abuse and for treatment of associated morbidity.

There is a limited number of articles that underscore the public health significance of clinical detection of school bullying[1-3] or that propose strategies for clinical[1,3,4] or nonclinical[5-6] screening. In contrast, there is a broader range of studies addressing the detection of other forms of victimization, such as cyberbullying,[7-17] intimate partner violence,[18-126] and childhood maltreatment.[127-136]

Clinical Detection of School Bullying

The notion of screening for exposure to, and/or participation in, school bullying during health assessment has been proposed[1-3] as an important public health tool in the process of secondary prevention of peer victimization incidents that were not averted through primary prevention strategies. In turn, detection could pave the way for intervention to halt ongoing episodes of bullying and/or for treatment of associated health problems.[1-3] Srabstein et al.[1] put forward preliminary recommendations to advance the detection of ongoing and recent (in the preceding two months) exposure to school bullying and associated health risks among children and adolescents evaluated by health practitioners in outpatient, emergency, or inpatient settings. The proposed ways of conducting such a screening could include:

- Explaining to the patient and family that everyone is asked questions about exposure to bullying to ensure everyone is safe
- Offering a developmental and culturally sensitive explanation of the notion of bullying
- Asking whether the patient has been recently subjected to bullying, and, if so, ascertaining the type of bullying, the place of occurrence, the identity of the perpetrators, and the experience of associated physical and/or emotional morbidity and/or psychosocial risks

Thus far, there is no published account of the development and implementation of a standardized and validated questionnaire that could be used by clinicians for detection of school bullying and associated health risks as part of a face-to face pediatric anamnesis.

Carr-Gregg and Manocha[4] underscored the need to detect bullying by general practitioners and suggested the use of HEADSS (Home, Education and Employment, Activities, Drug, Sexuality, Suicide/depression),[137-139] a psychosocial assessment strategy to provide a framework for clinical assessment of bullying. Yet, HEADSS,[137] an evaluation approach that is intended to create a meaningful connection between the health provider and the adolescent, only suggests inquiring about bullying in the context of ascertaining quality of peer relations, without providing or requiring a definition of bullying or details about it.

Artificial Intelligence to Detect School Bullying

Artificial intelligence methodology has been proposed[5,6] to detect school verbal[5] and/or physical[5,6] bullying. In a 2014 report, Ye et al.[6] put forward a physical bullying detection process built on motion identification; the process uses a Fuzzy multithreshold logarithm to differentiate physical bullying, such as pushing, hitting, and shaking, from nonbullying daily movements, such as standing up, sitting down, walking, running, doing push-ups, or falling. The hardware involved in the detection included an accelerometer and a gyroscope for movement data sampling, and they were linked to RAM for data and function storage, which in turn was connected to a central processing unit (CPU) that was used to run the algorithm, with a connection to a short message system (SMS) module in charge of sending alarm messages if bullying was detected. The research[6] attained an "average classification accuracy of 92%,"[6] establishing the potential for the development of "smartphone-based detection of physical bullying."[6]

Another study conducted by Ye et al.[5] advanced a model for detection of school bullying based on the recognition of both motor activity and speech emotion. To this end, the study[5] utilized movement sensors and a microphone to gather motion and voice data, while a back-propagation neural network (BPNN)[140] was trained to recognize bullying and to distinguish it from ordinary activities.[140] Ye et al.[5] documented that "motion-audio combined feature vector outperforms sole motion features and sole acoustic features, with accuracy of 82.4% and precision of 92.2%."[5]

Detection of Cyberbullying

There are a growing number of studies exploring the use of artificial intelligence strategies for the detection of cyberbullying.[7,8-17,141-145]

Al-Harigy et al.[12] provided a snapshot of the most modern technological advances in cyberbullying detection research by conducting a comparative analysis of 45 studies published in peer-reviewed journals and/or presented in conference proceedings between 2012 and 2020. Their review[12] examined the different cyberbullying techniques from different views, while it underscored the method of manual or automatic labeling of datasets, known as supervised learning (SL), as the most popular approach for cyberbullying detection.[12] Furthermore, the report[12] suggested that future research should consider the use of a self-supervised learning (SSL) approach "for labeling large-scale cyberbullying datasets by learning the features from the data without use of human intervention,"[12] as well as incorporating the use of emojis and analysis of victims' emotional behavior in future automated cyberbullying detection.

Screening and Detection of Intimate Partner Violence

Feltner et al.[30] were commissioned by the US Preventive Services Task Force[146] to review the evidence on screening for intimate partner violence (IPV). The researchers examined the accuracy of 10 screening tools in detecting past or current IPV and found that both the WAST (Woman Abuse Screening Tool)[147,148] and the OVAT (Ongoing Violence Assessment Tool)[149] have a greater than 80% sensitivity and specificity in identifying past-year or present exposure to IPV.

The WAST[150] aims to establish whether a female patient has ever, and with what frequency, been abused physically, sexually, or emotionally by her partner, and/or if she has been frightened by her partner's words or actions, and/or whether arguments with her partner have ever led to physical aggression or feeling down or bad about herself.

The OVAT[149] uses four questions that try to ascertain whether, in the previous month, a the patient's partner has threatened her with a weapon, beaten her badly enough to require medical care, disrespected her for her feelings, or acted in a life-threatening manner.

The efficacy of computer-assisted screening to detect IPV, as compared to other screening strategies, was investigated by several studies.[21,23,50,67,68,70,72,79,92,93,103] Hussain et al.[21] conducted a meta-analysis of six randomized controlled studies[95,151-155] and showed that computer-assisted self-administered screens leads to higher rates of IPV disclosure in comparison to both face-to-face interview and self-administered written screens.[21]

Many studies have reported on the experience of screening for IPV across clinical settings and/organizations, including emergency departments,[38,51,70,106] primary care system,[86,87,108,111,156] obstetrics and gynecology clinics,[28,48,115] veterans' health facilities,[35,49,68] dental clinics,[49] and workplaces,[114] as well as among members of a managed behavioral health organization.[24]

Universal Screening for IPV

The US Preventive Services Task Force[146] recommended "that clinicians screen for IPV in women of reproductive age and provide or refer women who screen positive to ongoing support services."[31] This recommendation has been supported by the American Academy of Pediatrics,[157] the American College of Obstetricians and Gynecologists,[158] and the American Academy of Family Phyisicians.[159]

As Wathen et al.[160] have described, there is an ongoing debate between advocates for universal IPV screening of all women attending healthcare clinics[158,161] and the proponents of a "case-finding approach," consisting of an "assessment of a patient based on risks for, and/or clinical signs or symptoms of, exposure."[162-164]

Barriers to, and Limited Extent of, IPV Screening

A study by Waalen et al.[124] identified, among the main barriers to IPV screening, the lack of provider education regarding IPV, as well as their lack of time, the lack of effective interventions, and providers' fear of offending patients. In 2014-2015, Daoud et al.[26] investigated the rate of women who have ever been screened for IPV, based on a cross-sectional survey of 1,401 Arab and Jewish Israeli women, age 16 to 48 years, who were either pregnant or up to 6 months postpartum and were attending 63 maternal and child health clinics in four geographical districts of Israel. The research showed that less than half of the participants (48.8%) reported that they were ever screened for IPV, despite Israeli policy mandating IPV screening for women attending maternal and child health clinics.[165] A similar limited extent of IPV screening was shown by Lawoko et al.[166] in a survey of 168 Swedish health providers who were practicing either at the women's clinic, emergency clinic, or ambulatory department of the Södersjukhuset Hospital. The study documented that only 50% of the participants reported that they had been screened for IPV at least once in the previous three months. Physicians and nurses who screened for IPV were more likely to be female, to perceive high efficiency in dealing with IPV issues, to have fewer worries about offending patients, to have better professional readiness on the subject, and to have access to support networks.[166]

Screening and Detection of Child Maltreatment

Lessons from the Dutch Universal Screening for Child Maltreatment

Since 2009, all emergency departments (EDs) in the Netherlands have been required by the Health and Youth Care Inspectorate[167] to screen every child being evaluated in an ED for child abuse, and to provide regular training on child abuse detection for ED staff.[168,169] A study led by van Konijnenburg et al.[170] surveyed almost all EDs (94%) in the Netherlands about their approach to screening for child maltreatment, and the survey documented that 100% used checklists, 41% utilized screening physical examinations, and 60% of the EDS applied a screening based on parental risk factors.[170] Twenty percent of the EDs utilized the SPUTOVAMO[171,172] and SPUTAVAMO-R[173] screening checklists, 6% employed the ESCAPE form[174] or an adaptation of the Berger-pediatric flowchart,[175] and most of the hospitals used modified versions of the above-mentioned checklists.[170]

The screening tools include items pertaining to three areas of concern relevant in the investigation of child maltreatment: an unclear history of physical trauma, unusual aspects of an injury, and/or odd parental behavior.

In 2010, the ED of the Academic Medical Center in Amsterdam added a complete physical examination, known as top–toe inspection (TTI), to the existing checklist screening protocol, with the goal of "identifying signs of child abuse and neglect in all children regardless of the mode of presentation."[176] The TTI provided another clinical strategy to identify unexplained injuries and scars, poor care and hygiene, failure to thrive, and other potential signs of child abuse and neglect.[176] Teeuw et al.[177] have documented that combining the TTI and the SPUTOVAMO screening test significantly increases the number of positive tests, resulting in more cases of child abuse detected.

The Dutch detection of child maltreatment based on parental risk factors[170] consisted of screening all adults visiting an ED because of IPV, substance abuse, or suicide attempt to ascertain whether they have children under their care; if so, the children were referred for further child maltreatment detection.

The ISPCAN Child Abuse Screening Tool (ICAST)

In 2004, the International Society for the Prevention of Child Abuse and Neglect (ISPCAN)[178] organized an international meeting in Brisbane, with participation of 31 countries, that led to the development of three internationally valid instruments[179-181] that could be applied to survey parents about their disciplinary strategies for dealing with their children's behavior in the previous year,[179] to retrospectively assess young adults about their exposure to childhood maltreatment,[180] and to allow "mature children" to report harsh treatment or maltreatment in their homes or institutions.[181]

With pilot work in six countries[182] and seven languages, Runyan et al.[179] documented details about the development of the ISPCAN Child Abuse Screening Tool–Parent version (ICAST-P), an instrument that ascertains parental behaviors aimed at their children. ICAST-P has 30 items pertaining to three types of violent discipline, three examples of neglect (unmet medical needs, inadequate food or liquid, or inadequate supervision when being hurt), two types of sexual abuse (sexual touch by an adult or sex with an adult), and five types of nonviolent disciplinary strategies, including use of explanation to children, telling the children to stop something, providing "time out," taking away privileges, or using distraction.[179]

An average of 95% of the 697 parents screened with the ICAST-P in the six countries[181] reported that they used nonviolent discipline strategies, with the most common (95%) being the use of explanation to children. Yet, 69% of the parents indicated they used moderate physical punishment, with more than one-third reporting that they applied spanking. Furthermore, almost 80% of parents surveyed reported the use of psychological discipline, with shouting being the most common form (72%).

Dunne et al.[180] reported on the development of the ISPCAN Child Abuse Screening Tool–Retrospective version (ICAST-R), its field testing in seven countries,[183] and its translation into six languages. ICAST-R contains 15 items, reflected in questions pertaining to exposure to physical, psychological, or sexual maltreatment that may have occurred before age 18. The researchers' field analysis showed that an average of almost 34% of young adults surveyed in seven countries reported having been hit or punched before age 18, 49% indicated that they were insulted or criticized as children or adolescents, and approximately 17% were subjected to someone who exposed or touched their genitals.[180]

Zolotor et al.[181] described the development of the ISPCAN Child Abuse Screening Tool–Children's version (ICAST-C), designed to ascertain the occurrence of childhood maltreatment, at home or in an institution, from the child's perspective. It consists of 36 items pertaining to five types of victimization or exposure to maltreatment at home, or at least 36 items concerning three kinds of maltreatment that could occur at an institution. The results of field testing[181] in four countries[184] showed that 51% of the 459 children and adolescents surveyed reported having been exposed to violence in their homes, with almost a third having witnessed adults shouting in a frightening way. Furthermore, 66% of the young people had experienced psychological victimization, primarily by being screamed at or insulted, while 37% felt neglected, mostly by being perceived as unimportant or feeling that inadequate support or help was being provided. Moreover, more than half of the respondents were subjected to physical punishment (being spanked with a hand, hit, pushed, grabbed, or kicked), while 18% of the youth surveyed reported having been subjected to sexual abuse, either by feeling that somebody talked to them in a "sexual way" or by being touched on private parts.

Of the children and adolescents surveyed about their exposure to maltreatment in an institution, more than half reported that they suffered physical victimization, most commonly by having somebody slap their hand or arm, by being hurt by someone, or by having an object thrown at them. Almost 60% of the youth experienced psychological victimization, primarily by being cursed at, insulted, or embarrassed by somebody, as well as being called hurtful names, while 22% were exposed to sexual maltreatment, mostly by being shown pornography or being given an unwanted kiss.

Future Directions

Universal Screening for Exposure to Victimization

For several years, I have advocated, along with some of my colleagues, for universal screening of patients by all health practitioners for exposure to bullying and related morbidity.[1,2] Furthermore, the concept of universal screening should be expanded to include the detection of all types of victimization according to age group and social setting.

In this context, exposure in the home or neighborhood to any form of victimization can affect individuals at all ages, while young people (ages 5 to 21) are also prone to be maltreated in school or during extracurricular activities. Furthermore, individuals who are adolescents or older should also be assessed for exposure to cyberbullying, while people who are late adolescents or older should be screened for maltreatment in intimate relationships and/or the workplace.

What Should Universal Screening for Victimization Look for?

Universal screening for victimization along the life span should ascertain, through physical examination and/or anamnesis, evidence suggesting exposure to physical, sexual, verbal, or relational abuse (including neglect), which may occur across social settings.

By Whom, Where, and When Should Exposure to Bullying and Other Forms of Victimization Be Identified?

All health professionals should inquire about patients' exposure to recent and/or ongoing bullying and other forms of victimization occurring in any social setting or circumstances. This inquiry should be conducted routinely during a first clinical encounter.

Explanation to the Patient about the Need to Inquire about Bullying and Other Forms of Victimization

The patient and/or family (depending on the patient's age and cognitive level) should be advised that the health professional is concerned about health problems that can result from being exposed to, or participating in, bullying and other forms of victimization. Thus, the professional regularly inquires whether patients are being bullied or mistreated in any environment or circumstances, and if they are suffering from related health problems.

Validation of Patient/Physician Concept of Bullying

The concept of bullying, as understood by the physician and the patient, should be sustained or clarified in a cultural/language and developmental context.[1] Thus, terms like being *bothered*, *hurt*, *offended*, *insulted*, or *harassed* could be used. The multifaceted aspects of bullying can be illustrated by using different categories and examples of mistreatment (verbal, physical, emotional, relational).

Ascertaining Exposure to Bullying and Other Forms of Victimization

After clarification of the patient and health provider's mutual understanding of bullying as a form of victimization, a semi-structured interview can be conducted to determine whether the patient has been bullied or maltreated during the preceding two months. An affirmative answer requires further clarification of the type of victimization, its frequency, its location or milieu, the perpetrators, and what is being done to stop it.

Screening for Health and Psychosocial Problems Related to Being Bullied or Victimized

Patients who report being exposed to current victimization should also be screened for current associated emotional or physical symptoms (occurring more than once a week), as well as psychosocial hazards (i.e., suicidal ideation).

Detection Outcomes and Clinical Management

Patients who are clinically determined to have maltreatment-associated mental health and/or psychosocial risks should be provided with a referral for an intervention to stop further victimization as well as for mental health treatment (see Chapter 9).[1]

Notes

1. Srabstein J, Joshi P, Due P, et al. Prevention of public health risks linked to bullying: a need for a whole community approach. *Int J Adolesc Med Health*. 2008;20(2):185–200.
2. Srabstein JC, Leventhal BL. Prevention of bullying-related morbidity and mortality: a call for public health policies. *Bull World Health Organ*. 2010;88(6):403.
3. Srabstein J. Working towards a detection of bullying related morbidity. *Int J Adolesc Med Health*. 2011;24(1):77–82.
4. Carr-Gregg M, Manocha R. Bullying: effects, prevalence, and strategies for detection. *Aust Fam Physician*. 2011;40(3):98.
5. Ye L, Wang P, Wang L, Ferdinando H, Seppänen T, Alasaarela E. A combined motion-audio school bullying detection algorithm. *Int J Pattern Recognit Artif Intell.* 2018;32(12):1850046.
6. Ye L, Ferdinando H, Seppänen T, Alasaarela E. Physical violence detection for preventing school bullying. *Adv Artif Intell*. 2014;2014(2014):1–9.
7. Van Hee C, Jacobs G, Emmery C, et al. Automatic detection of cyberbullying in social media text. *PLOS One*. 2018;13(10):e0203794.
8. Huang Q, Singh VK, Atrey PK. Cyber bullying detection using social and textual analysis. In: *Proceedings of the 3rd International Workshop on Socially Aware Multimedia.* Orlando, Florida, November 7, 2014. Association for Computing Machinery, New York, NY, USA; 2014:3–6.
9. Sanchez H, Kumar S. Twitter bullying detection. *ser NSDI*. 2011;12(2011):15.
10. Zhao R, Zhou A, Mao K. Automatic detection of cyberbullying on social networks based on bullying features. In: *Proceedings of the 17th International Conference on Distributed*

Computing and Networking. Singapore January 4–7, 2016. Association for Computer Machinery, NY New York, USA; 2016:1–6.

11. Nandhini BS, Sheeba JI. Online social network bullying detection using intelligence techniques. *Procedia Comput Sci.* 2015;45:485–492.
12. Al-Harigy LM, Al-Nuaim HA, Moradpoor N, Tan Z. Building towards automated cyberbullying detection: a comparative analysis. *Computat Intell Neurosci.* 2022;2022:4794227.
13. Di Capua M, Di Nardo E, Petrosino A. Unsupervised cyber bullying detection in social networks. *2016 23rd International Conference on Pattern Recognition (ICPR).* Cancun, Mexico: IEEE Computer Society; 2016:432–437.
14. Calvo-Morata A, Alonso-Fernández C, Freire M, Martínez-Ortiz I, Fernández-Manjón B. Serious games to prevent and detect bullying and cyberbullying: a systematic serious games and literature review. *Comput Educ.* 2020;157:103958.
15. Abdhullah-Al-Mamun and Akhter S. Social media bullying detection using machine learning on Bangla text. In: *2018 10th International Conference on Electrical and Computer Engineering (ICECE).* Dhaka, Bangladesh: IEEE; 2018:385–388.
16. AlHarbi BY, AlHarbi MS, AlZahrani NJ, Alsheail MM, Alshobaili JF, Ibrahim DM. Automatic cyber bullying detection in Arabic social media. *Int J Eng Res Technol.* 2019;12(12):2330–2335.
17. Wu J, Wen M, Lu R, Li B, Li J. Toward efficient and effective bullying detection in online social network. *Peer-to-Peer Netw Appl.* 2020;13(5):1567–1576.
18. McLaughlin L. Improving intimate partner violence detection in the primary care setting: review of the literature. *West J Nurs Res.* 2017;39(10):1369.
19. Guček NK, Petek D, Švab I. Barriers to screening and possibilities for active detection of family medicine attendees exposed to intimate partner violence. *Slovenian J Public Health.* 2016;55(1):11–20.
20. Dichter ME, Wagner C, Goldberg EB, Iverson KM. Intimate partner violence detection and care in the Veterans Health Administration: patient and provider perspectives. *Womens Health Issues.* 2015;25(5):555–560.
21. Hussain N, Sprague S, Madden K, Hussain FN, Pindiprolu B, Bhandari M. A comparison of the types of screening tool administration methods used for the detection of intimate partner violence: a systematic review and meta-analysis. *Trauma Violence Abuse.* 2015;16(1):60–69.
22. Soglin LF, Bauchat J, Soglin DF, Martin GJ. Detection of intimate partner violence in a general medicine practice. *J Interpers Violence.* 2009;24(2):338–348.
23. Rhodes KV, Lauderdale DS, He T, Howes DS, Levinson W. "Between me and the computer": increased detection of intimate partner violence using a computer questionnaire. *Ann Emerg Med.* 2002;40(5):476–484.
24. Matevia ML, Goldman W, McCulloch J, Randall PK. Best practices: detection of intimate-partner violence among members of a managed behavioral health organization. *Psychiatr Serv.* 2002;53(5):555–557.
25. Schrier MW, Rougas SC, Schrier EW, Elisseou S, Warrie S. Intimate partner violence screening and counseling: an introductory session for health care professionals. *MedEdPORTAL.* 2017;13.
26. Daoud N, Berger-Polsky A, Sergienko R, O'Campo P, Leff R, Shoham-Vardi I. Screening and receiving information for intimate partner violence in healthcare settings: a cross-sectional study of Arab and Jewish women of childbearing age in Israel. *BMJ Open.* 2019;9(2):e022996.
27. Soglin LF, Ragavan MI, Li JC, Soglin DF. A validated screening instrument for identifying intimate partner violence in South Asian immigrant women. *J Interpers Violence.* 2019:0886260518822344.

28. Halpern-Meekin S, Costanzo M, Ehrenthal D, Rhoades G. Intimate partner violence screening in the prenatal period: variation by state, insurance, and patient characteristics. *Matern Child Health J.* 2019:1–2.

29. Long AJ, Golfar A, Olson DM. Screening in the prenatal period for intimate partner violence and history of abuse: a survey of Edmonton obstetrician/gynaecologists. *J Obstet Gynaecol Can.* 2019;41(1):38–45.

30. Feltner C, Wallace I, Berkman N, et al. Screening for intimate partner violence, elder abuse, and abuse of vulnerable adults: evidence report and systematic review for the US Preventive Services Task Force. *JAMA.* 2018;320(16):1688–1701.

31. US Preventive Services Task Force, Curry SJ, Krist AH, Owens DK, et al. Screening for intimate partner violence, elder abuse, and abuse of vulnerable adults: US Preventive Services Task Force final recommendation statement. *JAMA.* 2018;320(16):1678–1687.

32. Miller E, Beach SR, Thurston RC. Addressing intimate partner violence and abuse of older or vulnerable adults in the health care setting—beyond screening. *JAMA Intern Med.* 2018;178(12):1583–1585.

33. Sharples L, Nguyen C, Singh B, Lin S. Identifying opportunities to improve intimate partner violence screening in a primary care system. *Fam Med.* 2018;50(9):702–705.

34. De PK, Murshid NS. Associations of intimate partner violence with screening for mental health disorders among women in urban Bangladesh. *Int J Public Health.* 2018;63(8):913–921.

35. Portnoy GA, Haskell SG, King MW, Maskin R, Gerber MR, Iverson KM. Accuracy and acceptability of a screening tool for identifying intimate partner violence perpetration among women veterans: a pre-implementation evaluation. *Womens Health Issues.* 2018;28(5):439–445.

36. Knox B. Screening women for intimate partner violence: creating proper practice habits. *Nurse Pract.* 2018;43(5):14–20.

37. Schwab-Reese LM, Renner LM. Screening, management, and treatment of intimate partner violence among women in low-resource settings. *Womens Health.* 2018;14:1745506518766709.

38. Randell KA, Sherman A, Walsh I, O'Malley D, Dowd MD. Intimate partner violence educational materials in the acute care setting: acceptability and impact on female caregiver attitudes toward screening. *Pediatr Emerg Care.* 2018;37(1):e37–e41.

39. Começanha R, Maia A. Screening tool for psychological intimate partner violence: Portuguese validation of the Psychological Maltreatment of Women Inventory. *Violence Vict.* 2018;33(1):75–90.

40. Dichter ME, Sorrentino AE, Haywood TN, et al. Women's healthcare utilization following routine screening for past-year intimate partner violence in the Veterans Health Administration. *J Gen Intern Med.* 2018;33(6):936–941.

41. Rasch V, Van TN, Nguyen HT, et al. Intimate partner violence (IPV): the validity of an IPV screening instrument utilized among pregnant women in Tanzania and Vietnam. *PLOS One.* 2018;13(2):e0190856.

42. Parish CL, Pereyra MR, Abel SN, Siegel K, Pollack HA, Metsch LR. Intimate partner violence screening in the dental setting: results of a nationally representative survey. *J Am Dent Assoc.* 2018;149(2):112–121.

43. Iverson KM, Sorrentino AE, Bellamy SL, et al. Adoption, penetration, and effectiveness of a secondary risk screener for intimate partner violence: evidence to inform screening practices in integrated care settings. *Gen Hospital Psychiatry.* 2018;51:79–84.

44. Clark CJ, Renner LM, Logeais ME. Intimate partner violence screening and referral practices in an outpatient care setting. *J Interpers Violence.* 2017:0886260517724253.

45. Stoler J, Verity J, Williams JR. Geodemographic disparities in availability of comprehensive intimate partner violence screening services in Miami-Dade County, Florida. *J Interpers Violence*. 2017:0886260517698283.
46. Crane CA, Rice SL, Schlauch RC. Development and psychometric evaluation of a rapid intimate partner violence perpetration screening tool. *Aggress Behav*. 2018;44(2):199–208.
47. Kim YJ, Montano NP. Validity of single question for screening intimate partner violence among urban Latina women. *Public Health Nurs*. 2017;34(6):569–575.
48. Chisholm CA, Bullock L, Ferguson JE II. Intimate partner violence and pregnancy: screening and intervention. *Am J Obstet Gynecol*. 2017;217(2):145–149.
49. Dichter ME, Haywood TN, Butler AE, Bellamy SL, Iverson KM. Intimate partner violence screening in the veterans' health administration: demographic and military service characteristics. *Am J Prev Med*. 2017;52(6):761–768.
50. Frazier T, Yount KM. Intimate partner violence screening and the comparative effects of screening mode on disclosure of sensitive health behaviours and exposures in clinical settings. *Public Health*. 2017;143:52–59.
51. Ahmad I, Ali PA, Rehman S, Talpur A, Dhingra K. Intimate partner violence screening in emergency department: a rapid review of the literature. *J Clin Nurs*. 2017;26(21-22):3271–3285.
52. Bender AK. Using the Consolidated Framework for implementation research to increase provider screening for intimate partner violence in rural health clinics. *Womens Health Issues*. 2016;26(4):384–392.
53. Al-Natour A, Qandil A, Gillespie GL. Nurses' roles in screening for intimate partner violence: a phenomenological study. *Int Nurs Rev*. 2016;63(3):422–428.
54. Tavrow P, Bloom BE, Withers MH. Intimate partner violence screening practices in California after passage of the Affordable Care Act. *Violence Against Women*. 2017;23(7):871–886.
55. Samandari G, Delamou A, Traore P, et al. Integrating intimate partner violence screening and counseling in a family planning clinic: evaluation of a pilot project in Conakry, Guinea. *Afr J Reprod Health*. 2016;20(2):86–93.
56. Bianchi AL, Cesario SK, McFarlane J. Interrupting intimate partner violence during pregnancy with an effective screening and assessment program. *J Obstet Gynecol Neonatal Nurs*. 2016;45(4):579–591.
57. Williams JR, Halstead V, Salani D, Koermer N. Intimate partner violence screening and response: policies and procedures across health care facilities. *Womens Health Issues*. 2016;26(4):377–383.
58. Alvarez C, Fedock G, Grace KT, Campbell J. Provider screening and counseling for intimate partner violence: a systematic review of practices and influencing factors. *Trauma Violence Abuse*. 2017;18(5):479–495.
59. Madden K, Bhandari M. Cochrane in *CORR*®: Screening women for intimate partner violence in healthcare settings. *Clin Orthop Relat Res*. 2016;474(9):1897–1903.
60. Arkins B, Begley C, Higgins A. Measures for screening for intimate partner violence: a systematic review. *J Psychiatr Ment Health Nurs*. 2016;23(3–4):217–235.
61. Heyman RE, Slep AM, Foran HM. Enhanced definitions of intimate partner violence for DSM-5 and ICD-11 may promote improved screening and treatment. *Fam Process*. 2015;54(1):64–81.
62. Ghandour RM, Campbell JC, Lloyd J. Screening and counseling for intimate partner violence: a vision for the future. *J Womens Health*. 2015;24(1):57–61.

63. O'Doherty LJ, Taft A, Hegarty K, Ramsay J, Davidson LL, Feder G. Screening women for intimate partner violence in healthcare settings: abridged Cochrane systematic review and meta-analysis. *BMJ*. 2014;348:g2913.
64. O'Doherty L, Hegarty K, Ramsay J, Davidson LL, Feder G, Taft A. Screening women for intimate partner violence in healthcare settings. *Cochrane Database Syst Rev*. 2015(7), Art. No.: CD007007. https://www.cochrane.org/CD007007/BEHAV_screening-women-intimate-partner-violence-healthcare-settings
65. Jewkes R. Intimate partner violence: the end of routine screening. *Lancet*. 2013;382(9888):190–191.
66. Sprague S, Madden K, Simunovic N, et al. Barriers to screening for intimate partner violence. *Women & Health*. 2012 Aug 1;52(6):587–605.
67. Chang JC, Dado D, Schussler S, et al. In person versus computer screening for intimate partner violence among pregnant patients. *Patient Educ Counsel*. 2012;88(3):443–448.
68. Gerlock AA, Grimesey JL, Pisciotta AK, Harel O. Documentation of screening for perpetration of intimate partner violence in male veterans with PTSD. *Am J Nurs*. 2011;111(11):26–32.
69. Ernst AA, Weiss SJ, Morgan-Edwards S, et al. Derivation and validation of a short emergency department screening tool for perpetrators of intimate partner violence: the Perpetrator Rapid Scale (PERPS). *J Emerg Med*. 2012;42(2):206–217.
70. Scribano PV, Stevens J, Marshall J, Gleason E, Kelleher KJ. Feasibility of computerized screening for intimate partner violence in a pediatric emergency department. *Pediatr Emerg Care*. 2011;27(8):710–716.
71. Todahl J, Walters E. Universal screening for intimate partner violence: a systematic review. *J Marital Fam Ther*. 2011;37(3):355–369.
72. Ahmad F, Hogg-Johnson S, Stewart DE, Skinner HA, Glazier RH, Levinson W. Computer-assisted screening for intimate partner violence and control: a randomized trial. *Ann Intern Med*. 2009;151(2):93–102.
73. Rabin RF, Jennings JM, Campbell JC, Bair-Merritt MH. Intimate partner violence screening tools: a systematic review. Am J Prev Med. 2009;36 (5):439–445.
74. Sormanti M, Smith E. Intimate partner violence screening in the emergency department: US medical residents' perspectives. *Int Q Community Health Educ*. 2010;30(1):21–40.
75. Klevens J, Saltzman LE. The controversy on screening for intimate partner violence: a question of semantics? *J Womens Health*. 2009;18(2):143–145.
76. Gottlieb AS. Intimate partner violence: a clinical review of screening and intervention. *Womens Health*. 2008;4(5):529–539.
77. Wathen CN, Jamieson E, MacMillan HL, McMaster Violence Against Women Research Group. Who is identified by screening for intimate partner violence? *Womens Health Issues*. 2008;18(6):423–432.
78. Koziol-McLain J, Giddings L, Rameka M, Fyfe E. Intimate partner violence screening and brief intervention: experiences of women in two New Zealand health care settings. *J Midwifery Womens Health*. 2008;53(6):504–510.
79. Renker PR. Breaking the barriers: the promise of computer-assisted screening for intimate partner violence. *J Midwifery Womens Health*. 2008;53(6):496–503.
80. Daugherty JD, Houry DE. Intimate partner violence screening in the emergency department. *J Postgrad Med*. 2008;54(4):301.

81. Jack SM, Jamieson E, Wathen CN, MacMillan HL. The feasibility of screening for intimate partner violence during postpartum home visits. *Can J Nurs Res*. 2008;40(2):150–170.
82. Jaeger JR, Spielman D, Cronholm PF, Applebaum S, Holmes WC. Screening male primary care patients for intimate partner violence perpetration. *J Gen Intern Med*. 2008;23(8):1152.
83. Wrangle J, Fisher JW, Paranjape A. Ha sentido sola? Culturally competent screening for intimate partner violence in Latina women. *J Womens Health*. 2008;17(2):261–268.
84. Houry D, Kaslow NJ, Kemball RS, et al. Does screening in the emergency department hurt or help victims of intimate partner violence? *Ann Emerg Med*. 2008;51(4):433–442.
85. Todahl JL, Linville D, Chou LY, Maher-Cosenza P. A qualitative study of intimate partner violence universal screening by family therapy interns: implications for practice, research, training, and supervision. *J Marital Fam Ther*. 2008;34(1):28–43.
86. Dubowitz H, Prescott L, Feigelman S, Lane W, Kim J. Screening for intimate partner violence in a pediatric primary care clinic. *Pediatrics*. 2008;121(1):e85–e91.
87. Falsetti SA. Screening and responding to family and intimate partner violence in the primary care setting. *Primary Care Clin Office Pract*. 2007;34(3):641–657..
88. Trabold N. Screening for intimate partner violence within a health care setting: a systematic review of the literature. *Soc Work Health Care*. 2007;45(1):1–8.
89. Snyder JE. The importance of screening for intimate partner violence (IPV). *NC Med J*. 2007;68(4):224.
90. Furniss K, McCaffrey M, Parnell V, Rovi S. Nurses and barriers to screening for intimate partner violence. *Am J Matern Child Nurs*. 2007;32(4):238–243.
91. Thackeray J, Stelzner S, Downs SM, Miller C. Screening for intimate partner violence: the impact of screener and screening environment on victim comfort. *J Interpers Violence*. 2007;22(6):659–670.
92. Trautman DE, McCarthy ML, Miller N, Campbell JC, Kelen GD. Intimate partner violence and emergency department screening: computerized screening versus usual care. *Ann Emerg Med*. 2007;49(4):526–534.
93. Paterno MT, Draughon JE. Screening for intimate partner violence. *J Midwifery Womens Health*. 2016;61(3):370–375.
94. Chan EK. Screening for intimate partner violence in emergency departments. *Hong Kong Med J*. 2006;12(4):323–324
95. MacMillan HL, Wathen CN, Jamieson E, et al.; Violence Against Women Research Group. Approaches to screening for intimate partner violence in health care settings: a randomized trial. *JAMA*. 2006;296(5):530–536. Cited by Hussain et al.[21]
96. MacMillan HL, Wathen CN, Jamieson E, et al. Screening for intimate partner violence in health care settings: a randomized trial. *JAMA*. 2009;302(5):493–501.
97. Williams KR, Grant SR. Empirically examining the risk of intimate partner violence: the Revised Domestic Violence Screening Instrument (DVSI-R). *Public Health Rep*. 2006;121(4):400–408.
98. Zeitler MS, Paine AD, Breitbart V, et al. Attitudes about intimate partner violence screening among an ethnically diverse sample of young women. *J Adolesc Health*. 2006;39(1):119.
99. Hindin PK. Intimate partner violence screening practices of certified nurse-midwives. *J Midwifery Womens Health*. 2006;51(3):216–221.
100. Bair-Merritt MH, Mollen CJ, Yau PL, Fein JA. Health care providers' opinions on intimate partner violence resources and screening in a pediatric emergency department. *Pediatr Emerg Care*. 2006;22(3):150–153.

101. Bair-Merritt MH, Mollen CJ, Yau PL, Fein JA. Health care providers' opinions on intimate partner violence resources and screening in a pediatric emergency department. *Pediatr Emerg Care.* 2006;22(3):150–153.
102. Bair-Merritt MH, Feudtner C, Mollen CJ, Winters S, Blackstone M, Fein JA. Screening for intimate partner violence using an audiotape questionnaire: a randomized clinical trial in a pediatric emergency department. *Arch Pediatr Adolesc Med.* 2006;160(3):311–316.
103. Knapp JF, Dowd MD, Kennedy CS, Stallbaumer-Rouyer J, Henderson DP. Evaluation of a curriculum for intimate partner violence screening in a pediatric emergency department. *Pediatrics.* 2006;117(1):110–116.
104. Jaffee KD, Epling JW, Grant W, Ghandour RM, Callendar E. Physician-identified barriers to intimate partner violence screening. *J Womens Health.* 2005;14(8):713–720.
105. McCloskey LA, Lichter E, Ganz ML, et al. Intimate partner violence and patient screening across medical specialties. *Acad Emerg Med.* 2005;12(8):712–722.
106. Newman JD, Sheehan KM, Powell EC. Screening for intimate-partner violence in the pediatric emergency department. *Pediatr Emerg Care.* 2005;21(2):79–83.
107. Hurley KF, Brown-Maher T, Campbell SG, Wallace T, Venugopal R, Baggs D. Emergency department patients' opinions of screening for intimate partner violence among women. *Emerg Med J.* 2005;22(2):97–98.
108. Ross J, Walther V, Epstein I. Screening risks for intimate partner violence and primary care settings: implications for future abuse. *Soc Work Health Care.* 2004;38(4):1–23.
109. US Preventive Services Task Force. Screening for family and intimate partner violence: recommendation statement. *Ann Fam Med.* 2004;2(2):156–160.
110. Nelson HD, Nygren P, McInerney Y, Klein J. Screening women and elderly adults for family and intimate partner violence: a review of the evidence for the US Preventive Services Task Force. *Ann Intern Med.* 2004;140(5):387–396.
111. Peralta RL, Fleming MF. Screening for intimate partner violence in a primary care setting: the validity of "feeling safe at home" and prevalence results. *J Am Board Fam Pract.* 2003;16(6):525–532.
112. Jonassen JA, Mazor KM. Identification of physician and patient attributes that influence the likelihood of screening for intimate partner violence. *Acad Med.* 2003;78(10):S20–S23.
113. Zink TM, Jacobson J. Screening for intimate partner violence when children are present: the victim's perspective. *J Interpers Violence.* 2003;18(8):872–890.
114. Malecha A, Wachs JE. Screening for and treating intimate partner violence in the workplace. *AAOHN J.* 2003;51(7):310–316.
115. Scholle SH, Buranosky R, Hanusa BH, Ranieri L, Dowd K, Valappil B. Routine screening for intimate partner violence in an obstetrics and gynecology clinic. *Am J Public Health.* 2003;93(7):1070–1072.
116. Heron SL, Kellermann AL. Screening for intimate partner violence in the emergency department: where do we go from here? *Ann Emerg Med.* 2002;40(5):493–495.
117. Borowsky IW, Ireland M. Parental screening for intimate partner violence by pediatricians and family physicians. *Pediatrics.* 2002;110(3):509–516.
118. Dowd MD, Kennedy C, Knapp JF, Stallbaumer-Rouyer J. Mothers' and health care providers' perspectives on screening for intimate partner violence in a pediatric emergency department. *Arch Pediatr Adolesc Med.* 2002;156(8):794–799.
119. Fogarty CT, Burge S, McCord EC. Communicating with patients about intimate partner violence: screening and interviewing approaches. *Fam Med.* 2002;34(5):369–375.

120. Glowa PT, Frasier PY, Newton WP. Increasing physician comfort level in screening and counseling patients for intimate partner violence: hands-on practice. *Patient Educ Couns.* 2002;46(3):213–220.
121. Koziol-McLain J, Campbell JC. Universal screening and mandatory reporting: an update on two important issues for victims/survivors of intimate partner violence. *J Emerg Nurs.* 2001;27(6):602–606.
122. Centers for Disease Control and Prevention (CDC). Role of victims' services in improving intimate partner violence screening by trained maternal and child health-care providers—Boston, Massachusetts, 1994–1995. *MMWR.* 2000;49(6):114.
123. Salber PR, McCaw B. Barriers to screening for intimate partner violence: time to reframe the question. *Am J Prev Med.* 2000;19(4):276–278..
124. Waalen J, Goodwin MM, Spitz AM, Petersen R, Saltzman LE. Screening for intimate partner violence by health care providers: barriers and interventions. *Am J Prev Med.* 2000;19(4):230–237.
125. Larkin GL, Hyman KB, Mathias SR, D'amico F, MacLeod BA. Universal screening for intimate partner violence in the emergency department: importance of patient and provider factors. *Ann Emerg Med.* 1999;33(6):669–675.
126. Sprague S, Swaminathan A, Slobogean GP, et al. A scoping review of intimate partner violence educational programs for health care professionals. *Women Health.* 2018;58(10):1192–1206.
127. Hornor G, Bretl D, Chapman E, et al. Child maltreatment screening and anticipatory guidance: a description of pediatric nurse practitioner practice behaviors. *J Pediatr Health Care.* 2017;31(6): e35–e44.
128. van der Put CE, Bouwmeester-Landweer MB, Landsmeer-Beker EA, et al. Screening for potential child maltreatment in parents of a newborn baby: the predictive validity of an Instrument for early identification of Parents at Risk for child Abuse and Neglect (IPARAN). *Child Abuse Negl.* 2017;70:160–168.
129. Teeuw AH, Sieswerda-Hoogendoorn T, Sangers EJ, Heymans HS, van Rijn RR. Results of the implementation of a new screening protocol for child maltreatment at the Emergency Department of the Academic Medical Center in Amsterdam. *Int Emerg Nurs.* 2016;24:9–15.
130. van Konijnenburg EM, Teeuw AH, Zwaard SA, van der Lee JH, van Rijn RR. Screening methods to detect child maltreatment: high variability in Dutch emergency departments. *Emerg Med J.* 2014;31(3):196–200.
131. Hornor G. Child maltreatment: screening and anticipatory guidance. *J Pediatr Health Care.* 2013;27(4):242–250.
132. Murry S, Lewin L. Parenting support needs assessment: screening for child maltreatment risk in young families. *J Pediatr Health Care.* 2014;28(3):208–216.
133. Murry SK, Baker AW, Lewin L. Screening families with young children for child maltreatment potential. *Pediatr Nurs.* 2000;26(1):47–54, 65.
134. Bolton FG, Charlton JK, Gai DS, Laner RH, Shumway SM. Preventive screening of adolescent mothers and infants: critical variables in assessing risk for child maltreatment. *J Primary Prev.* 1985;5(3):169–187.
135. Schertz M, Karni-Visel Y, Hershkowitz I, Flaisher M, Hershkowitz F. Child maltreatment identification rates in a child development center: suggestions for improved detection. *Eur J Pediatrics.* 2018;177(7):1081–1087..
136. Inkilä J, Flinck A, Luukkaala T, Åstedt-Kurki P, Paavilainen E. Interprofessional collaboration in the detection of and early intervention in child maltreatment: employees' experiences. *Nurs Res Pract.* 2013;2013:Article ID 186414.

137. Cerezo MA, Pons-Salvador G. Improving child maltreatment detection systems: a large-scale case study involving health, social services, and school professionals. *Child Abuse Negl.* 2004;28(11):1153–1169.
138. British Columbia Children's Hospital, Youth Health Program. HEADSS—An Interview and Assessment Guide for Adolescents. http://www.bcchildrens.ca/Youth-Health-Clinic-site/Documents/headss20assessment20guide1.pdf. Accessed October 19, 2022.
139. Cohen E, Mackenzie RG, Yates GL. HEADSS, a psychosocial risk assessment instrument: implications for designing effective intervention programs for runaway youth. *J Adolesc Health.* 1991;12(7):539–544.
140. Hecht-Nielsen R. Theory of the backpropagation neural network. In: Harry Wechsler (Ed.), *Neural Networks for Perception.* Academic Press; 1992:65–93.
141. Dadvar M, Jong FD, Ordelman R, Trieschnigg D. Improved cyberbullying detection using gender information. In: *Proceedings of the Twelfth Dutch-Belgian Information Retrieval Workshop (DIR 2012).* University of Ghent; 2012:23–25.
142. Akhter A, Acharjee UK, Polash MM. Cyber bullying detection and classification using multinomial Naïve Bayes and fuzzy logic. *Int J Math Sci Comput.* 2019;5(4):1–2.
143. Shekhar A, Venkatesan M. A bag-of-phonetic-codes model for cyber-bullying detection in Twitter. In: *2018 International Conference on Current Trends towards Converging Technologies (ICCTCT).* Coimbatore, India: IEEE; 2018:1–7.
144. Marathe S, Shirsat KP. Approaches for mining You Tube videos metadata in cyber bullying detection. *Int J Eng Res Technol.* 2015;4(5):680–684.
145. Zhong H, Li H, Squicciarini AC, et al. Content-driven detection of cyberbullying on the Instagram social network. Proceedings of the Twenty-Fifth International Joint Conference on Artificial Intelligence (IJCAI-16) New York, New York, USA 9–15 July 2016, Published by AAAI Press/International Joint Conferences on Artificial Intelligence, Palo Alto, California USA; 2016:3952–3958. https://www.ijcai.org/Proceedings/16/Papers/556.pdf. Accessed September 24, 2023.
146. US Preventive Services Task Force: "An independent, volunteer panel of national experts in disease prevention and evidence-based medicine. The Task Force works to improve the health of all Americans by making evidence-based recommendations about clinical preventive services." https://www.uspreventiveservicestaskforce.org/uspstf/about-uspstf. Accessed October 19, 2022.
147. Feldhaus KM, Koziol-McLain J, Amsbury HL, Lowenstein SR, Abbott JT. Accuracy of 3 brief screening questions for detecting partner violence in the emergency department. *JAMA.* 1997;277(17):1357–1361. Cited by Feltner.[30]
148. MacMillan HL, Wathen CN, Jamieson E, et al.; McMaster Violence Against Women Research Group. Approaches to screening for intimate partner violence in health care settings: a randomized trial. *JAMA.* 2006;296(5):530–536. Cited by Feltner.[30]
149. Ernst AA, Weiss SJ, Cham E, Hall L, Nick TG. Detecting ongoing intimate partner violence in the emergency department using a simple 4-question screen: the OVAT. *Violence Vict.* 2004;19(3):375. Cited by Feltner.[30]
150. Woman Abuse Screening Tool (WAST). Brown JB, Lent B, Schmidt CG. Application of the Woman Abuse Screening Tool (WAST) and WAST-Short in the family practice setting. *J Fam Pract.* 2000;49(10):896–903. http://womanabuse.webcanvas.ca/documents/wast.pdf. Accessed October 19, 2022.
151. Chen PH, Rovi S, Washington J, et al. Randomized comparison of 3 methods to screen for domestic violence in family practice. *Ann Fam Med.* 2007;5(5):430–435. Cited by Hussain et al.[21]

152. Furbee PM, Sikora R, Williams JM, Derk SJ. Comparison of domestic violence screening methods: a pilot study. *Ann Emerg Med.* 1998;31(4):495–501. Cited by Hussain et al.[21]

153. Kataoka Y, Yaju Y, Eto H, Horiuchi S. Self-administered questionnaire versus interview as a screening method for intimate partner violence in the prenatal setting in Japan: a randomised controlled trial. *BMC Pregnancy Childbirth.* 2010;10(1):84. Cited by Hussain et al.[21]

154. Klevens J, Sadowski L, Kee R, Trick W, Garcia D. Comparison of screening and referral strategies for exposure to partner violence. *Womens Health Issues.* 2012;22(1):e45–e52. Cited by Hussain et al.[21]

155. Bair-Merritt MH, Feudtner C, Mollen CJ, Winters S, Blackstone M, Fein JA. Screening for intimate partner violence using an audiotape questionnaire: a randomized clinical trial in a pediatric emergency department. *Arch Pediatr Adolesc Med.* 2006;160(3):311–316. Cited by Hussain et al.[21]

156. Sharples L, Nguyen C, Singh B, Lin S. Identifying opportunities to improve intimate partner violence screening in a primary care system. *Fam Med.* 2018;50(9):702–705.

157. Thackeray JD, Hibbard R, Dowd MD. Intimate partner violence: the role of the pediatrician. *Pediatrics.* 2010;125(5):1094–1100.

158. American College of Obstetricians and Gynecologists. Intimate partner violence. Committee opinion no. 518. *Obstet Gynecol.* 2012 Feb;119(2):412–417. Cited by Wathen et al. (see Note 160).

159. American Academy of Family Physicians. Intimate Partner Violence and Abuse of Vulnerable Adults. https://www.aafp.org/pubs/afp/issues/2019/0515/od1.html. Accessed October 19, 2022.

160. Wathen CN, MacGregor JC, Sibbald SL, MacMillan HL. Exploring the uptake and framing of research evidence on universal screening for intimate partner violence against women: a knowledge translation case study. *Health Res Policy Sys.* 2013;11(1):13.

161. James L, Schaeffer S. *Interpersonal and Domestic Violence Screening and Counselling: Understanding New Federal Rules and Providing Resources for Health Providers.* CA: Futures Without Violence; 2012. Cited by Wathen et al.[160]

162. Wathen CN, MacMillan HL. Interventions for violence against women: scientific review. *JAMA.* 2003;289(5):589–600. Cited by Wathen et al.[160]

163. Ramsay J, Carter Y, Davidson L, et al. Advocacy interventions to reduce or eliminate violence and promote the physical and psychosocial well-being of women who experience intimate partner abuse. *Cochrane Database Syst Rev.* 2009;8(3):CD005043. Cited by Wathen et al.[160]

164. Feder G, Ramsay J, Dunne D, et al. How far does screening women for domestic (partner) violence in different health-care settings meet criteria for a screening programme? Systematic reviews of nine UK National Screening Committee criteria. *Health Technol Assess.* 2009;13(16):iii-iv, xi-xiii, 1–113, 137–347. Cited by Wathen et al.[160]

165. Lavi-Zahar Z. *Laws and Procedures on Domestic Violence.* Jerusalem: Israel Ministry of Health; 2009. Cited by Daoud et al.[26]

166. Lawoko S, Sanz S, Helström L, Castren M. Screening for intimate partner violence against women in healthcare Sweden: prevalence and determinants. *ISRN Nurs.* 2011;2011, Article ID 510692, 7 pages doi:10.5402/2011/51069

167. The Health Care Inspectorate and the Inspectorate for Youth Care have become one organization since October 1, 2017: the Health and Youth Care Inspectorate. https://english.igj.nl/about-us. Accessed October 19, 2022.

168. Louwers EC, Korfage IJ, Affourtit MJ, De Koning HJ, Moll HA. Facilitators and barriers to screening for child abuse in the emergency department. *BMC Pediatrics.* 2012;12(1):167.
169. van der Wal G. Afdeling spoedeisende hulp van ziekenhuizen signaleert kindermishandeling nog onvoldoende: gebroken arm nog te vaak een ongelukje. *Inspectie voor de Gezondheidszorg.* 2008:1–48. Cited by Louwers et al.[168]
170. van Konijnenburg EM, Teeuw AH, Zwaard SA, van der Lee JH, van Rijn RR. Screening methods to detect child maltreatment: high variability in Dutch emergency departments. *Emerg Med J.* 2014;31(3):196–200.
171. Compernolle T. Eerste hulp bij kindermishandeling en het Struisarts-syndroom. *Tijdschrift voor kindergeneeskunde.* 1996;64:168–179. Cited by van Konijnenburg et al.[170]
172. Bleeker G, Vet NJ, Haumann TJ, Gemke RJ. Increase in the number of reported cases of child abuse following adoption of a structured approach in the VU Medical Centre, Amsterdam, in the period 2001–2004. *Nederlands tijdschrift voor geneeskunde.* 2005;149(29):1620–1624. Cited by van Konijnenburg et al.[170]
173. Sittig JS, Uiterwaal CS, Moons KG, Nieuwenhuis EE, van de Putte EM. Child abuse inventory at emergency rooms: CHAIN-ER rationale and design. *BMC Pediatrics.* 2011;11(1):91. Cited by van Konijnenburg et al.[170]
174. Louwers EC, Korfage IJ, Affourtit MJ, et al. Effects of systematic screening and detection of child abuse in emergency departments. *Pediatrics.* 2012;130(3):457–464. Cited by van Konijnenburg et al.[170]
175. Benger JR, Pearce AV. Simple intervention to improve detection of child abuse in emergency departments. *BMJ.* 2002;324(7340):780–782. Cited by van Konijnenburg et al.[170]
176. Teeuw AH, van Konijnenburg EM, Sieswerda-Hoogendoorn T, Molenaar S, Heymans HS, van Rijn RR. Parents' opinion about a routine head-to-toe examination of children as a screening instrument for child abuse and neglect in children visiting the emergency department. *J Emerg Nurs.* 2016;42(2):128–138.
177. Teeuw AH, Kraan RB, van Rijn RR, Bossuyt PM, Heymans HS. Screening for child abuse using a checklist and physical examinations in the emergency department led to the detection of more cases. *Acta Paediatr.* 2019;108(2):300–313.
178. International Society for the Prevention of Child Abuse and Neglect (ISPCAN). https://ispcan.org/. Accessed September 24, 2023.
179. Runyan DK, Dunne MP, Zolotor AJ, et al. The development and piloting of the ISPCAN Child Abuse Screening Tool–Parent Version (ICAST-P). *Child Abuse Negl.* 2009;33(11):826–832.
180. Dunne MP, Zolotor AJ, Runyan DK, et al. ISPCAN Child Abuse Screening Tool Retrospective Version (ICAST-R): Delphi study and field testing in seven countries. *Child Abuse Negl.* 2009;33(11):815–825.
181. Zolotor AJ, Runyan DK, Dunne MP, et al. ISPCAN Child Abuse Screening Tool Children's Version (ICAST-C): instrument development and multi-national pilot testing. *Child Abuse Negl.* 2009;33(11):833–841.
182. The ISPCAN Child Abuse Screening Tool–Parent version (ICAST-P) has been piloted in Colombia, Egypt, India, Lebanon, Malaysia, and Russia.[179]
183. The ISPCAN Child Abuse Screening Tool–Retrospective version (ICAST-R) has been piloted in Colombia, Egypt, India, Lebanon, Malaysia, Kyrgystan, and Russia.[180]
184. The ISPCAN Child Abuse Screening Tool–Children's version (ICAST-C) has been tested in Colombia, India, Russia, and Iceland.

9

Intervention and Treatment for Bullying and Other Forms of Victimization

The term *intervention,* as used in this chapter, relates to the process of halting ongoing victimization that was not averted at the level of primary prevention (as discussed in Chapter 7). In this context, a strategy of intervention to stop "in-progress" victimization is one of the elements in secondary prevention after detection (as discussed in Chapter 8).[1]

The chapter also examines the concept of *treatment* as a component of tertiary prevention, aimed at remedying morbidity resulting from, or preceding, victimization, as well as reducing the related mortality risk.

Although the chapter methodically explores the understanding of intervention and treatment for bullying and other forms of maltreatment as two distinct strategic constructs exemplifying different levels of maltreatment prevention, the two approaches may be implemented consecutively and/or concurrently, or they may be construed as being intertwined or having similar meaning.

Intervention to Prevent Further Victimization

Established Methods to Stop and/or Cope with Bullying

A review of prevalent strategies being applied to stop and/or cope with ongoing incidents of school bullying[2-3] highlighted the following methods:

- Direct sanctions (disciplinary consequences), as proposed by Olweus[4] and incorporated in many US statutes to prevent bullying[5]
- Restorative practice,[6-9] including the perpetrator's recognition of the harm inflicted and leading to an apology or an act of reparation to the victim
- Strengthening the victims[10] by helping them deal with the bullying more effectively through an assertive communication approach
- Mediation,[11] enabling students to work with a trained teacher or peer-mediator to settle their difficulty
- The support group method,[12,13] a nondisciplinary approach involving the perpetrators (without appearance of the victim) to confront them about the harm done and to require them to help in lessening the impact of the maltreatment
- Method of shared concern,[14] a multistep approach working first separately with the perpetrators and the victim and eventually jointly to agree on a solution.

Thompson and Smith[15] conducted a national survey of 1,378 schools in England to ascertain which strategies were used to deal with episodes of bullying from 2008 through 2010. The approach most used (92% of the schools) was direct sanctions, or negative consequences inflicted on perpetrators. The range of sanctions included verbal reprimands, meeting with parents, temporary removal from class, withdrawal of privileges, and school community service.[15]

The rate of success in preventing further bullying, based on reports from schools in England, ranged from 62%, through the implementation of direct sanctions, to 76% through use of the support group method.[15]

There is no documented benefit–risk assessment taking into consideration the likely stressful effects of any of these strategies on the potential emotional vulnerability of either the perpetrator or the victim.

Potential Limitations of Current Approaches

Discomfort of Victims in Interacting with Perpetrators

Clinical experience in working with young people who have been exposed to victimization has shown that they would like the mistreatment to stop, while wishing to avoid immediate contact with the offender. In this context, many victims may feel anxious about having to meet with the perpetrator, as may be required in mediation, restorative practice, and the method of shared concern.

Burden on the Victim

The method of strengthening the victim puts the burden on the injured party to cope with the maltreatment by developing resilience, without first addressing the immediate need for the perpetrator to halt further bullying.

Being Coerced to Stop Bullying

The coercive style of the direct sanctions method and required participation in either mediation, restorative practices, the support group method, or the method of shared concern could be intimidating and perhaps aggravating to perpetrators in view of their potential emotional vulnerability.

Treatment of Bullying and Other Forms of Victimization

A review[16] of published literature on the topic of "treatment of bullying" generated a considerable number of citations pertaining to other bullying-related areas, such as the need for prevention and intervention,[17-23] detection,[24,25] treatment of conditions associated with bullying,[26-32] and psychopharmacological treatment later in life.[33,34] In contrast, such a bibliographic search yielded a very small number of references covering evidence-based treatment, including psychopharmacological treatment of flashbacks,[35] therapies to develop coping skills[36-38] and empathy,[39] and therapeutic strategies to contend with anxiety[40] or aggression.[41,42]

The shortage of publications about treatment of bullying may reflect a lack of evidence-based research or clinical experience in the therapeutics of this type of victimization or maltreatment and its associated morbidity and psychosocial consequences. Therefore, the treatment of bullying needs to find answers or guidelines in the evidence derived from experience in treating victimization and psychological trauma.

Treatment within a Diagnostic Framework

Treatment of the morbidity (see Chapter 4) and psychosocial dysfunctions and risks (see Chapter 5) associated with recent and/or past exposure to bullying and/or other forms of victimization can be considered within the diagnostic context of disorders specifically associated with stress and/or harmful/traumatic events. Diagnoses in this framework include adjustment disorder,[43-44] acute stress disorder[45] (acute stress reaction[46]), posttraumatic stress disorder (PTSD),[47,48] and complex PTSD[49,50] (Table 9.1).

There is published[51] evidence that all these conditions[43-49] can manifest as depressed or negative mood, irritability, anxiety, sleep disturbance, nightmares, or intrusive memories (Table 9.2). However, symptoms like flashbacks, depersonalization, derealization, dissociation, inattention, hypervigilance, and nausea have been shown to be associated with acute stress disorder (ASD), PTSD, and complex PTSD. Furthermore, adjustment disorder and PTSD appear to be linked to suicidal ideation, hallucinations, headache, tinnitus, non-epileptic seizures, diabetes, inflammation, autoimmune disorders, and backaches (Table 9.2).

Among the psychosocial risks associated with disorders specifically linked with stress and/or harmful events[43-49] are absenteeism (which has been linked to adjustment disorder, ASD, and PTSD), as well as substance abuse, self-injury, and suicide attempts, which have been shown to be experienced by individuals with PTSD, complex PTSD, and adjustment disorder (Table 9.3).

Table 9.1. Disorders Associated with Stress or Traumatic Events by Onset/Cause and Duration

Diagnoses	Adjustment Disorder[43]	Acute Stress Disorder[45]	Posttraumatic Stress Disorder[47]	Complex Posttraumatic Stress Disorder[49,50**]
Onset/Cause and Duration	Within three months, response to an identifiable stressor. Condition does not persist beyond six months after the stressor or consequences ended.	Direct or indirect[a] exposure to threatened death or serious injury. Experiencing repeated or extreme exposure to the hard details of the traumatic episode. Duration of the condition is three days to one month after the trauma.	Direct or indirect[a] exposure to threatened death or serious injury. Condition of disturbance is more than one month.	Follows exposure to an extremely threatening or horrific event or series of events.[49] "Symptoms may result from prolonged, chronic exposure to traumatic experiences, especially in childhood."[50]

[a] Witnessing in person as the exposure happens to others, or learning that the exposure happened to somebody close.[47]

[b] This disorder is not included in DSM-V,[44] but it was incorporated to ICD-11.[49]

Table 9.2. Disorders Specifically Linked with Stress and/or Harmful Events,[43-49] by Associated Symptoms or Conditions

Symptoms or Conditions	Adjustment Disorder[43,44]	Acute Stress Disorder[45,46]	Posttraumatic Stress Disorder (PTSD)[47,48]	Complex PTSD[49,50]
Depressed/Negative mood	✓[44]	✓[45,46]	✓[48]	✓[49]
Irritability	✓[52a]	✓[45,46]	✓[48,53]	✓[54]
Anxiety	✓[43,44]	✓[45,55-57]	✓[47b]	✓[49b]
Sleep disturbance	✓[58]	✓[46]	✓[48]	✓[59]
Nightmares	✓[52]	✓[46]	✓[47,48]	✓[49]
Intrusive memories	✓[43,60,61]	✓[46]	✓[47,48]	✓[49]
Flashbacks	?	✓[46]	✓[47,48]	✓[49]
Depersonalization/derealization/dissociation	?	✓[62]	✓[48]	✓[63c]
Suicidal ideation	✓[64-66]	?	✓[67-70]	✓[71]
Hallucinations	✓[72]	?	✓[73-75]	?
Delusions	?	?	✓[76,77]	?
Inattention/Impaired executive function	?	✓[78]	✓[48]	✓[79]
Hypervigilance	?	✓[46]	✓[47,48]	✓[49]
Headaches	✓[80]	?	✓[81,82]	?
Dizziness/Vertigo	?	?	✓[83]	?
Tinnitus	✓[84]	?	✓[85,86]	?
Psychogenic non-epileptic seizures (PNES)	✓[87]	?	✓[88]	?
Hypertension/Cardiovascular reactivity	?	?	✓[89,90d]	✓[91]
Obesity	?	?	✓[92,93]	?
Diabetes	✓[94]	?	✓[95-97]	?
Inflammation	✓[98]	✓[99]	✓[100-103]	?
Autoimmune disorders	✓[104]	✓[104]	✓[105]	?
Stomachaches	?	?	✓[106,107]	✓[108]
Nausea	?	✓[109]	✓[110]	✓[111]
Backaches	✓[112]	?	✓[113,114]	?
Fibromyalgia	?	?	✓[115-117]	?

Symbols: ✓= published report; ? = No publish report.[51]

[a] The association between irritability and adjustment disorder was not statistically significant.

[b] Fear or horror, and strong physical sensations.

[c] Psychoform dissociation mediates the relationship between childhood complex trauma and complex PTSD.

[d] PTSD symptoms may increase risk for cardiovascular disease through depression.[90]

Table 9.3. Disorders Specifically Linked with Stress and/or Harmful Events,[43-49] by Associated Psychosocial Risks or Dysfunctions

Psychosocial Risks or Dysfunctions	Adjustment Disorder[43,44]	Acute Stress Disorder[46,47]	PTSD[47,48]	Complex PTSD[49,50]
Absenteeism	✓[118,119]	✓[120]	✓[121]	?
Alcohol/Drug abuse	✓[122]	?	✓[123,124]	✓[125]
Decline in academic or work performance	?	?	✓[126,127]	✓[128]
Self-injury	✓[129]	?	✓[130,131]	✓[132]
Suicide attempt	✓[133]	?	✓[134,135]	✓[136]

Symbols: ✓= published report; ? = No publish report.[51]

Association of Bullying and Other Forms of Victimization with Disorders Specifically Linked with Stress and/or Harmful Events

Several published studies have highlighted the link of bullying and other forms of victimization with the diagnoses of PTSD,[136-142] adjustment disorder,[143-145] and ASD.[146-149] Yet, there are few studies describing the association of repeated maltreatment and complex PTSD,[150,151] perhaps due to the evolving recognition of complex PTSD as a diagnostic entity.

Analysis of Trauma Symptoms as Part of a Structural Network (Symptomics)

The heterogeneity of symptoms and behavioral risks that are the expression of, or are associated with, disorders specifically linked to stress and trauma[44-49] (Tables 9.2 and 9.3) can be better understood within an integrated structural approach to psychopathology, as is being provided by the evolving methodology for network analysis of symptom structure.[152-161] This approach[152] is based on the premise that mental disorders are the "result of the causal interplay between symptoms (e.g., worry→insomnia→fatigue), possibly involving feedback loops (e.g., a person may engage in substance abuse to forget the problems that arose from substance abuse)."[152] Within this conceptual framework, a psychiatric condition is understood as a complex network of symptoms "mutually interacting, often reciprocally reinforcing [each other],"[152] while analysis techniques can be applied to ascertain the central symptoms in a person's network.[152]

The concept of centrality degree,[162] or importance of a symptom in a network, is determined by the number of connections that a symptom (node) has to other symptoms in the system. It has been hypothesized that network analysis could eventually be used to investigate whether it is more effective to treat the central symptom in a client's network.[163]

The concept of symptomics was highlighted by Armour et al.,[153] who underscored the detailed research on the network of psychiatric symptoms led by Fried et al.[164,165] The concept of symptomics[153] is based on:

- The relationships of symptoms with risk factors, biomarkers, impairment of functioning and treatment response[153,166]
- The analysis of the potentially causal relations among symptoms in symptom networks[152,153]
- Gaining better understanding of psychopathology by investigating personalized processes at the level of individuals instead of heterogeneous groups of patients[153,167]

An application of the network analysis approach to explore the grid structure and centrality of PTSD symptoms was led by Spiller et al.[160] in a study based on a cross-sectional clinical sample of 151 severely traumatized refugees, seen in outpatient units for victims of torture and war, in Zurich and Bern, Switzerland. This research[160] documented, albeit with the limitations of a small sample, the strong connections between hypervigilance and exaggerated startle response, intrusion of memories and difficulties in falling asleep, and irritability (outbursts of anger) and self-destructive and reckless behavior. Furthermore, no strong connection was found between nightmares and flashbacks, while emotional-cue reactivity had the highest centrality, and trauma-related amnesia had the lowest.[160]

Bryant et al.[156] conducted an investigation of the role of acute and chronic posttraumatic stress symptoms in the emergence of PTSD, in a study based on network analysis of symptoms presented by 1,138 patients. The research showed that intrusive memories and emotional-cue reactivity are centrally associated with symptoms in the acute phase, while fear circuitry and dysphoric PTSD symptoms appear as connected networks as time passes by after trauma.[156]

Using network analysis in alternative models of PTSD, McBride et al.[157] studied posttraumatic stress experiences of 473 Danish adults seeking psychological treatment for childhood sexual abuse. This research documented that, among individuals with a diagnosis of PTSD that met DSM-5 criteria,[43] strong associations were evident between the following pairs of experiences: (a) feeling as if they don't have future and feeling guilty for having survived, (b) blaming themselves for things that happened and feeling guilty for not doing enough, and (c) recurrent thoughts and flashbacks.[157] These three strong associations were outranked by the symptoms of depersonalization and derealization when the latter items were included in the analysis network.[157] Among patients with a network of complex PTSD symptoms, interpersonal problems and negative self-concept appeared to be the core elements of the posttraumatic experience, while difficulties in regulating mood were less central.[157]

Lazarov et al.[158] studied PTSD symptom structure among almost 1,800 male veterans from the Israeli Defense Forces who were seeking treatment for combat-related PTSD. The study showed that flashbacks and getting emotionally upset by trauma reminders were the core symptoms in the PTSD network, regardless of the inclusion of depressive symptoms.[158]

A significant advance in the implementation of network analysis to grasp the complexity of the interface between symptoms of PTSD was recently made by Papini et al.[159] in a second analysis using data[168] from a completed multisite trial of behavioral interventions for co-occurring PTSD and substance use disorders. Their results demonstrated that patients who showed greater decreases in highly central nodes or symptoms also showed greater decreases in the overall network of symptoms.

For the time being, until analysis of trauma symptoms as part of a structural network can be implemented in clinical practice, clinicians must rely on what is known about treatment of diagnostic categories related to trauma and stress.

Treatment of Adjustment Disorder

Casey[169] described elements of the psychological interventions for adjustment disorder, which include strategies to lessen or remove the stressor, to facilitate adaptation and/or to modify the response to the stressor by reduction of symptoms and/or behavioral change.

So far, there is only one published systematic review of treatments for adjustment disorder in adults, conducted in 2018 by O'Donnell et al.,[170] based on almost 30 studies published between 1980 and 2016 investigating psychological and pharmacological treatment for adjustment disorder. This review[171] has established that the evidence for positive effects of psychological treatments for symptoms of adjustment disorder "were ranked as low to very low"[170] (Table 9.4).

Greiner et al.[197] conducted analyzed the medication data of 4,235 psychiatric inpatients with a primary diagnosis of adjustment disorder from 2000 to 2016. Most of the pharmacotherapy the patients received was symptom-oriented, aimed at depressive mood, agitation, and anxiety[197]: 81% of the patients were medicated with antidepressants (60%), followed by antipsychotics (35%) and tranquilizers (almost 23%).

Treatment of ASD and PTSD

In 2004, the American Psychiatric Association (APA) published a practice guideline for the treatment of patients with ASD and PTSD[198] that underscored the essential elements of the disorders' psychiatric management:

- Evaluate the safety of the patient and others[198]
- Define of the most appropriate treatment setting, with the less restrictive setting also being the most effective and safe[198]
- Establish and maintain a therapeutic alliance[198]
- Coordinate the treatment effort[198]
- Monitor treatment response[198]
- Provide education about the natural course of, and interventions for, ASD and PTSD[198]
- Enhance adherence to treatment[198]
- Increase understanding of, and adaptation to, the psychosocial effects of the disorder[198]
- Evaluate and manage physical health and functional impairments[198]

According to the APA guidelines,[198] the goals of treatment of ASD and PTSD should include:

- Reduction in the severity of symptoms[198]
- Prevention or reduction of trauma-related comorbid conditions[198]
- Improvement of adaptive functioning[198]
- Protection against relapse[198]
- Integration of the danger experienced during trauma into a positive "schema of risk, safety, prevention, and protection"[198]

For the treatment of symptoms of ASD or PTSD, the APA guidelines[198] recognized three strategies—psychopharmacology, psychotherapy, and education/supportive measures—to be used independently or in combination.[198]

Table 9.4. Psychological and Pharmacological Treatments for Adjustment Disorder in Adults, by Quality of Evidence for Positive Effects[a]

Study	Quality of Evidence	Study	Quality of Evidence	Study	Quality of Evidence
Behavioral-based therapy vs. Active control[171]	Low (moderate quality)	Psychodynamic psychotherapy (no control)[182,183]	Very low (poor quality)	Trazodone[g] vs. Clorazepate[h,189,190]	Low
Behavioral-based therapy (no control)[172,173]	Very low (poor quality)	Relaxation-based therapy vs. Active control[184]	Low (poor quality)	Sertraline[e] followed by fluoxetine[f] no control[191]	Very low (poor quality)
Cognitive behavioral therapy (CBT) vs. work-focused CBT (W-CBT)[174]	Low (moderate quality)	Relaxation-based therapy (no control)[185]	Very low (poor quality)	Various SSRIs and some concurrent psychotherapy (no control)[192]	Very low (poor quality)
CBT vs Active control[175-177]	Low (moderate quality)	Euphytose[b] vs. Placebo control[186]	Low (moderate quality)	Viloxazine[i] vs. SAMe[j] vs. Lormetazepam[k] vs. supportive psychotherapy vs. placebo[193]	Very low (poor quality)
CBT (no control)[178-180]	Very low (poor quality)	Tianeptine[c] vs. Mianserin[d] vs. Alprazolam[e,187]	Low (moderate quality)	Etifoxine[l] vs. Alprazolam[e,194,195]	Low (moderate quality)
Brief psychodynamic psychotherapy vs. Intermediate psychodynamic psychotherapy[181]	Low (poor quality)	Gradual dose of paroxetine[f] vs. Full dose of paroxetine[188]	Low (moderate quality)	Combined pharmacotherapy and psychological therapy (no control)[196]	Very low (poor quality)

[a] Based on Donnell et al.[170]

[b] Combination of six plant extracts.

[c] Serotonin reuptake enhancer.

[d] Tetracyclic antidepressant.

[e] Anxiolytic.

[f] Selective serotonin reuptake inhibitor (SSRI).

[g] Serotonin antagonist and reuptake inhibitor (SARI).

[h] Benzodiazepine derivative.

[i] Selective norepinephrine reuptake inhibitor (NRI).

[j] S-Adenosyl-L-methionine.

[k] Benzodiazepine derivative.

[l] Nonbenzodiazepine anxiolytic.

Psychopharmacology of ASD and PTSD

The APA guidelines[198] include a comprehensive assessment of studies published before 2004 that address the efficacy of psychopharmacological interventions for the treatment of symptoms of ASD and PTSD. The topics covered include the usefulness of selective serotonin reuptake inhibitors (SSRIs) as a first-line medication treatment, followed by experience with the use of tricyclic antidepressants, monoamine oxidase inhibitors (MAOIs), benzodiazepines, anticonvulsants, second-generation antipsychotics, and adrenergic inhibitors (Table 9.5).

Table 9.5. Efficacy of Medications for Acute Stress Disorder and Posttraumatic Stress Disorder

Type of Medication	Efficacy/Comments
Selective serotonin reuptake inhibitors (SSRIs)	First-line medication treatment for both men and women with PTSD[198-205]: sertraline,[199,203] paroxetine,[200,204] fluoxetine,[201,202] fluvoxamine[205]
Tricyclic antidepressants and Monoamine oxidase inhibitors (MAOIs)	Efficacy shown for imipramine[206] and amitrytiline[207] but not for desipramine.[208] Efficacy shown for phenelzine[206] and brofaromine.[209,210] Most studies in male veterans.[198]
Benzodiazepines	Can reduce anxiety and improve sleep but their efficacy in preventing PTSD or treating the core symptoms of PTSD has been neither established nor adequately evaluated.[198,211,212]
Anticonvulsants	Carbamazepine,[213] valproic acid,[214,215] and lamictal[216] showed efficacy in preventing the re-experiencing of symptoms.[198]
Antipsychotics	Olanzapine,[217-219] quetiapine,[220] and risperidone[221] were shown to have a potential role when concomitant psychotic symptoms are present.[198]
Adrenergic inhibitors	Preliminary evidence has shown possible benefits with the α_1-antagonist prazosin[222] and with the α_2-agonist clonidine[223] in combination with imipramine. β-Adrenergic blockers like propranolol have been used after trauma to reduce some later symptoms of PTSD.[224-226]

[a] Based on Ursano et al.[198]

The updated *Practice Guideline for the Treatment of Patients with Acute Stress Disorder and Posttraumatic Stress Disorder*, published by the American Psychiatric Association in 2009,[227] sustained previous evidence[198] supporting "the superiority of SSRIs and serotonin-norepinephrine reuptake inhibitors (SNRIs) over placebo for non-combat-related PTSD."[227]

A meta-analysis conducted in 2006 by Stein et al.,[228] based on 35 short-term randomized controlled trials (RCTs), documented that in 50% of the trials the intensity of the symptoms was significantly decreased in the medication groups as compared to placebo. Indication of efficacy was most compelling for the SSRIs, "across all symptom clusters and for co-occurring depression and disability."[198]

In particular, the efficacy of paroxetine,[229] sertraline,[230] and fluoxetine[231] over placebo was documented in treatment trials of civilians with PTSD. Yet, by 2009, the APA Guidelines,[227] based on a review of studies conducted by Van der Kolk et al.,[232,233] Hertzberg et al.,[234] Friedman et al.,[235] and Zohar et al.,[236] indicated that there was no clear evidence that the use of SSRIs could be recommended with the same level of confidence for veterans with PTSD as for patients with non-combat-related PTSD.[227]

Among SNRIs, venlafaxine extended release was found to be "effective and well tolerated"[237] in the treatment of PTSD based on an international, 6-month, controlled trial involving 56 sites.[237]

By 2009, the α-adrenergic antagonist prazosin was regarded as one of the "most promising advances in the pharmacological treatment of PTSD,"[227] primarily for the management of nightmares and sleep disruption.[238,239]

Huemer et al.[240] reviewed studies conducted before 2010 on psychopharmacological treatment of PTSD in children and adolescents, and they highlighted the limited number of studies in this area.[241] Furthermore, most of the research lacked verification via RCTs, except for the studies using imipramine,[242] divalproex sodium,[241] and sertraline.[243]

A systematic review of psychopharmacological treatment for adults with PTSD published in 2018 by Forman-Hoffman et al.[244] documented that moderate strength of evidence[245] for the efficacy of fluoxetine, paroxetine, and venlafaxine compared with placebo,[244] yet a moderate increase of nausea was found in treatment with venlafaxine versus placebo.[244] Low strength of evidence[245] was documented in studies assessing the efficacy of sertraline, prazosin, topiramate, olanzapine, and risperidone in the treatment of PTSD.[244]

Above all, it should be noted that the Australian guidelines for the treatment of adults with ASD and PTSD have cautioned practitioners that, in the immediate aftermath of trauma, medication should not be used as a first choice; instead, preference should be given to "trauma-focused psychological therapy."[246]

Psychotherapy for ASD and PTSD

In 2004, the APA Guidelines[198] underscored the potential value of cognitive behavioral therapy (CBT), eye movement desensitization and reprocessing (EMDR), psychodynamic psychotherapy, and psychoeducation/support as interventions for patients with ASD and PTSD, while questioning the benefits of psychological debriefing "with groups of unknown individuals who have widely varying trauma exposures or when it is administered early after trauma exposure, before safety and decreased arousal are established."[198]

Five years later (2009), the revised APA Guidelines, authored by Benedek et al.,[227] gave special attention to the knowledge gained by six trials[247-252] of exposure-based CBT (Table 9.6), which may include elements of re-exposure, EMDR, group psychotherapy, psychoeducation, and/or breathing/relaxation techniques. The 2009 APA Guidelines also recognized two small studies[253,254] that suggest the efficacy of brief EMDR (Table 9.6).

Bryant et al.[56] conducted a treatment study of outpatient civilians with a diagnosis of ASD by randomly assigning them to receive either imaginal and in vivo exposure, cognitive restructuring, or being placed on a waiting list. The study's objective was to prevent PTSD, and the study documented that, on follow-up, the patients who underwent exposure treatment were more likely (OR = 2.1) to not meet criteria for PTSD than those who underwent cognitive restructuring.[56]

The efficacy of different therapeutic strategies to prevent PTSD in adults who were exposed to psychological trauma was analyzed by Gartlehner et al.,[262] who examined 19 trials published from 1980 until July 30, 2012. The analysis found that there was no evidence supporting "efficacy for the prevention of PTSD or for the reduction of PTSD-related symptom severity."[262] Yet, brief trauma-focused CBT "might be the preferable choice for reducing PTSD symptom severity in persons with acute stress disorder."[262]

In 2017, the APA developed a guideline[263] on treatments for PTSD in adults that strongly recommended the use of either CBT, cognitive processing therapy, cognitive therapy, or prolonged exposure therapy in psychotherapy for patients with PTSD.[263] Furthermore, the guideline[263] suggested or conditionally recommended the use of either brief eclectic therapy, EMDR, or narrative exposure therapy in treatment for PTSD. Yet, the guideline[263] found insufficient evidence to recommend for or against relaxation therapy or seeking-safety therapy for PTSD.

Table 9.6. Psychotherapy Trials for the Treatment of PTSD, by Characteristics and Outcome[227]

Study	Sample	Treatment	Outcome
Monson et al[247]	Veterans with military-related PTSD (N = 60)	CPT[a] Participants were randomized to receive treatment immediately or to wait for 10 weeks to receive treatment.	Participants receiving CPT, as compared to wait-list control participants, had a significant reduction in the severity of PTSD symptoms across time.
Chard[248]	Women victims of sexual abuse with diagnosis of PTSD (N = 71)	CPT for Sexual Abuse[b] Participants were randomly assigned to active treatment or to a wait-list control group.	Participants receiving active treatment showed significant improvement in PTSD, depression, and dissociation in comparison to wait-list controls.
Resick et al[249]	Women with PTSD associated with history sexual or physical assault (N = 150)	CPT[255,a] Participants were randomly assigned to CPT,[c] CPT-C,[c] or WA.[c]	Patients in all three treatments had substantial improvement in PTSD and depression. Yet, patients on CPT-C reported greater improvement in PTSD than those on WA.
Schnurr et al[250]	Female veterans (N = 277) and female active-duty personnel (N = 7) with PTSD	Patients were randomly assigned to 10 weeks of PE[256] or present-centered therapy.[d]	Women who received PE experienced greater reduction of PTSD symptoms than women who were treated with present-centered therapy.
Rothbaum et al[251]	Women with PTSD associated with history of having been raped (N = 74)	EMDR[e] vs. PE[256] as compared to nontreatment wait-list control (WAIT)	Improvements in PTSD, depression, dissociation, and anxiety were significantly greater in both the PE and EMDR group than in the WAIT group.
Başoğlu et al[252]	Survivors of an earthquake suffering from PTSD (N = 59)	Single-session modified behavioral treatment[257] compared to a wait-list control[f]	The was a 49% improvement after six weeks and 83% improvement at one- to two-year follow-up.
Van der Kolk et al[253]	Subjects with PTSD (N = 88)	Random selection for EMDR,[258] fluoxetine, or placebo	EMDR was more successful than fluoxetine in reducing PTSD and depression.[g]
Högberg et al[254]	Public transportation workers with PTSD (N = 24)	Random selection for EMDR[258] or wait list	EMDR was successful for 67% of the participants.

Abbreviations: CPT, cognitive processing therapy; EMDR, eye movement desensitization and reprocessing; PE, prolonged exposure; PTSD, posttraumatic stress disorder.

[a] Specific form of CPT for PTSD that has a primary focus on cognitive interventions (manualized 12-session course).[259]

[b] CPT-SA adaptation of CPT for rape victims.[260] Consists of manualized group and individual therapy for 17 weeks.

[c] CPT = full protocol of cognitive therapy + written accounts; CPT-C = cognitive therapy only; WA = written accounts.

[d] Prolonged exposure is aimed at enhancing emotional processing of one or more traumatic events by coping with traumatic memories and circumstances associated with them. It includes education, breathing retraining, recounting of trauma, homework, and discussion of thoughts and feelings.[250] Present-centered therapy focuses on current life problems as manifestations of PTSD.[250]

[e] EMDR[261] involves having the patient imagine a scene that represents the worst part of the trauma, focusing on body sensations of distress and rehearsing negative thoughts corresponding to the picture while following the therapist's fingers back and forth for roughly 18 minutes. Distress feelings are measured in a scale of 0 to 10, and when the degree of distress drops to 0 or 1, the patient is asked to follow the therapist's finger while rehearsing a new, preferred belief, until the new statement feels true to the patient.[251]

[f] Shorter version of CBT that focuses on reduction of fear and avoidance while shifting focus from habituation to anxiogenic stimuli to enhancement of sense of control over traumatic stressors.[252]

[g] For most childhood-onset trauma patients, neither treatment produced complete symptom remission.

A systematic review of psychotherapy for adults with PTSD by Forman-Hoffman et al.[244] showed a high strength of evidence[245] for the efficacy of CBT-exposure[264] and CBT-mixed[265] in the treatment of PTSD.

Psychological Treatment of Complex PTSD

A critical analysis of current treatment guidelines for complex PTSD in adults, conducted by De Jongh et al.[266] in 2016, recommended that "trauma-focused therapies should routinely be offered to individuals with complex presentations of PTSD, such as multiple or severe comorbidities, in an adequate dose, consistent with current general PTSD treatment guidelines."[266]

Psychological Treatment of PTSD in Children and Adolescents

In 2015, Gillies et al.[267] assessed the effects of psychological therapies in preventing PTSD and associated negative outcomes in children and adolescents who have suffered a traumatic episode. The study was based on the analysis of 51 RCTs[268] of psychological therapies[269] compared with a control, such as treatment as usual, waiting list, or no treatment. The results showed that there was a small effect favoring CBT over EMDR, play therapy, and supportive therapies for the reduction of PTSD symptoms in the short term (up to and including one month after therapy), with the quality of evidence for this outcome being regarded as moderate.[267]

In early 2020, Mavranezouli et al.[270] published results of a network meta-analysis of psychological and psychosocial treatment for children and young people with PTSD, based on 32 trials of 17 interventions involving 2,260 participants. The study[270] showed that trauma-focused CBT,[271] "in particular individual forms, appears to be most effective in the management of PTSD in youth,"[270] and furthermore that EMDR is effective, although to a lesser extent, while supportive counseling does not appear to be efficacious.

In a previous study, Mavranezouli et al.[272] assessed the cost-effectiveness of a variety of psychological treatments for children and young people with PTSD, and the assessment demonstrated that individual forms of trauma-focused CBT and, to a lesser degree, play therapy appeared to be the most cost-effective interventions for the treatment of PTSD in young people.

Future Directions for Intervention to Stop Bullying

Intervention to stop ongoing bullying and other forms of victimization is an integral part of a alleviating the morbidity associated with such victimization. This is a common-sense idea, as illustrated by the analogy of having to remove a foreign object in a shoe as part of an appropriate treatment for a toe that is being injured by such a foreign object. Thus, approaches to intervention need to be further thought through and validated.

Toward a Brief Health Intervention To Stop Ongoing Bullying and Other Forms of Mistreatment

In consideration of the morbidity (see Chapter 4) and psychosocial risks (see Chapter 5) associated with bullying and other forms of mistreatment, there is a need to stop victimization in progress, using a strategy that is comprised of public health and primary care elements. Such an intervention should be construed as a short-term and defined therapeutic procedure involving voluntary participation (without coercion). The process aims to assist the person who is mistreating others to stop further ill-treatment, while separately supporting the victim through regular monitoring of potential exposure to recurrent bullying and assessment for development of health problems and/or psychosocial hazards.

Elements of a Health Intervention to Stop Ongoing Bullying and Other Forms of Victimization

The notion of a health intervention to stop ongoing bullying and other forms of victimization, as previously described, is based on the principles that the process is:

- A health procedure, intended to stop a public health hazard, bullying, which is linked to biopsychosocial antecedents and consequences
- Optional, with voluntary participation and without coercion, yet involving the support and consent of parents of minors
- Short-term, limited to few sessions over three weeks, with two follow-up appointments to ensure a lack of relapse (Its brevity is justified due to the urgency of ensuring a halt to a very prevalent public health hazard despite limited availability of health professionals.)
- Therapeutic, because it is intended to remediate an ongoing psychosocial stressor and health risk, to restore physical and emotional environmental safety, and to care for the well-being both the victim and the perpetrator
- Comprised of public health and primary care components, including: periodic screening to detect participation and/or exposure to bullying and linked morbidity; procuring health assistance to stop ongoing bullying; facilitating a voluntary report to a health professional about ongoing bullying, for the purpose of halting it; providing public policy protection from civil or criminal liability for a good faith health report about ongoing bullying and other forms of victimization; preserving the health information privacy of victims and perpetrators; applying a psychotherapeutic strategy that deals with bullying from a strength-based perspective[273]; identifying contraindications; monitoring intercurrent risks; and defining criteria for mental health referral

Recommended Approach

A health intervention to stop on going bullying can be:

- Requested by a person who is being victimized or by the parent of a minor
- Offered to a person who is reported to be bullying others (offender), with the understanding, support, and consent of parents of a minor
- Provided by a school, workplace, or correctional health professional if the victimization occurs between people interacting with an organizational milieu or by a primary care provider if the maltreatment occurs among family members
- Unsuitable for an offender who is suffering from frequent physical or emotional symptoms and/or psychosocial hazards and/or has presented with a relapse of victimizing others despite receiving a health intervention to stop ongoing maltreatment

Suggested Steps

The victim is first seen by a health professional to report ongoing incidents of victimization and to request help. At this point, information[273] is gathered about the nature of maltreatment, dates, circumstances, and identity of offender. A brief clinical inquiry is conducted to ascertain whether the victim has also victimized the perpetrator and/or if the victim is currently suffering from symptoms and psychosocial dysfunctions linked to maltreatment.

The victim is informed that attempts will be made to help the perpetrator to stop ongoing abuse through a brief health intervention or a health referral if needed. Furthermore, the victim is invited to attend follow-up visits, to ensure that the maltreatment does not recur and that frequent symptoms or dysfunctions do not evolve. Evidence indicating that the victim is also mistreating the offender would also lead to an offer to participate in a brief health intervention to stop bullying. Indications that the victim is suffering from symptoms or psychosocial dysfunction should warrant referral to mental health consultation.

The perpetrator is invited to meet with the health professional and is advised about the report of his/her participation in victimization and about the potential health risks affecting people who are bullied and/or bully others. Furthermore, information is provided about available brief health support to stop bullying, and an invitation is offered to the perpetrator to receive such a service. If the perpetrator denies participation in bullying and/or declines any support to stop it, the perpetrator is advised that a referral for mental health support will be provided if further incidents are reported.

If the perpetrator confirms the reported incident/s of bullying and accepts the offer to be helped, a brief assessment should be conducted to determine whether the perpetrator is qualified to receive support at this level of mental healthcare or needs referral to a higher level of psychological intervention. Providing that the clinical requirements for a brief health intervention to stop bullying are met, the health provider could help the client to develop a bullying prevention plan[273] based on:

- Trying to develop a milieu that is less propitious to bullying,[273] by avoiding potential victims, by avoiding people with a history of bullying others, and/or staying away from physical locations, chat sites, and social networks that may provoke or induce an urge to maltreat somebody.
- Identifying prodromal signals of impending bullying, including feelings of anger or having urges to bully someone.[273]
- Applying a personal approach to avoid urges to bully, by using alternative, diverting, and/or self-calming strategies.[273]
- Interacting with people who may help to divert the wish to bully.[273]
- Avoiding retaliation if being bullied. If the perpetrator is also being bullied, this should be noted, and a health intervention to stop those incidents of mistreatment should be sought.[273]
- Seeking health professional support if the impulse to bully is very strong and the client worries that it will be difficult to elude it.[273]
- Understanding by the client (as well as the parents of a minor) that a relapse may occur, which would require ongoing intervention at a higher level of mental healthcare.

The initial appointment should be followed by clinical encounters to ascertain the development of bullying-related morbidity or psychosocial risks and/or the relapse of bullying, which could support referral to a higher level of mental health treatment.

The health intervention to stop ongoing bullying recommended in this chapter is based on therapeutic objectives primarily established in the Bullying Prevention Plan[273] and keeps to the goals introduced by solution-focused brief therapy.[13-15,274] It is geared toward helping people have a healthy cognitive ability, appropriate insight, judgment, and empathy as well as a lack of major impulsivity and/or mood instability. Adaptations accounting for the client's developmental stage and/or sociocultural or ecological background may be needed. The intervention requires further development, standardization, and assessment of its efficacy.

Finally, the intervention to stop bullying and other forms of victimization could be adapted for use by the lay public, as a form of psychological first aid that could be applied by parents to deter ongoing sibling bullying or by others when health providers are not available.

Future Treatment of Morbidity Arising from Victimization

Symptom-Targeted Treatment

Future treatment of morbidity stemming from victimization should considered targeting symptoms for remedy,[275,276] instead of treating established diagnostic categories. Toward this end, there will be a need to conduct longitudinal research to identify the clusters of symptoms that develop after exposure to different types of victimization. Furthermore, a network analysis strategy[152,153] should ascertain the hierarchical organization (degree of centrality[277]) of the symptoms as well as their active role in a dynamic network interaction. Moreover, it will be necessary to determine the interaction between central[278] symptoms with individual factors of resilience or vulnerability, including exposure to trauma, as well as environmental aspects of support, care, or respect versus neglect or abuse, which may dampen, sustain, or reinforce the dynamics and strength of the central[278] symptoms. In this context, interventions to stop ongoing stressful and/or traumatic events, as well as treatment strategies, will affect the dynamic interplay of the network by improving the central symptoms, worsening them, or having no significant therapeutic effect.

Fried et al.[162] have underscored the notion that a network analysis approach might provide unique therapeutic strategies for mental disorders, and yet there are no published studies showing how analysis of trauma symptoms as part of a structural network could be implemented in clinical practice. In the meantime, research is being conducted by Frumkin et al.[279] to ascertain the feasibility and utility of idiographic models in a clinic setting. In this pilot study, the individual (idiographic) patient's symptoms are monitored several times a day, concurrently with a brief ecological assessment, leading to a patient's generated prediction about the associative and directed relationships in the networks of symptoms. Preliminary results[279] indicate that although both patients and therapists found the personalized methods to be acceptable, the patients "tended to perceive more utility from these methods than therapists," and the pilot findings endorse previous results from other studies.[280]

Notes

1. Srabstein J. Working towards a detection of bullying related morbidity. *Int J Adolesc Med Health*. 2011;24(1):77–82..
2. Rigby K. How teachers address cases of bullying in schools: a comparison of five reactive approaches. *Educ Psychol Pract*. 2014;30(4):409–419.
3. Rigby K. What can schools do about cases of bullying? *Pastoral Care Educ*. 2011;29(4):273–285.
4. Olweus D. *Bullying at School*. Cambridge, MA: Blackwell Publishers; 1993. Cited in Rigby.[3]
5. Srabstein JC, Berkman BE, Pyntikova E. Antibullying legislation: a public health perspective. *J Adolesc Health*. 2008;42(1):11–20.
6. Bonell C, Allen E, Christie D, et al. Initiating change locally in bullying and aggression through the school environment (INCLUSIVE): study protocol for a cluster randomised controlled trial. *Trials*. 2014;15:381..
7. Hutchinson M. Restorative approaches to workplace bullying: educating nurses towards shared responsibility. *Contemp Nurse*. 2009;32(1-2):147–155.
8. Hopkins BA. *Whole School Approach to Restorative Justice*. New York, NY: Jessica Kingsley Publishers; 2004. Cited by Bonell et al.[6]
9. Morrison B. *Restoring Safe School Communities: A Whole School Response to Bullying, Violence and Alienation*. Annadale, NSW: Federation Press; 2007. Cited by Rigby.[3]
10. Savage R. Friendship and bullying patterns in children attending a language base in a mainstream school. *Educ Psychol Pract*. 2005;21(1):23–36. Cited by Rigby.[3]
11. Johnson DW, Johnson RT, Dudley B. Effects of peer mediation training on elementary school students. *Mediation Q*. 1992;10(1):89–99. Cited by Rigby.[3]
12. Robinson G, Maines B. *Bullying: A Complete Guide to the Support Group Method*. London, England: SAGE; 2008. Cited by Rigby.[2]
13. Young S, Holdorf G. Using solution focused brief therapy in individual referrals for bullying. *Educ Psychol Pract*. 2003;19(4):271–282. Cited by Rigby.[2]
14. Pikas A. New developments of the shared concern method. *Sch Psychol Int*. 2002;23(3):307–336. Cited by Rigby.[3]
15. Thompson F, Smith PK. *The Use and Effectiveness of Anti-Bullying Strategies in Schools*. Research Report DFE-RR098. London, England: Department of Education; 2011. Cited by Rigby.[2]
16. Bibliographic search under the terms *treatment of bullying* or *evidence based treatment for bullying* through PubMed. https://www.ncbi.nlm.nih.gov/pubmed. Accessed October 27, 2022.
17. Goncy EA, Sutherland KS, Farrell AD, Sullivan TN, Doyle ST. Measuring teacher implementation in delivery of a bullying prevention program: the impact of instructional and procedural adherence and competence on student responsiveness. *Prev Sci*. 2015;16(3):440–450.
18. Jenson JM, Dieterich WA. Effects of a skills-based prevention program on bullying and bully victimization among elementary school children. *Prev Sci*. 2007;8(4):285–296.
19. Kärnä A, Voeten M, Little TD, Poskiparta E, Kaljonen A, Salmivalli C. A large-scale evaluation of the KiVa antibullying program: grades 4–6. *Child Dev*. 2011;82(1):311–330.
20. Santos RG, Chartier MJ, Whalen JC, Chateau D, Boyd L. Effectiveness of school-based violence prevention for children and youth: a research report. *Healthcare Q (Toronto)*. 2011;14:80–91.

21. Wong DS, Cheng CH, Ngan RM, Ma SK. Program effectiveness of a restorative whole-school approach for tackling school bullying in Hong Kong. *Int J Offender Ther Comp Criminol.* 2011;55(6):846–862.
22. Pearce JB, Thompson AE. Practical approaches to reduce the impact of bullying. *Arch Dis Child.* 1998;79(6):528–531.
23. Twemlow SW, Fonagy P, Sacco FC. A developmental approach to mentalizing communities: II. The Peaceful Schools experiment. *Bull Menninger Clin.* 2005;69(4):282–304.
24. Waseem M, Ryan M, Foster CB, Peterson J. Assessment and management of bullied children in the emergency department. *Pediatr Emerg Care.* 2013;29(3):389.
25. Srabstein J. Working towards a detection of bullying related morbidity. *Int J Adolesc Med Health.* 2011;24(1):77–82.
26. Seehra J, Newton JT, DiBiase AT. Interceptive orthodontic treatment in bullied adolescents and its impact on self-esteem and oral-health-related quality of life. *Eur J Orthod.* 2012;35(5):615–621.
27. Puhl RM, Peterson JL, Luedicke J. Weight-based victimization: bullying experiences of weight loss treatment–seeking youth. *Pediatrics.* 2013;131(1):e1–e9.
28. Al-Omari IK, Al-Bitar ZB, Sonbol HN, Al-Ahmad HT, Cunningham SJ, Al-Omiri M. Impact of bullying due to dentofacial features on oral health–related quality of life. *Am J Orthod Dentofac Orthop.* 2014;146(6):734–739.
29. Alanko OM, Svedström-Oristo AL, Peltomäki T, Kauko T, Tuomisto MT. Psychosocial well-being of prospective orthognathic-surgical patients. *Acta Odont Scand.* 2014;72(8):887–897.
30. Seehra J, Fleming PS, Newton T, DiBiase AT. Bullying in orthodontic patients and its relationship to malocclusion, self-esteem and oral health-related quality of life. *J Orthod.* 2011;38(4):247–256.
31. Radhakishun NN, de Wit M, van Vliet M, et al. Impaired quality of life in treatment-seeking obese children of Dutch, Moroccan, Turkish and Surinamese descent. *Public Health Nutr.* 2016;19(5):796–803.
32. Straube A, Heinen F, Ebinger F, von Kries R. Headache in school children: prevalence and risk factors. *Dtsch Ärztebl Int.* 2013;110(48):811.
33. Sourander A, Gyllenberg D, Klomek AB, Sillanmäki L, Ilola AM, Kumpulainen K. Association of bullying behavior at 8 years of age and use of specialized services for psychiatric disorders by 29 years of age. *JAMA Psychiatry.* 2016;73(2):159–165.
34. Sourander A, Ronning J, Brunstein-Klomek A, et al. Childhood bullying behavior and later psychiatric hospital and psychopharmacologic treatment: findings from the Finnish 1981 birth cohort study. *Arch Gen Psychiatry.* 2009;66(9):1005–1112.
35. Sasaki T, Hashimoto K, Okawada K, et al. Ifenprodil for the treatment of flashbacks in adolescent female posttraumatic stress disorder patients with a history of abuse. *Psychother Psychosom.* 2013;82(5):344–345.
36. Panzer BM, Dhuper S. Designing a group therapy program for coping with childhood weight bias. *Soc Work.* 2014;59(2):141–147.
37. Murphy WP, Yaruss JS, Quesal RW. Enhancing treatment for school-age children who stutter: II. Reducing bullying through role-playing and self-disclosure. *J Fluency Disord.* 2007;32(2):139–162.
38. DeRosier ME. Building relationships and combating bullying: Effectiveness of a school-based social skills group intervention. *J Clin Child Adolesc Psychol.* 2004;33(1):196–201.
39. Garaigordobil M, Martínez-Valderrey V. Effects of Cyberprogram 2.0 on "face-to-face" bullying, cyberbullying, and empathy. *Psicothema.* 2015;27(1).

40. Stallard P, Taylor G, Anderson R, et al. The prevention of anxiety in children through school-based interventions: study protocol for a 24-month follow-up of the PACES project. *Trials.* 2014;15(1):77.
41. Santos RG, Chartier MJ, Whalen JC, Chateau D, Boyd L. Effectiveness of school-based violence prevention for children and youth: a research report. *Healthcare Q (Toronto).* 2011;14:80–91.
42. Fung AL. Intervention for aggressive victims of school bullying in Hong Kong: a longitudinal mixed-methods study. *Scand J Psychol.* 2012;53(4):360–367.
43. ICD-11 for Mortality and Morbidity Statistics (Version: 04/2019). Disorders specifically associated with stress, 6B 43 Adjustment Disorder. https://icd.who.int/browse11/l-m/en#/http://id.who.int/icd/entity/264310751. Accessed October 26, 2022.
44. American Psychiatric Association. Trauma and stress-related disorders, adjustment disorders, diagnostic criteria. In: *Diagnostic and Statistical Manual of Mental Disorders.* 5th ed. Arlington, VA: American Psychiatric Association; 2013: 286–289.
45. ICD-11 for Mortality and Morbidity Statistics (Version: 04/2019). Problems associated with harmful or traumatic events, QE84 Acute Stress Reaction. https://icd.who.int/browse11/l-m/en#/http://id.who.int/icd/entity/505909942. Accessed October 26, 2022.
46. American Psychiatric Association. Trauma and stress-related disorders, acute stress disorders, diagnostic criteria. In: *Diagnostic and Statistical Manual of Mental Disorders.* 5th ed. Arlington, VA: American Psychiatric Association; 2013: 280–286.
47. ICD-11 for Mortality and Morbidity Statistics (Version: 04/2019). Disorders specifically associated with stress, 6B40 Post-Traumatic Stress Disorder. https://icd.who.int/browse11/l-m/en#/http://id.who.int/icd/entity/2070699808. Accessed October 26, 2022.
48. American Psychiatric Association. Trauma and stress-related disorders, post traumatic stress disorder, diagnostic criteria. In: *Diagnostic and Statistical Manual of Mental Disorders.* 5th ed. Arlington, VA: American Psychiatric Association; 2013: 271–280.
49. ICD-11 for Mortality and Morbidity Statistics (Version: 04/2019). Disorders specifically associated with stress, 6B41Complex Post-Traumatic Stress Disorder. https://icd.who.int/browse11/l-m/en#http%3a%2f%2fid.who.int%2ficd%2fentity%2f585833559. Accessed October 26, 2022.
50. Rosenfield PJ, Stratyner A, Tufekcioglu S, Karabell S, Mckelvey J, Litt L. Complex PTSD in ICD-11: a case report on a new diagnosis. *J Psychiatr Pract.* 2018;24(5):364–370.
51. No available published report documented in the ICD-11,[20] DSM-5,[21] PubMed (https://pubmed.ncbi.nlm.nih.gov/), or Google Scholar (https://scholar.google.com/). Accessed October 26, 2022.
52. O'Donnell ML, Alkemade N, Creamer M, et al. A longitudinal study of adjustment disorder after trauma exposure. *Am J Psychiatry.* 2016;173(12):1231–1238.
53. Glück TM, Knefel M, Lueger-Schuster B. A network analysis of anger, shame, proposed ICD-11 post-traumatic stress disorder, and different types of childhood trauma in foster care settings in a sample of adult survivors. *Eur J Psychotraumatology.* 2017;8(suppl 3):1372543.
54. Dyer KF, Dorahy MJ, Hamilton G, et al. Anger, aggression, and self-harm in PTSD and complex PTSD. *J Clin Psychol.* 2009;65(10):1099–1114.
55. Bryant RA, Friedman MJ, Spiegel D, Ursano R, Strain J. A review of acute stress disorder in DSM-5. *Focus.* 2011;9(3):335–350. Cited in DSM-5.[46]
56. Bryant RA, Panasetis P. Panic symptoms during trauma and acute stress disorder. *Behav Res Ther.* 2001;39(8):961–966.
57. Sinclair E, Salmon K, Bryant RA. The role of panic attacks in acute stress disorder in children. *J Trauma Stress.* 2007;20(6):1069–1073.

58. Doherty AM, Lorenz L, Jabbar F, O'Leary E, Casey P. Sleep disturbance in adjustment disorder and depressive episode. *Int J Environ Res Public Health.* 2019;16(6):1083.
59. Grossman ES, Hoffman YS, Shrira A, et al. Preliminary evidence linking complex-PTSD to insomnia in a sample of Yazidi genocide survivors. *Psychiatry Res.* 2019;271:161–166.
60. Eberle DJ, Maercker A. Preoccupation as psychopathological process and symptom in adjustment disorder: a scoping review. *Clin Psychol Psychother.* 2022;29(2):455–468.
61. Levin Y, Bachem R, Karatzias T, Shevlin M, Maercker A, Ben-Ezra M. Network structure of ICD-11 adjustment disorder: a cross-cultural comparison of three African countries. *Br J Psychiatry.* 2021;219(4):557–564.
62. Harvey AG, Bryant RA. Dissociative symptoms in acute stress disorder. *J Trauma Stress.* 1999;12(4):673–680.
63. van Dijke A, Ford JD, Frank LE, Van der Hart O. Association of childhood complex trauma and dissociation with complex posttraumatic stress disorder symptoms in adulthood. *J Trauma Dissoc.* 2015;16(4):428–441.
64. Chung MS, Chiu HJ, Sun WJ, et al. Association among depressive disorder, adjustment disorder, sleep disturbance, and suicidal ideation in Taiwanese adolescent. *Asia-Pacific Psychiatry.* 2014;6(3):319–325.
65. Portzky G, Audenaert K, van Heeringen K. Adjustment disorder and the course of the suicidal process in adolescents. *J Affective Disord.* 2005;87(2-3):265–270.
66. Casey P, Jabbar F, O'Leary E, Doherty AM. Suicidal behaviours in adjustment disorder and depressive episode. *J Affective Disord.* 2015;174:441–446.
67. Florez IA, Allbaugh LJ, Harris CE, Schwartz AC, Kaslow NJ. Suicidal ideation and hopelessness in PTSD: spiritual well-being mediates outcomes over time. *Anxiety Stress Coping.* 2018;31(1):46–58.
68. Noor N, Pao C, Dragomir-Davis M, Tran J, Arbona C. PTSD symptoms and suicidal ideation in US female firefighters. *Occup Med.* 2019;69(8-9):577–585.
69. Law KC, Allan NP, Kolnogorova K, Stecker T. An examination of PTSD symptoms and their effects on suicidal ideation and behavior in non-treatment seeking veterans. *Psychiatry Res.* 2019;274:12–19.
70. Kimbrel NA, Johnson ME, Clancy C, et al. Deliberate self-harm and suicidal ideation among male Iraq/Afghanistan-era veterans seeking treatment for PTSD. *J Trauma Stress.* 2014;27(4):474–477.
71. Rosenfield PJ, Stratyner A, Tufekcioglu S, Karabell S, Mckelvey J, Litt L. Complex PTSD in ICD-11: a case report on a new diagnosis. *J Psychiatr Pract.* 2018;24(5):364–370.
72. Ohayon MM. Prevalence of hallucinations and their pathological associations in the general population. *Psychiatry Res.* 2000;97(2-3):153–164.
73. McCarthy-Jones S, Longden E. Auditory verbal hallucinations in schizophrenia and post-traumatic stress disorder: common phenomenology, common cause, common interventions? *Front Psychol.* 2015;6:1071.
74. Scott JG, Nurcombe B, Sheridan J, McFarland M. Hallucinations in adolescents with post-traumatic stress disorder and psychotic disorder. *Australasian Psychiatry.* 2007;15(1):44–48.
75. Crompton L, Lahav Y, Solomon Z. Auditory hallucinations, and PTSD in ex-POWS. *J Trauma Dissoc.* 2017;18(5):663–678.
76. Peach N, Alvarez-Jimenez M, Cropper SJ, Sun P, Bendall S. Testing models of post-traumatic intrusions, trauma-related beliefs, hallucinations, and delusions in a first episode psychosis sample. *Br J Clin Psychol.* 2019;58(2):154–172.

77. Norredam M, Jensen M, Ekstrøm M. Psychotic symptoms in refugees diagnosed with PTSD: a series of case reports. *Nordic J Psychiatry*. 2011;65(4):283–288.
78. Park S, Choi JS, Lee J, Lee JY, Lee S, Jung H. Impaired executive functioning of sexual assault survivors with acute stress disorder. *J Clin Med*. 2018;7(10):362.
79. Herzog JI, Niedtfeld I, Rausch S, et al. Increased recruitment of cognitive control in the presence of traumatic stimuli in complex PTSD. *Eur Arch Psychiatry Clin Neurosci*. 2019;269(2):147–159.
80. Fujita M, Fujiwara J, Maki T, Shibasaki K, Shigeta M, Nii J. Pediatric chronic daily headache associated with school phobia. *Pediatr Int*. 2009;51(5):621–625.
81. Peres JF, Gonçalves AL, Peres MF. Psychological trauma in chronic pain: implications of PTSD for fibromyalgia and headache disorders. *Curr Pain Headache Rep*. 2009;13(5):350–357.
82. Peterlin BL, Tietjen G, Meng S, et al. Post-traumatic stress disorder in episodic and chronic migraine. *Headache*. 2008;48:517–522. Cited by Peres et al.[81]
83. Haber YO, Chandler HK, Serrador JM. Symptoms associated with vestibular impairment in veterans with posttraumatic stress disorder. *PLOS One*. 2016;11(12):e0168803.
84. Carlson KF, Gilbert TA, O'Neil ME, et al. Health care utilization and mental health diagnoses among veterans with tinnitus. *Am J Audiol*. 2019;28(1S):181–190.
85. Gupta MA. Review of somatic symptoms in post-traumatic stress disorder. *Int Rev Psychiatry*. 2013;25(1):86–99.
86. Fagelson MA. The association between tinnitus and posttraumatic stress disorder. Am J Audiol. 2007 Cited by Gupta.[85]
87. Yi YY, Kim HD, Lee JS, Cheon KA, Kang HC. Psychological problems and clinical outcomes of children with psychogenic non-epileptic seizures. *Yonsei Med J*. 2014;55(6):1556–1561.
88. Fiszman A, Alves-Leon SV, Nunes RG, Isabella DA, Figueira I. Traumatic events and post-traumatic stress disorder in patients with psychogenic nonepileptic seizures: a critical review. *Epilepsy Behav*. 2004;5(6):818–825. Cited by Gupta.[85]
89. Lenane Z, Peacock E, Joyce C, et al. Association of post-traumatic stress disorder symptoms following Hurricane Katrina with incident cardiovascular disease events among older adults with hypertension. *Am J Geriatr Psychiatry*. 2019;27(3):310–321.
90. Hoerster KD, Campbell S, Dolan M, et al. PTSD is associated with poor health behavior and greater body mass index through depression, increasing cardiovascular disease and diabetes risk among US veterans. *Prev Med Rep*. 2019; 15:100930.
91. Ho GW, Karatzias T, Vallières F, et al. Complex PTSD symptoms mediate the association between childhood trauma and physical health problems. *J Psychosom Res*. 2021;142:110358.
92. Smith BN, Tyzik AL, Neylan TC, Cohen BE. PTSD and obesity in younger and older veterans: results from the Mind Your Heart study. *Psychiatry Res*. 2015;229(3):895–900.
93. Mitchell KS, Aiello AE, Galea S, Uddin M, Wildman D, Koenen KC. PTSD and obesity in the Detroit neighborhood health study. *Gen Hosp Psychiatry*. 2013;35(6):671–673.
94. Cline GD, Schwartz DD, Axelrad ME, Anderson B. A pilot study of acute stress symptoms in parents and youth following diagnosis of type I diabetes. *J Clin Psychol Med Settings*. 2011;18(4):416–422.
95. Agyemang C, Goosen S, Anujuo K, Ogedegbe G. Relationship between post-traumatic stress disorder and diabetes among 105,180 asylum seekers in the Netherlands. *Eur J Public Health*. 2011;22(5):658–662.
96. Arigo D, Juth V, Trief P, Wallston K, Ulbrecht J, Smyth JM. Unique relations between post-traumatic stress disorder symptoms and patient functioning in type 2 diabetes. *J Health Psychol*. 2017:1359105317727839.

97. Trief PM, Ouimette P, Wade M, Shanahan P, Weinstock RS. Post-traumatic stress disorder and diabetes: co-morbidity and outcomes in a male veterans sample. *J Behav Med.* 2006;29(5):411–418.
98. Klyushnik TP, Nikitina VB, Androsova LV, et al. Inflammatory factors and immunophenotypes in adjustment disorders. *Zh Nevrol Psikhiatr.* 2018;118(3):83–88.
99. Bielas H, Meister-Langraf RE, Schmid JP, et al. Acute stress disorder and C-reactive protein in patients with acute myocardial infarction. *Eur J Prev Cardiol.* 2018;25(3):298–305.
100. Miller MW, Lin AP, Wolf EJ, Miller DR. Oxidative stress, inflammation, and neuroprogression in chronic PTSD. *Harvard Rev Psychiatry.* 2018;26(2):57–69.
101. Lindqvist D, Mellon SH, Dhabhar FS, et al. Increased circulating blood cell counts in combat-related PTSD: associations with inflammation and PTSD severity. *Psychiatry Res.* 2017; 258:330–336.
102. Groer MW, Kane B, Williams SN, Duffy A. Relationship of PTSD symptoms with combat exposure, stress, and inflammation in American soldiers. *Biol Res Nurs.* 2015;17(3):303–310.
103. Heath NM, Chesney SA, Gerhart JI, et al. Interpersonal violence, PTSD, and inflammation: potential psychogenic pathways to higher C-reactive protein levels. *Cytokine.* 2013;63(2):172–178.
104. Song H, Fang F, Tomasson G, et al. Association of stress-related disorders with subsequent autoimmune disease. *JAMA.* 2018;319(23):2388–2400.
105. O'Donovan A, Cohen BE, Seal KH, et al. Elevated risk for autoimmune disorders in Iraq and Afghanistan veterans with posttraumatic stress disorder. *Biol Psychiatry.* 2015;77(4):365–374.
106. Moeller-Bertram T, Afari N, Mostoufi S, Fink DS, Wright LJ, Baker DG. Specific pain complaints in Iraq and Afghanistan veterans screening positive for post-traumatic stress disorder. *Psychosomatics.* 2014;55(2):172–178.
107. White DL, Savas LS, Daci K, et al. Trauma history and risk of the irritable bowel syndrome in women veterans. *Aliment Pharmacol Ther.* 2010;32(4):551–561.
108. Ottisova L, Smith P, Oram S. Psychological consequences of human trafficking: complex posttraumatic stress disorder in trafficked children. *Behav Med.* 2018;44(3):234–241.
109. Michopoulos V, Maples-Keller J, Roger EI, et al. Nausea in the peri-traumatic period is associated with prospective risk for PTSD symptom development. *Neuropsychopharmacology.* 2019;44(4):668–673.
110. Michopoulos V, Maples-Keller J, Roger EI, et al. Nausea in the peri-traumatic period is associated with prospective risk for PTSD symptom development. *Neuropsychopharmacology.* 2019;44(4):668.
111. Herman JL. Complex PTSD: a syndrome in survivors of prolonged and repeated trauma. *J Trauma Stress.* 1992;5(3):377–391.
112. Shoaib LC, Yaqoob N, Sharif A. Psychiatric co-morbidity in chronic pain disorder. *Pak Armed Forces Med J.* 2013;63(2):241–244.
113. Bilić M, Mičković V, Lončar Z. Quality and intensity of low back pain in chronic PTSD patients. *Coll Antropol.* 2013;37(4):1229–1236..
114. Suri P, Boyko EJ, Smith NL, et al. Post-traumatic stress disorder symptoms are associated with incident chronic back pain: a longitudinal twin study of older male veterans. *Spine.* 2019;44(17):1220–1227.
115. Cohen H, Neumann L, Haiman Y, Matar MA, Press J, Buskila D. Prevalence of post-traumatic stress disorder in fibromyalgia patients: overlapping syndromes or post-traumatic fibromyalgia syndrome? *Semin Arthritis Rheum.* 2002;32(1):38–50.

116. Coppens E, Van Wambeke P, Morlion B, et al. Prevalence and impact of childhood adversities and post-traumatic stress disorder in women with fibromyalgia and chronic widespread pain. *Eur J Pain*. 2017;21(9):1582–1590.
117. Conversano C, Carmassi C, Bertelloni CA, et al. Potentially traumatic events, post-traumatic stress disorder and post-traumatic stress spectrum in patients with fibromyalgia. *Clin Exp Rheumatol*. 2019;37(1):39–43.
118. Salomonsson S, Hedman-Lagerlöf E, Öst LG. Sickness absence: a systematic review and meta-analysis of psychological treatments for individuals on sick leave due to common mental disorders. *Psychol Med*. 2018;48(12):1954–1965.
119. van der Klink JJ, Blonk RW, Schene AH, van Dijk FJ. Reducing long term sickness absence by an activating intervention in adjustment disorders: a cluster randomised controlled design. *Occup Environ Med*. 2003;60(6):429–437. Cited by Salomonsson et al.[118]
120. Malt UF, Karlehagen S, Hoff H, et al. The effect of major railway accidents on the psychological health of train drivers—I. Acute psychological responses to accident. *J Psychosom Res*. 1993;37(8):793–805.
121. Belleville G, Marchand A, St-Hilaire MH, Martin M, Silva C. PTSD and depression following armed robbery: patterns of appearance and impact on absenteeism and use of health care services. *J Trauma Stress*. 2012;25(4):465–468.
122. Strain JJ, Smith GC, Hammer JS, et al. Adjustment disorder: a multisite study of its utilization and interventions in the consultation-liaison psychiatry setting. *Gen Hosp Psychiatry*. 1998;20(3):139–149.
123. McFarlane AC. Epidemiological evidence about the relationship between PTSD and alcohol abuse: the nature of the association. *Addict Behav*. 1998;23(6):813–825.
124. Shipherd JC, Stafford J, Tanner LR. Predicting alcohol and drug abuse in Persian Gulf War veterans: what role do PTSD symptoms play? *Addict Behav*. 2005;30(3):595–599.
125. Powers A, Fani N, Carter S, Cross D, Cloitre M, Bradley B. Differential predictors of DSM-5 PTSD and ICD-11 complex PTSD among African American women. *Eur J Psychotraumatology*. 2017;8(1):1338914.
126. Pereira JL, Guedes-Carneiro GM, Netto LR, et al. Types of trauma, posttraumatic stress disorder, and academic performance in a population of university students. *J Nerv Ment Dis*. 2018;206(7):507–512.
127. Adler DA, Possemato K, Mavandadi S, et al. Psychiatric status, and work performance of veterans of Operations Enduring Freedom and Iraqi Freedom. *Psychiatr Serv*. 2011;62(1):39–46.
128. Kokonya DA, Kuria WM, Ong'echa FA, Mburu JM, Ndetei DM. Complex post traumatic stress disorder (PTSD) in defilement: case report. *Open J Psychiatry*. 2014;4(3):Article ID: 47431, 6 pages doi:10.4236/ojpsych.2014.43023
129. Stewart SL, Baiden P, Theall-Honey L. Examining non-suicidal self-injury among adolescents with mental health needs, in Ontario, Canada. *Arch Suicide Res*. 2014;18(4):392–409.
130. Kimbrel NA, Gratz KL, Tull MT, et al. Non-suicidal self-injury as a predictor of active and passive suicidal ideation among Iraq/Afghanistan war veterans. *Psychiatry Res*. 2015;227(2-3):360–362.
131. Christoffersen MN, Møhl B, DePanfilis D, Vammen KS. Non-suicidal self-injury—does social support make a difference? An epidemiological investigation of a Danish national sample. *Child Abuse Negl*. 2015;44:106–116.
132. Dyer KF, Dorahy MJ, Hamilton G, et al. Anger, aggression, and self-harm in PTSD and complex PTSD. *J Clin Psychol*. 2009;65(10):1099–1114.

133. Gradus JL, Qin P, Lincoln AK, Miller M, Lawler E, Lash TL. The association between adjustment disorder diagnosed at psychiatric treatment facilities and completed suicide. *Clin Epidemiol.* 2010;2:23.
134. Miché M, Hofer PD, Voss C, et al. Mental disorders, and the risk for the subsequent first suicide attempt: results of a community study on adolescents and young adults. *Eur Child Adolesc Psychiatry.* 2018;27(7):839–848.
135. Selaman ZM, Chartrand HK, Bolton JM, Sareen J. Which symptoms of post-traumatic stress disorder are associated with suicide attempts? *J Anxiety Disord.* 2014;28(2):246–251.
136. Idsoe T, Dyregrov A, Idsoe EC. Bullying and PTSD symptoms. *J Abnorm Child Psychol.* 2012;40(6):901–911.
137. Schuster MA, Bogart LM. Did the ugly duckling have PTSD? Bullying, its effects, and the role of pediatricians. *Pediatrics.* 2013;131(1):e288–e291.
138. Ranney ML, Patena JV, Nugent N, et al. PTSD, cyberbullying and peer violence: prevalence and correlates among adolescent emergency department patients. *Gen Hosp Psychiatry.* 2016;39:32–38.
139. Plexousakis SS, Kourkoutas E, Giovazolias T, Chatira K, Nikolopoulos D. School bullying and post-traumatic stress disorder symptoms: the role of parental bonding. *Front Public Health.* 2019;7:75.
140. Lo T, De Stefano L, Lu S, et al. Post-traumatic stress disorder in resident physicians. *Cureus.* 2019;11(6):e4816. doi:10.7759/cureus.4816
141. Spence Laschinger HK, Nosko A. Exposure to workplace bullying and post-traumatic stress disorder symptomology: the role of protective psychological resources. *J Nurs Manage.* 2015;23(2):252–262.
142. Humphreys KL, Sauder CL, Martin EK, Marx BP. Tonic immobility in childhood sexual abuse survivors and its relationship to posttraumatic stress symptomatology. *J Interpers Violence.* 2010;25(2):358–373.
143. Tatar ZB, Yüksel Ş. Mobbing at workplace–psychological trauma and documentation of psychiatric symptoms. *Arch Neuropsychiatry.* 2019;56(1):57.
144. Bachem R, Maercker A. Self-help interventions for adjustment disorder problems: a randomized waiting-list controlled study in a sample of burglary victims. *Cogn Behav Ther.* 2016;45(5):397–413.
145. Signorelli MS, Costanzo MC, Cinconze M, Concerto C. What kind of diagnosis in a case of mobbing: post-traumatic stress disorder or adjustment disorder? *Case Rep.* 2013;bcr2013010080.
146. Brewin CR, Andrews B, Rose S. Diagnostic overlap between acute stress disorder and PTSD in victims of violent crime. *Am J Psychiatry.* 2003;160(4):783–785.
147. Brewin CR, Andrews B, Rose S, Kirk M. Acute stress disorder and posttraumatic stress disorder in victims of violent crime. *Am J Psychiatry.* 1999;156(3):360–366.
148. Meiser-Stedman R, Yule W, Smith P, Glucksman E, Dalgleish T. Acute stress disorder and posttraumatic stress disorder in children and adolescents involved in assaults or motor vehicle accidents. *Am J Psychiatry.* 2005;162(7):1381–1383.
149. Elklit A, Brink O. Acute stress disorder in physical assault victims visiting a Danish emergency ward. *Violence Vict.* 2003;18(4):461.
150. Cloitre M, Stolbach BC, Herman JL, et al. A developmental approach to complex PTSD: childhood and adult cumulative trauma as predictors of symptom complexity. *J Trauma Stress.* 2009;22(5):399–408.

151. Hull AM, Corrigan FM, Curran SA. Identifying patients with complex PTSD. *Practitioner.* 2016;260(1795):31–37.
152. Borsboom D, Cramer AO. Network analysis: an integrative approach to the structure of psychopathology. *Ann Rev Clin Psychol.* 2013;9:91–121.
153. Armour C, Fried EI, Olff M. PTSD symptomics: network analyses in the field of psychotraumatology. *Eur J Psychotraumatology.* 2017;8(suppl 3).
154. Rademaker AR, van Minnen A, Ebberink F, van Zuiden M, Hagenaars MA, Geuze E. Symptom structure of PTSD: support for a hierarchical model separating core PTSD symptoms from dysphoria. *Eur J Psychotraumatology.* 2012;3(1):17580.
155. Boschloo L, van Borkulo CD, Rhemtulla M, Keyes KM, Borsboom D, Schoevers RA. The network structure of symptoms of the diagnostic and statistical manual of mental disorders. *PLOS One.* 2015;10(9):e0137621.
156. Bryant RA, Creamer M, O'Donnell M, et al. Acute and chronic posttraumatic stress symptoms in the emergence of posttraumatic stress disorder: a network analysis. *JAMA Psychiatry.* 2017;74(2):135–142.
157. McBride O, Hyland P, Murphy J, Elklit A. Network analysis of posttraumatic stress experiences of adults seeking psychological treatment for childhood sexual abuse. *J Trauma Stress.* 2020;33(1):10–18.
158. Lazarov A, Suarez-Jimenez B, Levy O, et al. Symptom structure of PTSD and co-morbid depressive symptoms—a network analysis of combat veteran patients. *Psychol Med.* 2019:1–7.
159. Papini S, Rubin M, Telch MJ, Smits JA, Hien DA. Pretreatment posttraumatic stress disorder symptom network metrics predict the strength of the association between node change and network change during treatment. *J Trauma Stress.* 2020;33(1):64–71.
160. Spiller TR, Schick M, Schnyder U, Bryant RA, Nickerson A, Morina N. Symptoms of posttraumatic stress disorder in a clinical sample of refugees: a network analysis. *Eur J Psychotraumatology.* 2017;8(suppl 3):1318032.
161. Frewen PA, Schmittmann VD, Bringmann LF, Borsboom D. Perceived causal relations between anxiety, posttraumatic stress and depression: extension to moderation, mediation, and network analysis. *Eur J Psychotraumatology.* 2013;4(1):20656.
162. Fried EI, van Borkulo CD, Cramer AO, Boschloo L, Schoevers RA, Borsboom D. Mental disorders as networks of problems: a review of recent insights. *Soc Psychiatry Psychiatr Epidemiol.* 2017;52(1):1–0
163. Rodebaugh TL, Tonge NA, Piccirillo ML, et al. Does centrality in a cross-sectional network suggest intervention targets for social anxiety disorder? *J Consult Clin Psychol.* 2018;86(10):831.
164. Fried EI, Cramer AO. Moving forward: challenges and directions for psychopathological network theory and methodology. *Perspect Psychol Sci.* 2017;12(6):999–1020. Cited by Armour et al.[153]
165. Fried EI, van Borkulo CD, Cramer AO, Boschloo L, Schoevers RA, Borsboom D. Mental disorders as networks of problems: a review of recent insights. *Soc Psychiatry Psychiatr Epidemiol.* 2017;52(1):1–10. Cited by Armour et al.[153]
166. Fried EI, Nesse R. Depression sum-scores don't add up: why analyzing specific depression symptoms is essential. *BMC Med.* 2015;13(1):72. Cited by Armour et al.[153]
167. Fisher AJ, Boswell JF. Enhancing the personalization of psychotherapy with dynamic assessment and modeling. *Assessment.* 2016;23(4):496–506. Cited by Armour et al.[153]

168. National Institute on Drug Abuse (NIDA) Clinical Trials Network. https://datashare.nida.nih.gov/study/nida-ctn-0015. Accessed January 5, 2020. Cited by Papini et al.[159]
169. Casey P. Adjustment disorder. *CNS Drugs*. 2009;23(11):927–938.
170. O'Donnell ML, Metcalf O, Watson L, Phelps A, Varker T. A systematic review of psychological and pharmacological treatments for adjustment disorder in adults. *J Trauma Stress*. 2018;31(3):321–331.
171. Arends I, van der Klink JJ, Bültmann U. Prevention of recurrent sickness absence among employees with common mental disorders: design of a cluster-randomised controlled trial with cost-benefit and effectiveness evaluation. *BMC Public Health*. 2010;10(1):132. Cited in O'Donnell et al.[170]
172. Hosaka T, Sugiyama Y, Hirai K, Okuyama T, Sugawara Y, Nakamura Y. Effects of a modified group intervention with early-stage breast cancer patients. *Gen Hosp Psychiatry*. 2001;23(3):145–151. Cited in O'Donnell et al.[170]
173. Hosaka T, Sugiyama Y, Tokuda Y, Okuyama T. Persistent effects of a structured psychiatric intervention on breast cancer patients' emotions. *Psychiatry Clin Neurosci*. 2000;54(5):559–563. Cited in O'Donnell et al.[170]
174. Lagerveld SE, Blonk RW, Brenninkmeijer V, Wijngaards-de Meij L, Schaufeli WB. Work-focused treatment of common mental disorders and return to work: a comparative outcome study. *J Occup Health Psychol*. 2012;17(2):220–234. Cited in O'Donnell et al.[170]
175. Carta MG, Petretto D, Adamo S, et al. Counseling in primary care improves depression and quality of life. *Clin Pract Epidemiol Ment Health*. 2012;8: 152. Cited in O'Donnell et al.[170]
176. Moorey S, Greer S, Bliss J, Law M. A comparison of adjuvant psychological therapy and supportive counselling in patients with cancer. *Psycho-Oncology*. 1998;7(3):218–228. Cited in O'Donnell et al.[170]
177. van der Klink JJ, Blonk RW, Schene AH, van Dijk FJ. Reducing long term sickness absence by an activating intervention in adjustment disorders: a cluster randomised controlled design. *Occup Environ Med*. 2003;60(6):429–437. Cited in O'Donnell et al.[170]
178. Halford WK. Cognitive behavioural treatment of adjustment disorder with depressed mood following marital breakdown. *Behav Change*. 1987;4(1):28–33. Cited in O'Donnell et al.[170]
179. Powell S, McCone D. Treatment of adjustment disorder with anxiety: a September 11, 2001, case study with a 1-year follow-up. *Cogn Behav Pract*. 2004;11(3):331–336. Cited in O'Donnell et al.[170]
180. van der Heiden C., Melchior K. Cognitive-behavioral therapy for adjustment disorder: a preliminary study. *Behav Therapist*. 2012;35:57–60. Cited in O'Donnell et al.[170]
181. Ben-Itzhak S, Bluvstein I, Schreiber S, et al. The effectiveness of brief versus intermediate duration psychodynamic psychotherapy in the treatment of adjustment disorder. *J Contemp Psychother*. 2012;42(4):249–256. Cited in O'Donnell et al.[170]
182. Halford WK. Cognitive behavioural treatment of adjustment disorder with depressed mood following marital breakdown. *Behav Change*. 1987;4(1):28–33. Cited in O'Donnell et al.[170]
183. Kramer U, Despland JN, Michel L, Drapeau M, de Roten Y. Change in defense mechanisms and coping over the course of short-term dynamic psychotherapy for adjustment disorder. *J Clin Psychol*. 2010;66(12):1232–1241. Cited in O'Donnell et al.[170]
184. Hsiao FH, Lai YM, Chen YT, et al. Efficacy of psychotherapy on diurnal cortisol patterns and suicidal ideation in adjustment disorder with depressed mood. *Gen Hosp Psychiatry*. 2014;36(2):214–219. Cited in O'Donnell et al.[170]

185. Bos EH, Merea R, van den Brink E, Sanderman R, Bartels-Velthuis AA. Mindfulness training in a heterogeneous psychiatric sample: outcome evaluation and comparison of different diagnostic groups. *J Clin Psychol.* 2014;70(1):60–71. Cited in O'Donnell et al.[170]
186. Bourin M, Bougerol T, Guitton B, Broutin E. A combination of plant extracts in the treatment of outpatients with adjustment disorder with anxious mood: controlled study versus placebo. *Fundam Clin Pharmacol.* 1997;11(2):127–132. Cited in O'Donnell et al.[170]
187. Ansseau M, Bataille M, Briole G, et al. Controlled comparison of tianeptine, alprazolam and mianserin in the treatment of adjustment disorders with anxiety and depression. *Hum Psychopharmacol Clin Exp.* 1996;11(4):293–298 Cited in O'Donnell et al.[170]
188. Amodeo L, Castelli L, Leombruni P, Cipriani D, Biancofiore A, Torta R. Slow versus standard up-titration of paroxetine for the treatment of depression in cancer patients: a pilot study. *Support Care Cancer.* 2012;20(2):375–384. Cited in O'Donnell et al.[170]
189. De Wit S, Cremers L, Hirsch D, Zulian C, Clumeck N, Kormoss N. Efficacy, and safety of trazodone versus clorazepate in the treatment of HIV-positive subjects with adjustment disorders: a pilot study. *J Int Med Res.* 1999;27(5):223–232. Cited in O'Donnell et al.[170]
190. Razavi D, Kormoss N, Collard A, Farvacques C, Delvaux N. Comparative study of the efficacy and safety of trazodone versus clorazepate in the treatment of adjustment disorders in cancer patients: a pilot study. *J Int Med Res.* 1999;27(6):264–272. Cited in O'Donnell et al.[170]
191. Özten E, Sayar GH, Gül IG, Ceylan ME. Sertraline induced galactorrhea. *Nöro Psikiyatri Arşivi.* 2015;52(2):202. Cited in O'Donnell et al.[170]
192. Hameed U, Schwartz TL, Malhotra K, West RL, Bertone F. Antidepressant treatment in the primary care office: outcomes for adjustment disorder versus major depression. *Ann Clin Psychiatry.* 2005;17(2):77–81. Cited in O'Donnell et al.[170]
193. De Leo D. Treatment of adjustment disorders: a comparative evaluation. *Psycholog Rep.* 1989;64(1):51–54. Cited in O'Donnell et al.[170]
194. Nguyen N, Fakra E, Pradel V, et al. Efficacy of etifoxine compared to lorazepam monotherapy in the treatment of patients with adjustment disorders with anxiety: a double-blind controlled study in general practice. *Hum Psychopharmacol Clin Exp.* 2006;21(3):139–149. Cited in O'Donnell et al.[170]
195. Stein DJ. Etifoxine versus alprazolam for the treatment of adjustment disorder with anxiety: a randomized controlled trial. *Adv Ther.* 2015;32(1):57–68. Cited in O'Donnell et al.[170]
196. Ichitovkina EG, Zlokazova MV, Solov'ev AG. Efficacy of medical-psychological rehabilitation of combatants. *Neurosci Behav Physiol.* 2014;8(44):933–938. Cited in O'Donnell et al.[170]
197. Greiner T, Haack B, Toto S, et al. Pharmacotherapy of psychiatric inpatients with adjustment disorder: current status and changes between 2000 and 2016. *Eur Arch Psychiatry Clin Neurosci.* 2020;270:107–117.
198. Ursano RJ, Bell C, Eth S, et al. Practice guideline for the treatment of patients with acute stress disorder and posttraumatic stress disorder. *Am J Psychiatry.* 2004;161(11 suppl):3–31. https://psychiatryonline.org/pb/assets/raw/sitewide/practice_guidelines/guidelines/acutestressdisorderptsd.pdf. Accessed October 26, 2022.
199. Davidson J, Pearlstein T, Londborg P, et al. Efficacy of sertraline in preventing relapse of posttraumatic stress disorder: results of a 28-week double-blind, placebo-controlled study. *Am J Psychiatry.* 2001;158(12):1974–1981. Cited by Ursano et al.[198]
200. Marshall RD, Beebe KL, Oldham M, Zaninelli R. Efficacy and safety of paroxetine treatment for chronic PTSD: a fixed-dose, placebo-controlled study. *Am J Psychiatry.* 2001;158(12):1982–1988. Cited by Ursano et al.[198]

201. Connor KM, Sutherland SM, Tupler LA, Malik ML, Davidson JR. Fluoxetine in posttraumatic stress disorder: randomised, double-blind study. *Br J Psychiatry.* 1999;175:17–22. Cited by Ursano et al.[198]
202. van der Kolk BA, Dreyfuss D, Michaels M, et al. Fluoxetine in posttraumatic stress disorder. *J Clin Psychiatry.* 1994;55(12):517–522. Cited by Ursano et al.[198]
203. Brady K, Pearlstein T, Asnis GM, et al. Efficacy and safety of sertraline treatment of posttraumatic stress disorder: a randomized controlled trial. *JAMA.* 2000;283(14):1837–1844. Cited by Ursano et al.[198]
204. Tucker P, Zaninelli R, Yehuda R, Ruggiero L, Dillingham K, Pitts CD. Paroxetine in the treatment of chronic posttraumatic stress disorder: results of a placebo-controlled, flexible-dosage trial. *J Clin Psychiatry.* 2001;62(11):860–868. Cited by Ursano et al.[198]
205. Neylan TC, Metzler TJ, Schoenfeld FB, et al. Fluvoxamine and sleep disturbances in posttraumatic stress disorder. *J Trauma Stress.* 2001;14(3):461–467. Cited by Ursano et al.[198]
206. Kosten TR, Frank JB, Dan E, McDougle CJ, Giller EL. Pharmacotherapy for posttraumatic stress disorder using phenelzine or imipramine. *J Nerv Ment Dis.* 1991;179(6):366–370. Cited by Ursano et al.[198]
207. Davidson J, Kudler H, Smith R, et al. Treatment of posttraumatic stress disorder with amitriptyline and placebo. *Arch Gen Psychiatry.* 1990;47(3):259–266. Cited by Ursano et al.[198]
208. Reist C, Kauffmann CD, Haier RJ, et al. A controlled trial of desipramine in 18 men with posttraumatic stress disorder. *Am J Psychiatry.* 1989;146(4):513–516. Cited by Ursano et al.[198]
209. Katz RJ, Lott MH, Arbus P, et al. Pharmacotherapy of post-traumatic stress disorder with a novel psychotropic. *Anxiety.* 1994;1(4):169–174. Cited by Ursano et al.[198]
210. Baker DG, Diamond BI, Gillette G, et al. A double-blind, randomized, placebo-controlled, multi-center study of brofaromine in the treatment of post-traumatic stress disorder. *Psychopharmacology.* 1995;122(4):386–389. Cited by Ursano et al.[198]
211. Mellman MD, Thomas A, Bustamante V, David D, Fins AI. Hypnotic medication in the aftermath of trauma. *J Clin Psychiatry.* 2002;63(12):1183. Cited by Ursano et al.[198]
212. Gelpin E, Bonne O, Peri-T, Brandes D, Shalev AY. Treatment of recent trauma survivors with benzodiazepines: a prospective study. *J Clin Psychiatry.* 1996;57(9):390–394. Cited by Ursano et al.[198]
213. Lipper S, Davidson JR, Grady TA, et al. Preliminary study of carbamazepine in posttraumatic stress disorder. *Psychosomatics.* 1986;27(12):849–854. Cited by Ursano et al.[198]
214. Clark RD, Cañive JM, Calais LA, Qualls CR, Tuason VB. Divalproex in posttraumatic stress disorder: an open-label clinical trial. *J Trauma Stress.* 1999;12(2):395–401. Cited by Ursano et al.[198]
215. Fesler FA. Valproate in combat-related posttraumatic stress disorder. *J Clin Psychiatry.* 1991;52(9):361–364. Cited by Ursano et al.[198]
216. Hertzberg MA, Butterfield MI, Feldman ME, et al. A preliminary study of lamotrigine for the treatment of posttraumatic stress disorder. *Biol Psychiatry.* 1999;45(9):1226–1229. Cited by Ursano et al.[198]
217. Butterfield MI, Becker ME, Connor KM, Sutherland S, Churchill LE, Davidson JR. Olanzapine in the treatment of post-traumatic stress disorder: a pilot study. *Int Clin Psychopharmacol.* 2001;16(4):197–203. Cited by Ursano et al.[198]
218. Petty F, Brannan S, Casada J, et al. Olanzapine treatment for post-traumatic stress disorder: an open-label study. *Int Clin Psychopharmacol.* 2001;16(6):331–337. Cited by Ursano et al.[198]

219. Stein MB, Kline NA, Matloff JL. Adjunctive olanzapine for SSRI-resistant combat-related PTSD: a double-blind, placebo-controlled study. *Am J Psychiatry.* 2002;159(10):1777–1779. Cited by Ursano et al.[198]

220. Hamner MB, Deitsch SE, Brodrick PS, Ulmer HG, Lorberbaum JP. Quetiapine treatment in patients with posttraumatic stress disorder: an open trial of adjunctive therapy. *J Clin Psychopharmacol.* 2003;23(1):15–20. Cited by Ursano et al.[198]

221. Hamner MB, Faldowski RA, Ulmer HG, Frueh BC, Huber MG, Arana GW. Adjunctive risperidone treatment in post-traumatic stress disorder: a preliminary controlled trial of effects on comorbid psychotic symptoms. *Int Clin Psychopharmacol.* 2003;18(1):1–8. Cited by Ursano et al.[198]

222. Raskind MA, Peskind ER, Kanter ED, et al. Reduction of nightmares and other PTSD symptoms in combat veterans by prazosin: a placebo-controlled study. *Am J Psychiatry.* 2003;160(2):371–373. Cited by Ursano et al.[198]

223. Kinzie JD, Leung P. Clonidine in Cambodian patients with posttraumatic stress disorder. *J Nerv Ment Dis.* 1989;177(9):546–550. Cited by Ursano et al.[198]

224. Faustman WO, White PA. Diagnostic and psychopharmacological treatment characteristics of 536 inpatients with posttraumatic stress disorder. *J Nerv Ment Dis.* 1989;177(3):154–159. Cited by Ursano et al.[198]

225. Pitman RK, Sanders KM, Zusman RM, et al. Pilot study of secondary prevention of posttraumatic stress disorder with propranolol. *Biol Psychiatry.* 2002;51(2):189–192. Cited by Ursano et al.[198]

226. Vaiva G, Ducrocq F, Jezequel K, et al. Immediate treatment with propranolol decreases posttraumatic stress disorder two months after trauma. *Biol Psychiatry.* 2003;54(9):947–949. Cited by Ursano et al.[198]

227. Benedek DM, Friedman MJ, Zatzick D, Ursano RJ. Guideline watch (March 2009): *Practice Guideline for the Treatment of Patients with Acute Stress Disorder and Posttraumatic Stress Disorder.* https://psychiatryonline.org/pb/assets/raw/sitewide/practice_guidelines/guidelines/acutestressdisorderptsd-watch.pdf. Accessed October 26, 2022.

228. Stein DJ, Ipser JC, Seedat S, Sager C, Amos T. Pharmacotherapy for post-traumatic stress disorder (PTSD). *Cochrane Database Syst Rev.* 2006;(1):CD002795. Cited by Benedek et al.[227]

229. Marshall RD, Lewis-Fernandez R, Blanco C, et al. A controlled trial of paroxetine for chronic PTSD, dissociation, and interpersonal problems in mostly minority adults. *Depress Anxiety.* 2007;24(2):77–84. Cited by Benedek et al.[227]

230. Stein DJ, Van Der Kolk BA, Austin C, Fayyad R, Clary C. Efficacy of sertraline in posttraumatic stress disorder secondary to interpersonal trauma or childhood abuse. *Ann Clin Psychiatry.* 2006;18(4):243–249. Cited by Benedek et al.[227]

231. Davidson JR, Connor KM, Hertzberg MA, Weisler RH, Wilson WH, Payne VM. Maintenance therapy with fluoxetine in posttraumatic stress disorder: a placebo-controlled discontinuation study. *J Clin Psychopharmacol.* 2005;25(2):166–169. Cited by Benedek et al.[227]

232. Dreyfuss D, Michaels M, Shera D, Berkowitz R, Fisler R, Saxe G. Fluoxetine in posttraumatic stress disorder. *J Clin Psychiatry.* 1994;55(12):517–522. Cited by Benedek et al.[227]

233. van der Kolk BA, Spinazzola J, Blaustein ME, Hopper JW, Hopper EK. A randomized clinical trial of eye movement desensitization and reprocessing (EMDR), fluoxetine, and pill

placebo in the treatment of posttraumatic stress disorder: treatment effects and long-term maintenance. *J Clin Psychiatry*. 2007;68(1):37–46. Cited by Benedek et al.[227]

234. Hertzberg MA, Feldman ME, Beckham JC, Kudler HS, Davidson JR. Lack of efficacy for fluoxetine in PTSD: a placebo-controlled trial in combat veterans. *Ann Clin Psychiatry*. 2000;12:101–105. Cited by Benedek et al.[227]
235. Friedman MJ, Marmar CR, Baker DG, Sikes CR, Farfel GM. Randomized, double-blind comparison of sertraline and placebo for posttraumatic stress disorder in a Department of Veterans Affairs setting. *J Clin Psychiatry*. 2007;68(5):711–720. Cited by Benedek et al.[227]
236. Zohar J, Amital D, Miodownik C, et al. Double-blind placebo-controlled pilot study of sertraline in military veterans with posttraumatic stress disorder. *J Clin Psychopharmacol*. 2002;22(2):190–195. Cited by Benedek et al.[227]
237. Davidson J, Baldwin D, Stein DJ, et al. Treatment of posttraumatic stress disorder with venlafaxine extended release: a 6-month randomized controlled trial. *Arch Gen Psychiatry*. 2006;63(10):1158–1165. Cited by Benedek et al.[227]
238. Raskind MA, Peskind ER, Hoff DJ, et al. A parallel group placebo-controlled study of prazosin for trauma nightmares and sleep disturbance in combat veterans with post-traumatic stress disorder. *Biol Psychiatry*. 2007;61(8):928–934. Cited by Benedek et al.[227]
239. Taylor FB, Martin P, Thompson C, et al. Prazosin effects on objective sleep measures and clinical symptoms in civilian trauma posttraumatic stress disorder: a placebo-controlled study. *Biol Psychiatry*. 2008;63:629–632. Cited by Benedek et al.[227]
240. Huemer J, Erhart F, Steiner H. Posttraumatic stress disorder in children and adolescents: A review of psychopharmacological treatment. *Child Psychiatry Hum Dev*. 2010;41(6):624–640.
241. Steiner H, Saxena KS, Carrion V, Khanzode LA, Silverman M, Chang K. Divalproex sodium for the treatment of PTSD and conduct disordered youth: a pilot randomized controlled clinical trial. *Child Psychiatry Hum Dev*. 2007;38(3):183–193. Cited by Huemer et al.[240]
242. Robert R, Blakeney PE, Villarreal C, Rosenberg L, Meyer WJ III. Imipramine treatment in pediatric burn patients with symptoms of acute stress disorder: a pilot study. *J Am Acad Child Adolesc Psychiatry*. 1999;38(7):873–882. Cited by Huemer et al.[240]
243. Cohen JA, Mannarino AP, Perel JM, Staron V. A pilot randomized controlled trial of combined trauma-focused CBT and sertraline for childhood PTSD symptoms. *J Am Acad Child Adolesc Psychiatry*. 2007;46(7):811–819. Cited by Huemer et al.[240]
244. Hoffman V, Middleton JC, Feltner C, et al. *Psychological and Pharmacological Treatments for Adults with Posttraumatic Stress Disorder: A Systematic Review Update*. Comparative Effectiveness Review No. 207. Rockville, MD: Agency for Healthcare Research and Quality; 2018. https://effectivehealthcare.ahrq.gov/sites/default/files/pdf/cer-207-ptsd-update-2018.pdf. Accessed October 26, 2022.
245. High strength of evidence means that one can be confident that the estimate of effect lies close to the true effect for the outcome, that the body of evidence has few or no deficiencies, and that the findings are stable (i.e., another study would not change the conclusions). Moderate strength of evidence implies that there is moderate confidence that the estimate of effect comes close to the true effect for the outcome. Furthermore, although the body of evidence may have some deficiencies, the findings are likely to be stable, albeit with some doubt remaining. Low strength of evidence indicates that there is limited certainty that the estimate of effect lies close to the true effect for this outcome. The body of evidence has major or numerous deficiencies (or both). Furthermore, it signifies that additional evidence is needed before concluding either that the findings are stable or that the estimate of effect is close to

the true effect. See Berkman ND, Lohr KN, Ansari M, et al. *Grading the Strength of a Body of Evidence When Assessing Health Care Interventions for the Effective Health Care Program of the Agency for Healthcare Research and Quality: An Update.* Methods Guide for Comparative Effectiveness Reviews. AHRQ Publication No. 13(14)-EHC130-EF. Rockville, MD: Agency for Healthcare Research and Quality; 2013. https://effectivehealthcare.ahrq.gov/sites/default/files/pdf/methods-guidance-grading-evidence_methods.pdf. Accessed October 26, 2022.

246. Forbes D, Creamer M, Phelps A, et al. Australian guidelines for the treatment of adults with acute stress disorder and post-traumatic stress disorder. *Aust NZ J Psychiatry.* 2007;41(8):637–648.
247. Monson CM, Schnurr PP, Resick PA, Friedman MJ, Young-Xu Y, Stevens SP. Cognitive processing therapy for veterans with military-related posttraumatic stress disorder. *J Consult Clin Psychol.* 2006;74(5):898. Cited by Benedek et al.[227]
248. Chard KM. An evaluation of cognitive processing therapy for the treatment of posttraumatic stress disorder related to childhood sexual abuse. *J Consult Clin Psychol.* 2005;73(5):965. Cited by Benedek et al.[227]
249. Resick PA, Galovski TE, Uhlmansiek MO, Scher CD, Clum GA, Young-Xu Y. A randomized clinical trial to dismantle components of cognitive processing therapy for posttraumatic stress disorder in female victims of interpersonal violence. *J Consult Clin Psychol.* 2008;76(2):243. Cited by Benedek et al.[227]
250. Schnurr PP, Friedman MJ, Engel CC, et al. Cognitive behavioral therapy for posttraumatic stress disorder in women: a randomized controlled trial. *JAMA.* 2007;297(8):820–830. Cited by Benedek et al.[227]
251. Rothbaum BO, Astin MC, Marsteller F. Prolonged exposure versus eye movement desensitization and reprocessing (EMDR) for PTSD rape victims. *J Trauma Stress*: 2005; 18(6):607–616. Cited by Benedek et al.[227]
252. Başoğlu M, Şalcıoğlu E, Livanou M, Kalender D, Acar G. Single-session behavioral treatment of earthquake-related posttraumatic stress disorder: a randomized waiting list-controlled trial. *J Trauma Stress*: 2005;18(1):1–11. Cited by Benedek et al.[227]
253. van der Kolk BA, Spinazzola J, Blaustein ME, et al. A randomized clinical trial of eye movement desensitization and reprocessing (EMDR), fluoxetine, and pill placebo in the treatment of posttraumatic stress disorder: treatment effects and long-term maintenance. *J Clin Psychiatry.* 2007;68(1):37. Cited by Benedek et al.[227]
254. Högberg G, Pagani M, Sundin Ö, et al. On treatment with eye movement desensitization and reprocessing of chronic post-traumatic stress disorder in public transportation workers–a randomized controlled trial. *Nordic J Psychiatry.* 2007;61(1):54–61. Cited by Benedek et al.[227]
255. Resick PA, Schnicke MK. Cognitive processing therapy for sexual assault victims. *J Consult Clin Psychol.* 1992;60(5):748. Cited by Resick et al.[249]
256. Foa EB, Rothbaum BO. *Treating the Trauma of Rape: Cognitive-Behavioral Therapy for PTSD.* New York, NY: Guilford, 1998. Cited by Schnurr et al.[250]
257. Başoğlu M, Livanou M, Şalcioğlu E, Kalender D. A brief behavioural treatment of chronic post-traumatic stress disorder in earthquake survivors: results from an open clinical trial. *Psychol Med.* 2003;33(4):647–654. Cited by Başoğlu et al.[252]
258. Shapiro F. *Eye Movement Desensitization and Reprocessing (EMDR): Basic Principles, Protocols, and Procedures.* New York, NY: Guilford; 1995. Cited by van der Kolk et al.[253]

259. Resick PA. *Cognitive Processing Therapy: Generic Version*. St. Louis: University of Missouri-St. Louis; 2001. Cited by Monson et al.[247]

260. Resick PA, Schnicke MK. *Cognitive Processing Therapy for Rape Victims: A Treatment Manual*. Newbury Park, CA: SAGE; 1993. Cited by Chard.[248]

261. Chemtob CM, Tolin DF, Van Der Kolk BA, Pitman RK. Guidelines for treatment of PTSD: eye movement desensitization and reprocessing. *J Trauma Stress*. 2000;13:569–570. Cited by Rothbaum et al.[251]

262. Gartlehner G, Forneris CA, Brownley KA. Interventions for the prevention of posttraumatic stress disorder (PTSD) in adults after exposure to psychological trauma. Comparative Effectiveness Review No 109. Rockville, MD: Agency for Healthcare Research and Quality; 2013.

263. American Psychological Association. *Clinical Practice Guideline for the Treatment of Posttraumatic Stress Disorder (PTSD) in Adults*. https://www.apa.org/ptsd-guideline/ptsd.pdf. Accessed October 26, 2022.

264. Resick PA, Nishith P, Weaver TL, et al. A comparison of cognitive-processing therapy with prolonged exposure and a waiting condition for the treatment of chronic posttraumatic stress disorder in female rape victims. *J Consult Clin Psychol*. 2002;70(4):867–879. Cited by Hoffman et al.[244]

265. Foa EB, Dancu CV, Hembree EA, Jaycox LH, Meadows EA, Street GP. A comparison of exposure therapy, stress inoculation training, and their combination for reducing posttraumatic stress disorder in female assault victims. *J Consult Clin Psychol*. 1999;67(2):194–200. Cited by Hoffman et al.[244]

266. De Jongh A, Resick PA, Zoellner LA, et al. Critical analysis of the current treatment guidelines for complex PTSD in adults. *Depress Anxiety*. 2016;33(5):359–369.

267. Gillies D, Maiocchi L, Bhandari AP, Taylor F, Gray C, O'Brien L. Psychological therapies for children and adolescents exposed to trauma. *Cochrane Database Syst Rev*. 2016;10. https://www.ncbi.nlm.nih.gov/pmc/articles/PMC6457979/pdf/CD012371.pdf

268. Randomized controlled trials registered in the Cochrane Library by May 29, 2015.

269. The interventions analyzed in this study included CBT, EMDR, exposure-based therapy, family therapy, narrative therapy, posttrauma interventions (including debriefing and psychological first aid), psychodynamic psychotherapy (including play therapy), psychoeducation, and supportive therapy (including nondirective counseling). Gillies D, Maiocchi L, Bhandari AP, Taylor F, Gray C, O'Brien L. Psychological therapies for children and adolescents exposed to trauma. *Cochrane Library*. 2016. http://onlinelibrary.wiley.com/doi/10.1002/14651858.CD012371/epdf

270. Mavranezouli I, Megnin-Viggars O, Daly C, et al. Research review: psychological and psychosocial treatments for children and young people with post-traumatic stress disorder: a network meta-analysis. *J* Child Psychol Psychiatry Allied Disciplines. 2020;61(1):18.

271. Cohen JA, Mannarino AP, Deblinger E. *Treating Trauma and Traumatic Grief in Children and Adolescents*. New York, NY: Guilford Press; 2006. Cited by Mavranezouli et al.[270]

272. Mavranezouli I, Megnin-Viggars O, Trickey D, et al. Cost-effectiveness of psychological interventions for children and young people with post-traumatic stress disorder. *J Child Psychol Psychiatry*. 2020;61(6):699–710.

273. Klomek AB, Stanley A, Sourander A. Bullying prevention plan. *Adolesc Psychiatry*. 2014;4(3):185–193.

274. Bond C, Woods K, Humphrey N, Symes W, Green L. Practitioner review: the effectiveness of solution focused brief therapy with children and families: a systematic and critical evaluation of the literature from 1990–2010. *J Child Psychol Psychiatry*. 2013;54(7):707–723.

275. Epskamp S, van Borkulo CD, van der Veen DC, et al. Personalized network modeling in psychopathology: the importance of contemporaneous and temporal connections. *Clin Psychol Sci*. 2018;6(3):416–427.

276. Fried EI, Epskamp S, Nesse RM, Tuerlinckx F, Borsboom D. What are 'good'depression symptoms? Comparing the centrality of DSM and non-DSM symptoms of depression in a network analysis. *J Affective Disord*. 2016;189:314–320. Cited by Epskamp et al.[275]

277. The concept of centrality degree[162] or importance of a symptom within a network is determined by the number of connections that a symptom (node) has to other symptoms within the system.

278. A central symptom or node is the one that has the highest number of connections to other symptoms or nodes in a system.

279. Frumkin M, Piccirillo M, Beck ED, Grossman J, Rodebaugh T. Feasibility and utility of idiographic models in the clinic: a pilot study. *Psychother Res*. 2019;31(4):520–534. doi:10.31234/osf.io/m34aw.

280. Zimmermann J, Woods W, Ritter S, et al. Integrating structure and dynamics in personality assessment. *Psychol Assess*. 2018;31(4):516–531. Cited by Frumkin et al.[279]

10
National Initiatives for the Prevention of Bullying and Other Forms of Maltreatment

This chapter examines national efforts to prevent bullying and other forms of victimization through legislation and research-based initiatives.

What Is Known?

In the past three decades, more than 300 laws have been enacted around the world[1-356] to prevent the occurrence of bullying and other forms of victimization in different social environments.

School Bullying Prevention Laws

School bullying prevention laws[1-115] have been passed in 20 countries, by either the national or the state/provincial legislatures (Table 10.1).

A review[357] of the statutes[1-115] indicated that 70% of them called for the development and implementation of programs to avert the onset of school bullying or victimization, an approach defined as primary prevention (see Chapter 7). Such a legislative requirement has been conveyed by some laws without stipulations,[94,95,106,115] but most of the laws put forward some specifics about the methods and by whom bullying primary prevention programs or strategies should be selected or developed, as well as the distinctive elements or features that should characterize them (Table 10.2).

Prohibition of bullying, as a possible strategy to deter the occurrence of this form of victimization, was mandated in antibullying laws enacted in at least seven countries or in some of their provinces or states (Table 10.3).

Elements of secondary prevention to stop ongoing bullying from recurring, are found in at least 50% of the laws reviewed and involve strategies aimed at detection and intervention (Table 10.4).

The need to prevent and/or treat the serious physical and emotional morbidity associated with school bullying (tertiary prevention) seems to be considered in some of the laws reviewed,[357] as manifested by a legislative call for the support of mental health resources and for the role and participation of public health officials, as well legislative requirements for data collection and research to ascertain the health impact of bullying (Table 10.5).

Table 10.1. Countries That Have Enacted School Bullying Prevention Laws[a]

Argentina[1-11]	Lithuania[32]
Brazil[12-19]	Mexico[33-54]
Canada[20-24]	Norway[55]
Colombia[25]	Paraguay[56]
Costa Rica[26]	Peru[57]
Denmark[27]	Philippines[58]
El Salvador[28]	Sweden[59]
Honduras[29]	Ukraine[60]
India[30]	United States[61-114]
Japan[31]	Uruguay[115]

[a] Countries for which legislative texts were found.[357]

Table 10.2. Characteristics of Primary Prevention, as Required by Various Laws

Responsible Agents	Type of Approach	Specific Requirements for a Bullying Prevention Program
All school and community segments[114] Student participation[27,37,43,53,58,102]	Development of programs or training/discussion of available programs[2,4,7,8,10-13,16-19,25,26,28,31,33-36,38,42-45,47-54,65,70,71,72,74-77,82,83,90,101-103,105,107,108]	Needs to be evidence-based[83]
Coexistence council[a,2-6,11,25,26,42,43,45]	Promotion of safe school environment or climate[c,1-5,17,20,22-26,28,29,32,33,35,37,39.46,54 67,85,87,90,109]	Must be developmentally appropriate[83]
Committee or task force[b,68,69,84,109,112]	Public education campaign[d,2,3,12-16,18-20,26,33,39-45,48,49,52,87,113]	Should recognize vulnerability of special groups[e,83]

[a] A committee with representation of all segments of the school community, formed to foster coexistence.

[b] To develop a schoolwide bullying prevention program.

[c] Promotion of orderly, civil, and positive learning milieu. Fostering coexistence and respect while facilitating positive human relations and behavior.

[d] To disseminate knowledge about bullying and its ill-effects

[e] Actual or perceived differentiating characteristics, including race, color, religion, ancestry, national origin, sex, socioeconomic status, homelessness, academic status, gender identity or expression, physical appearance, pregnancy or parenting status, sexual orientation, mental, physical, and developmental or sensory disability, or by association with a person who has, or is perceived to have, one or more of these characteristics.[83]

Table 10.3. Countries with Laws Prohibiting Bullying among School Peers

Canada[20,21]	El Salvador[28]	India[30]	Japan[31]
Mexico[36,37,44,53]	Peru[57]		United States[61-65,67-88,90-99,101-106,108-114]

Table 10.4. Elements of Secondary Prevention, as Required by Various Laws

Detection	Intervention
Reporting to school authorities[1,3,24,28,30,32,36-43,45,49-51,53,55,57-65,67-77,79-99,101-106,108-114]	Application of consequences[1-3,8,11,16,17,20,21,24,30,36,37,39,42-45,47,52,53,55,57,58,61-74,76,77,79-88,90-106,108-114]
Reporting online or to an ombudsman[1,2,30,39,42,68,]	Conflict resolution[1-4,8,13,34-36,46,86,107]
	Restorative justice[66,75,84]

Table 10.5. Countries with Antibullying Laws Requiring Mental Health Resources and/or Public Health Involvement

Country	Legislative Requirement for Mental Health Support	Legislative Requirement for Public Health Involvement
Argentina	✓[2,3,9]	NDE
Brazil	✓[12-19]	NDE
Costa Rica	✓[26]	NDE
Japan	✓[31]	NDE
Lithuania	✓[32]	NDE
Mexico	✓[33-39,41-51,54]	✓[35-37,43,45-52,54]
Peru	✓[57]	NDE
Philippines	✓[58]	NDE
Ukraine	✓[60]	NDE
United States	✓[61,65,68-70,74-76,80-94,96,98,99,101,102,105,106,111,112]	✓[83]

Abbreviations: ✓, documented evidence found in the review of antibullying laws[357]; NDE, no documented evidence found in the review of antibullying laws.[357]

Laws for the Prevention of Cyberbullying and Other Forms of Cybervictimization

At least 23 countries have enacted laws to stop the occurrence of cyberbullying and other forms of computer-generated victimization (Table 10.6). An examination of the statutes[357] showed that almost 30% of them encompass part of a wide range of distinct types of cybervictimization or misconduct, while rarely[133,136] including the notion of cyberbullying (Table 10.7).

The prevention of cyberbullying or cyberharassment is uniquely addressed in legislation enacted in Italy[128] and the United States[138-158] or is considered in some of the United States' laws regarding school bullying prevention (Table 10.8).

Cyberbullying as contemplated in US laws concerning school bullying (Table 10.8) is not considered an illegal offense, and strategies for one or more levels of prevention are provided by the statutes. However, as is evident in the statute review,[357] cyberbullying and/or other forms of cybervictimization are regarded as criminal offenses by most the legislative initiatives enacted around the world,[116-127,129-158] and they subject the perpetrators to penalties as the only strategy for prevention.

Laws for the Prevention of Bullying and Other Forms of Victimization in the Workplace

Legislation[159-205] concerning the occurrence of bullying and other forms of victimization in the workplace has passed in 34 countries (Table 10.9).

A review[357] of the text of these laws revealed a wide range of terms for types of victimization in the workplace, with *harassment* and *discrimination* the most widely used, while occasionally the terms *bullying* or *mobbing* are used (Table 10.10). Notably, Japanese law has

Table 10.6. Countries That Have Enacted Laws for Prevention of Cyberbullying and/or Other Forms of Computer-Generated Victimization[a]

Albania[116]	Grenada[124]	Palestine[132]
Antigua and Barbuda [117]	Guyana[125]	Papua New Guinea[133]
Argentina[118]	India[126]	Paraguay[134]
Bahamas[119]	Iran[127]	St. Vincent and Grenadines[135]
Barbados[120]	Italy[128]	Tanzania[136]
Bostwana[121]	Jamaica[129]	Uganda[137]
El Salvador[122]	New Zealand[130]	United States[61,65,67,68,70,71,73,75,76,80-85,87,88,91,92,94,95,98,102,104-106,108,109,114,138-158]
Fiji[123]	Nigeria[131]	

[a] Countries for which legislative texts were found.[357]

Table 10.7. Forms of Cybervictimization[a] or Cybermisconduct Considered in Legislative Initiatives

Assisting or inciting crimes against humanity[132,136]	Electronic espionage[133]	Intimidation[158]	Tampering with critical infrastructure[131]
Building a fake Web site or impersonating a minor[148]	False Web site or spam[117]	Misuse of encryption[117,124,132]	Theft[117,133]
Child[b] or adult pornography[117,120,124,125,133,135-137,148]	Follow a minor online or in a chat room[148]	Offenses against critical national information infrastructure[131]	Threat[158]
Child grooming[133]	Forgery[117,124,125,127,129,131,133,135,136]	Posting electronic messages to cause harm[131]	Unauthorized eavesdroping[127,132]
Copy of any data pertaining to a minor to intimidate[148]	Fraud[117,121,122,124,125,127,129,131,133,135-137]	Posting or encouraging others to post personal or sexual information about a minor[148]	Unauthorized access to a computer/computer sabotage[131,132,134-137]
Crime against chastity and morality[127]	Hacking[126,133]	Posting an intimate visual recording[123,140,143]	Unauthorized interception of computer function or service[c,116,129,132,133,135,136,137]
Defamation and spreading lies[127,133]	Harassment[137-140,143-145,149-152,154-156,158]	Posting an offensive or obscene message[117,126,132,137,139,149]	Unauthorized modification of computer program or data[116,118-122,129,137]
Cyber extortion[121]	Identity theft[124]	Spoof/spam[135,144]	Use of illegal devices[133]
Electronic terrorism[117,124,131]	Inciting racial or religious hatred or discrimination[132,135]	Stalking[124]	Violation of privacy[117,124]

[a] In addition to cyberbullying.

[b] Signing up a minor for a pornographic Internet.

[c] Includes obstruction of operation and interference with data or the system.

introduced the concept of overwork as a type of workplace maltreatment, represented by the term *Karoshi* (Table 10.10).

The primary prevention of workplace victimization is addressed by its prohibition, as a form of deterrence, and, to a lesser degree, by legal stimulus for the identification of psychosocial risks in the workplace (Table 10.11). In fact, most of the workplace victimization laws reviewed[357] emphasized the prevention of ongoing maltreatment (secondary prevention), through such mechanisms as reporting, intervention, and sanctions or penalty, while very few laws addressed treatment of victims and/or perpetrators (tertiary prevention; Table 10.11).

Table 10.8. Prevention[a] of Cyberbullying Addressed by US State Laws on School Bullying Prevention

Alabama[61]	Illinois[75]	Minnesota[85]	Oklahoma[98]
Arkansas[65]	Indiana[76]	Missouri[87]	Rhode Island[102]
Connecticut[67]	Louisiana[80]	Montana[88]	South Dakota[104]
Delaware[68]	Maine[81]	New Hampshire[91]	Tennessee[105]
Florida[70]	Maryland[82]	New Jersey[92]	Texas[106]
Georgia[71]	Massachusetts[83]	New York[94]	Utah[108]
Hawaii[73]	Michigan[84]	North Carolina[95]	Vermont[109]
			Wyoming[114]

[a] Prevention may include primary, secondary, or tertiary elements (see Chapter 7).

Table 10.9. Countries[a] That Have Enacted Laws for the Prevention of Bullying and/or Other Forms of Victimization in the Workplace

Albania[159]	Malaysia[188]
Argentina[160]	Malta[189]
Australia[161-168]	Mexico[190]
Austria[169]	New Zealand[191]
Belgium[170]	Norway[192]
Bosnia and Hertzegovina[171]	Poland[193]
Brazil[172]	Portugal[194]
Bulgaria[173]	Serbia[195]
Canada[174-179]	Slovakia[196]
Chile[180]	Slovenia[197]
Colombia[181]	Spain[198]
Croatia[182]	Sweden[199]
Czechia[183]	Switzerland[200]
Finland[184]	Taiwan[201]
France[185]	The Netherlands[202]
India[186]	United Kingdom[203]
Japan[187]	United States[204,205]

[a] Countries for which legislative texts were found.[357]

Table 10.10. Types of Workplace Victimization Addressed in Legislative Preventive Initiatives

Bullying[174,181,193]	Incitement to discriminate[171]	Mobbing[171]	Racial harassment[191]
Coercion[161-163,165-167]	Labor abuse[181]	Moral or psychological harassment[170,179,185]	Segregation[171]
Discrimination[159-169, 171-173,182,183,185,188-194, 196-198]	Labor inequality[181]	Overwork[a,187]	Sexual harassment[170,173,180,182, 185,186,190,191,194]
Duress[191]	Labor persecution[181]	Physical violence[170]	Teasing[174]
Harassment[171,176,178,181, 182,184,190,192,194,195]	Labor slowdown[181]	Psychological violence[170]	Threat of violence[184]
Improper activity or behavior[175]	Lack of protection[181]	Psychosocial risk at work[170]	Workplace violence[174-178]

[a] In Japanese, *Karoshi.*

Table 10.11. Prevention Components Proposed or Mandated by Workplace Victimization Laws

Development of a safe, healthy, and violence-free workplace[a,174,195]	Research development[a,187]	Mediation[b,195]	Prevention of death and injury[c,187]
Identification of psychosocial risks in the workplace[a,170,174,175,177,178]	Training of workers in victimization prevention policy[a,176,177]	Reporting[b,171,175-178, 180-182,186,188,189,191, 195-197]	Role of counselor or occupational physician[c,170,175]
Prohibition of victimization in the workplace[a,159-169, 171-173,175,182,183,185,186, 188-192,194-197]	Violence prevention policy[a,175-178]	Role of the ombudsman[b,171]	Role of public health[c,187]
Raising awareness[a,171,187]	Intervention/ correction and/or legal protection[b,170,174,181,182,184]	Sanctions/penalty[b,171, 172,181,189,190]	Support for the victim[c,174]

[a] Element of primary of prevention.

[b] Element of secondary prevention.

[c] Element of tertiary prevention.

Laws for the Prevention of Domestic or Family Maltreatment

At least 65 countries have developed legislative initiatives for the prevention of abuse in the family milieu, with the enactment of more than 120 statutes[357] (Table 10.12).

The titles of the laws use different terms to refer to maltreatment among family members, with the most common terms being *domestic* or *family violence*, followed by *domestic* or *family abuse* (Table 10.13).

Table 10.12. Countries[a] That Have Enacted Laws for the Prevention of Domestic or Family Maltreatment

Albania[206]	El Salvador[227]	Naminbia[248]
Andorra[207]	Fiji[228]	Nepal[249]
Antigua and Barbuda[208]	Ghana[229]	New Zealand[250]
Argentina[209]	Grenada[230]	Paraguay[251]
Azerbaijan[210]	Guatemala[231]	Peru[252]
Bahamas[211]	Guyana[232]	Romania[253]
Bangladesh[212]	Honduras[233]	St. Christopher and Nevis[254]
Barbados[213]	India[234]	St. Vincent and the Grenadines[255]
Belize[214]	Indonesia[235]	Sierra Leone[256]
Bolivia[215]	Iraq[b,236]	Solomon Islands[257]
Bosnia and Herzegovina[216]	Ireland[237]	Thailand[258]
Bostwana[217]	Israel[238]	Timor Leste[259]
Bulgaria[218]	Jamaica[239]	Trinidad and Tobago[260]
Canada[358-364]	Kenya[240]	Turkey[261]
Chile[219]	Kyrgyz Republic[241]	Tuvalu[262]
China[220]	Lithuania[242]	Uganda[263]
Costa Rica[221]	Malaysia[243]	Ukraine[264]
Croatia[222]	Maldives[244]	United States[265-315]
Cyprus[223]	Mauritius[245]	Uruguay[316]
Czechia[224]	Mexico[365]	Vanuatu[317]
Dominican Republic[225]	Moldova[246]	Vietnam[318]
Ecuador[226]	Mongolia[247]	Zimbabwe[319]

[a] Countries for which legislative texts were found.[357]

[b] Iraq had a bill for the prevention of domestic violence drafted in 2019, but there is no evidence[357] that it has yet been enacted.[236]

Table 10.13. Terms Used in the Titles of Laws for the Prevention of Family or Domestic Maltreatment

Cohabitant abuse[309]	Family or intrafamily violence[209,219,223,226,227,250,252,261,271,273,275,283,296,308,318,358,360,362,364,365]
Domestic battery[279,281]	Intimate partner violence[359]
Domestic violence[207.209-218,220-222,224-225,228-234,237-249,251,253-260,262-270,272,274,277,278,282,285,294,295,297-300,312,313,315-317,319,363]	Spouse or domestic assault[291,292]
Domestic or family abuse[207,276,280,284,286,288-290,300,302-307,310,311,314,361]	Violence in the household[235]

The laws' definitions include a range of types of victimization, with the most common being physical, psychological, sexual, or economic abuse, as well as harassment (Table 10.14). It is of note that the Kenyan law for the prevention of domestic violence[240] addresses forms of domestic abuse found more commonly in non-Western countries, such as child marriage,[366] virginity testing,[367] and widow cleansing[368] (Table 10.14).

The primary prevention of domestic or family abuse is tackled by legislation requiring the development of awareness campaigns and public education (Table 10.15). Most of the laws addressing family victimization give specific attention to strategies aimed at the deterrence of ongoing maltreatment (secondary prevention), primarily through reporting, protective orders, and social support services, as well as protectives shelters. Finally, almost one-third of the laws address the need for treatment of physical and emotional problems associated with domestic violence (tertiary prevention; Table 10.15).

Table 10.14. Conceptual Elements of Victimization in Laws for the Prevention of Family or Domestic Maltreatment

Child abuse[265,307,310]	Emotional, psychological, or verbal abuse or violence[208,210-213, 215-217,220-222,226-233,235, 240-242,244,245,247,249,250, 252-254,256,257,259-261, 263,264,319]	Interference from in-laws[240]	Physical abuse or threat to harm someone[208,210-213, 215-217,220-222,226-229, 231-233, 235,240,242-245,247-250,252-254, 256,257,259-261,263,264,294,305,319]
Child marriage[240,319]	Entry into the victim's residence[a] without consent[208,217,228,240, 248]	Intimidation[208,218,220, 240,244]	Sexual abuse or threats of sexual abuse[208,210-212,215-217, 221,222,226-229,231-233,235, 240, 241,243-245,247-250,252-254,256, 257,259-261,263,264,294,305,319]
Cruelty to pets or injury/killing an animal[266,293,294]	Female genital mutilation[240,319]	Minor witnessing or hearing an act of domestic violence[244]	Spiritual violence[246]
Damage to or destruction of property[208,217,221,228, 230,240,243,245,246]	Forced marriage[240,319]	Moral damage[246]	Stalking[208,211,217,228,230,240, 244,265,293,319,361]
Defilement[240]	Forced wife inheritance[240]	Neglect[222,230]	Virginity testing[240]
Economic abuse[208, 210-212,215-217,222,227, 229-233,240,244,247-250,252, 256,257,259-261,264,319]	Harassment[208,211.213, 217,228-230,232,240,244,248, 254,256,260,262,265,294,319]	Parental kidnapping[273]	Widow cleansing[240]

[a] When the parties do not share the same residence.

Table 10.15. Prevention Components Proposed or Mandated by Domestic Victimization Laws

Awareness campaign/Public education[a,210,215,220,221,223,227,235,242,246,252,254,259,268,297,317,318,365]	Legal support for the victim[b,206,209,224,234,235,237,241,244,252,261]	Protective shelter and/or financial aid[b,209,215,220,223,225,226,234,241,244,247,252,254,257,259,261,265,276,283289,290,297,298,300,306,307,309,313,318,319,366]	Training for officials[b,216,219,226,227,231,235,242,244,247,252,257,266,268,271,273,278,280,284,295,297,300,313,317]
Courses about peaceful resolution of domestic conflict[a,242,247,365]	Mediation/Resolution[b,220,266,302,318]	Removal of perpetrator[b,206,208,213-216,224,225,230]	Medical or psychological evaluation/report and/or treatment[c,206,210,212,215,20,221,223,224,234,235,245-247,251,252,254,259,264,266,271,274,278,296,297,316,318]
Education activities for parents and families about family violence[a,226]	National database/registry[b,226,247,252,261,270,295,317]	Reporting[b,111.206,209,209,210,212,220,222-224,227,229,231,233,235,238,241,244,246,252,258,261,273,308,318]	Programs for children affected by family violence[c,271]
Prohibition or unlawfulness of domestic violence[a,220,229,235,244,247,249,257,263,318]	National strategy to protect victims[b,206]	Risk assessment[b,209,253,264]	Rehabilitation/counseling of victims and perpetrators[c,206,208,210,237,241,246,261,262,277,288,290,365]
Promotion of family relations based on mutual respect[a,210]	Penalties[b,207,215,219,220,222,223,225,233,258,277,281,287,291,292,312,317]	Social support services for domestic violence/Crisis center[b,206,209,210,212,222,223,233, 235,241,243,253,264,265,297,298,313,318]	Research on domestic violence's impact on health[c,215,221,223,227,243,244,247,319,365]
School curriculums that foster respect and avoidance of behaviors that promote family violence[a,215,219,220,227,247,252,253,259,268,318,365]	Professional training in domestic violence[b,300]	Specialized police corps or police units[b,207,209,227,252,259]	Spiritual guidance[c,235]
Psychosocial treatment of perpetrator[b,222,233,237,244,246,252, 254,261,265,267,271,272,274,277,282,284,286, 288,289,297,306,311]	Protective orders[b,206,208,210,212-225,227-257,260-271,273-278,280-286,288-290,293-300,302-313,315,317-319,358-364]	Support line (24 hours)[b,246,253,265,305,307]	Statistics and fatality review[c,210,233,241,242,246,265,266,271,273,274,280,284,290,297,299,311,358]

[a] Element of primary prevention.

[b] Element of secondary prevention.

[c] Element of tertiary prevention.

Table 10.16. Countries[a] That Have Enacted Laws Prohibiting, and/or Protecting Children from, Corporal Punishment

Albania[320]	Denmark[328]	Latvia[336]	Peru[b,344]
Austria[321]	Estonia[329]	Moldova[337]	Poland[345]
Benin[322]	Finland[330]	Mongolia[338]	Republic of Congo[346]
Bolivia[323]	France[331]	Netherlands[339]	Romania[347]
Brazil[324]	Georgia[332]	Nicaragua[340]	Slovenia[348]
Cabo Verde[325]	Germany[333]	North Macedonia[341]	South Sudan[349]
Costa Rica[326]	Hungary[334]	Norway[342]	Sweden[350]
Croatia[327]	Iceland[335]	Paraguay[b,343]	Ukraine[351]
			Uruguay[352]

[a] Countries for which legislative texts were found.[357]

[b] Law that exclusively addresses the prohibition of corporal punishment.

Laws Prohibiting Corporal Punishment

In at least 33 countries, legislation prohibits the use of corporal punishment, at least by parents (Table 10.16). All these decrees are included in laws that focus on the rights of children and adolescents,[320-326,332,336,338] family relationships and parental responsibilities,[327,328,330,331,333,337,339,340] or child protection.[329,334,335,341,343] The only statute that exclusively addresses the protection of children and adolescents against physical punishment or any other type of violence as a method of correction and discipline was enacted in Paraguay, in 2016, and is known as Law 5659.[343] This act prohibits physical punishment and demeaning treatment of children and adolescents as a "method of correction or discipline." Its primary prevention approach incorporates a call for public awareness, inclusion of positive parental guidelines in school curriculums, and development of programs to foster positive parenting and effective treatment of children.[343] Furthermore, the law deters the ongoing use of corporal punishment by ensuring a reporting system to an ombudsman for children, by supporting the role of a child protective unit that can provide further secondary prevention steps, by assessing risk, and by recommending further prevention measures, including parental training, counseling, or therapy, as well as rehabilitation and reintegration programs and services. The law apparently lacks provision for treatment of physical or emotional consequences of corporal punishment.

Laws for the Prevention of Harassment in the Street and Other Public Places

It is noteworthy that laws[353-356] are being developed and enacted to prevent exposure to sexual harassment in public places[353-355] or street harassment[356] (Table 10.17). Almost identical and

Table 10.17. Countries/Cities[a] That Have Enacted Laws to Prevent Harassment in Public Places, by strategies proposed or mandated

Preventive Strategy Proposed or Mandated	Argentina, City of Buenos Aires[353]	Chile[354]	Peru[355]	United States, Washington, DC[356]
Epidemiologic survey				✓
Penalty[c]	✓	✓	✓	
Public awareness[b]			✓	✓
Reporting[d]			✓	✓
School curriculum about harassment in public places[b]			✓	
Training of police officers[c]			✓	
Treatment of mental health problems associated with street harassment[d]			✓	

[a] Countries for which legislative texts were found.[357]

[b] Primary prevention.

[c] Secondary prevention.

[d] Tertiary prevention.

very comprehensive descriptions of sexual harassment in public places are found in related legislation enacted in Peru[355] and the City of Buenos Aires, Argentina.[353] This form of victimization is legally understood as

> physical or verbal behaviors of a sexual nature or connotation, based on gender, identity and/or sexual orientation, carried out by one or more persons against other or others, who do not want or reject these behaviors as they affect their dignity, their fundamental rights such as freedom, integrity and free movement, creating in them intimidation, hostility, degradation, humiliation or an offensive environment in public spaces and in the private spaces with public access.[353]

Sexual harassment in the public environment can include the following behaviors[353,355]:

- Direct or indirect comments about the victim's body
- Nonconsensual photographs and recordings
- Improper or nonconsensual physical contact
- Intimidation or cornering
- Masturbation or exhibitionism and obscene gestures or other expressions

The Peruvian law[355] to prevent and punish sexual harassment in public places, passed in 2015, distinguishes itself from the few similar statutes passed in other countries[353,354,356] in that it fully mandates deterrence strategies at all three levels of prevention (Table 10.17).

National Strategies for the Prevention of Bullying and Other Forms of Victimization

National Strategies for the Prevention of School Bullying and Cyberbullying

The *Global Status Report on Violence Prevention 2014*,[370] developed by the World Health Organization (WHO), provides insight into government efforts made to prevent diverse types of maltreatment in the 113 countries surveyed for the report. The report indicates that, in 2014, only 62 countries and territories had reported that they had implemented school antibullying programs[369] (Table 10.18). There are no data identifying the types of antibullying strategies implemented by each of the 62 countries, but a literature review[386] showed that least six nations had put into practice programs to prevent peer victimization and had published the outcomes[371-385] (Table 10.18).

Norway took a leading role in bullying prevention through the first national implementation of an antibullying strategy, the Olweus Bullying Prevention Program, as part of the First Bergen Project Against Bullying.[377] The Norwegian experience led the way for other countries to develop national strategies: Finland put into practice the KiVa Antibullying Program[374,375] and Austria implemented the Viennese Social Competence (VISC) training.[371,372] In the United States, the efficacy of bullying prevention was ascertained through trials with the Olweus Program,[381-383,385] Second Step: Student Success Through Prevention (SS-SSTP),[384] and Steps to Respect (STR).[380]

The US Department of Health and Human Services has been promoting public awareness about bullying and cyberbullying through a Web site known as StopBullying.gov.[387] The Web

Table 10.18. Countries and Territories[a] That Had Reported Implementation of Large-Scale School Antibullying Programs by 2014[370]

Afghanistan	Canada	Ghana	Kazakhstan	Nigeria	Singapore
Albania	China	Guatemala	Kuwait	Norway[377]	Slovakia
Australia	Colombia[373]	Iceland	Laos	Panama	South Africa
Austria[371,372]	Costa Rica	India	Lithuania	Peru	Spain
Bahrain	Croatia	Iran	Malawi	Qatar	Sweden
Belarus	Czech Rep	Iraq	Mexico	Romania	Thailand
Benin	Egypt	Israel	Montenegro	Rwanda	Trinidad and Tobago
Brazil	Finland[374,375]	Italy	Morocco	Samoa	Turkey
Bulgaria	Georgia	Japan	Netherlands	Serbia	United Kingdom[378,379]
Burundi	Germany[376]	Jordan	Nicaragua	Seychelles	United States[380-385]
					Vietnam
					West Bank and Gaza Strip

[a] Note numbers indicate study/studies related to school antibullying programs implemented in the country.

site provides information from different government agencies about the nature of bullying and cyberbullying and strategies for prevention and intervention.

In Canada, initiatives for bullying and cyberbullying prevention advocacy and research have been fostered by PREVNET,[388] a "national research and knowledge mobilization hub," founded in 2006 by Pepler and Craig. The network includes more than 100 researchers from different academic institutions in Canada, as well as more than 60 national organizations serving young people.[388]

Elsewhere, Colombia introduced the Classrooms in Peace (Aulas en Paz) program[373]; Germany has utilized *Medienhelden* ("Media Heroes"),[376] a classroom-based intervention to promote empathy and reduced cyberbullying; and the United Kingdom has implemented the KiVa program in Wales[378] and a trial of the INCLUSIVE program (initiating change locally in bullying aggression through the school environment) in secondary schools.[379]

The prevention of cyberbullying among adolescent students in Cordoba, Spain, was examined by Del Rey et al. in a study[389] using the ConRed Program,[390] and more recently with a research project[391] based on an intervention known as Asegúrate.[392]

A strategy to reduce the prevalence of cybervictimization among more than 3,000 adolescents in the city of Perth, Australia, was developed by Cross et al.[393] through a longitudinal study utilizing the Cyber Friendly Schools Program.[394]

National Initiatives for the Prevention of Workplace Bullying

Some of the national initiatives for the prevention of workplace bullying in Europe have been summarized in a report[395] published in 2010 by the European Agency for Safety and Health at Work (EU OSHA). This study[395] points out to the development, in the United Kingdom, of the National Occupational Standards for the Management and Prevention of Work-Related Violence.[396] These guidelines should provide employers with a framework in their development of policies and procedures to prevent workplace violence.[396]

The EU OSHA report on workplace harrasment[395] refers to the responsibility assigned to the Danish Working Environment Authority in receiving information, or a complaint, about harassment, assessing the case and issuing injunctions to the employer, if necessary. Another national strategy for the prevention of workplace victimization mentioned in the EU OSHA report[395] relates to the nationwide campaign known as "Working without bullying," launched by the government of Norway during 2005 to 2007, during which knowledge and guidelines about bullying were disseminated. This included a TV promotion, a wide-range training program for union members and managers, as well as the development of a webpage by the Norwegian Labor Inspection Authority (Arbeidstilsynet).[397]

The EU OSHA review[395] highlighted the international initiatives for the prevention of workplace victimization developed by the International Labour Organization (ILO) and WHO. ILO has released several publications[398-402] about violence at work and recommended some strategies[398] to tackle this form of victimization, including:

- Commitment of all participants to a prevention program and a written policy to apply it
- Use of screening tools to select the right individual for a job
- Training in communication and interpersonal skills to avert a hostile situation and to identify a potential violent situation, as well as training in how to respond

- Open communication and guidance to reduce the risk of violence at work
- Design of physical environment and layout to prevent violence
- Work organization and job design to reduce tensions
- Development of guidelines and procedures to defuse violent confrontations
- Recording and reporting of incidents
- Therapeutic support of the victim
- Monitoring and evaluation of the effectiveness of preventive measures

WHO has led an initiative to raise awareness about psychological harassment at work,[403] while also proposing preventive approaches to be used at the primary, secondary, and tertiary level of prevention.

National Strategies and Programs for the Prevention of Dating Violence

According to the 2014 WHO assessment of violence prevention, only 24 countries reported having developed strategies for the prevention of dating violence by 2014. At least six of these countries have published reports about their research in progress[404,405] or have completed studies[406-408] (Table 10.19).

In Brazil, an ongoing study protocol[404] worked to develop an online intervention, identified as Dating SOS (SOS Namoro), aimed to prevent victimization in dating relationships among people 15 to 29 years old. In Europe, an investigation known as Lights4Violence[405] promoted protective factors against gender violence among adolescents. This research[405] involves a longitudinal, "quasi-experimental" educational intervention geared to adolescents (age 13 to 17) of all genders who attend secondary schools in Alicante (Spain), Rome (Italy), Cardiff (Wales), Iasi (Romania), Poznan (Poland), and Matosinhos (Portugal).

In Canada, a strategy to prevent abuse between adolescent dating partners was implemented by Wolfe et al.[406] through a community-based intervention focused on 14- to 16-year-old teens who had a history of child maltreatment. The intervention was based on the Youth Relationships Project (YRP)[409] and consists of 18 sessions to prevent dating violence,

Table 10.19. Countries[a] That Had Reported Implementation of Dating Violence Prevention in Schools by 2014[370]

Australia	Canada[406]	Guinea	Romania[408]
Austria	Colombia	Israel	Rwanda
Belarus	Costa Rica	Italy[408]	Singapore
Belize	Croatia	Kazakhstan	Spain[405,408]
Benin	Cuba	Mexico[407]	Sweden
Botswana	Czech Republic	Mozambique	Thailand
Brazil[404]	Germany	Nicaragua	Vietnam

[a] Note numbers indicate study/studies related to dating violence school prevention programs implemented in the country.

involving education and awareness about abuse and power dynamics in intimate relationships, skill development, and social action.

Prevention of dating violence in Mexico City was pioneered by Sosa-Rubi et al.[407] through a pilot study among high school students. The students were exposed to a program known as "True Love" ("Amor... pero del Bueno"), which consists of a school-climate enhancement strategy component, based on schoolyard activities, and a classroom-based curriculum that aims to foster critical thinking about gender and dating norms, understanding of the sequelae of dating abuse, and learning of useful interaction skills to reduce conflicts.

In Southern Spain, Muñoz-Fernández et al.[408] investigated the efficacy of a school-based prevention program to reduce dating aggression and victimization among 2,050 adolescents. The research utilized a multicomponent program known as "Date-e-Adolescence," which involves seven one-hour sessions conducted during school hours, with the goals, among others, of providing understanding about healthy relationships, fostering recognition of emotional regulation, stimulation of better self-esteem, improvement in interaction abilities, and promotion of the recognition of violent behavior.

Efforts to avert violence among dating adolescents in the United States have been led by the Centers for Disease Control and Prevention (CDC) through the development and implementation of Dating Matters: Strategies to Promote Healthy Teen Relationships (DM),[410] "an evidence-based teen dating violence prevention model that includes prevention strategies for individuals, peers, families, schools, and neighborhoods."[410] From 2011 to 2016, the CDC piloted a DM demonstration project in Baltimore, Chicago, Oakland, and Fort Lauderdale. A study conducted in those cities by Niolon et al.[411] showed that the DM comprehensive model was more effective in reducing teen dating violence than the standard of care provided by the Safe Dates[412,413] evidence-based curriculum.

National Strategies for the Prevention of Sexual Violence

According to the WHO report[370] on violence prevention, 47 countries have implemented strategies for the prevention of sexual violence in schools and colleges, and related articles have been published in at least five countries (Table 10.20).

In Cuba, the responsibility of primary care settings and mental health centers for tackling the risk of violence against women has been underscored[414] with recommendations to provide appropriate training to health practitioners in the prevention, detection, and treatment of gender violence.

In 2019, a study[416] was developed in Mumbai, India, to provide community interventions to prevent violence against women and girls living in informal settlements. The project[416] is part of the SNEHA[419] (Society for Nutrition, Education and Health Action) program, and it evaluates the effects of community mobilization activities[416] on the prevalence of violence against women, as well as its disclosure.

An investigation led by Moor[417] assessed the efficacy of a rape prevention program for adolescent students provided in Israel by its Association of Rape Crisis Centers. The research involved almost 400 eleventh graders in the Sharon area of Israel. The students participated in three mandatory two-hour workshops that provided awareness about sexual violence (including sexual coercion), dismissed rape untruths, reinforced the ability to tolerate peer pressure, and taught respectful sexual behavior "based on mutuality and proper

Table 10.20. Countries[a] That Had Reported Implementation of Sexual Violence Prevention Programs in Schools and Colleges by 2014[370]

Australia	Kazakhstan
Bahrain	Malaysia
Belarus	Maldives
Belgium	Mexico
Belize	Montenegro
Benin	Morocco
Botswana	Netherlands
Brazil	Nicaragua
Cameroon	Philippines
Canada	Poland
China	Qatar
Colombia	Romania
Costa Rica	Rwanda
Croatia	Saudi Arabia
Cuba[414]	Senegal
Czech Republic	Seychelles
Ecuador	Singapore
Finland	Slovakia
Germany	Spain
Ghana[415]	Sudan
India[416]	Sweden
Iraq	Tuvalu
Israel[417]	United Kingdom
	United States[418]

[a] Note number indicates a study pertaining to sexual violence prevention programs implemented in the country.

communication."[417] The project[417] led to awareness of how to differentiate rape from mutually consensual relationships, as well as a notable change in "rape-supportive attitudes."

In the central region of Ghana, a research project[415] was conducted to prevent or reduce violence against women, using a community response model known as COMBAT, an acronym for Community-Based Action Teams.[420] The program sensitizes the community by raising awareness about the "harmful effects of violence as well as the benefits of a relationship based on equality."[415]

Since 2000, initiatives for the prevention of sexual violence in the United States have been advanced by the Division of Violence Prevention (DVP) within the CDC's Injury Center.[421]

A summary of its activities from 2000 to 2010 can be found in a review published by DeGue et al.,[418] which highlights the DVP's efforts to advance the profile of sexual violence as a public health question, to focus on primary prevention of perpetration, and to use a public health framework for sexual violence research and prevention strategies. The DVP has published a "technical package"[422] that includes a compilation of strategies to help communities and states prevent sexual violence and its consequences.

A survey[423] of sexual violence prevention activities implemented in non-Māori and bicultural communities in New Zealand has shown that the main emphasis of prevention efforts was on sexual violence education, followed by public policy advocacy and sexual awareness-raising activities. There was less focus on the implementation of youth sexual violence primary prevention programs, prevention strategies with specific communities or cultural groups, and child abuse primary prevention programs.

National Initiatives for the Prevention of Family Violence

Australia,[424-427] Canada,[428,429] and the United States[430-434] have implemented national programs for the prevention of family violence.

The Australian government has put into action the National Plan to Reduce Violence against Women and Their Children 2010–2022[424] ("National Plan"), coordinating the efforts of states and territories to reduce domestic or family violence, through four three-year action plans. In August 2019, the Council of Australian Governments released the Fourth Action Plan 2019–2022.[425] This plan has, among its national priorities, a focus on primary prevention, support for First Australian Nations women and children, consideration of the lived experience and knowledge of women and their children affected by violence, response to sexual violence and sexual harassment, and improved responses of support and service systems. As part of the National Plan,[424] the Australian government approved funding for "developing innovative ways of using technology to keep women safe (GPS trackers for perpetrators, safe phones and safety devices for homes), extending support services in remote Indigenous communities, as well as education resources to teach young people about respectful relationships."[426] The National Plan[424] also helped to support a 24-hour counseling service as 1800RESPECT,[427] a national 24-hour sexual assault and domestic/family violence counseling service.

In 1988, the Public Health Agency of Canada developed the Family Violence Initiative,[428] a collaborative forum of 12 governmental agencies, aimed to prevent and respond to family violence. The objectives included increasing public awareness of the risk factors for family violence, improvement of government agencies' ability to respond to the problem, and support of data collection, research, and evaluation strategies to identify effective interventions. Canada's Family Violence Initiative has facilitated the development of a Web site, known as Stop Family Violence,[429] that promotes public awareness of the problem, facilitates referrals to support and service programs, and provides resources to professionals as well as information about federal funding.

In the United States, the national effort to address family violence began in 1984, with the passage of the Family Violence Prevention and Services Act (FVPSA).[430] Responsibility for administration of US federal funding of assistance for victims of family violence and their children has been delegated to the Family Violence Prevention and Services Program

(FVPSA Program[431]), which oversees provision of shelters and other support services and coordination of state programs for the prevention of, and intervention for, domestic violence. Furthermore, the FVPSA Program is responsible for promoting public awareness of the prevalence of family violence and for supporting local programs with technical assistance in areas like trauma-informed care, co-occurrence of domestic violence and child maltreatment, culturally specific domestic violence services, and effective interventions for children exposed to domestic violence.[431] The FVPSA Program funds grants to states, territories, Tribal Nations, state domestic violence coalitions,[432] national resource centers,[433] and the national domestic violence hotline.[434]

An important initiative for the prevention of family violence in New Zealand was the development, in 2005, of the New Zealand Family Violence Clearinghouse (NZFVC),[435,436] a national center for family and Whānau[437] violence research and information. The NZFVC, which is operated by the University of Auckland under a contract funded by the Ministry of Justice, provides, among other services, a very extensive library (with some of material available online), news updated several times a week, lists of upcoming professional events and community activities, bibliographies, and data summaries.

The government of New Zealand has issued a document[438] proposing a framework for screening, assessing, and managing family violence, which includes practice guidelines specifically aimed at general services providers (who don't specialize in family violence), statutory service providers (individuals whose core activity is partly involved in family violence), and specialist service providers (providers working in specialist family violence agencies or organizations).

Future Directions

Future national or regional legislative initiatives for the prevention of bullying and other forms of maltreatment should be developed within a public health framework that recognizes the evolving understanding of the nature, prevalence, and co-occurrence of different forms of victimization across social settings and along the life span, as well as their associated health risks. The laws should make available funding for programs to foster and provide:

- Mutual respect, support, and sensitivity to others, across social settings and all age groups, as a principle of public safety and well-being
- Awareness about the nature and toxicity of diverse types of victimization and ways of preventing them, by incorporating this knowledge into educational curriculums from pre-K thru graduate school, workplace forums, and public campaigns
- Understanding of the need to report incidents of bullying and other forms of maltreatment as part of the public health aim to stop ongoing victimization
- Development of a reporting system, through an ombudsman for victims and with 24- hour online availability, to receive and rapidly examine reports about incidents of victimization, while promptly procuring and facilitating victims' access to available agencies and strategies to ensure their support and safety
- Establishment of assistance programs for the delivery of medical, psychological, social, and/or legal support to victims, as well as settings for providing psychosocial help to perpetrators, to stop ongoing victimization of others
- Treatment services for sequelae of victimization

- Training of health practitioners in the detection of victimization and related health problems, as well as providing mental health professionals with continuing medical education in the treatment of acute and chronic conditions associated with victimization
- Programs to train educators, workplace managers, lawyers, police officers, and judges about the potential cognitive, memory, perceptual, and performance impairment affecting victims
- Programs to help lawyers, police officers, and judges understand the emotional distress that may be experienced by a victim due to the need to recall traumatic details (e.g., place or circumstances linked to the victimization) or to encounter the victimizer for the purpose of an investigation or judicial testimony
- Research programs to monitor the prevalence of different forms of victimization and associated health risks, to ensure ongoing monitoring of the efficacy of present and future national prevention efforts

Notes

1. Argentina, Law 26,892. Law for the promotion of coexistence and the approach to social conflict in educational institutions, 2013. https://www.argentina.gob.ar/normativa/nacional/ley-26892-220645/texto?_x_tr_sl+=+es&_x_tr_tl+=+en&_x_tr_hl+=+en&_x_tr_pto+=+sc. Accessed September 22, 2023. [Title and text translation from Google]
2. Argentina, Province of Buenos Aires, Law 14750. Law for the promotion of coexistence and the approach to social conflict in educational institutions, 2015. https://normas.gba.gob.ar/documentos/BKav4Co0.html#:~:text=%2D%20Esta%20Ley%20tiene%20por%20objeto,la%20Ley%20Nacional%20N%C2%BA%2026892. Accessed September 14, 2022. [Title and text translation from Google]
3. Argentina, Provincia of Catamarca, Ley 5402. Exclusion del maltrato y promoción de la cultura de paz en la comunidad educative andomize, 2015. Boletin Official y Judicial, No 9, 30/04/2015, Páginas 243–248. https://web.catamarca.edu.ar/sitio/images/documentos/normativas/nuevas/ley_provincial_5.416_educacion_uso_del_guardapolvo_blanco_nivel_primario.pdf. Accessed September 15, 2022. [Text in Spanish, English translation not available from Google]
4. Argentina, Province of Chaco, Law 4986. Provincial Plan for the Prevention of Violence in Schools, 2010. https://todosobremediacion.com.ar/planprovincial/?_x_tr_sl = es&_x_tr_tl = en&_x_tr_hl = en&_x_tr_pto = sc. Accessed September 15, 2022. [Title and text translation from Google]
5. Argentina, Province of Corrientes, Ley No 6212, 2013. http://www.hcdcorrientes.gov.ar/Leyes-texto/Ley6212.pdf?_x_tr_sch = http&_x_tr_sl = es&_x_tr_tl = en&_x_tr_hl = en&_x_tr_pto = sc&_x_tr_sl = auto&_x_tr_tl = en&_x_tr_hl = en&_x_tr_pto = nui. Accessed September 15, 2022. [Text in Spanish, English translation not available from Google]
6. Argentina, Provincia de Entre Rios, Ley 9655, 2005. https://www.senadoer.gob.ar/descargas/3666. Accessed September 22, 2023. [Text in Spanish, no English translation available from Google]
7. Argentina, Provincia de Neuquen, Ley 2635, 2008. http://www.legislaturaneuquen.gob.ar/svrfiles/Neuleg/normaslegales/pdf/LEY2635.pdf?var = 1092762507&_x_tr_sch = http&_x_tr_sl = es&_x_tr_tl = en&_x_tr_hl = en&_x_tr_pto = sc. Accessed September 15, 2022. [Text in Spanish, no English translation available from Google]

8. Argentina, Provincia de Rio Negro, Ley 4977, 2014. https://web.legisrn.gov.ar/legislativa/legislacion/documento?id=9127. Accessed September 22, 2023. [Text in Spanish, no English translation available from Google]
9. Argentina, Provincia de San Luis, Ley Nº II-0858-2013. https://diputados.sanluis.gob.ar/diputadosweb/Contenido/Pagina120/File/Legajo%20Ley%20II-0858-2013.pdf. Accessed September 15, 2022. [Text in Spanish, English translation not available from Google]
10. Argentina, Province of Santa Fe, Law 13674, 2017. https://www.santafe.gov.ar/boletinoficial/recursos/boletines/19-06-2018ley13674-2018.html. Accessed September 15, 2022. [Title and text translation from Google]
11. Argentina, Provincia de Tierra del Fuego, Ley 937, 2012. http://www.legistdf.gob.ar/lp/leyes/Provinciales/LEYP937.pdf. Accessed September 22, 2023 [Text in Spanish, English translation not available from Google]
12. Brazil, Brasilia, Law 13185, 2015. https://www.planalto.gov.br/ccivil_03/_ato2015-2018/2015/lei/l13185.htm. Accessed September 22, 2023. [Title and text translation from Google]
13. Brazil, State of Goias, Law 17,151, 2010. https://legisla.casacivil.go.gov.br/pesquisa_legislacao/89139/lei-17151. Accessed September 16, 2022. [Title and text translation from Google]
14. Brazil, State of Maranhao, Law 9297, 2010. https://www.legisweb.com.br/legislacao/?id=130691. Accessed September 22, 2023. [Title and text translation from Google]
15. Brazil, State of Mato Grosso, Law 9724, 2012. https://www.legisweb.com.br/legislacao/?id=240539. Accessed September 22, 2023. [Title and text translation from Google]
16. Brazil, State of Mato Grosso do Sul, Law 3887, 2010. https://www.legisweb.com.br/legislacao/?id=139239. Accessed September 22, 2023. [Title and text translation from Google]
17. Brazil, State of Parana, Law 17355, 2012. https://www.legisweb.com.br/legislacao/?id=246061. Accessed September 22, 2023. [Title and text translation from Google]
18. Brazil, State of Pernambuco, Law 13995, 2009. https://www.legisweb.com.br/legislacao/?id=150119. Accessed September 22, 2023. [Title and text translation from Google]
19. Brazil, State of Rio de Janeiro, Law 6084, 2011. https://www.jusbrasil.com.br/legislacao/1030039/lei-6084-11. Accessed September 22, 2023. [Title and text translation from Google]
20. Canada, Province of Alberta, Education Act, Statutes of Alberta, 2012 Chapter E-0.3. Current as of January 1, 2020. §31 (c; d; e); §32 (d); §33(d; k); §35(1); §35.1(1); §36(1) (a)(b); §37(1)(a)(b). http://www.qp.alberta.ca/documents/Acts/e00p3.pdf. Accessed September 16, 2022.
21. Canada, Province of Manitoba, C.C.S.M. c. P250 The Public Schools Act 47.1(2);47.1.1;47.1.2. https://web2.gov.mb.ca/laws/statutes/ccsm/_pdf.php?cap=p250. Accessed September 22, 2023.
22. Canada, Province of Nova Scotia, Education (CSAP) Act Chapter 1 of the Acts of 1995–96 Subsection 64(2) (f) (ra);(rb). https://www.canlii.org/en/ns/laws/stat/sns-1995-96-c-1/latest/sns-1995-96-c-1.html. Accessed September 16, 2022.
23. Canada, Province of Ontario, Education Act R.S.O. 1990, Chapter E.2 169.1 (1;2;2.1;3;4;5). https://www.ontario.ca/laws/statute/90e02#BK144. Accessed September 16, 2022.
24. Canada, Province of Quebec, chapter I-13.3 Education Act 18.1;75.1;75.2;75.3;77;83.1;96.6;96.7.1. http://legisquebec.gouv.qc.ca/en/showdoc/cs/I-13.3?langCont = en#ga:l_i-gb:l_iii-h1. Accessed September 16, 2022.
25. Colombia, Law 1620, 2013. https://www.icbf.gov.co/cargues/avance/docs/ley_1620_2013.htm. Accessed September 22, 2023. [Title and text translation from Google]
26. Costa Rica, Law 9404, 2016. http://www.pgrweb.go.cr/scij/Busqueda/Normativa/Normas/nrm_texto_completo.aspx?param1=NRTC&nValor1=1&nValor2=83200&nValor3=106726&strTipM=TC. Accessed September 22, 2023. [Title and text translation from Google]

27. Denmark, Act No 166 of March 14, 2001, on the teaching environment of pupils and students. https://www.retsinformation.dk/eli/lta/2001/166. Accessed September 16, 2022. [Title and text translation from Google]
28. El Salvador, Reformas a la Ley de Protección Integral de la Niñez y Adolescencia Artículo 85-A.- Del acoso en el ámbito escolar. https://www.asamblea.gob.sv/sites/default/files/documents/decretos/800157B0-B762-4304-82AD-9A3833078585.pdf. Accessed September 22, 2023. [Text in Spanish, English translation not available from Google]
29. Honduras, Decreto No. 96-2014. https://www.tsc.gob.hn/web/leyes/Ley_contra_acoso_escolar.pdf. Accessed September 16, 2022. [Text in Spanish, English translation not available from Google]
30. India, UGC Regulations on Curbing the Menace of Ragging in Higher Educational Institutions, 2009. https://www.nitt.edu/home/students/UGC_Regulations.pdf. Accessed September 16, 2022. [Title and text translation from Google]
31. Japan, Bullying Prevention Measures Promotion Act (Act No. 71 of 2013). https://www.japaneselawtranslation.go.jp/en/laws/view/3748/en. Accessed September 26, 2023. [Title and text translation from Google]
32. Lithuania, Education Law I-1489 Amending Articles 1, 2, 19, 23, 43, 46, 47, 49, 56, 58, 59 and Supplementing Article 23 2016 October Dec. https://e-seimas.lrs.lt/portal/legalAct/lt/TAD/17d94ea2976411e68adcda1bb2f432d1. Accessed September 16, 2022. [Title and text translation from Google]
33. Mexico, State of Aguascalientes, Ley para Prevenir, Tratar y Erradicar la Violencia Escolar en el Estado de Aguascalientes, 2019. https://eservicios2.aguascalientes.gob.mx/NormatecaAdministrador/archivos/EDO-18-100.pdf. Accessed September 26, 2023. [Text in Spanish, English translation not available from Google]
34. Mexico, State of Baja California Ley para Prevenir y Evitar el Acoso Escolar en el Estado de Baja California, 2014. http://dceg.bajacalifornia.gob.mx/Sasip/documentos/archivos/cec51201872152047974_24.pdf?_x_tr_sch = http&_x_tr_sl = es&_x_tr_tl = en&_x_tr_hl = en&_x_tr_pto = sc. Accessed September 16, 2022. [Text in Spanish, English translation not available from Google]
35. Mexico, State of Baja California Sur, Ley para Prevenir, Atender y Erradicar la Violencia y el Maltrato Escolar del Estado de Baja California Sur, 2015. http://www.ordenjuridico.gob.mx/Documentos/Estatal/Baja%20California%20Sur/wo120353.pdf. Accessed September 26, 2023. [Text in Spanish, English translation not available from Google]
36. Mexico, State of Coahulla, Ley para la Prevención, Atención y Control del Acoso Escolar para el Estado de Coahula de Zaragoza, 2015 https://www.congresocoahuila.gob.mx/transparencia/03/Leyes_Coahuila/coa228.pdf. Accessed September 26, 2023. [Text in Spanish, English translation not available from Google]
37. Mexico, State of Colima, Decreto No 310 Ley de Seguridad Integral Escolar para el Estado de Colima. https://www.secolima.gob.mx/doctos/juridico/NORMATECA%20INTERNA%20COMPLETA/(02)%20NORMAS%20ESTATALES/(39).pdf. Accessed September 16, 2022. [Text in Spanish, English translation not available from Google]
38. Mexico, State of Guanajauto, Ley para una Convivencia Libre de Violencia en el Entorno Escolar para el Esatdo de Gunajato y sus Municipios, 2017. https://www.poderjudicial-gto.gob.mx/pdfs/Ley%20para%20una%20Convivencia%20Libre%20de%20Violencia%20en%20el%20Entorno%20Escolar%20para%20el%20Estado%20de%20Guanajuato%20y%20sus%20Municipios%2022-jul-20.pdf. Accessed September 18, 2022. [Text in Spanish, English translation not available from Google]

39. Mexico, State of Guerrero, Ley Número 1256 para la Promoción de la Convivencia Libre de Violencia en el Entorno Escolar del Estado de Guerrero, 2012. https://oce.uaq.mx/docs/Marcos_CE/Marcos_estatales/Guerrero/GUERRERO_Ley_1256_para_la_promocion_de_la_convivencia_libre_de_violencia_en_el_entorno_escolar_2015.pdf?_x_tr_sl = es&_x_tr_tl = en&_x_tr_hl = en&_x_tr_pto = sc. Accessed September 18, 2022. [Text in Spanish, English translation not available from Google]
40. Mexico, State of Hidalgo, Ley para la Prevención, Atención y Erradicación de la Violencia Escolar en el Estado de Hidalgo, 2013. http://www.congreso-hidalgo.gob.mx/biblioteca_legislativa/leyes_cintillo/Ley%20para%20la%20Prevencion%20Atencion%20y%20Erradicacion%20de%20Violencia%20Escolar%20en%20el%20Estado%20de%20Hidalgo.pdf. Accessed September 18, 2022. [Text in Spanish, English translation not available from Google]
41. Mexico, State of Mexico, Ley para Prevenir y Atender el Acosos Escolar en el Estado de Mexico, 2018. https://legislacion.edomex.gob.mx/sites/legislacion.edomex.gob.mx/files/files/pdf/ley/vig/leyvig249.pdf. Accessed September 18, 2022. [Text in Spanish, English translation not available from Google]
42. Mexico, State of Michoacan, Ley para la Atención de la Violencia Escolar en el Estado de Michoacán, 2011. http://congresomich.gob.mx/file/Ley-para-la-Atenci%C3%B3n-de-la-Violencia-Escolar-en-el-Estado-de-Michoac%C3%A1n..pdf. Accessed September 26, 2023. [Text in Spanish, English translation not available from Google]
43. Mexico, State of Nueva Leon, Law to Prevent, Treat and Eradicate Harassment and School Violence, 2013. https://www.hcnl.gob.mx/trabajo_legislativo/leyes/leyes/ley_para_prevenir_atender_y_erradicar_el_acoso_y_la_violencia_escolar_del_estado_de_nuevo_leon/#:~:text = La%20presente%20Ley%20es%20de,de%20manera%20directa%20o%20indirecta%2C. Accessed September 18, 2022. [Title and text translation from Google]
44. Mexico, State of Oaxaca, Ley contra la Violencia y el Acoso entre Iguales para el Estado de Oaxaca, 2014. https://docs64.congresooaxaca.gob.mx/documents/legislacion_estatals/193.pdf. Accessed September 18, 2022. [Text in Spanish, English translation not available from Google]
45. Mexico, State of Quintana Roo, Ley para Prevenir, Atender y Erradicar la Violencia entre Estudiantes del Estado de Quintana Roo, 2013. http://documentos.congresoqroo.gob.mx/leyes/educacion/ley142/L1320130619285.pdf?_x_tr_sch = http&_x_tr_sl = es&_x_tr_tl = en&_x_tr_hl = en&_x_tr_pto = sc. Accessed September 18, 2022. [Text in Spanish, English translation not available from Google]
46. Mexico, State of San Luis Potosi, Ley de Prevención y Seguridad Escolar del Estado y Municipios de San Luis de Potosi, 2013. http://www.cegaipslp.org.mx/HV2019Tres.nsf/nombre_de_la_vista/1678812453C210AF862584790066672D/$File/21-Ley_de_Prevencion_y_Seguridad_Escolar_del_Estado_y_Municipios_+01_Jun_2019.pdf. Accessed September 26, 2023. [Text in Spanish, English translation not available from Google]
47. Mexico, State of Sinaloa, Ley para Prevenir, Atender y Erradicar la Violencia Escolar del Estado de Sinaloa, 2016. http://www.ordenjuridico.gob.mx/Documentos/Estatal/Sinaloa/wo120496.pdf. Accessed September 18, 2022. [Text in Spanish, English translation not available from Google]
48. Mexico, State of Tamaulipas, Ley para la Prevención de la Violencia en el Entorno Escolar del Estado de Tamaulipas, 2013. https://vlex.com.mx/vid/ley-prevencion-violencia-ento

rno-575244326. Accessed September 26, 2023. [Text in Spanish, English translation not available from Google]

49. Mexico, State of Tlaxcala, Ley para Prevenir y Cobatir la Violencia Escolar en el Estado de Tlaxcala, 2015. https://ofstlaxcala.gob.mx/doc/Legislacion/locales/leyes/LEY%20PARA%20PREVENIR%20Y%20COMBATIR%20LA%20VIOLENCIA%20ESCOLAR%20EN%20EL%20ESTADO%20DE%20TLAXCALA.pdf. Accessed September 18, 2022. [Text in Spanish, English translation not available from Google]
50. Mexico, State of Nayarit, Ley de Seguridad Integral Escolar para el Estado de Nayarit, Relativa al Acoso Escolar, 2010. https://vlex.com.mx/vid/ley-seguridad-integral-escolar-575273770. Accessed September 26, 2023. [Text in Spanish, English translation not available from Google]
51. Mexico, Federal District, Ley para la Promoción de la Convivencia Libre de Violencia en el Entorno Escolar del Distrito Federal, 2012. https://www.cndh.org.mx/sites/default/files/doc/Programas/VIH/LeyesNormasReglamentos/Leyes/LeyesEspecificasVIH/Ley_PCLVEE_DF.pdf. Accessed October 15, 2023. [Text in Spanish, English translation not available from Google]
52. Mexico, State of Puebla, Ley de Seguridad Integral Escolar para el Estado Libre y Soberano de Puebla, 2011. http://www.ordenjuridico.gob.mx/Documentos/Estatal/Puebla/wo105242.pdf?_x_tr_sch = http&_x_tr_sl = es&_x_tr_tl = en&_x_tr_hl = en&_x_tr_pto = sc. Accessed September 19, 2022. [Text in Spanish, English translation not available from Google]
53. Mexico, State of Veracruz, Ley Número 303 Contra el Acoso Escolar para el Estado de Veracruz de Ignacio De La Llave, 2011. https://www.sev.gob.mx/educacion-primaria-estatal/files/2013/04/LEYCONTRAELACOSOESCOLAR.pdf. Accessed September 19, 2022. [Text in Spanish, English translation not available from Google]
54. Mexico, State of Yucatan, Ley para la prevención, combate y erradicación de la violencia en el entorno escolar del Estado de Yucatán, 2012. http://oce.uaq.mx/docs/Marcos_CE/Marcos_estatales/Yucatan/YUCATAN_Ley_prevencion_combate_erradicacion_violencia_entorno_escolar_2013.pdf. Accessed September 19, 2022. [Text in Spanish, English translation not available from Google]
55. Norway, Amendment Act to the Education Act on amendments to the Act of July 17, 1998, No. 61 on primary and secondary education LOV-2002-12-20-112 Changing LOV-1998-07-17-61. https://lovdata.no/dokument/LTI/lov/2002-12-20-112. Accessed September 18, 2022. [Title and text translation from Google]
56. Paraguay, Law No 4633, Against School Harassment in Public, Private or Private Subsidized Educational Institutions, 2015. https://www.bacn.gov.py/leyes-paraguayas/3112/contra-el-acoso-escolar-en-instituciones-educativas-publicas-privadas-o-privadas-subvencionadas. Accessed September 26, 2023. [Title and text translation from Google]
57. Peru, Ley que promueve la convivencia andomized sin violencia en las instituciones educativas, Ley N° 29719, 2011. https://cdn.www.gob.pe/uploads/document/file/105175/_29719_-_11-10-2012_11_42_55_-LEY_29719.pdf. Accessed September 19, 2022. [Text in Spanish, English translation not available from Google]
58. Philippines, Republic Act No. 10627, An Act Requiring All Elementary and Secondary Schools To Adopt Policies To Prevent and Address the Acts of Bullying in Their Institutions, 2012. https://www.officialgazette.gov.ph/2013/09/12/republic-act-no-10627/. Accessed September 20, 2022.

59. Sweden, Sweden School Act (2010: 800) ch 6. Measures against abusive treatment. https://www.riksdagen.se/sv/dokument-och-lagar/dokument/svensk-forfattningssamling/skollag-2010800_sfs-2010-800/#K6. Accessed September 26, 2023. [Title and text translation from Google]
60. Ukraine, Law of Ukraine on Amendments to Some Legislative Acts of Ukraine on Countering Bullying (Information of the Verkhovna Rada (VVR), 2019, No. 5, Article 33). https://zakon.rada.gov.ua/laws/show/2657-19#Text. Accessed September 26, 2023. [Title and text translation from Google]
61. Ala. Code §16-28B-5. https://www.alabamaachieves.org/wp-content/uploads/2021/06/Harassment-Section-16-28B-3-Information.pdf. Accessed October 15, 2023.
62. Alaska Stat. §14.33.200. https://education.alaska.gov/tls/safeschools/Docs/AS_14.33.200_14.33.250.pdf. Accessed September 20, 2022.
63. Territory of American Samoa, American Samoa Compilation of School Discipline Laws and Regulations, Student Policy Handbook. §22. Control of dangerous and anti-social behavior—Bullying. Student Policy Handbook. §55. Use of technology. https://safesupportivelearning.ed.gov/sites/default/files/discipline-compendium/American%20Samoa%20School%20Discipline%20Laws%20and%20Regulations.pdf. Accessed September 20, 2022.
64. Ariz. Rev. Stat. 15-341-40 (2005). https://codes.findlaw.com/az/title-15-education/az-rev-st-sect-15-341.html. Accessed September 20, 2022.
65. Ark. Code Ann. §6-18-514. https://law.justia.com/codes/arkansas/2012/title-6/subtitle-2/chapter-18/subchapter-5/section-6-18-514. Accessed September 20, 2022.
66. Colo. Rev. Stat. 22-32-109.1. https://codes.findlaw.com/co/title-22-education/co-rev-st-sect-22-32-109-1.html. Accessed September 20, 2022.
67. Conn. Gen. Stat. §10-222d. https://law.justia.com/codes/connecticut/2014/title-10/chapter-170/section-10-222d. Accessed September 21, 2022.
68. Del. Code-§4112A-E. https://law.justia.com/codes/delaware/2014/title-14/chapter-41/section-4112. Accessed September 20, 2022.
69. D.C. Code §2–1535.03. https://code.dccouncil.us/dc/council/code/sections/2-1535.02.html. Accessed September 20, 2022.
70. Fla. Stat. §1006.147. https://codes.findlaw.com/fl/title-xlviii-k20-education-code/fl-st-sect-1006-147.html. Accessed September 20, 2022.
71. Ga. Code §20-2-751.4. https://codes.findlaw.com/ga/title-20-education/ga-code-sect-20-2-751-5.html. Accessed September 20, 2022.
72. Territory of Guam, Guam 17 GCA §3112.1. http://www.guamcourts.org/CompilerofLaws/GCA/17gca/17gc003.pdf#xml = http://www.guamcourts.org/JusticeDocs/dtSearch/dtisapi6.dll?cmd = getpdfhits&u = 1146fb25&DocId = 619&Index=%252a35e832c666b950bea561c27fb68c949f&HitCount = 77&hits = 7b + ef+102 + 103+104 + 2e9+303 + 3a7+402 + b69+caf + d0d+1091 + 1582+1635 + 1636+1637 + 166a+16c7 + 1716+171b + 1724+. Accessed September 20, 2022.
73. Haw. Admin. R. §8-19. http://boe.hawaii.gov/policies/AdminRules/Pages/AdminRule19.aspx. Accessed September 20, 2022.
74. Idaho Stat. 33-1631. https://legislature.idaho.gov/statutesrules/idstat/Title33/T33CH16/SECT33-1631/. Accessed September 20, 2022.
75. Ill. Comp. Stat.105 5/27-23.7. https://www.ilga.gov/legislation/ilcs/fulltext.asp?DocName=010500050K27-23.7. Accessed September 26, 2023.

76. Ind. Code 20-33-8-13.5. https://codes.findlaw.com/in/title-20-education/in-code-sect-20-33-8-13-5.html. Ind. Code 20-26-5-34.2. Accessed September 20, 2022. https://law.justia.com/codes/indiana/2019/title-20/article-26/chapter-5/section-20-26-5-34-2/. Ind. Code 20-33-8-13.5. Accessed September 20, 2022. https://law.justia.com/codes/indiana/2019/title-20/article-33/chapter-8/section-20-33-8-13-5/. Accessed September 20, 2022.
77. Iowa Code 280.28. https://www.legis.iowa.gov/docs/code/280.28.pdf. Accessed September 20, 2022.
78. Kan. Stat. 72-6147. https://www.ksrevisor.org/statutes/chapters/ch72/072_061_0047.html. Accessed September 20, 2022.
79. Ky. Rev. Stat. Ann. §158.148. https://apps.legislature.ky.gov/law/statutes/statute.aspx?id = 45145. Accessed September 20, 2022.
80. La. Rev. Stat. §17:416.13. https://law.justia.com/codes/louisiana/2011/rs/title17/rs17-416-13/. Accessed September 20, 2022.
81. Me. Rev. Stat. Title 20-A §6554. http://www.mainelegislature.org/legis/statutes/20-a/title20-Asec6554.html. Accessed September 20, 2022.
82. Md. Code §7-424.1. https://law.justia.com/codes/maryland/2019/education/division-ii/title-7/subtitle-4/sect-7-424-1/. Accessed September 20, 2022. Md. Code §7-424.3. https://law.justia.com/codes/maryland/2018/education/division-ii/title-7/subtitle-4/section-7-424.3/. Accessed September 20, 2022.
83. Mass. Gen. Laws, Part I, Title XII, ch 71, §370. https://malegislature.gov/Laws/GeneralLaws/PartI/TitleXII/Chapter71/Section37O#:~:text="Bullying"%2C%20the%20repeated,a%20written%2C%20verbal%20or%20electronic. Accessed September 27, 2023.
84. Mich. Comp. Laws §380.1310b. http://www.legislature.mi.gov/(S(skc2d4gzcl3h2z21a3mj2wts))/mileg.aspx?page=GetObject&objectname=mcl-380-1310b. Accessed September 27, 2023.
85. Minn. Stat. 121A.031. https://www.revisor.mn.gov/statutes/cite/121A.031. Accessed September 22, 2022.
86. Miss. Code §37-11-54. https://law.justia.com/codes/mississippi/2020/title-37/chapter-11/section-37-11-57/. Accessed September 27, 2023. Miss. Code §37-11-67. https://codes.findlaw.com/ms/title-37-education/ms-code-sect-37-11-67.html. Accessed September 22, 2022.
87. Mo. Rev. Stat. 160.775. https://law.justia.com/codes/missouri/2016/title-xi/chapter-160/section-160.775. Accessed September 20, 2022.
88. Mont. Code 20-5-207 through 20-5-210 https://law.justia.com/codes/montana/2022/title-20/chapter-5/part-2/. Accessed September 28, 2023. Mont. Admin. R. 10.55.801. School climate. https://rules.mt.gov/gateway/ruleno.asp?RN=10.55.801. Accessed September 28, 2023.
89. Neb. Rev. Stat. 79-2,137. https://law.justia.com/codes/nebraska/2016/chapter-79/statute-79-2-137. Accessed September 28, 2023.
90. Nev. Rev Stat. §388.133(2011). https://law.justia.com/codes/nevada/2011/chapter-388/statute-388.133/. Accessed September 20, 2022.
91. N.H. Rev. Stat. §193-F:4 (2014). https://law.justia.com/codes/new-hampshire/2014/title-xv/chapter-193-f/section-193-f-4/. Accessed September 20, 2022.
92. N.J. Rec. Stat. §18a:37-15 (2018). https://law.justia.com/codes/new-jersey/2018/title-18a/chapter-37/section-18a-37-15/. Accessed September 22, 2022.
93. N.M. Code §6.12.7.1-8. https://regulations.justia.com/states/new-mexico/title-6/chapter-12/part-7/. Accessed September 20, 2022.

94. N.Y. Educ. Law §12, §13, and §14. https://www.nysenate.gov/legislation/laws/EDN/12. Accessed September 20, 2022. https://www.nysenate.gov/legislation/laws/EDN/13. Accessed September 20, 2022. https://www.nysenate.gov/legislation/laws/EDN/14. Accessed September 20, 2022.
95. N.C. Gen. Stat. §115C-407.15-17. https://law.justia.com/codes/north-carolina/2015/chapter-115c/article-29c/section-115c-407.15/. Accessed September 22, 2022. https://law.justia.com/codes/north-carolina/2015/chapter-115c/article-29c/section-115c-407.16/. Accessed September 22, 2022. https://law.justia.com/codes/north-carolina/2015/chapter-115c/article-29c/section-115c-407.17/. Accessed September 22, 2022.
96. N.D. Cent. Code 15.1-19-17 through 15.1-19-22. https://www.ndlegis.gov/cencode/t15-1c19.pdf. Accessed September 22, 2022.
97. Ohio Rev. Code 3313.666-667. https://law.justia.com/codes/ohio/2011/title33/chapter3313/section3313-666. Accessed September 28, 2023.
98. Okla. Admin. Code §210:10-1-20. Implementation of policies prohibiting bullying. https://sde.ok.gov/sites/ok.gov.sde/files/Rules-3.29.12Ch.10Bullying.pdf. Accessed September 22, 2022.
99. Or. Stat. 339.356 District policy required. https://www.oregonlaws.org/ors/339.356. Accessed September 22, 2022.
100. Pa. Stat. Title 24 P.S. Educ. §13-1303. https://codes.findlaw.com/pa/title-24-ps-education/pa-st-sect-24-13-1303-1-a.html. Accessed September 22, 2022.
101. PR Laws tit. 1, § 9809f (2020). https://law.justia.com/codes/puerto-rico/2020/titulo-3/capitulo-133/subcapitulo-ix/9809f/. Accessed September 28, 2023.
102. RI Gen L § 16-21-33. (2022). https://law.justia.com/codes/rhode-island/2022/title-16/chapter-16-21/section-16-21-33/. Accessed September 28, 2023; RI Gen L § 16-21-34. (2022). https://law.justia.com/codes/rhode-island/2022/title-16/chapter-16-21/section-16-21-34/. Accessed September 28, 2023.
103. S.C. Code §59-63-130, §59-63-140 (2016). https://law.justia.com/codes/south-carolina/2019/title-59/chapter-63/. Accessed September 23, 2022.
104. S.D. Codified Laws §13-32-15, §13-32-16, §13-32-17, §13-32-18, §13-32-19. https://law.justia.com/codes/south-dakota/2019/title-13/chapter-32/. Accessed September 28, 2023.
105. Tenn. Code Ann. §49-6-4502 to §49-6-4506. https://law.justia.com/codes/tennessee/2014/title-49/chapter-6/part-45/. Accessed September 23, 2022.
106. Tex. Educ. Code §37.0832. https://codes.findlaw.com/tx/education-code/educ-sect-37-0832.html. Accessed September 23, 2022.
107. Virgin Islands Code 17 VIC §780–784. https://law.justia.com/codes/virgin-islands/2019/title-17/chapter-42b/. Accessed September 23, 2022.
108. Utah Code 53G-9-601-608. https://le.utah.gov/xcode/Title53G/Chapter9/53G-9-P6.html?v=C53G-9-P6_2018012420180124. Accessed September 23, 2022.
109. Vt. Stat. §570c. https://legislature.vermont.gov/statutes/section/16/009/00570c. Accessed September 23, 2022.
110. Va. Code §22.1-279.6. https://law.justia.com/codes/virginia/2019/title-22-1/chapter-14/section-22-1-279-6/. Accessed September 23, 2022.
111. Wash. RCW 28A.600.477; RCW 28A.600.480. https://law.justia.com/codes/washington/2020/title-28a/chapter-28a-600/section-28a-600-477/. Accessed September 29, 2023. https://app.leg.wa.gov/rcw/default.aspx?cite=28A.600.480#:~:text=RCW%2028A.600.480-,Reporting%20of%20harassment%2C%20intimidation%2C%20or%20bullying%E2%80%94Reta

liation%20prohibited%E2%80%94,harassment%2C%20intimidation%2C%20or%20bully ing. Accessed September 29, 2023.

112. W. Va. Code Educ. §18-2C-1 to §18-2C-6. https://law.justia.com/codes/west-virginia/2022/chapter-18/article-2c/. Accessed September 29, 2023.
113. Wis. Stat. §118.46 (2019). https://law.justia.com/codes/wisconsin/2019/chapter-118/sect ion-118-46/. Accessed September 23, 2022.
114. Wyo. Stat. §21-4-313; Wyo. Stat. §21-4-314. https://law.justia.com/codes/wyoming/2013/title-21/chapter-4/article-3/section-21-4-313/. https://law.justia.com/codes/wyoming/2013/title-21/chapter-4/article-3/section-21-4-314/. Accessed September 23, 2022.
115. Uruguay, Law 19098, 2013. https://www.impo.com.uy/bases/leyes/19098-2013. Accessed September 29, 2023. [Title and text translation from Google]
116. Albania, Law No. 8888, April 25, 2002. https://www.cybercrimelaw.net/Albania.html. Accessed September 23, 2022.
117. Antigua and Barbuda, Electronic Crimes (Amendment) Act, 2018 No. 25 of 2018. http://laws.gov.ag/wp-content/uploads/2019/02/No.-25-of-2018-Electronic-Crimes-Amendm ent-Act-2018.pdf. Accessed September 23, 2022.
118. Argentina, Law 26,388, 2008. http://servicios.infoleg.gob.ar/infolegInternet/anexos/140 000-144999/141790/norma.htm. Accessed September 23, 2022. [Title and text translation from Google]
119. Bahamas Computer Misuse Act, 2006. http://laws.bahamas.gov.bs/cms/images/LEGISLAT ION/PRINCIPAL/2003/2003-0002/ComputerMisuseAct_1.pdf. Accessed September 23, 2022.
120. Barbados, Computer Misuse Act 2005. http://www.oas.org/juridico/spanish/cyb_bbs_c omputer_misuse_2005.pdf. Accessed September 23, 2022.
121. Botswana, Laws of Botswana Chapter 08:06 Cybercrime and Computer Related Crimes. http://www.itu.int/ITU-D/projects/ITU_EC_ACP/hipssa/Activities/SA/docs/SA-1_Legis lations/Botswana/CYBERCRIMES.pdf. Accessed September 23, 2022.
122. El Salvador, Ley Especial Contra los Delitos Informáticos y Conexos. https://www.jurispr udencia.gob.sv/DocumentosBoveda/D/2/2010-2019/2016/02/B6B74.PDF. Accessed September 23, 2022. [Text in Spanish, English translation not available from Google]
123. Fiji, Online Safety Act 2018. http://www.parliament.gov.fj/wp-content/uploads/2018/03/Bill-7-Online-Safety-.pdf. Accessed September 23, 2022.
124. Grenada, Electronic Crimes Bill, 2013. https://nowgrenada.com/wp-content/uploads/2013/07/Electronic-Crimes-Bill.pdf. Accessed September 23, 2022.
125. Guyana, Cibercrime Act 2018. https://officialgazette.gov.gy/images/gazettes-files/Extra_1 3AUG2018Act16of2018.pdf. Accessed September 23, 2022.
126. India, The Information Technology Act, 2000. https://www.wipo.int/edocs/lexdocs/laws/en/in/in024en.pdf. Accessed September 23, 2022.
127. Iran, Islamic Republic of Iran: Computer Crimes Law, 2012. https://www.article19.org/data/files/medialibrary/2921/12-01-30-FINAL-iran-WEB%5B4%5D.pdf. Accessed September 23, 2022.
128. Italy, Law 29 May 2017, n. 71. https://www.gazzettaufficiale.it/eli/id/2017/06/3/17G00085/sg. Accessed September 29, 2023. [Title and text translation from Google]
129. Jamaica, The Cybercrimes Act, 2015. https://www.japarliament.gov.jm/attachments/339_The%20Cybercrimes%20Acts,%202015.pdf. Accessed September 23, 2022.
130. New Zealand, Harmful Digital Communications Act 2015. http://www.legislation.govt.nz/act/public/2015/0063/latest/whole.html. Accessed September 23, 2022.

131. Nigeria, Cybercrimes (Prohibition, Prevention, etc.) Act, 2015. https://cert.gov.ng/ngcert/resources/CyberCrime__Prohibition_Prevention_etc__Act__2015.pdf. Accessed September 23, 2022.
132. Palestine, Resolution No. (10) of 2018 on cybercrime. https://cyrilla.org/en/entity/thzylydj0c?page=1. Accessed September 29, 2023. [Title and text translation from Google]
133. Papua New Guinea, Cybercrime Code 2016. http://www.parliament.gov.pg/uploads/acts/16A_35.pdf. Accessed September 23, 2022.
134. Paraguay, Codigo Penal del Paraguay, Ley Numero. 1,160–97. http://www.oas.org/juridico/spanish/cyb_par_cod_penal.pdf?_x_tr_sch=http&_x_tr_sl=es&_x_tr_tl=en&_x_tr_hl=en&_x_tr_pto=sc. Accessed September 29, 2023. [Text in Spanish, English translation not available from Google]
135. St. Vincent and the Grenadines, Cybercrime Act 2016. https://www.gov.vc/images/PoliciesActsAndBills/SVG_Cybercrime_Act_2016.pdf. Accessed September 29, 2023.
136. Tanzania, The Cybercrimes Act, 2015. https://rsf.org/sites/default/files/the_cyber_crime_act_2015.pdf. Accessed September 23, 2022.
137. Uganda, Computer Misuse Act 2011. https://ict.go.ug/wp-content/uploads/2019/12/UGANDA-Computer-Misuse-Act-No.-2-of-2011-1.pdf. Accessed September 29, 2023.
138. Guam, Guam Code Ann. Tit. 9 §19.69. https://law.justia.com/codes/guam/2022/title-9/chapter-19/. Accessed September 29, 2023.
139. Ill. 720 ILCS 5/12-7.5- and 720 ILCS 135/1-3-. http://www.ilga.gov/legislation/ilcs/documents/072000050K12-7.5.htm. Accessed September 23, 2022. https://law.justia.com/codes/illinois/2010/chapter720/1883.html. Accessed September 23, 2022.
140. Iowa Code §708.7. https://www.legis.iowa.gov/docs/code/708.7.pdf. Accessed September 23, 2022.
141. Kan. Stat. Ann. §21-3438 (f) (2). https://law.justia.com/codes/kansas/2011/Chapter21/Article34/21-3438.html. Accessed September 23, 2022.
142. La. Rev. Stat. Ann. §14:40.3-. https://law.justia.com/codes/louisiana/2011/rs/title14/rs14-40-3/. Accessed September 23, 2022.
143. Me. Rev. Stat. Ann. Tit. 17 §506-. https://www.mainelegislature.org/legis/statutes/17-A/title17-Asec506.html. Accessed September 23, 2022.
144. Md. Code Ann. Crim. Law §3-805-. https://law.justia.com/codes/maryland/2013/article-gcr/section-3-805/. Accessed September 23, 2022.
145. Mass. Ann. Laws ch 265 §43A. https://malegislature.gov/Laws/GeneralLaws/PartIV/TitleI/Chapter265/section43A. Accessed September 23, 2022.
146. Mich. Comp Laws Serv. §750.411s. http://www.legislature.mi.gov/(S(twihilfdsqbtjtkfmpnibnup))/mileg.aspx?page=GetObject&objectname=mcl-750-411s. Accessed September 29, 2023.
147. Miss. Code Ann. §97-45-15. https://law.justia.com/codes/mississippi/2013/title-97/chapter-45/section-97-45-15. Accessed September 30, 2022.
148. N.C. Gen. Stat. ch 14. Criminal Law §14-458.1. https://www.ncleg.gov/EnactedLegislation/Statutes/HTML/BySection/Chapter_14/GS_14-458.1.html. Accessed September 23, 2022.
149. Okla. Stat. Ann. Tit 21 1172. https://law.justia.com/codes/oklahoma/2014/title-21/section-21-1172. Accessed September 23, 2022.
150. Or. Rev. Stat. §166.065. https://www.oregonlaws.org/ors/166.065. Accessed September 23, 2022.
151. Pa. 18 PA. Cons. Stat. Ann. §2709- (a.1) Cyber harassment of a child. https://law.justia.com/codes/pennsylvania/2022/title-18/chapter-27/section-2709/. Accessed October 1, 2023.

152. S.C. Code Ann. §16-3-1700. https://law.justia.com/codes/south-carolina/2013/title-16/chapter-3/section-16-3-1700. Accessed September 29, 2022.
153. SD Codified L § 22-19A-1 (2013). https://law.justia.com/codes/south-dakota/2013/title-22/chapter-19a/section-22-19a-1/. Accessed October 1, 2023.
154. Tenn. Code Ann. §39-17-308. https://law.justia.com/codes/tennessee/2010/title-39/chapter-17/part-3/39-17-308. Accessed October 2, 2020.
155. Tex. Penal Code Ann. §42.07. https://law.justia.com/codes/texas/2021/penal-code/title-9/chapter-42/section-42-07/. Accessed October 1, 2023.
156. Va. Code Stat. §18.2-152.7:1. https://law.lis.virginia.gov/vacode/title18.2/chapter5/section18.2-152.7:1/. Accessed September 23, 2022.
157. Wash. Rev. Code Ann. §9.61.260. https://app.leg.wa.gov/RCW/default.aspx?cite = 9.61.260. Accessed September 23, 2022.
158. Wis. Stat. Ann. §947.0125. https://docs.legis.wisconsin.gov/statutes/statutes/947/0125. Accessed September 23, 2022.
159. Albania, Law 7961 Code of Labor of the Republic of Albania, articles 9 and 32. https://www.wipo.int/edocs/lexdocs/laws/en/al/al066en.pdf. Accessed September 23, 2022.
160. Argentina, Employment Contract Law, No 20.744, 1974 known as Labor contract law, Article 17. https://www.argentina.gob.ar/normativa/nacional/ley-20744-25552/actualizacion. Accessed October 1, 2023. [Title and text translation from Google]
161. Australia, Fair Work Act 2009, ch 3, Division 3-Workplace Rights. https://www.legislation.gov.au/Details/C2018C00512/Html/Volume_1. Accessed September 25, 2022.
162. Australia, Australian Capital Territory, Work Health and Safety Act 2011, Part 6 Discriminatory, coercive, or misleading conduct. https://www.legislation.act.gov.au/View/a/2011-35/current/PDF/2011-35.PDF. Accessed September 25, 2022.
163. Australia, New South Wales, Work Health and Safety Act 2011, Part 6 Discriminatory, coercive, and misleading conduct. https://www.legislation.nsw.gov.au/#/view/act/2011/10/part6. Accessed September 25, 2022.
164. Australia, Northern Territory, Anti-Discrimination Act 1992, Part 4, Division 3, Work. https://legislation.nt.gov.au/Legislation/ANTIDISCRIMINATION-ACT-1992. Accessed September 25, 2022.
165. Australia, Queensland, Work Health and Safety Act 2011, Part 6 Discriminatory, coercive, and misleading conduct. https://www.legislation.qld.gov.au/view/html/inforce/current/act-2011-018#pt.6. Accessed September 25, 2022.
166. Australia, South Australia, Work Health and Safety Act 2012, Part 6–Discriminatory, coercive, and misleading conduct. https://www.legislation.sa.gov.au/__legislation/lz/c/a/work%20health%20and%20safety%20act%202012/current/2012.40.auth.pdf. Accessed October 2, 2023.
167. Australia, Tasmania, Work Health and Safety Act 2012, Part 6–Discriminatory, Coercive and Misleading Conduct. https://www.legislation.tas.gov.au/view/whole/html/inforce/current/act-2012-001. Accessed September 25, 2022.
168. Australia, Victoria, Occupational Health and Safety Act 2004–§76. http://www5.austlii.edu.au/au/legis/vic/consol_act/ohasa2004273/s76.html. Accessed September 25, 2022.
169. Austria, Federal Equal Treatment Act, §13B-GIBG. https://www.ilo.org/dyn/natlex/natlex4.detail?p_lang=en&p_isn=42823. Accessed October 2, 2023. [Title and text translation from Google]
170. Belgium, Royal Decree of April 10, 2014, on Prevention of Psychosocial Risks at Work. https://www.eurofound.europa.eu/en/resources/article/2014/belgium-preventing-psychosocial-risks-work. Accessed October 2, 2023. [Title and text translation from Google]

171. Bosnia and Herzegovina, Law on the Prohibition of Discrimination 2009. https://arsbih.gov.ba/wp-content/uploads/2014/02/002-Anti-Discrimination-Law-.pdf. Accessed October 2, 2023.
172. Brazil, Federal Law 9029/95 Labour Code 1943, as amended 1999, art 1. https://www.planalto.gov.br/ccivil_03/leis/l9029.htm. Accessed October 2, 2023. [Title and text translation from Google]
173. Bulgaria, Health and Safety at Work Act, 1997, articles 12–24. https://lex.bg/laws/ldoc/2134178305. Accessed October 2, 2023 [Title and text translation from Google]
174. Workplace Harassment and Violence Prevention Regulations, SOR/2020-130. https://www.canlii.org/en/ca/laws/regu/sor-2020-130/latest/sor-2020-130.html. Accessed October 3, 2023.
175. Canada, Province of British Columbia, BC Occupational Health and Safety Regulation B.C Reg. 296/97 as amended 2012, Workplace Conduct (4.24 to 4.26); Violence in the Workplace (4.27 to 4.31). https://www.canlii.org/en/bc/laws/regu/bc-reg-296-97/latest/bc-reg-296-97.html. Accessed September 25, 2022.
176. Canada, Province of Manitoba, The Workplace Safety and Health Act, Workplace Safety and Health Regulation, 217/2006, Part 10 (Harassment) and Part 11 (Violence in the Workplace). https://www.canlii.org/en/mb/laws/regu/man-reg-217-2006/latest/man-reg-217-2006.html. Accessed October 3, 2023.
177. Canada, Province of Nova Scotia, Violence in the Workplace Regulations made under Section 82 of the Occupational Health and Safety Act S.N.S. 1996. https://novascotia.ca/just/regulations/regs/ohsviolence.htm. Accessed September 25, 2022.
178. Canada, Province of Ontario, Ontario Occupational Health and Safety Act 2010, Part III.0.1 Violence and Harassment, 32.0.1–32.0.8. https://www.ontario.ca/laws/statute/90o01#BK56. Accessed September 25, 2022.
179. Canada, Province of Quebec, Quebec Act Respecting Labor Standards 2004, Division V.2 Psychological Harassment 81.18; 81.19. http://legisquebec.gouv.qc.ca/en/showdoc/cs/N-1.1?langCont = fr#se:81_18. Accessed September 25, 2022.
180. Chile, Labor Code 2003 Title IV Article 211A-E. https://www.bcn.cl/leychile/navegar?idNorma=207436. Accessed October 3, 2023. [Title and text translation from Google]
181. Colombia, Work Harassment Law 1010 of 2006. https://www.arlsura.com/index.php?option=com_content&view=article&id=232:ley-1010-de-2006&catid=50:leyes-y-normas&Itemid=33. Accessed October 3, 2023. [Title and text translation from Google]
182. Croatia, Labor Act, Articles 2-6 and 30. http://www.vsrh.hr/CustomPages/Static/HRV/Files/Legislation__Labour-Act.pdf. Accessed September 25, 2022.
183. Czech Republic, Labor Code, 2012, Part 1, ch 4; Part 5, ch 1. https://www.mpsv.cz/documents/625317/625915/Labour_Code_2012.pdf/a66525f7-0ddf-5af7-4bba-33c7d7a8bfdf. Accessed September 25, 2022.
184. Finland, Occupational Safety and Health Act §27 and §28. https://www.ilo.org/dyn/natlex/docs/ELECTRONIC/62320/60971/F1688833574/FIN62320%20English.pdf. Accessed September 25, 2022.
185. France, Labor Code/Code du Travail 2008 with further amendments, Part 1: Individual labor relations, Title III Discrimination, Title V Harassment. https://www.legifrance.gouv.fr/codes/texte_lc/LEGITEXT000006072050?init=true&page=1&query=Code+du+Travail+2008+&searchField=ALL&tab_selection=all. Accessed October 3, 2023.
186. India, Sexual Harassment of Women at the Workplace (Prevention, Prohibition and Redressal) Act, 2013. https://www.iitk.ac.in/wc/data/Sexual-Harassment-at-Workplace-Act.pdf. Accessed October 4, 2023.

187. Japan, Act Promoting Measures to Prevent Death and Injury from Overwork. https://www.japaneselawtranslation.go.jp/en/laws/view/3258/en. Accessed September 25, 2022.
188. Malaysia, Occupational Safety and Health Act, 1994, 27. Discrimination against employee, etc. https://www.dosh.gov.my/index.php/legislation/acts-legislation/23-02-occupational-safety-and-health-act-1994-act-514/file. Accessed October 4, 2020.
189. Malta, Employment and Industrial Relations Act, 2002, Part IV, Protection against Discrimination related to Employment, Articles 26–32. https://legislation.mt/eli/cap/452/eng. Accessed October 4, 2023.
190. Mexico, Federal Labor Law Articles 3 and 3b. https://mexico.justia.com/federales/leyes/ley-federal-del-trabajo/titulo-primero//#articulo-3o. Accessed October 4, 2023. [Title and text translation from Google]
191. New Zealand, Employers Relations Act 2000, Part 9. http://www.legislation.govt.nz/act/public/2000/0024/112.0/DLM58317.html. Accessed September 25, 2022.
192. Norway, Working Environment Act, 2006, Section 4.3, Requirements regarding the psychosocial working environment; Section 13-1 Prohibition against discrimination. https://lovdata.no/dokument/NLE/lov/2005-06-17-62#KAPITTEL_14. Accessed September 25, 2022.
193. Poland, Labor Code 1974 Art. 94-2b; 94^3. https://www.ilo.org/dyn/natlex/docs/ELECTRONIC/45181/91758/F1623906595/The-Labour-Code%20consolidated%201997.pdf. Accessed September 25, 2022.
194. Portugal, Labor Code articles 23–29. https://files.dre.pt/diplomastraduzidos/7_2009_CodigoTrabalho_EN_publ.pdf. Accessed September 25, 2022. [Title and text translation from Google]
195. Serbia, Law of Prevention of Abuse at Work 2010. https://doklestic.law/files/2020/08/law_on_prevention_of_harassment_at_work.pdf. Accessed September 25, 2022.
196. Slovakia, Labor Code Article §13 Prohibition of discrimination. https://www.employment.gov.sk/files/praca-zamestnanost/vztah-zamestnanca-zamestnavatela/zakonnik-prace/zakonnik-prace-anglicka-verzia-labour-code-full-wording-2012.pdf. Accessed September 25, 2022.
197. Slovenia, Employment Relationships Act, 2013; The Health and Safety Work Act, 2011, §13. http://ilo.org/dyn/natlex/docs/ELECTRONIC/89470/102799/F2013305698/Slovenia%20Health%20and%20Safety%20at%20Work.pdf. Accessed September 25, 2022.
198. Spain, Ley del Estatuto de los Trabajadores Artículo 17. No discriminación en las relaciones laborales. https://www.boe.es/eli/es/rdlg/2015/10/23/2. Accessed September 25, 2022. [Text in Spanish, English translation not available from Google]
199. Sweden, AFS 1993:17, Ordinance of the Swedish National Board of Occupational Safety and Health containing Provisions on measures against Victimization at Work, 1993. https://www.kth.se/polopoly_fs/1.527926.1550157127!/Provisions%20on%20measures%20against%20Victima.pdf. Accessed September 25, 2022.
200. Switzerland, Federal Act on Gender Equality §2; Equality at Work Articles 2–7. https://www.admin.ch/opc/en/classified-compilation/19950082/index.html#a4. Accessed September 25, 2022.
201. Taiwan, Sexual harassment prevention act. https://law.moj.gov.tw/ENG/LawClass/LawAll.aspx?pcode=D0050074. Accessed October 4, 2023.
202. The Netherlands, Working Conditions Acts (WCA) 2007, as amended ch 1, Article 3 (e); ch 2, Article 3 (2). https://www.ilo.org/dyn/natlex/docs/ELECTRONIC/68800/67767/F386275802/NLD68800.pdf. Accessed September 25, 2022.

203. United Kingdom, Protection from Harassment Act 1997, §1, Prohibition of Harassment. http://www.legislation.gov.uk/ukpga/1997/40/section/1. Accessed September 25, 2022. United Kingdom, Equality Act 2010, ch 2, Discrimination. http://www.legislation.gov.uk/ukpga/2010/15/part/2/chapter/2. Accessed September 25, 2022.
204. Utah Code 34A-5-106. https://le.utah.gov/xcode/Title34A/Chapter5/34A-5-S106.html?v = C34A-5-S106_2015051220150512. Accessed September 25, 2022.
205. Tenn. Code §50-1-503 (2016), ch 1, pt 5, Healthy Workplace Act. https://law.justia.com/codes/tennessee/2016/title-50/chapter-1/part-5/section-50-1-503/. Accessed September 25, 2022.
206. Albania, Law No. 9669, dated 18.12.2006 on Measures against Violence in Family Relation. https://www.osce.org/files/f/documents/4/6/30436.pdf. Accessed October 4, 2023.
207. Andorra, Nouveau Code Pénal Article 114 Sévices dans le domaine domestique. https://legislationline.org/sites/default/files/documents/2e/Andorra_CC_2005_fr.pdf. Accessed September 25, 2022. [Text in French, English translation not available from Google]
208. Antigua and Barbuda, Domestic Violence Act 2015 No. 27 of 2015. https://oig.cepal.org/sites/default/files/2015_atg_domesticviolenceact.pdf. Accessed September 25, 2022.
209. Argentina, Protección contra la Violencia Familiar Decreto 235/96 Reglamentase la Ley No. 24,417. http://servicios.infoleg.gob.ar/infolegInternet/anexos/30000-34999/34210/norma.htm#:~:text = Decreto%20Nacional%20235%2F96&text = Reglam%C3%A9ntase%20la%20Ley%20N%C2%BA%2024.417.&text = CONSIDERANDO%3A&text = Que%20dicha%20Ley%20ha%20creado,grupo%20familiar%20al%20que%20pertenecen. Accessed September 25, 2022. [Text in Spanish, English translation not available from Google]
210. Azerbaijan, On the prevention of domestic violence. Law of The Republic of Azerbaijan. https://evaw-global-database.unwomen.org/-/media/files/un%20women/vaw/full%20text/asia/law%20on%20prevention%20of%20domestic%20violence%20(2010)/law%20on%20prevention%20of%20domsetic%20violence%202010.pdf?vs = 5250. Accessed September 25, 2022.
211. Bahamas, Statute Law of the Bahamas Chapter 99A, Domestic Violence (Protection Orders). http://laws.bahamas.gov.bs/cms/images/LEGISLATION/PRINCIPAL/2007/2007-0024/DomesticViolenceProtectionOrdersAct_1.pdf. Accessed September 25, 2022.
212. Bangladesh, Family Violence (Prevention and Protection) Act, 2010 (Act No. 56 of 2010). https://www.refworld.org/docid/5d4994364.html. Accessed October 4, 2023. [Title and text translation from Google]
213. Barbados, L.R.O. 1993 Domestic Violence (Protection Orders) CAP. 130A. https://oig.cepal.org/sites/default/files/1993_brb_domesticviolence.pdf. Accessed September 25, 2022.
214. Belize, Domestic Violence Act 2007. https://oig.cepal.org/sites/default/files/2007_blz_act19.pdf. Accessed September 25, 2022.
215. Bolivia, Ley No. 1674 Ley Contra la Violencia en la Familia o Domestica, 15 de Diciembre de 1995. http://scm.oas.org/pdfs/2010/CIM02724T-B.pdf. Accessed September 25, 2022. [Text in Spanish, English translation not available from Google]
216. Bosnia and Herzegovina, Law No.03/L –182 on Protection Against Domestic Violence, Assembly of Republic of Kosovo. http://old.kuvendikosoves.org/common/docs/ligjet/2010-182-eng.pdf. Accessed October 4, 2023. [Title and text translation from Google]
217. Botswana, Laws of Botswana ch 28:05 Domestic Violence. https://evaw-global-database.unwomen.org/-/media/files/un%20women/vaw/full%20text/africa/dv%20act%202008.pdf?vs = 1945. Accessed September 25, 2022.

218. Bulgaria, PROTECTION AGAINST DOMESTIC VIOLENCE ACT, Promulgated, State Gazette, issue 27 of 29 March 2005. https://evaw-global-database.unwomen.org/-/media/files/un%20women/vaw/full%20text/europe/protection%20against%20domestic%20violence%20act%20state%20gazette%2027%20of%2029%20march%202005/protection%20against%20domestic%20violence%20act%202005.pdf?vs=1337. Accessed October 4, 2023.
219. Chile, Law 20066, Establishes Law of Intrafamily Violence. https://www.bcn.cl/leychile/navegar?idNorma=242648. Accessed October 4, 2023. [Title and text translation from Google]
220. People's Republic of China, Anti-Domestic Violence Law of the People's Republic of China (Chairman Order No. 37). http://www.lawinfochina.com/display.aspx?id=20841&lib=law&EncodingName=big5. Accessed October 4, 2023. [Title and text translation from Google]
221. Costa Rica, LEY No. 7586, LEY CONTRA LA VIOLENCIA DOMESTICA. https://www.ciem.ucr.ac.cr/IMG/pdf/ley-7586_contra_la_violencia_domestica-2.pdf. Accessed October 5, 2023 [Text in Spanish, English translation not available from Google]
222. Croatia, Law on Protection from Domestic Violence NN 70/17, 126 19, in force from January 1, 2023. https://www.zakon.hr/z/81/Zakon-o-za%C5%A1titi-od-nasilja-u-obitelji. Accessed October 5, 2023. [Title and text translation from Google]
223. Cyprus, Law which provides for the Prevention of Violence in the Family and Protection of Victims 119 (1) of 2000 and 212(1) of 2004. http://www.familyviolence.gov.cy/upload/legislation/laws_2000_and_2004_en.pdf. Accessed October 5, 2023.
224. Czech Republic, Law on protection against domestic violence, NN 70/17, 26/19, 84/21. 114/22, in force from 01.01.2023. https://www.zakon.hr/z/81/Zakon-o-za%C5%A1titi-od-nasilja-u-obitelji. Accessed October 5, 2023 [Title and text translation from Google]
225. Dominican Republic, Ley No. 24-97 que introduce modificaciones al Código Penal y al Código para la Protección de Niños, Niñas y Adolescentes. https://www.oas.org/dil/esp/Ley%2024-97,%20sobre%20Violencia%20Intrafamiliar%20Republica%20Dominicana.pdf. Accessed October 5, 2023. [Text in Spanish, English translation not available from Google]
226. Ecuador, Ley N° 103/1995. Ley Contra la Violencia a la Mujer y a la Familia. https://siteal.iiep.unesco.org/sites/default/files/sit_accion_files/siteal_ecuador_0231.pdf. Accessed October 5, 2023 [Text in Spanish, English translation not available from Google]
227. El Salvador, Decreto N° 902/1996. Ley contra la Violencia Intrafamiliar. https://siteal.iiep.unesco.org/sites/default/files/sit_accion_files/sv_0196.pdf#:~:text=Establece%20los%20mecanismos%20adecuados%20para%20prevenir%2C%20sancionar%20y,%28mujeres%2C%20ni%C3%B1os%2C%20personas%20con%20discapacidad%2C%20y%20adultos%20mayores%29. Accessed October 5, 2023. [Text in Spanish, English translation not available from Google]
228. Fiji, The Domestic Violence Decree 2018. http://www.fijileaks.com/uploads/1/3/7/5/13759434/naz_on_the_domesticviolence-decree2009.pdf. Accessed September 25, 2022.
229. Ghana, The Domestic Violence Act. https://evaw-global-database.unwomen.org/-/media/files/un%20women/vaw/full%20text/africa/ghana%20-%20domestic%20violence%20act%20(2007).pdf?vs = 3618. Accessed September 25, 2022.
230. Grenada, Domestic Violence Act 19 of 2010. https://www.ilo.org/dyn/natlex/docs/ELECTRONIC/98277/116882/F-962113168/GRD98277.pdf. Accessed September 25, 2022.
231. Guatemala, Decreto N° 97/1996. Ley para Prevenir, Sancionar y Erradicar la Violencia Intrafamiliar. https://siteal.iiep.unesco.org/sites/default/files/sit_accion_files/gt_0744.pdf. Accessed October 5, 2023. [Text in Spanish, English translation not available from Google]

232. Guyana, Laws of Guyana, Domestic Violence, ch 11:09 Domestic Violence Act. http://badaj.org/wp-content/uploads/2014/07/Domestic%20Violence%20Act.pdf. Accessed September 25, 2022.
233. Honduras, Ley Contra la Violencia Doméstica con sus Reformas. https://www.oas.org/dil/esp/Ley_contra_la_violencia_domestica_Honduras.pdf. Accessed October 5, 2023. [Text in Spanish, English translation not available from Google]
234. India, THE PROTECTION OF WOMEN FROM DOMESTIC VIOLENCE ACT, 2005. https://www.indiacode.nic.in/bitstream/123456789/2021/1/200543.pdf. Accessed October 5, 2023.
235. Indonesia, Law of the Republic of Indonesia Number 23 of Year 2004 Regarding Elimination of Violence in Household. https://www.wcwonline.org/pdf/lawcompilation/Indonesia-Regarding-Elimination-of-Violence-in-Household.pdf. Accessed September 25, 2022.
236. Iraq, Law Combating Domestic violence, drafted in 2019, no evidence[357] of having yet been enacted. See EASO, COI query, Iraq, Situation of women who suffered domestic violence. Legislation on domestic violence in Iraq and the Kurdistan Region of Iraq (KRI), Date of completion, October 14, 2021, Query-Code 35-2021. https://www.ecoi.net/en/file/local/2062237/2021_10_Q35_EASO_COI_Query_Response_IRAQ_domestic_violence.pdf. Accessed September 25, 2022.
237. Ireland, Domestic Violence Act 2018. http://www.irishstatutebook.ie/eli/2018/act/6/enacted/en/html. Accessed September 25, 2022.
238. Israel, Domestic Violence Prevention Law, 1991. https://www.icj.org/wp-content/uploads/2013/05/Israel-Prevention-of-Family-Violence-Law-5751-1991-eng.pdf. Accessed September 25, 2022.
239. Jamaica, The Domestic Violence Act. https://evaw-global-database.unwomen.org/-/media/files/un%20women/vaw/full%20text/americas/domestic%20violence%20act%202004/domestic%20violence%20act%202004.pdf?vs = 3103. Accessed September 27, 2022.
240. Kenya, The Protection against Domestic Violence Act No. 2 of 2015. https://ke.boell.org/sites/default/files/uploads/2015/08/protectionagainstdomesticviolenceact_2015_1.pdf. Accessed September 25, 2022.
241. Kyrgyz Republic, Law of The Kyrgyz Republic On Social and Legal Protection from Domestic Violence. https://legislationline.org/taxonomy/term/18252. Accessed September 25, 2022.
242. Lithuania, Law on Protection Against Domestic Violence, 2011. https://legislationline.org/sites/default/files/documents/f1/Lithuania_law_protection_against_DV_2011_en.pdf. Accessed September 25, 2022.
243. Malaysia, Domestic Violence Act 1994. https://www.wcwonline.org/pdf/lawcompilation/malaysia_DVact1994.pdf. Accessed September 25, 2022.
244. Maldives, Domestic Violence Act Number 3/2012. https://maldives.unfpa.org/sites/default/files/pub-pdf/the_domestic_violence_act_2012_maldives_english_translation_unofficial.pdf. Accessed September 25, 2022.
245. Mauritius, Protection from Domestic Violence Act 1997. https://cyber.harvard.edu/population/domesticviolence/MAURITIU1.htm. Accessed September 25, 2022.
246. Moldova, Law No 45 from 01/03/2007 on preventing and combating domestic violence. https://www.legis.md/cautare/getResults?doc_id=122068&lang=ro. Accessed October 5, 2023. [Title and text translation from Google]
247. Mongolia, Law of Mongolia Against Domestic Violence. https://evaw-global-database.unwomen.org/-/media/files/un%20women/vaw/full%20text/asia/law%20to%20combat%20d

omestic%20violence%20-%202005/law%20to%20combat%20domestic%20violence%20-%202005.pdf?vs = 5302. Accessed September 25, 2022.

248. Namibia, Combating of Domestic Violence Act, 2003. https://evaw-global-database.unwomen.org/-/media/files/un%20women/vaw/full%20text/africa/namibia%20-%20domestic%20violence%20act.pdf?vs = 5411. Accessed September 25, 2022.
249. Nepal, Domestic Violence (Crime and Punishment) Act, 2008. https://www.wcwonline.org/pdf/lawcompilation/Nepal_Domestic%20Violence%20(Crime%20and%20Punishment)%20.pdf. Unofficial translation by Forum for Women, Law and Development (FWLD). Accessed September 25, 2022.
250. New Zealand, Family Violence Act 2018. http://legislation.govt.nz/act/public/2018/0046/latest/DLM7159322.html. Accessed September 25, 2022.
251. Paraguay, Ley 1600 Ley contra la Violencia Domestica. https://www.pj.gov.py/images/contenido/secretariadegenero/marcolegal/LEY-1600-2000.pdf. Accessed September 25, 2022. [Text in Spanish, English translation not available from Google]
252. Peru, Ley No 30364 Ley para Prevenir, Sancionar y Erradicar la Violencia contra las Mujeres y los Integrantes del Grupo Familiar. https://www.defensoria.gob.pe/deunavezportodas/wp-content/uploads/2019/02/Ley3036_erradicarviolencia.pdf. Accessed September 25, 2022. [Text in Spanish, English translation not available from Google]
253. Romania, Law No. 174/2018 to prevent and combat domestic violence. https://legislatie.just.ro/Public/DetaliiDocumentAfis/202718. Accessed October 6, 2023. [Title and text translation from Google]
254. St. Christopher and Nevis, ch 12.04 Domestic Violence Act. https://oig.cepal.org/sites/default/files/2005_kna_domesticviolenceact.pdf. Accessed September 25, 2022.
255. St. Vincent and the Grenadines, Domestic Violence (Summary Proceedings) Act, 1995 (Act No. 13 of 1995), October 17, 1995. https://oig.cepal.org/sites/default/files/1995_vct_act13.pdf. Accessed September 25, 2022.
256. Sierra Leone, The Domestic Violence Act, 2007. https://evaw-global-database.unwomen.org/-/media/files/un%20women/vaw/full%20text/africa/sierra%20leone%20-%20domestic%20violence%20act%202007.pdf?vs = 2145. Accessed September 25, 2022.
257. Solomon Islands, Family Protection Act 2014. https://www.ilo.org/dyn/natlex/docs/ELECTRONIC/98705/117521/F1967801277/SLB98705.pdf. Accessed September 25, 2022.
258. Thailand, Domestic Violence Victim Protection Act B.E 2550 (2007). https://evaw-global-database.unwomen.org/-/media/files/un%20women/vaw/full%20text/asia/protection%20of%20domestic%20violence%20victims%20act%20be%202550%20(2007)/dv%20ptc%20act%202550%20-%202007.pdf?vs=3211. Accessed October 6, 2023. [Translated by Wikisource]
259. Timor-Leste, Law Against Domestic Violence, 2010. https://jsmp.tl/wp-content/uploads/2013/08/LeiKontraViolensiaDomestika-No-7-2010-Eng.pdf. Accessed October 6, 2023. [Title and text translation from Google]
260. Trinidad and Tobago, Laws of Trinidad and Tobago, Domestic Violence Act, ch 45:56 Act 27 of 1999 Amended by 8 of 2006. https://rgd.legalaffairs.gov.tt/laws2/alphabetical_list/lawspdfs/45.56.pdf. Accessed September 25, 2022.
261. Turkey, Family Protection and Violence Against Women Law on Prevention. Law Number 6284 8/3/2012. http://www.lawsturkey.com/law/law-to-protect-family-and-prevent-violence-against-woman-6284. Accessed September 25, 2022.

262. Tuvalu, Family Protection and Domestic Violence Act 2014. https://www.ilo.org/dyn/natlex/docs/ELECTRONIC/98665/117481/F-1823765879/TUV98665.pdf. Accessed September 25, 2022.
263. Uganda, Domestic Violence Act, 2010. https://media.ulii.org/files/legislation/akn-ug-act-2010-3-eng-2010-04-09.pdf. Accessed October 6, 2023.
264. Ukraine, Law of Ukraine on the prevention and counteraction to domestic violence. https://www.legal-tools.org/doc/a81e53/pdf/. Accessed September 25, 2022.
265. Ala. Code Title 30, ch 5 through ch 9. https://codes.findlaw.com/al/title-30-marital-and-domestic-relations/#!tid = NC02D27B0BAC511DB8E46AD894CF6FAAB. Accessed September 28, 2022.
266. Alaska Stat. 2019 ch 18.66. Domestic Violence and Sexual Assault. https://law.justia.com/codes/alaska/2022/title-18/chapter-66/. Accessed October 6, 2023.
267. Ariz. Rev. Stat. Ann. Title 13, ch 36 §13-3601 through §13-3602. https://law.justia.com/codes/arizona/2022/title-13/section-13-3601/, https://law.justia.com/codes/arizona/2022/title-13/section-13-3601-01/, https://law.justia.com/codes/arizona/2022/title-13/section-13-3601-02/, https://law.justia.com/codes/arizona/2022/title-13/section-13-3602/. Accessed October 6, 2023.
268. Ark. Code, Title 9, Subtitle 2, ch 15, Subchapters 1 through 4 (2018). https://law.justia.com/codes/arkansas/2019/title-9/subtitle-2/chapter-15/. Accessed September 28, 2022.
269. Cal. Fam. Code §6200-6409. https://law.justia.com/codes/california/2011/fam/division-10. Accessed October 6, 2023.
270. Colo. Rev. Stat. Ann. §18-6-800.3 through §18-6-803.9. https://law.justia.com/codes/colorado/2022/title-18/article-6/part-8/. Accessed October 6, 2023.
271. Conn. Stat. §46b-38a through §46b-38m. https://law.justia.com/codes/connecticut/2018/title-46b/chapter-815e/. Accessed September 28, 2022.
272. Del. Stat. tit 13 ch 7A. https://delcode.delaware.gov/title13/c007a/sc01/index.shtml. Accessed September 28, 2022. Del. Stat. tit 13 ch 21. https://delcode.delaware.gov/title13/c021/index.shtml. Accessed September 28, 2022.
273. D.C. Code §16-1001 through §16-1058. https://law.justia.com/codes/district-of-columbia/2022/title-16/chapter-10/subchapter-v/. Accessed October 6, 2023.
274. Fla. Stat. §741.28 through §741.325. https://law.justia.com/codes/florida/2015/title-xliii/chapter-741. Accessed October 6, 2023.
275. Ga. Stat. Ann. §19-13-1 through §19-13-56. https://law.justia.com/codes/georgia/2018/title-19/chapter-13/. Accessed September 28, 2022.
276. Haw. Rev. Stat. §586-1 through §586-26. https://law.justia.com/codes/hawaii/2019/title-31/chapter-586/. Accessed September 28, 2022.
277. Idaho Code §18-918. https://law.justia.com/codes/idaho/2019/title-18/chapter-9/section-18-918/. Accessed September 28, 2022.
278. Ill. Stat. ch 750, §60/101 through §60/401. https://law.justia.com/codes/illinois/2019/chapter-750/act-750-ilcs-60/. Accessed September 28, 2022.
279. Ind. Code §35-42-2-1.3. https://law.justia.com/codes/indiana/2019/title-35/article-42/chapter-2/section-35-42-2-1-3/. Accessed September 28, 2022.
280. Iowa Stat. §236.1 through §236.20. https://law.justia.com/codes/iowa/2019/title-vi/chapter-236/. Accessed September 28, 2022.
281. Kan. Stat. §21-5414. https://law.justia.com/codes/kansas/2018/chapter-21/article-54/section-21-5414/. Accessed September 28, 2022.

282. Ky. Stat. §403.720 through §403.785. https://law.justia.com/codes/kentucky/2019/chapter-403/. Accessed September 28, 2022.
283. La. Rev. Stat. §46:2121 to §46:2148. https://law.justia.com/codes/louisiana/2018/code-revisedstatutes/title-46/. Accessed September 28, 2022.
284. Me. Stat. tit. 19-A, §4001 through §4014. https://law.justia.com/codes/maine/2019/title-19-a/part-4/chapter-101/. Accessed September 29, 2022.
285. Md. Fam. Law §4-501 through §4-531. https://law.justia.com/codes/maryland/2019/family-law/title-4/. Accessed September 28, 2022.
286. Mass. Stat. §209A, §1 to §209A, §11. https://law.justia.com/codes/massachusetts/2012/partii/titleiii/chapter209a/section1/. Accessed October 6, 2023.
287. Mich. Stat. §750.81. https://law.justia.com/codes/michigan/2019/chapter-750/statute-act-328-of-1931/division-328-1931-xi/section-750-81/. Accessed September 28, 2022.
288. Minn. Stat. §518B.01-02. https://www.revisor.mn.gov/statutes/cite/518B. Accessed September 28, 2022.
289. Miss. Code Ann. §93-21-3 through §93-21-123. https://law.justia.com/codes/mississippi/2019/title-93/chapter-21/article-1/. Accessed October 6, 2023.
290. Mo. Stat. §455.010 through §455.305 and Mo. Stat. §455.543 through §455.560. https://law.justia.com/codes/missouri/2019/title-xxx/chapter-455/. Accessed September 28, 2022.
291. Mont. Code §45-5-206. https://law.justia.com/codes/montana/2019/title-45/chapter-5/part-2/section-45-5-206/. Accessed September 28, 2022.
292. Neb. Rev. Stat. §28-323. https://law.justia.com/codes/nebraska/2019/chapter-28/statute-28-323/. Accessed September 28, 2022.
293. Nev. Rev. Stat. §33.018 though §33.152. https://law.justia.com/codes/nevada/2019/chapter-33/. Accessed September 28, 2022.
294. N.H. Stat. §173-B:1 through §173-B:25. https://law.justia.com/codes/new-hampshire/2019/title-xii/chapter-173-b/. Accessed September 28, 2022.
295. N.J. Stat. §2C:25-19 through §2C:25-35. https://law.justia.com/codes/new-jersey/2019/title-2c/. Accessed September 28, 2022.
296. N.M. Stat. §40-13-1 through §40-13-13. https://law.justia.com/codes/new-mexico/2019/chapter-40/article-13/. Accessed September 28, 2022.
297. N.Y. Soc. Serv. Law §459-A. https://law.justia.com/codes/new-york/2019/sos/article-6-a/459-a/. Accessed September 28, 2022. N.Y. Exec. Law §575. https://law.justia.com/codes/new-york/2019/exc/article-21/575/. Accessed September 28, 2022. N.Y. Exec. Law §576. https://law.justia.com/codes/new-york/2019/exc/article-21/576/. Accessed September 28, 2022. N.Y. Soc. Serv. Law §131-U. https://law.justia.com/codes/new-york/2019/sos/article-5/title-1/131-u/. Accessed September 28, 2022. N.Y. Pub. Health Law §2137. https://law.justia.com/codes/new-york/2019/pbh/article-21/title-3/2137/. Accessed September 28, 2022.
298. N.C. Gen. Stat. §50B-1. https://law.justia.com/codes/north-carolina/2019/chapter-50b/. Accessed September 28, 2022.
299. N.D. Cent. Code §14-07.1-01, N.D. Cent. Code §14-07.1-03 through §14-07.1-05. https://law.justia.com/codes/north-dakota/2019/title-14/. Accessed September 28, 2022.
300. Ohio Stat. §3113.31 through §3113.40. https://law.justia.com/codes/ohio/2019/title-31/chapter-3113/. Accessed September 28, 2022.
301. Okla. Stat. tit 22, §60.0 through §60.31 and Okla. Stat. tit 22, §70. https://law.justia.com/codes/oklahoma/2019/title-22/. Accessed September 28, 2022.

302. Or. Stat. §107.700 through §107.735. https://law.justia.com/codes/oregon/2019/volume-03/chapter-107/. Accessed September 28, 2022.
303. Penn. Cons. Stat. tit 23, §6101 through §6122. https://law.justia.com/codes/pennsylvania/2019/title-23/chapter-61/. Accessed September 28, 2022.
304. R.I. Gen. Laws §15-15-1 through §15-15-7. https://law.justia.com/codes/rhode-island/2019/title-15/chapter-15-15/. Accessed September 28, 2022.
305. S.C. Code §20-4-10 through §20-4-160. https://law.justia.com/codes/south-carolina/2019/title-20/chapter-4/. Accessed September 28, 2022.
306. S.D. Codified Laws §25-10-1 through §25-10-44. https://law.justia.com/codes/south-dakota/2019/title-25/chapter-10/. Accessed September 28, 2022.
307. Tenn. Code §36-3-601 through §36-3-626. https://law.justia.com/codes/tennessee/2019/title-36/chapter-3/part-6/. Accessed September 28, 2022.
308. Tex. Fam. Code Title 4 Protective Orders and Family Violence Subtitles A, B, and C. https://law.justia.com/codes/texas/2019/family-code/title-4/. Accessed September 28, 2022.
309. Utah Code §78B-7-102 through §78B-7-116. https://law.justia.com/codes/utah/2019/title-78b/chapter-7/part-1/. Accessed September 28, 2022.
310. Vt. Stat. Ann. Tit 15, §1101 through §1173. https://law.justia.com/codes/vermont/2019/title-15/chapter-21/. Accessed September 28, 2022.
311. Va. Code §16.1-228. https://law.justia.com/codes/virginia/2019/title-16-1/chapter-11/section-16-1-228-d-1/. Accessed September 28, 2022. Va. Code §18.2-57.2. https://law.justia.com/codes/virginia/2019/title-18-2/chapter-4/section-18-2-57-2/. Accessed September 28, 2022.
312. Wash. Stat. 10.99.020 through 10.99.100. https://law.justia.com/codes/washington/2018/title-10/chapter-10.99/. Accessed September 28, 2022.
313. W. Va. Code §48-27-101 through W.V. Code §48-27-1104. https://law.justia.com/codes/west-virginia/2019/chapter-48/article-27/. Accessed September 28, 2022.
314. Wis. Stat. §968.075. https://law.justia.com/codes/wisconsin/2019/chapter-968/section-968-075/. Accessed September 28, 2022.
315. Wyo. Stat. 35-21-101 through 35-21-112. https://law.justia.com/codes/wyoming/2019/title-35/chapter-21/. Accessed September 28, 2022.
316. Uruguay, Law No 19580 Law of Violence against Women. https://www.impo.com.uy/bases/leyes/19580-2017. Accessed October 6, 2023. [Title and text translation from Google]
317. Vanuatu, Republic of Vanuatu Family Protection Act No. 28 of 2008. http://www.paclii.org/cgi-bin/sinodisp/vu/other/VUGovGaz/2009/8.html?stem=&synonyms=&query = vanuatu andomi%20family%20protection%20act. Accessed September 29, 2022.
318. Vietnam, Law on Prevention and Control of Domestic Violence 2007. https://evaw-global-database.unwomen.org/-/media/files/un%20women/vaw/full%20text/asia/viet%20nam%20-%20law%20on%20domestic%20violence%20prevention%20and%20control%202007/viet%20nam%20-%20law%20on%20domestic%20violence%20prevention%20and%20control%202007.pdf?vs=1748. Accessed October 6, 2023.
319. Zimbabwe, Domestic Violence Act [ch 5:16] Act 14/2006. https://www.ilo.org/dyn/natlex/docs/ELECTRONIC/85410/95626/F1439238254/ZWE85410.pdf. Accessed September 29, 2022.
320. Albania, Law No. 18/2017 on the Rights and Protection of the Child Article 23.4. https://observator.org.al/wp-content/uploads/2017/06/Layout-A5-english_18May2017.pdf. Accessed September 29, 2022.

321. Austria, The Federal Constitutional Act on the Rights of Children 2011 Article 5(1). https://www.ilo.org/dyn/natlex/docs/ELECTRONIC/90242/103907/F-1423464726/ERV_2011_1_4.pdf. Accessed September 29, 2022.
322. Benin, Loi n° 2015-08 portant code de l'enfant en République du Benin, Article 130: Châtiments corporels. https://faolex.fao.org/docs/pdf/ben161458.pdf. Accessed October 8, 2023. [Text in French, no English translation available from Google]
323. Bolivia, Ley 548, 2014, Articulos 146;153. https://www.comunicacion.gob.bo/sites/default/files/dale_vida_a_tus_derechos/archivos/LEY%20548%20ACTUALIZACION%202018%20WEB.pdf. Accessed September 29, 2022. [Text in Spanish, no English translation available from Google]
324. Brazil, Law 8069, 1990, Articles 18A and 18B. https://www.planalto.gov.br/ccivil_03/leis/l8069.htm. Accessed October 8, 2023. [Title and text translation from Google]
325. Cabo Verde, Lei n.° 50/VIII/2013 de 26 de Dezembro, Artigo 31.° (2). https://www.dol.gov/sites/dolgov/files/legacy-files/submissions/CaboVerde20141204.pdf. Accessed October 8, 2023. [Text in Portuguese, no English translation available from Google]
326. Costa Rica, Law 8654, Rights of children and adolescents to discipline without physical punishment or humiliating treatment. http://www.pgrweb.go.cr/scij/Busqueda/Normativa/Normas/nrm_texto_completo.aspx?param1=NRTC&nValor1=1&nValor2=63842&nValor3=73689&strTipM=TC. Accessed October 8, 2023. [Title and text translation from Google]
327. Croatia, Family Law, in force from 25.4.2020 until 31.12.2023, Article 94(2). https://www.zakon.hr/z/88/Obiteljski-zakon. Accessed October 8, 2023. [Title and text translation from Google]
328. Denmark, Danish Act on Parental Responsibility 2007 article 2(2). https://boernebortfoerelse.dk/Media/637608190977168495/Danish_Act_on_Parental_Responsibility_transl2021.pdf. Accessed September 29, 2022.
329. Estonia, Child Protection Act 2014, Article 31. https://www.riigiteataja.ee/en/eli/531102014002/consolide#:~:text=(1)%20The%20Republic%20of%20Estonia,of%20Estonia%20concerning%20child%20protection. Accessed October 8, 2023. [Title and text translation from Google]
330. Finland, Child Custody and Right of Access Act Chapter 1 §1 paragraph 3. https://www.congreso.es/docu/docum/ddocum/dosieres/sleg/legislatura_10/spl_78/pdfs/39.pdf. Accessed October 8, 2023. [Title and text translation from Google]
331. France, Civil Code Article 371-1. https://www.legifrance.gouv.fr/codes/article_lc/LEGIARTI000038749626. Accessed October 8, 2023. [Title and text translation from Google]
332. Georgia, Code on the Rights of the Child 2019 Article 53-2. https://matsne.gov.ge/en/document/view/4613854?publication=4. Accessed October 8, 2023. [Title and text translation from Google]
333. Germany, German Civil Code article 1631(2). https://www.gesetze-im-internet.de/englisch_bgb/englisch_bgb.html#p6489. Accessed October 8, 2023.
334. Hungary, Child Protection Act 1997 Article 6(5). https://www.gesetze-im-internet.de/englisch_bgb/englisch_bgb.html#p6489. Accessed October 8, 2023. [Title and text translation from Google]
335. Iceland, Child Protection Act No. 80/2002 articles 82 and 99. https://www.government.is/media/velferdarraduneyti-media/media/acrobat-enskar_sidur/Child-Protection-Act-as-amended-2016.pdf. Accessed September 29, 2022.

336. Latvia, Law on Protection of the Rights of the Child 1998 Article 9(2) and Article 24 (4). https://www.vestnesis.lv/ta/id/49096-bernu-tiesibu-aizsardzibas-likums. Accessed October 8, 2023. [Title and text translation from Google]
337. Moldova, Family Code, Articles 53(4) and 62(2). https://www.legis.md/cautare/getResults?doc_id=112685&lang=ro. Accessed October 8, 2023. [Title and text translation from Google]
338. Mongolia, Law on the Rights of Children 2016, Article 7.1. https://lawforum.parliament.mn/draft/51/. Accessed October 8, 2023.
339. The Netherlands, Civil Code Title 1.14 Authority over minor children Article1:247(2). http://www.dutchcivillaw.com/civilcodebook01.htm. Accessed September 29, 2022. [Title and text translation from Google]
340. Nicaragua, Código de Familia Ley No. 870, Aprobada el 24 de junio de 2014 Articulo 280. https://www.ilo.org/dyn/natlex/docs/ELECTRONIC/102158/123413/F39376266/LEY%20870%20NICARAGUA.pdf. Accessed September 29, 2022. [Text in Spanish, English translation not available from Google]
341. North Macedonia, Law on Child Protection 2013 Article 12 (2). https://endcorporalpunishment.org/wp-content/uploads/country-reports/NorthMacedonia.pdf. Accessed October 8, 2023.
342. Norway, Parent and Child Act §30 3rd paragraph. https://www.regjeringen.no/en/dokumenter/the-children-act/id448389/. Accessed September 29, 2022.
343. Paraguay, Law 5659, Article 1. https://www.bacn.gov.py/leyes-paraguayas/5176/ley-n-5659-promocion-del-buen-trato-crianza-positiva-y-de-proteccion-a-ninos-ninas-y-adolescentes-contra-el-castigo-fisico-o-cualquier-tipo-de-violencia-como-metodo-de-correccion-o-disciplina. Accessed October 8, 2023 [Title and text translation from Google]
344. Peru, Law 30403 Article 1. https://www.mimp.gob.pe/webs/mimp/pnaia/pdf/Ley-30403-Prohibe-Castigo-Fisico.pdf. Accessed September 29, 2022. [Text in Spanish, English translation not available from Google]
345. Poland, Family and Guardianship Code, Article 96. https://przepisy.gofin.pl/przepisy,3,9,9,215,277675,20230926,art-92-112-wladza-rodzicielska.html. Accessed October 8, 2023 [Title and text translation from Google]
346. Republic of Congo, Loi N° 4-2010 du 14 Juin, portant protection de l'enfant en République du Congo2010, Article 53. http://www.unesco.org/education/edurights/media/docs/8827c7298af156a49466bc30f61b03fa980b92dc.pdf?_x_tr_sch = http&_x_tr_sl = fr&_x_tr_tl = en&_x_tr_hl = en&_x_tr_pto = sc. Accessed September 29, 2022. [Text in French, no English translation available from Google]
347. Romania, Law No. 272/2004 on the Protection and Promotion of the Rights of the Child Article 28 (1) (2). https://childhub.org/sites/default/files/library/attachments/92_177_en_original.pdf. Accessed September 29, 2022.
348. Slovenia, Law on the Prevention of Domestic Violence Article 3 A. http://pisrs.si/Pis.web/pregledPredpisa?id=ZAKO5084. Accessed October 8, 2023. [Title and text translation from Google]
349. South Sudan, Constitution of South Sudan Article 17 f. https://www.constituteproject.org/constitution/South_Sudan_2011.pdf. Accessed September 29, 2022.
350. Sweden, Children and Parents Code, ch 6(1). http://ceflonline.net/wp-content/uploads/Sweden-Parental-Responsibilities-Legislation.pdf. Accessed September 29, 2022.
351. Ukraine, Family Code 2003 Article 150 (7). https://www.refworld.org/cgi-bin/texis/vtx/rwmain/opendocpdf.pdf?reldoc=y&docid=5d667af64. Accessed October 8, 2023.

352. Uruguay, Código de la Niñez y la Adolescencia No 17823, Artículo 12 bis. https://www.impo.com.uy/bases/codigo-ninez-adolescencia/17823-2004. Accessed September 29, 2022. [Text in Spanish, English translation not available from Google]
353. Argentina, City of Buenos Aires Law 5742, 2016, Prevention of Sexual Harassment in Public Spaces. https://www.argentina.gob.ar/normativa/provincial/ley-5742-123456789-0abc-defg-247-5000xvorpyel/actualizacion. Accessed September 30, 2022. [Title and text translation from Google]
354. Chile, Ley Núm. 21.153 Modifica el Código Penal para Tipificar el Delito de Acoso Sexual en Espacios Públicos. https://oig.cepal.org/sites/default/files/2019_chl_ley21.153.pdf. Accessed September 30, 2022. [Text in Spanish, English translation not available from Google]
355. Peru, Law 30314 to prevent and sanction sexual harassment in public places. http://observatoriolegislativocele.com/wp-content/uploads/LEYES/Peru/30314.pdf. Accessed October 8, 2023 [Text in Spanish, English translation not available from Google]
356. D.C. Code §7–2421 through §7–2424. https://code.dccouncil.us/dc/council/code/titles/7/chapters/24B/. Accessed September 30, 2022.
357. For the development of this chapter, the author conducted a search and review of laws for the prevention of school bullying, cyberbullying, workplace bullying, domestic violence, physical punishment, and street harassment that have been enacted by country and/or regional jurisdiction (state or province). The search and review were supported with the use of Google and Google Translate. Data about enacted antibullying laws in the United States were derived from StopBullying.gov (a federal government Web site managed by the US Department of Health and Human Services), specifically at https://www.stopbullying.gov/resources/laws (accessed September 22, 2022). Search for workplace bullying laws by country was also supported with references listed in Cobb EP. *Workplace Bullying and Harassment: New Developments in International Law*. Taylor & Francis; 2017.
358. Canada, Province of Alberta, Protection Against Family Violence Act, RSA 2000, cP27. https://www.canlii.org/en/ab/laws/stat/rsa-2000-c-p-27/latest/rsa-2000-c-p-27.html. Accessed September 22, 2022.
359. Canada, Province of New Brunswick, Intimate Partner Violence Intervention Act. https://www.canlii.org/en/nb/laws/stat/snb-2017-c-5/latest/snb-2017-c-5.html. Accessed September 22, 2022.
360. Canada, Province of Newfoundland, and Labrador, Family Violence Protection Act, SNL 2005, c F-3.1. https://www.canlii.org/en/nl/laws/stat/snl-2005-c-f-3.1/latest/snl-2005-c-f-3.1.html. Accessed September 22, 2022.
361. Canada, Northwest Territories, Consolidation of Family Abuse Prevention Act. https://www.canlii.org/en/nu/laws/stat/snu-2006-c-18/latest/snu-2006-c-18.html. Accessed September 22, 2022.
362. Canada, Province of Prince Edward Island, Victims of Family Violence Act, RSPEI 1988. https://www.canlii.org/en/pe/laws/stat/rspei-1988-c-v-3.2/latest/rspei-1988-c-v-3.2.html. Accessed September 22, 2022.
363. Canada, Province of Saskatchewan, The Victims of Domestic Violence Act, SS 1994, c V-6.02. https://www.canlii.org/en/sk/laws/stat/ss-1994-c-v-6.02/latest/ss-1994-c-v-6.02.html. Accessed 09/30/2020
364. Canada, Yukon Territory, Family Violence Prevention Act, RSY 2002, c 84. https://www.canlii.org/en/yk/laws/stat/rsy-2002-c-84/latest/rsy-2002-c-84.html. Accessed September 22, 2022.

365. Mexico, State of Mexico, Ley para la Prevención y Erradicación de la Violencia Familiar del Estado de México. https://legislacion.edomex.gob.mx/sites/legislacion.edomex.gob.mx/files/files/pdf/ley/abr/leyabr138.pdf. Accessed October 8, 2023. [Text in Spanish, English translation not available from Google]
366. Child marriage is defined as marriage before age 18 that is a "fundamental violation of human rights." https://data.unicef.org/topic/child-protection/child-marriage/. Accessed September 22, 2022.
367. Virginity testing is "an inspection of female genitalia designed to determine whether a woman or girl has had vaginal intercourse." There "is no scientific or clinical basis" for this examination and furthermore is regarded as a "violation of human rights." See WHO "Interagency statement calls for the elimination of virginity-testing." https://www.who.int/news/item/17-10-2018-interagency-statement-calls-for-the-elimination-of-virginity-testing. Accessed September 22, 2022.
368. Widow cleansing is a cultural tradition in some areas of Africa by which "widows are expected to engage in sexual intercourse with a 'cleanser,' without the use of a condom, in order to remove the impurity ascribed to her after her husband's death." See Perry B, Oluoch L, Agot K, et al. Widow cleansing and inheritance among the Luo in Kenya: the need for additional women-centered HIV prevention options. *J Int AIDS Soc.* 2014;17(1):19010.
369. School-based bullying prevention programs could include anger management, social skills, and assertiveness training; basic skills for active listening, empathy, problem-solving and supportiveness; development of antibullying policies, increased adult supervision on school grounds; the establishment of an antibullying committee; and involvement of parents (see Butchart and Mikton, Note 370).
370. Butchart A, Mikton C. *Global Status Report on Violence Prevention, 2014.* https://www.who.int/publications/i/item/9789241564793. Accessed on September 22, 2022.
371. Spiel C, Strohmeier D. National strategy for violence prevention in the Austrian public school system: development and implementation. *Int J Behav Dev.* 2011;35(5):412–418..
372. Strohmeier D, Hoffmann C, Schiller EM, Stefanek E, Spiel C. ViSC social competence program. *New Dir Stud Leadersh.* 2012;2012(133):71–84.
373. Chaux E, Barrera M, Molano A, et al. Classrooms in peace within violent contexts: field evaluation of Aulas en Paz in Colombia. *Prev Sci.* 2017:1–1.
374. Salmivalli C, Poskiparta E. Making bullying prevention a priority in Finnish schools: the KiVa Antibullying Program. *New Dir Stud Leadersh.* 2012;2012(133):41–53.
375. Kärnä A, Voeten M, Little TD, Poskiparta E, Kaljonen A, Salmivalli C. A large-scale evaluation of the KiVa Antibullying Program: grades 4–6. *Child Dev.* 2011;82(1):311–330.
376. Schultze-Krumbholz A, Schultze M, Zagorscak P, Wölfer R, Scheithauer H. Feeling cybervictims' pain—the effect of empathy training on cyberbullying. *Aggress Behav.* 2016;42(2):147–156.
377. Olweus D, Limber SP. Bullying in school: evaluation and dissemination of the Olweus Bullying Prevention Program. *Am J Orthopsychiatry.* 2010;80(1):124.
378. Clarkson S, Axford N, Berry V, et al. Effectiveness, and micro-costing of the KiVa school-based bullying prevention programme in Wales: study protocol for a pragmatic definitive parallel group cluster randomized controlled trial. *BMC Public Health.* 2016;16(1):104.
379. Bonell C, Fletcher A, Fitzgerald-Yau N, et al. Initiating change locally in bullying and aggression through the school environment (INCLUSIVE): a pilot randomized controlled trial. *Health Technol Assess.* 2015;19(53):1–10.

380. Low S, Van Ryzin MJ, Brown EC, Smith BH, Haggerty KP. Engagement matters: lessons from assessing classroom implementation of steps to respect: a bullying prevention program over a one-year period. *Prev Sci*. 2014;15(2):165–176.
381. Schroeder BA, Messina A, Schroeder D, et al. The implementation of a statewide bullying prevention program: preliminary findings from the field and the importance of coalitions. *Health Promot Pract*. 2012;13(4):489–495.
382. Bowllan NM. Implementation and evaluation of a comprehensive, school-wide bullying prevention program in an urban/suburban middle school. *J Sch Health*. 2011;81(4):167–173.
383. Black S, Washington E, Trent V, Harner P, Pollock E. Translating the Olweus Bullying Prevention Program into real-world practice. *Health Promot Pract*. 2010;11(5):733–740.
384. Espelage DL, Low S, Polanin JR, Brown EC. The impact of a middle school program to reduce aggression, victimization, and sexual violence. *J Adolesc Health*. 2013;53(2):180–186.
385. Bauer NS, Lozano P, Rivara FP. The effectiveness of the Olweus Bullying Prevention Program in public middle schools: a controlled trial. *J Adolesc Health*. 2007;40(3):266–274.
386. PubMed review using the terms *national implementation of bullying prevention program* OR *implementation of bullying prevention program* AND [name of country]. https://www.ncbi.nlm.nih.gov/pubmed/. Accessed September 22, 2022.
387. StopBullying.gov. https://www.stopbullying.gov/.Accessed October 9, 2023.
388. PREVNET, Promoting relationships and eliminating violence network. https://www.prevnet.ca. Accessed September 22, 2022.
389. Del Rey R, Casas JA, Ortega R. Impact of the ConRed program on different cyberbulling roles. *Aggress Behav*. 2016;42(2):123–135.
390. European Commission, Employment, Social Affairs, and Inclusion. The ConRed cyberbullying prevention program. https://ec.europa.eu/social/main.jsp?catId=1252&langId=en&reviewId=164. Accessed October 15, 2023.
391. Del Rey R, Ortega-Ruiz R, Casas JA. Asegúrate: an intervention program against cyberbullying based on teachers' commitment and on design of its instructional materials. *Int J Environ Res Public Health*. 2019;16(3):434.
392. Del Rey R, Mora-Merchán JA, Casas JA, Ortega-Ruiz R, Elipe P. 'Asegúrate' program: effects on cyber-aggression and its risk factors. *Comunicar*. 2018;26(56):39–48. https://files.eric.ed.gov/fulltext/EJ1183308.pdf. Accessed September 25, 2022.
393. Cross D, Shaw T, Hadwen K, et al. Longitudinal impact of the Cyber Friendly Schools program on adolescents' cyberbullying behavior. *Aggress Behav*. 2016;42(2):166–180.
394. Edith Cowan University, Cyber Friendly Schools Project 2010-2012: Introduction. Video by Donna Cross. https://www.youtube.com/watch?v=KflKP5QCSoI&t=26s&ab_channel=EdithCowanUniversity. Accessed October 9, 2023.
395. Milczarek M. *Workplace Violence and Harassment: A European Picture*. Luxembourg: Publications Office of the European Union; 2010:99–14. https://osha.europa.eu/en/publications/workplace-violence-and-harassment-european-picture. Accessed September 22, 2022.
396. The Prevention and Management of Violence in the Workplace, National Occupational Standards, January 2013, Skills CFA, 6 Graphite Square, Vauxhall Walk, London SE11 5EE. https://fs.hubspotusercontent00.net/hubfs/8304001/Prevention-Management-of-Work-Related-Violence.pdf. Accessed October 9, 2023.
397. Arbeidstilsynet. Bullying. https://www.arbeidstilsynet.no/tema/mobbing/. Accessed September 22, 2022. [Title and text translation from Google]

398. Chappell D, Di Martino V. *Violence at Work*. Geneva, Switzerland: International Labour Office. Cited by Milczarek.[395]
399. International Labour Office. *Code of Practice on Workplace Violence in Services Sectors and Measures to Combat this Phenomenon*. Geneva, Switzerland: International Labour Office; 2003. Cited by Milczarek.[395]
400. International Labour Office/ICN/World Health Organization/PSI. Framework guidelines for addressing workplace violence in the health sector. Geneva, Switzerland: International Labour Office; 2002. Cited by Milczarek.[395]
401. Cooper CL, Swanson N. *Workplace Violence in the Health Sector: State of the Art*. Geneva, Switzerland: International Labour Office; 2002. Cited by Milczarek.[395]
402. Essenberg B. *Violence and Stress in the Transport Sector*. Geneva, Switzerland: International Labour Office; 2003. Cited by Milczarek.[395]
403. World Health Organization. *Raising Awareness of Psychological Harassment at Work*. Protecting Workers' Health Series, No 4. Geneva, Switzerland: WHO; 2003. Cited by Milczarek.[395]
404. Murta SG, de Oliveira Parada P, da Silva Meneses S, et al. Dating SOS: a systematic and theory-based development of a web-based tailored intervention to prevent dating violence among Brazilian youth. *BMC Public Health*. 2020;20(1):1–4.
405. Vives-Cases C, Davó-Blanes MC, Ferrer-Cascales R, et al. Lights4Violence: a quasi-experimental educational intervention in six European countries to promote positive relationships among adolescents. *BMC Public Health*. 2019;19(1):389.
406. Wolfe DA, Wekerle C, Scott K, Straatman AL, Grasley C, Reitzel-Jaffe D. Dating violence prevention with at-risk youth: a controlled outcome evaluation. *J Consult Clin Psychol*. 2003;71(2):279.
407. Sosa-Rubi SG, Saavedra-Avendano B, Piras C, Van Buren SJ, Bautista-Arredondo S. True love: effectiveness of a school-based program to reduce dating violence among adolescents in Mexico City. *Prev Sci*. 2017;18(7):804–817.
408. Muñoz-Fernández N, Ortega-Rivera J, Nocentini A, Menesini E, Sánchez-Jiménez V. The efficacy of the "Dat-e Adolescence" prevention program in the reduction of dating violence and bullying. *Int J Environ Res Public Health*. 2019;16(3):408.
409. Wolfe DA, Wekerle C, Gough R, et al. *The Youth Relationships Manual: A Group Approach with Adolescents for the Prevention of Woman Abuse and the Promotion of Healthy Relationships*. Thousand Oaks, CA: SAGE; 1996. Cited in Wolfe et al.[406]
410. Centers for Disease Control and Prevention, National Center for Injury Prevention and Control, Division of Violence Prevention. What Is Dating Matters? https://www.cdc.gov/violenceprevention/intimatepartnerviolence/datingmatters/index.html. Accessed September 22, 2022.
411. Niolon PH, Vivolo-Kantor AM, Tracy AJ, et al. An RCT of Dating Matters: effects on teen dating violence and relationship behaviors. *Am J Prev Med*. 2019;57(1):13–23.
412. Foshee VA, Linder GF, Bauman KE, Langwick SA, Arriaga XB, Heath JL, ... Bangdiwala S. The Safe Dates Project: Theoretical basis, evaluation design, and selected baseline findings. *Am J Prev Med*. 1996;12(5):39–47.
413. Foshee VA, Bauman KE, Arriaga XB, et al. An evaluation of Safe Dates, an adolescent dating violence prevention program. *Am J Public Health*. 1998;88(1):45–50. Cited in Niolon et al.[411]

414. Torralbas-Fernández A, Calcerrada-Gutiérrez M. Using primary care to address violence against women in intimate partner relationships: professional training needs. *MEDICC Rev.* 2016;18:38–41.
415. Addo-Lartey AA, Ogum Alangea D, Sikweyiya Y, et al. Rural response system to prevent violence against women: methodology for a community randomized controlled trial in the central region of Ghana. *Glob Health Action.* 2019; 12(1):1612604.
416. Daruwalla N, Machchhar U, Pantvaidya S, et al. Community interventions to prevent violence against women and girls in informal settlements in Mumbai: the SNEHA-TARA pragmatic cluster randomized controlled trial. *Trials.* 2019; 20(1):743.
417. Moor A. The efficacy of a high school rape prevention program in Israel. *Violence Vict.* 2011;26(3):283–295.
418. DeGue S, Simon TR, Basile KC, Yee SL, Lang K, Spivak H. Moving forward by looking back: reflecting on a decade of CDC's work in sexual violence prevention, 2000–2010. *J Womens Health.* 2012;21(12):1211–1218.
419. SNEHA (Society for Nutrition, Education and Health Action). https://snehamumbai.org/our-story/. Accessed September 20, 2022.
420. COMBAT'ing violence against women: a success story from rural Ghana. https://prevention-collaborative.org/resource/combating-violence-against-women-a-success-story-from-rural-ghana/. Accessed September 22, 2022.
421. Centers for Disease Control and Prevention, National Center for Injury Prevention and Control, Division of Violence Prevention. Sexual Violence. https://www.cdc.gov/violenceprevention/sexualviolence/index.html. Accessed September 22, 2022.
422. Basile KC, DeGue S, Jones K, et al. (2016). *STOP SV: A Technical Package to Prevent Sexual Violence.* Atlanta, GA: National Center for Injury Prevention and Control. https://www.cdc.gov/violenceprevention/pdf/SV-Prevention-Technical-Package.pdf. Accessed September 22, 2022.
423. Dickson S, Willis GM. Primary prevention of sexual violence in Aotearoa New Zealand: a survey of prevention activities. *Sex Abuse.* 2017;29(2):128–147.
424. Australian Government. National Plan to Reduce Violence Against Women and Their Children. https://plan4womenssafety.dss.gov.au/the-national-plan/what-is-the-national-plan/. Accessed September 22, 2022.
425. Fourth Action Plan, National Plan to Reduce Violence Against Women and Their Children, © Commonwealth of Australia (Department of Social Services) 2019. https://www.dss.gov.au/sites/default/files/documents/08_2019/fourth_action-plan.pdf. Accessed September 22, 2022.
426. Australian Government, Department of Social Services, Women's Safety, Women's Safety Package. https://www.dss.gov.au/women-programs-services-reducing-violence/womens-safety-package. Accessed September 22, 2022.
427. 1800RESPECT. https://www.1800respect.org.au/about-us. Accessed September 22, 2022.
428. Government of Canada, Public Health Agency. Family Violence Initiative. https://www.canada.ca/en/public-health/services/health-promotion/stop-family-violence/initiative.html. Accessed September 22, 2022.
429. Government of Canada, Public Health Agency. Stop Family Violence. https://www.canada.ca/en/public-health/services/health-promotion/stop-family-violence.html. Accessed September 22, 2022.

430. Congressional Research Service. Family Violence Prevention and Services Act (FVPSA): Background and Funding. https://fas.org/sgp/crs/misc/R42838.pdf. Updated April 4, 2019. Accessed September 22, 2022.
431. US Department of Health and Human Services, Administration for Children and Families, Family and Youth Services Bureau. Family Violence and Services Program. https://www.acf.hhs.gov/fysb/programs/family-violence-prevention-services/about. Accessed September 23, 2022.
432. US Department of Health and Human Services, Administration for Children and Families, Family and Youth Services Bureau. Family Violence and Services Program, State Domestic Violence Coalitions. https://www.acf.hhs.gov/ofvps/programs/fvpsa/fvpsa-grants-state-and-territorial-domestic-violence-coalitions. Accessed October 9, 2023.
433. US Department of Health and Human Services, Administration for Children and Families, Family and Youth Services Bureau. Family Violence and Services Program, Resource Centers. https://www.acf.hhs.gov/ofvps/programs/fvpsa/family-violence-prevention-services-resource-centers. Accessed October 9, 2023.
434. US Department of Health and Human Services, Administration for Children and Families, Family and Youth Services Bureau. Family Violence and Services Program, National Domestic Violence Hotline. https://www.acf.hhs.gov/fysb/programs/family-violence-prevention-services/programs/ndvh. Accessed September 23, 2022.
435. New Zealand Family Violence Clearinghouse, Overview and Highlights, 2016–17. https://nzfvc.org.nz/sites/nzfvc.org.nz/files/NZFVC-Overview-and-Highlights-2016-17.pdf. Accessed September 22, 2022.
436. New Zealand Family Violence Clearinghouse. https://nzfvc.org.nz/. Accessed September 22, 2022.
437. *Whānau* is defined as "extended family, family group, a familiar term of address to a number of people—the primary economic unit of traditional Māori society. In the modern context the term is sometimes used to include friends who may not have any kinship ties to other members." From Māori Dictionary. https://maoridictionary.co.nz/. Accessed October 9, 2023.
438. New Zealand Government, Ministry of Justice, Family Violence Risk Assessment and Management Framework. A Common Approach to Screening, Assessing and Management Risk. https://www.justice.govt.nz/assets/family-violence-ramf.pdf. Accessed October 9, 2023.

11

Bullying and Other Forms of Maltreatment in the School Milieu

What Is Known?

Scholarly articles on bullying published through 2022 predominantly[1] focused on its occurrence in the school environment, rather than the workplace or cyberspace.[2] Also, until 2008, public interest in bullying mostly concentrated on its occurrence in the school milieu, followed by its occurrence in cyberspace and workplace, as evidenced by Internet search trends[3] from 2004 to the present.[4] However, since 2008, public interest in cyberbullying has surpassed public interest in school and workplace bullying.[4]

Olweus' seminal work on the nature and prevention of school bullying[5-18] inspired the body of research published in the past two decades that examines the ecology[19-80] and prevalence[81-96] of this form of maltreatment, as well as developing strategies for its prevention.[97-132]

Concept

What is currently understood as school bullying follows the same notion of peer victimization occurring in an educational setting initially outlined by Olweus.[133-134] Bullying is still recognized as "unwanted aggressive behavior(s) by another youth or group of youths who are not siblings or current dating partners that involves an observed or perceived power imbalance and is repeated multiple times or is highly likely to be repeated."[135] The uniform definition of bullying[135] includes the same forms of maltreatment described by Olweus,[133-134] such as violent physical force (i.e., hitting, kicking, punching, spitting, tripping, and pushing), hostile oral or written communication (i.e., taunting, name-calling, threatening or offensive written notes or hand gestures, inappropriate sexual comments, or oral threats), or antagonistic relational behavior (i.e., ignoring or isolating somebody, spreading false and/or harmful rumors, publicly writing derogatory comments, or posting embarrassing images in a physical or electronic space without the target person's permission or knowledge).

Participants' Roles

Olweus' original research on students who play a part in school bulling focused on the role and characteristics of victims and bullies,[136] and it hinted at the situation of students in the dual role of victim and bully.[136] Beyond consideration of these three groups of participants, attention is turning to the direct or indirect role or influence of bystanders[137,138] and, to a lesser degree, teachers[19,46,47,1139,140] and family.[141-145]

Victims

Olweus discussed what could be characterized as a "typical victim" of bullying, describing them as "more anxious and insecure than students in general" and as being "often cautious, sensitive, and quiet."[136] Moreover, they were described as having low self-esteem and as being anxious, lonely, and insecure.[136] Olweus identified these characteristics as belonging to a "passive or submissive victim,"[136] while conversely he recognized the lesser number of victims who were both anxious and aggressive, whom he designated "provocative victims,"[136] thus introducing the notion of bully/victims.

In a cross-sectional study, Al Ali and colleagues[146] surveyed 913 Jordanian eighth-grade students to examine, among other issues, students' perceptions of the characteristics of participants in bullying. The research showed that two-thirds of students perceived victims as having low self-esteem, at least half felt that victims talked or sounded different than others, and one-third viewed victims as being shy and having no friends.[146]

Based on a second analysis of the 2009–2010 US Health Behavior in School-aged Children (HBSC) survey, 15.5% of US students in grades 5 to 10 reported having been bullied by peers at least once or more times in the preceding two months.[147] Females were very slightly more frequently victims (52.5%) than nonvictims. Furthermore, the frequency of victimization was found to gradually decline from fifth and sixth to tenth grade.[147]

Bullies

According to Olweus, aggression toward peers typifies a bully, together with impulsivity, little empathy, and a "hard need to dominate."[136] In the study by Al Ali et al.,[146] students perceived a bully mostly as one who is a coward underneath, lacks respect for other people, and wants to show power, to impress others, and to feel superior.

According to the 2009–2010 US HBSC survey, 15.6% of students reported bullying others, with a significantly higher proportion of male bullies (58%).[147] Furthermore, bullies were more prevalent in the eighth grade.[147]

Bully/Victims

Among US students, 12% reported being both bullied and bullying others at least once in the previous couple of months.[147] There was a slightly higher, but statistically significant, percentage of males (55%).[147]

A longitudinal study by Lereyra et al.[148] of a cohort of 4,101 British students showed that the largest fraction (42%) of bully/victims at age 13 were previously victims at age 10, while 35% and 20% were, respectively, nonparticipants in bullying or were bully/victims at age 10.[148]

Berkowitz and Benbenishty[149] surveyed a nationally representative sample of 13,262 Israeli students in grades 7 to 11, showing that bully/victims reported the lowest levels of teacher support and feelings of security as well as the most frequent school absenteeism because of fears.[149]

Bully/victims, as distinguished from students who only bully others and those who are not involved in bullying, have been recognized as showing higher levels of hyperactivity[150] and achieving lower levels of educational aptitude, social approval, and overall self-confidence.[137] Anecdotally, I have learned that school staff and, to some extent, parents may misunderstand bully/victims as being responsible for their victimization because of their roles as perpetrators.

Bystanders

A discussed in Chapter 20, witnesses to bullying have been categorized by Salmivali et al.[137] in four types, based on group dynamics: the assistant, who is the bully's helper; the reinforcer, who encourages the bully's actions by making fun of the victim; the outsider, who keeps away from the victimization; and the defender, who tries to stop the maltreatment and/or helps the victim.[137]

Empathy, problem-solving ability, and attitude toward bullying have been found to be major factors significantly associated with bystander support for the victim,[138] while concern about being bullied[138] is a significant element associated with being a bully follower or an outsider (neutral bystander).

Teachers' Role in Bullying

Some studies[19,46,47,139,140] have explored the influence of teachers' attributes in responding to, or failing to respond to, peer victimization.

The effect of teachers' trait empathy and years of study in reacting to bullying was investigated by Huang et al.[139] in research using 242 female university undergraduate students majoring in preschool education, during their last school term spent in practice. The research demonstrated that the participants' emotional empathy played a complex role in their reactions to bullying by moderating the relationship between years of study and responses to this form of maltreatment, while "personal distress negatively predicted the participant's responses to all types of bullying."[139]

In a study by Kochenderfer-Ladd and Pelletier[140] based on 34 second and fourth grade teachers and 363 ethnically diverse students, teachers' views and beliefs about bullying were found to be associated with their responses to peer victimization. The study showed that teachers were not likely to intervene if they viewed bullying as "normative behavior" (i.e., "teasing other children is just part of growing up"), but they were more likely to get involved if they held either an assertion belief ("children who stand up for themselves will not be victimized") or an avoidant view ("children who avoid aggressors will not be victimized").[140]

Similar findings were documented by Troop-Gordon and Ladd,[47] who showed that "teachers who held more normative views of peer victimization were less likely to report reprimanding aggressive students and were more likely to utilize passive response strategies."[47]

A study led by Banzon-Librojo et al.,[19] involving 401 first- to fourth-year high school students at an urban public school in the Philippines, documented that "experiences of harsh teacher discipline predicted higher bullying victimization and students' negative perception of teacher support."[19]

Lenzi et al.[46] also provided evidence that perceived teacher unfairness, manifested as the students' perceptions of being treated with dishonesty or disrespect by their teachers, is positively linked to bullying, and that this association is partially mediated by the students' endorsement of social goals or norms that model and allow disrespectful behaviors.[46]

Family's Role in School Bullying

Several studies have investigated the association of parental styles and psychological characteristics with peer victimization.[141-145]

Duncan[141] reviewed the limited research that has examined the parent and family characteristics of children involved in bullying. The review highlighted that families of male victims tend to be cohesive and warm, while female victims are more likely to live in families with low affect and communication and poor functioning.[141] Furthermore, bullies are more likely to live in a family with an absent father, harsh physical punishment, low cohesion, negative affect, and/or authoritarian parenting, while bully/victims are likely to come from families with domestic violence, a hostile mother, uninvolved parents, inconsistent discipline, and a negative environment.[141]

Lereyra et al.[142] conducted a systematic review of the literature on parenting behavior and peer victimization, showing that victims and bully/victims were more likely to be subjected to parental abuse and neglect or "maladaptive parenting," with effects being small to moderate for victims (Hedges' g range = 0.10–0.31) but moderate for bully/victims (g = 0.13–0.68).[142] Good parent–child communication, a kind and loving relationship, and parental involvement, support, and care were found to be safeguards against school bullying, with protective influences being small to moderate for both victims (Hedges' g range = -0.12 to -0.22) and bully/victims (Hedges' g range= -0.17 to -0.42).[142]

Zotis et al.[143] investigated the association of child disciplinary practices and bullying behavior in a cross-sectional study of 275 Brazilian children and adolescents. The research documented that parental power-assertive and punitive discipline (corporal punishment, psychological aggression, deprivation of privileges, and penalty tasks) is significantly linked to a child's becoming a bully.[143] Mothers who frequently used this type of discipline were 4.36 times more likely to have a child who bullies others.[143]

The parents' history of peer victimization has been found to be associated with an increased risk for their children to be bullied, as shown in research by Allison et al.,[144] which was based on face-to face interviews of 1,895 Australian parents. The study showed that parental history of previous peer victimization was a significant predictor [adjusted odds ratio (AOR) = 2.00] for their children's victimization at school.[144] These findings should be relevant in trying to understand the impact of a student's being bullied on his/her parents' potential reactivation of traumatic memories.[144]

Hale et al.[145] recounted the experiences of parents in dealing with school when their child is bullied through the stories of 21 parents living in the Northwest of England. The themes and concerns emerging from the narratives highlight the parental perception "that the teachers did not communicate with them and appeared to do very little"; a mistrust of teachers when they indicated that did not know about the bullying problem; a wariness that the teacher failed to deal with the problem because of "other priorities"; feelings of not being believed by the school when reporting their child's victimization; and the school's attitude that the situation was not "as serious as the parent perceived it to be." Overall, the narratives underscore the parents' feelings of helplessness, self-blame, frustration, anger, resentment, and aggression toward the bully.

Ecological Aspects of School Bullying

Beyond the role of the participants, teachers and families should consider other ecological aspects of school bullying, including the impact of classroom environment,[151] the effects of school climate,[152] and social conditions.[73,74]

Classroom Environment

Doll et al.[151] examined the classroom aspects and strategies that can discourage peer bullying; promote peer inclusion; improve the relationships between teachers and students and the parents with the classroom; foster behavioral self-control through self-monitoring, self-evaluation, and self-reinforcement; establish clear rules that disallow bullying; and encourage the development of self-efficacy and self-determination.[151]

School Climate

The qualities of the social and emotional school climate that deter peer victimization, as reviewed by Kasen et al.,[152] encompassed a school environment characterized by low conflict, high levels of organization and harmony, priority of learning, and discouragement of competition among students.[152]

Social Conditions

The association between income inequality and school bullying was ascertained by Elgar et al.[73] in a study based on 66,190 11-year-old students in 37 countries. The study findings revealed that each standard deviation increase in income inequality was significantly linked to more frequent bullying by males (relative OR = 1.17) and females (relative OR = 1.24).[73]

Chaux et al.[74] conducted a study based on 53,316 Colombian fifth and ninth grade students in order to determine the sociopolitical and economic factors that predict school bullying. The research demonstrated, through a multilevel analysis, that the presence of an armed conflict was the only municipality-level (community-level) variable explaining variance in frequency of bullying among fifth graders, while inequality was the only explanatory variable among ninth graders. Yet, in both cases, the percentage of variance explained was less than 1%.[74]

Prevalence of School Bullying

As discussed in Chapter 2, and based on surveys[153,154] of national representative samples of adolescent students in 77 countries and territories around the world, 48% of students reported being bullied at least once in the preceding 30 days, and 9% were bullied at least twice in the previous two months.[155]

Prevention of School Bullying

As examined in Chapter 7, after three decades of multiple international efforts to develop and implement bullying intervention strategies, the Olweus[132-134] and KiVA[105] programs are the most widely recognized and implemented programs so far.[156]

Teachers as Victims of Bullying

Several reports have addressed the victimization of teachers by students through verbal bullying, such as lewd and badly chosen statements, insults, intentional disrespect, and taunting, as well as nonverbal communication like insulting gestures and laughter.[157-160] Furthermore, teachers can be the object of indirect bullying, such as their work being sabotaged; students' refusal to cooperate; students' lying, cheating, ignoring the teacher, hiding from the teacher, or coming late to class; and students' dissemination of unfounded gossip or unjust criticism of the teacher's professional skills.[157-160] Moreover, teachers can be mistreated through intimidation, sexual harassment, physical violence, vandalism, theft of their property and/or cyberbullying.[157-160]

Teachers' Mistreatment of Students

Several published reports focus on teacher's victimization of students through bullying and other forms of maltreatment.[141,161-175]

Teachers Bullying Students

The literature on teachers' mistreatment of students that fits the concept of bullying is so far extremely limited.[161-163]

During the academic year of 1996–97, Twemlow et al.[161] conducted an anonymous survey of 116 elementary school teachers in seven urban schools in an effort to ascertain, in part, the extent of teachers' bullying of students as well as the teachers' perceptions of the causes of such bullying.[161] This study defined a bullying teacher as "a teacher who uses his/her power to punish, manipulate or disparage a student beyond what would be a reasonable disciplinary procedure."[161] The survey results showed that at least 70% of the teachers bully students in isolated cases and almost 18% bully students frequently.[161] Respondents revealed that 30% of them had bullied a student a few times, and 2.6% had done it frequently.[161]

Teachers who bullied students frequently were significantly more likely to have been bullied as students themselves and were more likely to be bullied in classrooms by their own students. A study by Twenlow and Fonagy[162] that was based on 214 teachers from eight elementary schools, four middle schools, and three high schools in the Midwest of the United States documented "that teachers from schools with high rates of suspensions reported that they themselves bullied more students."[162]

Other Forms of Teachers' Victimization of Students

Whitted and Dupper[163] explored the extent to which 50 US students (age 11 to 18) attending alternative schools for behavioral problems reported being physically or psychologically victimized by teachers or other adults in school during the 2004–2005 school year. The investigation found that 86% of the students reported at least once incident of being physically mistreated by an adult in school; examples included being locked up in a closet, locker, or small room; being slapped, punched, pushed, or hit with an object; being grabbed; being shaken; having one's hair or ear pulled; not being allowed to go to the bathroom, or the adult's allowing others to hit the student.[163] Furthermore, 88% of the students indicated that they were psychologically victimized at least once by an adult in school; examples included being ignored; being yelled at; being made to stay alone or away from everyone else; being made fun of, teased, or called names; being racially ridiculed; not being allowed to participate in special activities; not being given help when it was asked for; or being picked/chosen last.[163]

Research by Khoury-Kassabri,[175] based on a nationally representative sample of 17,465 students in grades 4 to 11 in 319 schools across Israel, aimed at studying student victimization by educational staff and documented that 30.9% of students reported that they were emotionally abused, 24.5% indicated that they were physically maltreated, and 8% reported being sexually victimized.[175]

Sexual Abuse by Teachers

Several published reports have highlighted the problem of sexual abuse by teachers in various parts of the world.[164-168]

A 2001 nonclinical retrospective case series by Nhundu and Shumba[164] documented a total of 110 child sexual abuse cases perpetrated by schoolteachers in six administrative jurisdictions of Zimbabwe from 1990 through 1997.[164] Almost all (98%) of the victims were females, and 69% were between 11 and 13 years old. All the perpetrators were males, with 68% of them being beginning teachers (none to 5 years of experience).[164]

A 1998 cross-sectional study by Jewkes et al.,[165] based on a nationally representative sample of 11,735 South African women 15 to 49 years old, showed that 1.6% of the women reported being raped before age 15 years, with schoolteachers being responsible of one-third of the rapes.[165]

Moulden et al.[166] analyzed the reports of 113 adult male teachers who had come to the attention of the Royal Canadian Mountain Police for a sexual offense against a child or adolescent under their care between 1995 and 2002. The reports indicated that 99% of the offenders were sexually motivated, with only 1% reported as being culturally or religiously motivated.[166] Only 4% to 5% of the offenders received treatment for alcohol, psychological, or sexual problems.[166] The age of the victims ranged from 3 to 16 years, and they were slightly more likely to be female (56%). The most common sexual acts perpetrated included fondling or hugging the victim, masturbation, and kissing.[166]

Gallagher[167] estimated there were 185 cases of substantiated institutional abuse in England and Wales for the period of 1988 to 1992, and approximately 46% (85 cases per year) occurred in schools (including special and boarding educational facilities).

Knoll[168] reviewed the literature on female teacher sexual misconduct, which highlights different "typologies," with the most common being the "heterosexual nurturer, who was least likely to have an arrest for sexual assault."[176] A classification of teacher/lover was suggested "for the adult female who views herself as emotionally equal to her teenage male victim (or female [victim] if the perpetrator is homosexual)."[177]

School Corporal Punishment

School corporal punishment is paddling, spanking, or other forms of physical punishment imposed on a student.[178] Other forms of harsh punishment include pinching, pulling one's ears or hair, being slapped, being forced to stand in painful positions, exercise without rest or water, and ingestion of noxious substances.[171-174]

During the academic year 2017–2018, 0.34% of students in the United States were subjected to corporal punishment, with males being more frequently (0.22%) disciplined in this way than females (0.05%), and black people, Native Americans, and Alaska Natives (0.3%) being more frequently disciplined than whites (0.15%), Hispanics (0.04%), and Pacific Islanders (0.04%).[178]

In the United States, school corporal punishment is not prohibited at the federal level.[179] In 1997, the United States Supreme Court established that "the Eighth Amendment, which prohibits cruel and unusual punishment, did not apply to school students, and that teachers could punish children without parental permission."[180]

Corporal punishment is not illegal or is partly prohibited in public and private schools in only 19 of the 50 US states[169,179] (Table 11.1).

As of April 2021, worldwide, there were 49 countries/territories where school corporal punishment was not fully prohibited[181] (Table 11.2).

According to Gershoff,[170] the range of prevalence of school corporal punishment, as reported by students, widely varied among countries, from 1% in the United States to rates of over 90% in Botswana, Cameroon, Jamaica, St. Kitts and Nevis, Republic of Korea, Trinidad and Tobago, Uganda, and Yemen. It is noteworthy that school corporal punishment continues to be reported even in countries where it has been banned (Table 11.3)

Future Directions

Future research and clinical efforts should contribute to the evolving notion of bullying and other forms of maltreatment occurring in the school milieu by:

- Regarding the school environment as a workplace milieu
- Considering all school stakeholders

Table 11.1. States Where School Corporal Punishment Is Not Illegal or Is Partially Prohibited[169,179]

Alabama	Idaho	New Hampshire[b]
Arizona	Indiana	North Carolina[c]
Arkansas	Kansas	Oklahoma[a]
Colorado	Kentucky	South Carolina
Florida	Mississippi[a]	Tennessee
Georgia	Missouri	Texas
		Wyoming

[a] Illegal to use on students with disabilities.[179]

[b] Law allows the use of force for the maintenance of discipline.[179]

[c] Paddling is prohibited by all district school boards, but a legislative provision still allows it.

Table 11.2. Countries/Territories Where School Corporal Punishment Was Not Fully Prohibited, as of April 2021[181]

Angola	Equatorial Guinea	Palau
Antigua and Barbuda	Eritrea	Qatar
Australia	Eswatini†	Samoa
Bahamas	Gambia	Saudi Arabia
Barbados	Grenada	Senegal
Bhutan	Guatemala	Singapore
Botswana	Guyana	Solomon Islands
Brunei Darussalam	India	Somalia*
Burkina Faso	Iran	St. Kitts and Nevis
Central African Republic	Iraq	St. Lucia
Comoros	Jamaica	St. Vincent and Grenadines
Cote d'Ivoire	Malaysia	State of Palestine[182]
		Suriname
Dominica	Maldives	Syrian Arab Republic
		Tuvalu
DPR Korea	Mauritania	Republic of North Macedonia Tanzania
		United States
Egypt	Morocco	Western Sahara
		Zimbabwe

† The name of Kingdom of Swaziland was changed to Kingdom of Eswatini in 2018. https://www.bbc.com/news/world-africa-43821512. Accessed September 9, 2022.

Table 11.3. Corporal Punishment Reported in Country/Territory Where It Has Been Banned[170]

Afghanistan	Czech Republic	Kenya	Taiwan
Bangladesh	Djibouti	Malawi	TFYR Macedonia
Belgium	Ethiopia	Mali	Togo
Benin	Fiji	Peru	Trinidad & Tobago
Cambodia	Hong Kong	Philippines	Uganda
Cameroon	Jordan	Serbia	Vietnam
China	Kazakhstan	South Africa	Yemen

- Attending to overwork as a form of maltreatment in the school
- Covering all types of maltreatment among school stakeholders
- Bearing in mind the range of potential perceived stressful circumstances affecting school stakeholders

The School Environment as a Workplace: Overwork in the Educational Setting

Regarding the school environment as a workplace[183,184] is indirectly reflected in the Swedish Work Environment Act[185] and the Finnish Occupational Safety and Health Act.[186] These laws,[185,186] which are intended to prevent occupational illnesses and accidents while ensuring a good working environment, regard students or trainees as employees, in the same way that people working for an employer, individuals in "institutional care performing work that they have been assigned,"[185] and persons working in the military are employees.

In the context of considering the school milieu as a workplace for both students and school staff, we can incorporate into the notion of school bullying or maltreatment instances of mismanagement, abuse, or neglect that are beyond physical aggression. These include psychological harassment or indirect bullying and are uniquely related to the work environment[187] (Box 11.1).

These instances of work mistreatment or mismanagement may represent a failure, inattention, or neglect in the development and implementation of educational policies and/or availability of services. They also reflect a lack of resources to recognize and attend to the individual sociocultural, developmental, physical, emotional, and/or cognitive needs of students, educational staff, and parents.

Overwork as a Form of School Maltreatment

Some of the patterns of work mistreatment in the educational milieu may lead to the problem of overwork, a concept already recognized more than 150 years ago as a concern in both the workplace[188,189] and the school environment.[190,191]

The role of school hygiene as a type of occupational health discipline was reflected in a paper published by Lundy[190] in 1883. In this article,[190] Lundy addressed his concerns about

Box 11.1. Examples of Workplace Abuse or Neglect Applied to the Educational Milieu

Being compelled to do tasks that are harmful to one's health
Denial of a request for appropriate assistance
Exposure to an unmanageable workload
Being given tasks above one's skill or ability
Being given tasks or assignments beyond school working hours and/or with unreasonable deadlines

the notion of overwork in public schools, as manifested by the excessive number of subjects included in the programs and the extraordinary number of hours required for school learning, resulting in additional study time at home. In addition to the "cramming process,"[190] the author underscored significant competition among students, which may have been imprudently boosted by the teacher to demonstrate how his/her instruction fostered the rapid advance of students. Lundy[190] argued that the cramming process[190] together with the students' competition would result in mental strain leading to absenteeism. Beyond avoiding overwork, Lundy advocated for a suitable working environment, as manifested by proper room temperatures, ventilation, and light; appropriately constructed and arranged seats and desks that fostering good posture; correction of refractive disorders; and provision for physical education.

If we consider the school milieu a workplace, we should recognize the evolving understanding of the notion of overwork[192] as a form occupational abuse or maltreatment linked to health risks[193-194] and apply it to the educational setting. In this context, we should ascertain potential health problems linked with the requirement for long school days and/or home assignments as well as intensely competitive exams.

Encompassing All Types of Maltreatment among Educational Stakeholders

The view of school bullying can be expanded beyond the notion of victimization among peers, to encompass all types of abuse or neglect that can occur among the stakeholders[195] involved in the work in a safe educational environment. The stakeholders include students, educators, support staff, administrators, parents, and families, as well as officials tasked with the development and implementation of educational policies, programs, and resources.

Perceived Stressful Circumstances That May Affect School Stakeholders

A wide range of stressful circumstances or events may be experienced or perceived by school stakeholders (Table 11.4), and studies are needed to ascertain their frequency and health impact.

Table 11.4. Perceived Stressful Circumstances That May Affect School Stakeholders

Experiencing a lack of school physical security	Experiencing the spread of rumors about oneself	Being reprimanded, criticized, or put down in front of others
Anxiety about competitive academic grades and/or test scores	Feeling glared at in a hostile manner	Being shouted at or yelled at
Being hit, pushed, slapped, spanked, shoved, kicked, or pinched	Feeling apprehensive about having to give an oral presentation in front of the class or being called on in class	Being the object of sexual allusions or proposals
Being refused or denied a request for assistance or help	Feeling of being ignored, excluded, rejected, unnoticed, regarded as non-existent, or discriminated against	Being treated with sarcasm, teased, disrespected, made fun of, ridiculed, mimicked, insulted, or degraded
Being sexually assaulted	Feeling of being intimidated by finger pointing or by having one's way being blocked or one's space invaded	Being criticized about one's competence or intelligence
Experiencing deficient school physical environmental conditions (chemical or biological hazards, poor ventilation, poor air conditioning, malfunctioning heating, or poor lighting)	Feeling of being harassed or threatened	Feeling overwhelmed with home assignments, unmanageable workload, or tasks with unreasonable deadlines
Experiencing distress about loud noises, crowded areas, or packed sitting arrangements	Feeling of being compelled to do tasks that are harmful to one's health	Feeling stressed by long school days (beyond 8 hours), early school schedule, or early bus schedule

Notes

1. Articles "predominantly" focusing on bullying in school have a factor of preponderance of at least 1.8, as compared to publications published during the same period that concentrated on either workplace bullying or cyberbullying.
2. A review of articles containing the Medical Subject Headings (MeSH; https://www.ncbi.nlm.nih.gov/mesh/) term *school bullying* was conducted on Pubmed (https://pubmed.ncbi.nlm.nih.gov/, accessed September 7, 2022) and was compared to a search of articles containing the MeSH terms *workplace bullying* or *cyberbullying*.
3. Search made with Google Trends. https://trends.google.com/trends/. Accessed September 22, 2023.
4. Graphic display of global interest, from 2004 to 2022, in searching the Web about the term *school bullying* as compared to either *workplace bullying* or *cyberbullying*. https://trends.google.com/trends/. Accessed September 22, 2023.
5. Olweus D. Aggression and peer acceptance in adolescent boys: two short-term longitudinal studies of ratings. *Child Dev.* 1977:1301–1313.
6. Olweus D. Aggression in the schools: bullies and whipping boys. *Hemisphere*; 1978.

7. Ekblad S, Olweus D. Applicability of Olweus 'aggression inventory in a sample of Chinese primary school children. *Aggress Behav*. 1986;12(5):315–325.
8. Olweus D. Victimization among school children. *Adv Psychol*. 1991;76:45–102.
9. Olweus D. Bully/victim problems among schoolchildren: basic facts and effects of a school-based intervention program. *Dev Treat Child Aggress*. 1991; 17:411–418.
10. Olweus D. Bullying at school: basic facts and effects of a school-based intervention program. *J Child Psychol Psychiatry*. 1994;35(7):1171–1190..
11. Olweus D. Bullying or peer abuse at school: facts and intervention. *Curr Dir Psychol Sci*. 1995;4(6):196–200.
12. Olweus D. Bullying at school: knowledge base and an effective intervention program. *Ann NY Acad Sci*. 1996;794(1):265–276.
13. Kallestad JH, Olweus D, Alsaker F. School climate reports from Norwegian teachers: a methodological and substantive study. *Sch Eff Sch Improv*. 1998;9(1):70–94.
14. Olweus D. Bullying at school: tackling the problem. *OECD Observer*. 2001(225):24.
15. Olweus D. A profile of bullying at school. *Educ Leadersh*. 2003;60(6):12–17.
16. Solberg ME, Olweus D. Prevalence estimation of school bullying with the Olweus Bully/Victim Questionnaire. *Aggress Behav*. 2003;29(3):239–268..
17. Olweus D. The Olweus Bullying Prevention Programme: design and implementation issues and a new national initiative in Norway. In: Smith PK, Pepler D, Rigby K, eds. *Bullying in Schools: How Successful Can Interventions Be?* Cambridge, United Kingdom: Cambridge University Press; 2004:13–36.
18. Olweus D. A useful evaluation design, and effects of the Olweus Bullying Prevention Program. *Psychol Crime Law*. 2005;11(4):389–402.
19. Banzon-Librojo LA, Garabiles MR, Alampay LP. Relations between harsh discipline from teachers, perceived teacher support, and bullying victimization among high school students. *J Adolescence*. 2017;57:18–22.
20. Wood L, Smith J, Varjas K, Meyers J. School personnel social support and nonsupport for bystanders of bullying: exploring student perspectives. *J Sch Psychol*. 2017;61:1–7.
21. Mujiks D. Can schools reduce bullying? The relationship between school characteristics and the prevalence of bullying behaviors. *Br J Educ Psychol*. 2017;87(2):255–272.
22. Wang C, Ryoo JH, Swearer SM, Turner R, Goldberg TS. Longitudinal relationships between bullying and moral disengagement among adolescents. *J Youth Adolesc*. 2017;46:1304–1317.
23. Alizadeh Maralani F, Mirnasab M, Hashemi T. The predictive role of maternal parenting and stress on pupils' bullying involvement. *J Interpers Violence*. 2019;34(17):3691–3710.
24. Kollerová L, Smolík F. Victimization and its associations with peer rejection and fear of victimization: moderating effects of individual-level and classroom-level characteristics. *Br J Educ Psychol*. 2016;86(4):640–656.
25. Moon SS, Kim H, Seay K, Small E, Kim YK. Ecological factors of being bullied among adolescents: a classification and regression tree approach. *Child Indic Res*. 2016;9(3):743–756.
26. Sampasa-Kanyinga H, Chaput JP, Hamilton HA, Larouche R. School bus travel is associated with bullying victimization among Canadian male, but not female, middle, and high school students. *Child Abuse Negl*. 2016;58:141–148.
27. Sharma B, Nam EW, Kim HY. The influence of witnessing inter-parental violence and bullying victimization in involvement in fighting among adolescents: evidence from a school-based cross-sectional survey in Peru. *J Lifestyle Med*. 2016;6(1):27.

28. Shukla K, Konold T, Cornell D. Profiles of student perceptions of school climate: relations with risk behaviors and academic outcomes. *Am J Community Psychol.* 2016;57(3-4):291–307.
29. Jackson V, Chou S, Browne K. Protective factors against child victimization in the school and community: an exploratory systematic review of longitudinal predictors and interacting variables. *Trauma Violence Abuse.* 2015;18(3):303–321.
30. Erhard RL, Ben-Ami E. The schooling experience of lesbian, gay, and bisexual youth in Israel: falling below and rising above as a matter of social ecology. *J Homosex.* 2016;63(2):193–227.
31. Berg JK, Cornell D. Authoritative school climate, aggression toward teachers, and teacher distress in middle school. *Sch Psychol Q.* 2016;31(1):122.
32. Gómez-Ortiz O, Romera EM, Ortega-Ruiz R. Parenting styles and bullying. The mediating role of parental psychological aggression and physical punishment. *Child Abuse Negl.* 2016;51:132–143.
33. Konold TR, Cornell D. Measurement, and structural relations of an Authoritative School Climate model: a multi-level latent variable investigation. *J Sch Psychol.* 2015;53(6):447–461.
34. Gower AL, McMorris BJ, Eisenberg ME. School-level contextual predictors of bullying and harassment experiences among adolescents. *Soc Sci Med.* 2015;147:47–53.
35. Elledge LC, Elledge AR, Newgent RA, Cavell TA. Social risk and peer victimization in elementary school children: the protective role of teacher-student relationships. *J Abnorm Child Psychol.* 2016;44(4):691–703.
36. Espelage DL, Hong JS, Rao MA, Thornberg R. Understanding ecological factors associated with bullying across the elementary to middle school transition in the United States. *Violence Vict.* 2015;30(3):470–487.
37. Casas JA, Ortega-Ruiz R, Del Rey R. Bullying: the impact of teacher management and trait emotional intelligence. *Br J Educ Psychol.* 2015;85(3):407–423.
38. Rajendran K, Kruszewski E, Halperin JM. Parenting style influences bullying: a longitudinal study comparing children with and without behavioral problems. *J Child Psychol Psychiatry.* 2016;57(2):188–195.
39. Mann MJ, Kristjansson AL, Sigfusdottir ID, Smith ML. The role of community, family, peer, and school factors in group bullying: implications for school-based intervention. *J Sch Health.* 2015;85(7):477–486.
40. Swearer SM, Hymel S. Understanding the psychology of bullying: moving toward a social-ecological diathesis–stress model. *Am Psychol.* 2015;70(4):344.
41. Cozma I, Kukaswadia A, Janssen I, Craig W, Pickett W. Active transportation and bullying in Canadian schoolchildren: a cross-sectional study. *BMC Public Health.* 2015;15(1):99.
42. Springer AE, Cuevas Jaramillo MC, Ortiz Gómez Y, Case K, Wilkinson A. School social cohesion, student-school connectedness, and bullying in Colombian adolescents. *Glob Health Promot.* 2016;23(4):37–48.
43. Gage NA, Prykanowski DA, Larson A. School climate and bullying victimization: a latent class growth model analysis. *Sch Psychol Q.* 2014;29(3):256.
44. Leadbeater B, Sukhawathanakul P, Smith D, Bowen F. Reciprocal associations between interpersonal and values dimensions of school climate and peer victimization in elementary school children. *J Clin Child Adolesc Psychol.* 2015;44(3):480–493.
45. Thornberg R, Jungert T. School bullying and the mechanisms of moral disengagement. *Aggress Behav.* 2014;40(2):99–108.
46. Lenzi M, Vieno A, Gini G, et al. Perceived teacher unfairness, instrumental goals, and bullying behavior in early adolescence. *J Interpers Violence.* 2014;29(10):1834–1849.

47. Troop-Gordon W, Ladd GW. Teachers' victimization-related beliefs and strategies: associations with students' aggressive behavior and peer victimization. *J Abnorm Child Psychol.* 2015;43(1):45–60.
48. Serdiouk M, Rodkin P, Madill R, Logis H, Gest S. Rejection, and victimization among elementary school children: the buffering role of classroom-level predictors. *J Abnorm Child Psychol.* 2015;43(1):5–17.
49. Gini G, Pozzoli T, Hymel S. Moral disengagement among children and youth: a meta-analytic review of links to aggressive behavior. *Aggress Behav.* 2014;40(1):56–68.
50. Goldweber A, Waasdorp TE, Bradshaw CP. Examining the link between forms of bullying behaviors and perceptions of safety and belonging among secondary school students. *J Sch Psychol.* 2013;51(4):469–485.
51. Troop-Gordon W, Kuntz KJ. The unique and interactive contributions of peer victimization and teacher-child relationships to children's school adjustment. *J Abnorm Child Psychol.* 2013;41(8):1191–1202.
52. Bowes L, Maughan B, Ball H, et al. Chronic bullying victimization across school transitions: the role of genetic and environmental influences. *Dev Psychopathol.* 2013;25(02):333–346.
53. Lereya ST, Samara M, Wolke D. Parenting behavior and the risk of becoming a victim and a bully/victim: a meta-analysis study. *Child Abuse Negl.* 2013;37(12):1091–1108.
54. Erginoz E, Alikasifoglu M, Ercan O, et al. The role of parental, school, and peer factors in adolescent bullying involvement: results from the Turkish HBSC 2005/2006 study. *Asia Pac J Public Health.* 2015;27(2):NP1591–NP1603.
55. Menesini E, Nocentini A, Camodeca M. Morality, values, traditional bullying, and cyberbullying in adolescence. *Br J Dev Psychol.* 2013;31(1):1–4.
56. Chui WH, Chan HC. Association between self-control and school bullying behaviors among Macanese adolescents. *Child Abuse Negl.* 2013;37(4):237–242.
57. Foster H, Brooks-Gunn J. Neighborhood, family, and individual influences on school physical victimization. *J Youth Adolescence.* 2013;42(10):1596–1610.
58. Klein J, Cornell D, Konold T. Relationships between bullying, school climate, and student risk behaviors. *Sch Psychol Q.* 2012;27(3):154.
59. Pozzoli T, Gini G, Vieno A. Individual and class moral disengagement in bullying among elementary school children. *Aggress Behav.* 2012; 38(5):378–388.
60. Donat M, Umlauft S, Dalbert C, Kamble SV. Belief in a just world, teacher justice, and bullying behavior. *Aggress Behav.* 2012;38(3):185–193.
61. Kendrick K, Jutengren G, Stattin H. The protective role of supportive friends against bullying perpetration and victimization. *J Adolescence.* 2012;35(4):1069–1080.
62. Lee CH, Song J. Functions of parental involvement and effects of school climate on bullying behaviors among South Korean middle school students. *J Interpers Violence.* 2012;27(12):2437–2464.
63. Salmivalli C, Voeten M, Poskiparta E. Bystanders matter: associations between reinforcing, defending, and the frequency of bullying behavior in classrooms. *J Clin Child Adolesc Psychol.* 2011;40(5):668–676.
64. Farmer TW, Hamm JV, Leung MC, Lambert K, Gravelle M. Early adolescent peer ecologies in rural communities: bullying in schools that do and do not have a transition during the middle grades. *J Youth Adolescence.* 2011;40(9):1106..
65. Obermann ML. Moral disengagement in self-reported and peer-nominated school bullying. *Aggress Behav.* 2011;37(2):133–144..

66. Harel-Fisch Y, Walsh SD, Fogel-Grinvald H, et al. Negative school perceptions and involvement in school bullying: a universal relationship across 40 countries. *J Adolescence*. 2011;34(4):639–652..
67. Eliot M, Cornell D, Gregory A, Fan X. Supportive school climate and student willingness to seek help for bullying and threats of violence. *J Sch Psychol*. 2010;48(6):533–553.
68. Scholte R, Sentse M, Granic I. Do actions speak louder than words? Classroom attitudes and behavior in relation to bullying in early adolescence. *J Clin Child Adolesc Psychol*. 2010;39(6):789–799.
69. Jacobson G, Riesch SK, Temkin BM, Kedrowski KM, Kluba N. Students feeling unsafe in school: fifth graders' experiences. *J Sch Nurs*. 2011;27(2):149–159.
70. Jolliffe D, Farrington DP. Empathy and offending: a systematic review and meta-analysis. *Aggress Violent Behav*. 2004;9(5):441–476.
71. Sapouna M. Collective efficacy in the school context: does it help explain victimization and bullying among Greek primary and secondary school students? *J Interpers Violence*. 2010;25(10):1912–1927.
72. Fox CL, Elder T, Gater J, Johnson E. The association between adolescents' beliefs in a just world and their attitudes to victims of bullying. *Br J Educ Psychol*. 2010;80(2):183–198.
73. Elgar FJ, Craig W, Boyce W, Morgan A, Vella-Zarb R. Income inequality and school bullying: multilevel study of adolescents in 37 countries. *J Adolesc Health*. 2009;45(4):351–359.
74. Chaux E, Molano A, Podlesky P. Socio-economic, socio-political, and socio-emotional variables explaining school bullying: a country-wide multilevel analysis. *Aggress Behav*. 2009;35(6):520–529.
75. Barboza GE, Schiamberg LB, Oehmke J, Korzeniewski SJ, Post LA, Heraux CG. Individual characteristics and the multiple contexts of adolescent bullying: an ecological perspective. *J Youth Adolescence*. 2009;38(1):101–121.
76. Correia I, Kamble SV, Dalbert C. Belief in a just world and well-being of bullies, victims, and defenders: a study with Portuguese and Indian students. *Anxiety Stress Coping*. 2009;22(5):497–508.
77. Bowes L, Arseneault L, Maughan B, Taylor A, Caspi A, Moffitt TE. School, neighborhood, and family factors are associated with children's bullying involvement: a nationally representative longitudinal study. *J Am Acad Child Adolesc Psychiatry*. 2009;48(5):545–553.
78. Due P, Merlo J, Harel-Fisch Y, et al. Socioeconomic inequality in exposure to bullying during adolescence: a comparative, cross-sectional, multilevel study in 35 countries. *Am J Public Health*. 2009; 99(5):907–914.
79. Woods S, Done J, Kalsi H. Peer victimisation and internalising difficulties: the moderating role of friendship quality. *J Adolescence*. 2009;32(2):293–308.
80. Idsoe T, Solli E, Cosmovici EM. Social psychological processes in family and school: more evidence on their relative etiological significance for bullying behavior. *Aggress Behav*. 2008;34(5):460–474.
81. Elgar FJ, McKinnon B, Walsh SD, et al. Structural determinants of youth bullying and fighting in 79 countries. *J Adolesc Health*. 2015;57(6):643–650.
82. Maïano C, Normand CL, Salvas MC, Moullec G, Aimé A. Prevalence of school bullying among youth with autism spectrum disorders: a systematic review and meta-analysis. *Autism Res*. 2016;9(6):601–615.
83. Maïano C, Aime A, Salvas MC, Morin AJ, Normand CL. Prevalence and correlates of bullying perpetration and victimization among school-aged youth with intellectual disabilities: A systematic review. *Res Dev Disabil*. 2016;49:181–195.

84. Zhu Y, Chan KL. Prevalence and correlates of school bullying victimization in Xi'an, China. *Violence Vict*. 2015;30(4):714–732.
85. Chester KL, Callaghan M, Cosma A, et al. Cross-national time trends in bullying victimization in 33 countries among children aged 11, 13 and 15 from 2002 to 2010. *Eur J Public Health*. 2015;25(suppl 2):61–64..
86. Perlus JG, Brooks-Russell A, Wang J, Iannotti RJ. Trends in bullying, physical fighting, and weapon carrying among 6th- through 10th-grade students from 1998 to 2010: findings from a national study. *Am J Public Health*. 2014;104(6):1100–1106.
87. Kubwalo HW, Muula AS, Siziya S, Pasupulati S, Rudatsikira E. Prevalence, and correlates of being bullied among in-school adolescents in Malawi: results from the 2009 Global School-Based Health Survey. *Malawi Med J*. 2013;25(1):12–14.
88. Fleming LC, Jacobsen KH. Bullying among middle-school students in low- and middle-income countries. *Health Promot Int*. 2010;25(1):73–84.
89. Wang J, Iannotti RJ, Nansel TR. School bullying among adolescents in the United States: physical, verbal, relational, and cyber. *J Adolesc Health*. 2009;45(4):368–375.
90. Craig W, Harel-Fisch Y, Fogel-Grinvald H, et al. A cross-national profile of bullying and victimization among adolescents in 40 countries. *Int J Public Health*. 2009;54:216–224.
91. Molcho M, Craig W, Due P, et al. Cross-national time trends in bullying behaviour 1994–2006: findings from Europe and North America. *Int J Public Health*. 2009;54(suppl 2):225–234.
92. Due P, Merlo J, Harel-Fisch Y, et al. Socioeconomic inequality in exposure to bullying during adolescence: a comparative, cross-sectional, multilevel study in 35 countries. *Am J Public Health*. 2009;99(5):907–914.
93. Due P, Holstein BE, Soc MS. Bullying victimization among 13 to 15-year-old school children: results from two comparative studies in 66 countries and regions. *Int J Adolesc Med Health*. 2008;20(2):209–221.
94. Hazemba A, Siziya S, Muula AS, Rudatsikira E. Prevalence and correlates of being bullied among in-school adolescents in Beijing: results from the 2003 Beijing Global School-Based Health Survey. *Ann Gen Psychiatry*. 2008;7(1):6.
95. Kim YS, Koh YJ, Leventhal BL. Prevalence of school bullying in Korean middle school students. *Arch Pediatrics Adolesc Med*. 2004;158(8):737–741.
96. Nansel TR, Overpeck M, Pilla RS, Ruan WJ, Simons-Morton B, Scheidt P. Bullying behaviors among US youth: prevalence and association with psychosocial adjustment. *JAMA*. 2001;285(16):2094–2100.
97. Garandeau CF, Vartio A, Poskiparta E, Salmivalli C. School bullies' intention to change behavior following teacher interventions: effects of empathy arousal, condemning of bullying, and blaming of the perpetrator. *Prev Sci*. 2016;17(8):1034–1043.
98. Trip S, Bora C, Sipos-Gug S, et al. Bullying prevention in schools by targeting cognitions, emotions, and behavior: evaluating the effectiveness of the REBE-ViSC program. *J Couns Psychol*. 2015;62(4):732.
99. Bonell C, Fletcher A, Fitzgerald-Yau N, et al. Initiating change locally in bullying and aggression through the school environment (INCLUSIVE): a pilot randomised controlled trial. *Health Technol Assess*. 2015;19(53):1–10.
100. Watson H, Rapee R, Todorov N. Forgiveness reduces anger in a school bullying context. *J Interpers Violence*. 2017;32(11):1642–1657.
101. Jantzer V, Haffner J, Parzer P, Resch F, Kaess M. Does parental monitoring moderate the relationship between bullying and adolescent nonsuicidal self-injury and suicidal behavior?

A community-based self-report study of adolescents in Germany. *BMC Public Health.* 2015;15(1):583.

102. Bradshaw CP. Translating research to practice in bullying prevention. *Am Psychol.* 2015;70(4):322.

103. Haataja A, Voeten M, Boulton AJ, Ahtola A, Poskiparta E, Salmivalli C. The KiVa antibullying curriculum and outcome: does fidelity matter? *J Sch Psychol.* 2014;52(5):479–493.

104. National Research Council. *Building Capacity to Reduce Bullying: Workshop Summary.* Washington, DC, USA: National Academies Press; 2014.

105. Garandeau CF, Poskiparta E, Salmivalli C. Tackling acute cases of school bullying in the KiVa Anti-bullying Program: a comparison of two approaches. *J Abnorm Child Psychol.* 2014;42(6):981–991.

106. Lee S, Kim CJ, Kim DH. A meta-analysis of the effect of school-based anti-bullying programs. *J Child Health Care.* 2015;19(2):136–153.

107. Domino M. Measuring the impact of an alternative approach to school bullying. *J Sch Health.* 2013;83(6):430–437.

108. Low S, Van Ryzin MJ, Brown EC, Smith BH, Haggerty KP. Engagement matters: lessons from assessing classroom implementation of Steps to Respect, a bullying prevention program over a one-year period. *Prev Sci.* 2014; 15(2):165–176.

109. Flanagan KS, Hoek KK, Ranter JM, Reich HA. The potential of forgiveness as a response for coping with negative peer experiences. *J Adolescence.* 2012;35(5):1215–1223.

110. Scheithauer H, Hess M, Schultze-Krumbholz A, Bull HD. School-based prevention of bullying and relational aggression in adolescence: the fairplayer.manual. *New Dir Stud Leadersh.* 2012;2012(133):55–70.

111. Salmivalli C, Poskiparta E. Making bullying prevention a priority in Finnish schools: the KiVa Antibullying Program. *New Dir Youth Dev.* 2012;2012(133):41–53..

112. Roland E, Midthassel UV. The Zero program. *New Dir Stud Leadersh.* 2012;2012(133):29–39.

113. Alsaker FD, Valkanover S. The Bernese program against victimization in kindergarten and elementary school. *New Dir Stud Leadersh.* 2012;2012(133):15–28.

114. Waasdorp TE, Bradshaw CP, Leaf PJ. The impact of schoolwide positive behavioral interventions and supports on bullying and peer rejection: a randomized controlled effectiveness trial. *Arch Pediatrics Adolesc Med.* 2012; 166(2):149–156.

115. Santos RG, Chartier MJ, Whalen JC, Chateau D, Boyd L. Effectiveness of school-based violence prevention for children and youth: a research report. *Healthcare Q (Toronto).* 2010;14:80–91.

116. Bowllan NM. Implementation and evaluation of a comprehensive, school-wide bullying prevention program in an urban/suburban middle school. *J Sch Health.* 2011;81(4):167–173.

117. Kärnä A, Voeten M, Little TD, Poskiparta E, Kaljonen A, Salmivalli C. A large-scale evaluation of the KiVa Antibullying Program: grades 4–6. *Child Dev.* 2011;82(1):311–330.

118. Wong DS, Cheng CH, Ngan RM, Ma SK. Program effectiveness of a restorative whole-school approach for tackling school bullying in Hong Kong. *Int J Offender Ther.* 2011;55(6):846–862..

119. Black S, Washington E, Trent V, Harner P, Pollock E. Translating the Olweus Bullying Prevention Program into real-world practice. *Health Promot Pract.* 2010;11(5):733–740.

120. Rigby K, Slee P. Interventions to reduce bullying. *Int J Adolesc Med Health.* 2008;20(2):165.

121. Houlston C, Smith PK. The impact of a peer counselling scheme to address bullying in an all-girl London secondary school: a short-term longitudinal study. *Br J Educ Psychol.* 2009;79(1):69–86.

122. Leadbeater B, Hoglund W. Changing the social contexts of peer victimization. *J Can Acad Child Adolesc Psychiatry*. 2006;15(1):21.
123. Pepler DJ. Bullying interventions: a binocular perspective. *J Can Acad Child Adolesc Psychiatry*. 2006;15(1):16.
124. Bauer NS, Lozano P, Rivara FP. The effectiveness of the Olweus Bullying Prevention Program in public middle schools: a controlled trial. *J Adolesc Health*. 2007;40(3):266–274.
125. Twemlow SW, Fonagy P, Sacco FC. A developmental approach to mentalizing communities: II. The Peaceful Schools experiment. *Bull Menninger Clin*. 2005;69(4):282–304.
126. Salmivalli C, Kaukiainen A, Voeten M. Anti-bullying intervention: implementation and outcome. *Br J Educ Psychol*. 2005;75(3):465–487..
127. Fonagy P, Twemlow SW, Vernberg E, Sacco FC, Little TD. Creating a peaceful school learning environment: the impact of an antibullying program on educational attainment in elementary schools. *Med Sci Monitor*. 2005;11(7):CR317–CR325.
128. Frey KS, Hirschstein MK, Snell JL, Edstrom LV, MacKenzie EP, Broderick CJ. Reducing playground bullying and supporting beliefs: an experimental trial of the steps to respect program. *Dev Psychol*. 2005;41(3):479.
129. Stevens V, De Bourdeaudhuij I, Van Oost P. Anti-bullying interventions at school: aspects of programme adaptation and critical issues for further programme development. *Health Promot Int*. 2001;16(2):155–167.
130. Twemlow SW, Fonagy P, Sacco FC, Gies ML, Evans R, Ewbank R. Creating a peaceful school learning environment: a controlled study of an elementary school intervention to reduce violence. *Am J Psychiatry*. 2001;158(5):808–810..
131. Stevens V, Bourdeaudhuij I, Van Oost P. Bullying in Flemish schools: an evaluation of anti-bullying intervention in primary and secondary schools. *Br J Educ Psychol*. 2000;70(2):195–210.
132. Olweus D. Bullying at school: basic facts and effects of a school based intervention program. *J Child Psychol Psychiatry*. 1994;35(7):1171–1190.
133. Olweus D. *Bullying at School: What We Know and What We Can Do*. Malden, MA: Blackwell Publishers; 1993:9.
134. Olweus D. Sweden. In: Smith PK, Morita Y, Junger-Tas J, Olweus D, Catalano R, Slee P, eds. *The Nature of School Bullying: A Cross-National Perspective*. London, England: Routledge; 1969:11.
135. Gladden RM, Vivolo-Kantor AM, Hamburger ME, Lumpkin CD. Bullying Surveillance among Youth: Uniform Definitions for Public Health and Recommended Data Elements, Version 1.0. Atlanta, GA: National Center for Injury Prevention and Control; 2014. https://www.cdc.gov/violenceprevention/pdf/bullying-definitions-final-a.pdf. Accessed September 8, 2022.
136. Olweus D. *Bullying at School: What We Know and What We Can Do*. Malden, MA: Blackwell Publishers; 1993:31–38.
137. Salmivalli C, Lagerspetz K, Björkqvist K, Österman K, Kaukiainen A. Bullying as a group process: participant roles and their relations to social status within the group. *Aggress Behav*. 1996;22(1):1–5. Cited in Rivers I. Morbidity among bystanders of bullying behavior at school: concepts, concerns, and clinical/research issues. *Int J Adolesc Med Health*. 2012;24(1):11–16.
138. Yang SA, Kim DH. Factors associated with bystander behaviors of Korean youth in school bullying situations: a cross-sectional study. *Medicine*. 2017; 96(32):e7757.

139. Huang H, Liu Y, Chen Y. Preservice preschool teachers' responses to bullying scenarios: the roles of years of study and empathy. *Front Psychol.* 2018;9:175.

140. Kochenderfer-Ladd B, Pelletier ME. Teachers' views and beliefs about bullying: influences on classroom management strategies and students' coping with peer victimization. *J Sch Psychol.* 2008;46(4):431–453.

141. Duncan RD. The impact of family relationships on school bullies and victims. In: Espelage DL, Swearer SM, eds. *Bullying in American Schools: A Social-Ecological Perspective on Prevention and Intervention.* Mahwah, NJ, United States: Lawrence Erlbaum Associates; 2004:227–244.

142. Lereya ST, Samara M, Wolke D. Parenting behavior and the risk of becoming a victim and a bully/victim: a meta-analysis study. *Child Abuse Negl.* 2013;37(12):1091–1108.

143. Zottis GA, Salum GA, Isolan LR, Manfro GG, Heldt E. Associations between child disciplinary practices and bullying behavior in children and adolescents. *J Pediatria.* 2014;90(4):408–414.

144. Allison S, Roeger L, Smith B, Isherwood L. Family histories of school bullying: implications for parent-child psychotherapy. *Australas Psychiatry.* 2014;22(2):149–153.

145. Hale R, Fox CL, Murray M. "As a parent you become a tiger": parents talking about bullying at school. *J Child Fam Stud.* 2017;26(7):2000–2015.

146. Al Ali NM, Gharaibeh M, Masadeh MJ. Students' perceptions of characteristics of victims and perpetrators of bullying in public schools in Jordan. *Nurs Res.* 2017;66(1):40–48.

147. Iannotti RJ. *Health Behavior in School-Aged Children (HBSC), 2009–2010.* ICPSR34792-v1. Ann Arbor, MI: Inter-university Consortium for Political and Social Research [distributor]; 2013. https://www.icpsr.umich.edu/web/NAHDAP/studies/34792/versions/V1. Accessed September 8, 2022.

148. Lereya ST, Copeland WE, Zammit S, Wolke D. Bully/victims: a longitudinal, population-based cohort study of their mental health. *Eur Child Adolesc Psychiatry.* 2015;24(12):1461–1471.

149. Berkowitz R, Benbenishty R. Perceptions of teachers' support, safety, and absence from school because of fear among victims, bullies, and bully-victims. *Am J Orthopsychiatry.* 2012;82(1):67.

150. Austin S, Joseph S. Assessment of bully/victim problems in 8 to 11 year-olds. *Br J Educ Psychol.* 1996;66(4):447–456. Cited by Haynie DL, Nansel T, Eitel P, et al. Bullies, victims, and bully/victims: distinct groups of at-risk youth. *J Early Adolescence.* 2001;21(1):29–49.

151. Doll B, Song S, Siemers E. Classroom ecologies that support or discourage bullying. In: Espelage DL, Swearer SM, eds. *Bullying in American Schools: A Social-Ecological Perspective on Prevention and Intervention.* Mahwah, NJ, United States: Lawrence Erlbaum Associates; 2004:161–183.

152. Kasen S, Berenson K, Cohen P, Johnson JG. The effects of school climate on changes in aggressive and other behaviors related to bullying. In: Espelage DL, Swearer SM, eds. *Bullying in American Schools: A Social-Ecological Perspective on Prevention and Intervention.* Mahwah, NJ, United States: Lawrence Erlbaum Associates; 2004.

153. Health Behavior in School-aged Children Survey, conducted in 2017–2018 among students age 11 to 15 living in 36 countries and regions.

154. Global School-based Students Health Survey (GSHS), which assessed students age 13 to 17 living in 41 countries or regions, at a specific year between 2010 and 2019.

155. For more detailed tables, see Chapter 2.

156. For more details on school bullying prevention, see Chapter 7.

157. Kauppi T, Pörhölä M. School teachers bullied by their students: teachers' attributions and how they share their experiences. *Teach Teach Educ.* 2012;28(7):1059–1068.
158. Kauppi T, Pörhölä M. Teachers bullied by students: forms of bullying and perpetrator characteristics. *Violence Vict.* 2012;27(3):396–413. Cited by Kauppi and Pörhölä.[157]
159. Terry AA. Teachers as targets of bullying by their pupils: a study to investigate incidence. *Br J Educ Psychol.* 1998;68(2):255–268. Cited by Kauppi and Pörhölä.[157]
160. Wet CD. Victims of educator-targeted bullying: a qualitative study. *S Afr J Educ.* 2010;30(2):189–201. Cited by Kauppi and Pörhölä.[157]
161. Twemlow SW, Fonagy P, Sacco FC, Brethour JR Jr. Teachers who bully students: a hidden trauma. *Int J Soc Psychiatry.* 2006;52(3):187–198.
162. Twemlow SW, Fonagy P. The prevalence of teachers who bully students in schools with differing levels of behavioral problems. *Am J Psychiatry.* 2005;162(12):2387–2389.
163. Whitted KS, Dupper DR. Do teachers bully students? Findings from a survey of students in an alternative education setting. *Educ Urban Soc.* 2008;40(3):329–341.
164. Nhundu TJ, Shumba A. The nature and frequency of reported cases of teacher perpetrated child sexual abuse in rural primary schools in Zimbabwe. *Child Abuse Negl.* 2001;25(11):1517–1534.
165. Jewkes R, Levin J, Mbananga N, Bradshaw D. Rape of girls in South Africa. *Lancet.* 2002;359(9303):319–320.
166. Moulden HM, Firestone P, Kingston DA, Wexler AF. A description of sexual offending committed by Canadian teachers. *J Child Sex Abuse.* 2010;19(4):403–418.
167. Gallagher B. The extent and nature of known cases of institutional child sexual abuse. *Br J Soc Work.* 2000;30(6):795–817.
168. Knoll J. Teacher sexual misconduct: grooming patterns and female offenders. *J Child Sex Abuse.* 2010;19(4):371–386.
169. Anderson MD. Where teachers are still allowed to spank students. *The Atlantic*, December 15, 2015. https://www.theatlantic.com/education/archive/2015/12/corporal-punishment/420420/. Accessed September 8, 2022.
170. Gershoff ET. School corporal punishment in global perspective: prevalence, outcomes, and efforts at intervention. *Psychol Health Med.* 2017;22(suppl 1):224–239.
171. ABa Saddik AS, Hattab AS. Physical abuse in basic-education schools in Aden governorate, Yemen: a cross-sectional study. *East Mediterr Health J.* 2013;19(4):333–339. Cited by Gershoff.[170]
172. Beazley HS, Bessell L, Ennew J, Waterson R. What children say: Results of comparative research on physical and emotional punishment of children in Southeast Asia, East Asia, and the Pacific. Sweden: Save the Children; 2005. Cited by Gershoff.[170]
173. Feinstein S, Mwahombela L. Corporal punishment in Tanzania's schools. *Int Rev Educ.* 2010;56(4):399–410. Cited by Gershoff.[170]
174. Hyman IA. Corporal punishment, psychological maltreatment, violence, and punitiveness in America: research, advocacy, and public policy. *Appl Prev Psychol.* 1995;4(2):113–130. Cited by Gershoff.[170]
175. Khoury-Kassabri M. Student victimization by educational staff in Israel. *Child Abuse Negl.* 2006;30(6):691–707.
176. Vandiver DM, Kercher G. Offender and victim characteristics of registered female sexual offenders in Texas: a proposed typology of female sexual offenders. *Sex Abuse.* 2004;16(2):121–137. Cited by Knoll.[168]

177. Matthews JK, Mathews RU, Speltz K. Female sexual offenders: a typology. *Fam Sex Abuse.* 1991:199–219. Cited by Knoll.[168]
178. US Department of Education, National Center of Education Statistics. Digest of Education Statistics, Table 233.28. Percentage of students receiving selected disciplinary actions in public elementary and secondary schools, by type of disciplinary action, disability status, sex, and race/ethnicity: 2017–10. https://nces.ed.gov/programs/digest/d21/tables/dt21_233.28.asp. Accessed September 8, 2022.
179. Global Initiative to End All Corporal Punishment of Children. Country Report for USA. http://www.endcorporalpunishment.org/wp-content/uploads/country-reports/USA.pdf. Accessed September 22, 2023.
180. Ingraham v Wright, 430 U.S. 651 (1977). Cited by Global Initiative to End All Corporal Punishment of Children, Country Report for USA. https://supreme.justia.com/cases/federal/us/430/651/. Accessed September 22, 2023.
181. Global Partnership to End Violence Against Children. Prohibiting All Corporal Punishment of Children: Laying the Foundations for Non-Violent Childhoods, States without a Clear Commitment to Law Reform, pp, 21-27, April 2021. https://endcorporalpunishment.org/wp-content/uploads/2021/04/Prohibiting-all-corporal-punishment-of-children-laying-the-foundations-for-nonviolent-childhoods.pdf. Accessed September 9, 2022.
182. The designation of "State of Palestine," as cited by Global Initiative to End All Corporal Punishment of Children,[181] is based on the official term used by UNICEF and other UN Agencies, and is also known as "Palestinian Territories," according to the US Department of State. https://www.state.gov/countries-areas/palestinian-territories/. Accessed September 9, 2022.
183. Newman D. The school as a workplace. In: Zucchermaglio C, Bagnara S, Stucky SU, eds. *Organizational Learning and Technological Change.* NATO ASI Series (Series F: Computer and Systems Sciences), vol 141. Berlin, Germany: Springer; 1995.
184. Griffin GA. The school as a workplace and the master teacher concept. *Elem Sch J.* 1985;86(1):1–6.
185. The Government of Sweden, Arbetsmiljölagen, The Work Environment Act [Non-official translation]. https://www.government.se/government-policy/labour-law-and-work-environment/19771160-work-environment-act-arbetsmiljolagen/. Accessed September 22, 2023.
186. Finland, Occupational Safety and Health Act §27, §28. https://www.ilo.org/dyn/natlex/docs/ELECTRONIC/62320/60971/F1688833574/FIN62320%20English.pdf. Accessed September 11, 2022.
187. See Chapter12, Table 12.1.
188. Routh CH. *On Overwork and Premature Mental Decay: Its Treatment.* London, UK: Baillière, Tindall, and Cox; 1876.
189. Oldright W. Overwork and unrest. *Public Health Papers Rep.* 1893; 19:210..
190. Lundy CJ. School hygiene. *Public Health Papers Rep.* 1883; 9:137. https://www.ncbi.nlm.nih.gov/pmc/articles/PMC2272445/pdf/pubhealthpap00020-0142.pdf. Accessed September 11, 2022.
191. Dukes C. *Work and Overwork in Relation to Health in Schools.* Percival; 1893. https://iiif.wellcomecollection.org/pdf/b28078378. Accessed September 22, 2023.
192. Rhoads JM. Overwork. *JAMA.* 1977;237(24):2615–2618..

193. Wong K, Chan AH, Ngan SC. The effect of long working hours and overtime on occupational health: a meta-analysis of evidence from 1998 to 2018. *Int J Environ Res Public Health*. 2019;16(12):2102.
194. Nishiyama K, Johnson JV. Karoshi—death from overwork: occupational health consequences of Japanese production management. *Int J Health Serv*. 1997;27(4):625–641.
195. Great School Partnership, The Glossary of Education Reform, Stakeholder. https://www.edglossary.org/stakeholder/#:~:text = In%20education%2C%20the%20term%20stakeholder,as%20school%20board%20members%2C%20city. Accessed September 11, 2022.

12
Workplace Bullying and Other Forms of Maltreatment

What Is Known?

The notion of workplace bullying emerged in the biomedical literature[1-2] in the second half of the 1990s,[3-11] and since then almost 2,000 articles have dealt with the concept.[1-2] Aspects of the same notion have been previously, and are presently, studied and published using the terms *workplace harassment*,[12-15] *workplace violence*,[16-18] and *mobbing*.[19-20]

Two decades of research on bullying at work has run parallel to the investigation on school bullying. Yet there is only one published study that has documented a link between the two forms of mistreatment.[21]

The Notion of Workplace Bullying

The original research in workplace bullying was pioneered by Heinz Leymann,[19,22] who identified the concept with the elements of physical, psychological, and verbal "negative actions," as formerly applied by Olweus[23] to the school setting, and added aspects of victimization that are unique to the workplace milieu (i.e., being assigned humiliating tasks, being obliged to do harmful work in spite of poor health, being given only new tasks without previous experience, or being assigned to jobs far above one's skill level).[22]

Einarsen et al.[24] suggested a definition of bullying at work, stating that it represents "harassing, offending, socially excluding someone or negatively affecting someone's work tasks." Furthermore, they indicated that for an interaction to be considered bullying, "it has to occur repeatedly and regularly (e.g., weekly) and over a period of time (e.g., about six months)." This book has already taken exception, based on a clinical perspective, to the research requirements that the concept of bullying entails elements of intentionality, recurrence, and imbalance of power (see Chapter 1).

Bullying at the workplace can be characterized by a wide range of patterns of victimization exemplified in the items of the research survey questionnaires[22,24-27] utilized to investigate this form of maltreatment, such as the Leymann Inventory of Psychological Terror (LIPT),[22,25] the Negative Acts Questionnaire (NAQ),[24,26] the Workplace Aggression Questionnaire (WAQ),[27] and the Malaysian Workplace Bullying Index (MWB).[28] These instances of workplace bullying can be grouped into two categories either pertaining to maltreatment specifically related to the work milieu or not specific to the labor environment.

Instances of Bullying Specific to the Work Environment

Some of the examples of workplace bullying are specific to the labor environment and represent many types of maltreatment including, among others, coercion, corruptness, denigration, endangerment, misguidance, unfairness, and overwork (Table 12.1).

Overwork

The notion of overwork and its association with health problems was initially documented in 1977 by Rhoads[29] in a report of several clinical cases of patients who engaged in self-induced work beyond their "endurance and recuperative capacities"[29] and who exhibited an array of physical and emotional symptoms.[29] Subsequently, Netterstrøm and Juel[30] demonstrated a significant link between the development of ischemic heart disease and the mental burden of working in heavy traffic among Danish urban bus drivers who were followed prospectively from 1978 to 1985.

For more than a decade, reports have been originating from East Asia that highlight the problem of overwork and its link to deaths from suicide, cardiovascular disease, or stroke.[31-39] The concept of overwork, understood as working "long hours," was systematically examined by Bannai and Tamakoshi[40] to ascertain its association with health problems. The study[40]

Table 12.1. Examples of Workplace Maltreatment Specifically Related to the Work Milieu[22,24-27]

Being requested to do overtime work without pay (Exploitation)	Being requested to do work outside of the job scope (Noncompliance)	Being prevented from expressing oneself or prohibited from talking to colleagues (Repression)	Exposed to unmanageable or excessive workload or with unreasonable deadlines (Overwork)
Being coerced, forced, or threatened to do work (Coercion)	Being humiliated or ridiculed in connection to work (Denigration)	Being refused a request for assistance (Abandonment)	Having information withheld that affects one's performance (Misguidance)
Being compelled to do tasks that are harmful to one's health (Endangerment)	Being instructed to do work without guidance (Misguidance)	Being requested to do work that is supposed to be done by others (Misuse)	Having one's contributions or opinions ignored by others or having someone else take credit for one's work or ideas (Disregard)
Being given little or no feedback about one's performance (Misguidance)	Not being entrusted with any task (Mistrust)	Being required to do work against one's conscience (Corruptness)	Having one's work be judged in an unjust and hurtful way (Unfairness)
Being given tasks above one's skill level (Mismanagement)	Being pressured not to claim something that one is entitled to (vacations, sick leave, travel expenses) (Coercion)	Exposed to attempts to turn other employees against somebody (Treachery)	Having somebody interfere with one's activities (Hampering)

defined working long hours as work time exceeding 40 hours per week (eight hours per day), including hours spent on work brought home.

The causes for overwork, as discussed in this section, go beyond an individual predisposition to "rigid perfectionism" leading to compulsive overwork.[41] Primarily, overwork is caused by organizational maltreatment of the employee, such as by requiring the attainment of job goals that are beyond the individual's capabilities.[41]

Examples of Workplace Bullying Not Specific to the Work Environment

A wide range of bullying or other forms of maltreatment occur in the workplace that are not specific to the work environment., including physical/sexual aggression, verbal harassment, and indirect bullying (Table 12.2).

Epidemiology of Workplace Bullying

Europe

The 2005 European Survey of Working Conditions,[42] conducted among almost 30,000 workers in 31 European countries, documented that an average of 5% of the employees

Table 12.2. Examples of Workplace Maltreatment Not Specifically Related to the Work Milieu[22,24-27]

Attacking or mocking somebody's origins or political or religious opinions	Made fun of because of disability
Being constantly criticized about private matters	Mimicking and/or ridiculing someone's appearance, voice, or attitude
Being glared at in a hostile manner	Object of sexual allusions or proposals
Being ignored or excluded	Physical abuse (hit, punched, slapped, kicked)
Being mocked with disrespectful or sarcastic gestures	Reprimanded or "put down" in front of others
Being given a silent treatment or not being spoken to	Saying mean things behind someone's back
Being unnoticed or regarded as non-existent	Sexually assaulted
Failing to return one's telephone calls or emails	Shouted at or target of spontaneous anger
Having offensive or insulting remarks about oneself, attitude, or personal life	Subjected to derogatory name-calling
Having rumors spread about someone	Subjected to negative comments about one's intelligence or competence
Insulted with obscene or degrading words	Teased or treated with sarcasm
Interrupted frequently when speaking	Threats of violence
Intimidating behaviors (finger-pointing, shoving, blocking one's way, invasion of personal space)	Telephone or online harassment

surveyed felt bullied or harassed at work in the preceding 12 months. There was a wide difference in the reported prevalence of exposure to bullying or harassment among European nations, varying from 17% in Finland to 2% in Italy and Bulgaria.[43] The geographical variance could be partly due to different levels of cultural awareness.[43]

Women were more exposed to bullying and harassment than men (6% vs. 4%), with younger women (< 30 years old) at greatest risk (8%), while employees were more vulnerable than self-employed people (6% vs. 3%).[43] In general, workers in the public sector reported higher frequency of bullying or harassment (6%) than employees of the private sector reported (4%).[43] There were considerable differences in the incidence of bullying and harassment by company size, with people working in larger establishments (over 250 workers) reporting the highest levels (8%).

Sexual harassment during the previous 12 months was reported by less than 2% of workers, but again female workers were three times more exposed than their male counterparts.[43] Sexual harassment was highly reported by female workers in Czechia, Norway, Turkey, Croatia, Denmark, Sweden, Lithuania, and the United Kingdom (5%–10%), while it was rarely disclosed in Italy, Spain, Malta, and Cyprus (less than 1%).[43] Again, it is not clear whether the differences in reporting were in some way associated with cultural variances in the recognition of the significance of sexual harassment.

Physical violence in the previous 12 months was reported by 5% of European workers,[43] with more risk of physical violence from people outside the workplace (4%) than from coworkers (2%), and greater risk among white collar workers (6%) than among blue collar employees (4%).[43]

It is important to note the significant differences in the reported frequency of harassment and violence depending on the labor area, with the highest risk found in the health sector, trailed by education, public administration, defense, transport, communication, and hotels and restaurants. The lowest prevalence rates were reported by workers in agriculture, construction, and manufacturing.[43]

The 5th European Working Conditions Survey, conducted in 34 countries during 2010, documented that 15% of workers reported that they were subject to "adverse social behavior."[44] Adverse social behavior was defined as one or more of the following types of maltreatment: verbal abuse, unwanted sexual attention, threats, or humiliation during the previous month, and/or physical violence, bullying, harassment, or sexual harassment during the previous year. The highest prevalence of adverse social behavior was faced by employees in the health sector, with the lowest frequency experienced among agricultural workers.[44]

United States

Data analysis of the 2010 National Health Interview Survey[45] documented that 7.8% of a US national representative sample of more than 17,000 adults reported that they suffered from a hostile working environment, characterized by being threatened, bullied, or harassed by anyone on the job in the previous 12 months.[45]

The highest rates of exposure to a hostile working environment were experienced by people employed in protective services (24.6%), public administration (16.2%), community and social services (15.7%), and healthcare support (11.1%).[45]

Canada

A self-report survey[46] of 180 adults from diverse occupations and industries in the Canadian prairies found that 40% had experienced one or more acts of bullying or aggressive behaviors, at least once per week, in the previous six months, and 10% of the sample had experienced five or more such acts, with the same frequency and within the same period of time.[46] The workers who were sampled were employed in public service, an elementary school, a hospital, and a potash mine. About 40% of the respondents were clerical workers, 30% were professionals, and 16% were managers, with the remaining employed in miscellaneous areas.[46]

According to the Canadian 2004 General Social Survey[47] on victimization, 17% of self-reported incidents of violent victimization occurred in the workplace. Certain workers were more likely to have been affected: in the survey, 33% of the victims worked in social assistance or healthcare, 14% in accommodation or food services, and 11% in education.[47]

Measuring Workplace Bullying

In general, the prevalence of bullying has been ascertained either by a subjective approach,[48] in which participants indicate whether they felt bullied at work based on a given operational definition, or by an operational approach, which determines "the frequency at which respondents have been subjected to various types of negative acts during the previous six months."[49] The operational methodology has been based on the use of the LIPT,[50] which includes 45 types of workplace bullying that may have occurred in the previous 12 months, and the NAQ, which is based on 22 negative acts.[26]

Petrović et al.[51] utilized a receiver operating characteristics (ROC) analysis to ascertain the NAQ–Revised (NAQ-R)[52] cutoff scores, applying a "lower" and "higher" threshold, in the context of a one-item self-labeling approach, while gold standards were developed as a combination of self-labeling with life satisfaction, intention to leave work, and perceived health.[51] Their research, using 1,998 Serbian employees, showed that the gold standard of self-labeling as being bullied at least "now and then" and thinking of leaving from "time to time" identified employees in a "preliminary stage of bullying" (corresponding to an NAQ-R of at least 34).[51] Furthermore, the study documented that the most precise recognition of victims could be established using the most complex gold standard of self-labeling as being bullied at least several times a week, indicating a "bad" or "very bad" health status, being dissatisfied or very dissatisfied with life, and very often thinking of leaving, corresponding to a NAQ-R of at least 80.[51]

Antecedents and Consequences of Workplace Bullying

Bowling and Beehr[53] conducted a meta-analysis of 90 studies to determine the potential antecedents and consequences of workplace harassment, and they showed that role conflict, role ambiguity, role overload, and work constraints were associated with workplace harassment.[54] Additionally, this form of victimization was found to be positively associated with anxiety, depression, burnout, frustration, and physical symptoms, while it was negatively linked with self-esteem, life satisfaction, organizational commitment, and perceptions of organizational justice.[53]

Wheeler et al.[55] highlighted common antecedents of workplace bullying, including "an unsupportive social and competitive environment," "task-oriented, autocratic, and laissez-faire managers," "hierarchical and changing organizations," and organizations that "lack formal employee behavioral policies and strong communication practices."[55]

Nielsen and Einarsen[54] reported results from two meta-analyses of the potential effects on individuals exposed to workplace bullying. The first meta-analysis, based on a review of 54 cross-sectional studies involving a total of 77,721 participants in 13 countries, showed that workplace bullying was positively associated with anxiety, depression, symptoms of post-traumatic stress, somatization, burnout, physical health problems, intent to leave the job, and absenteeism.[54] Furthermore, there was a significant negative association with job satisfaction and organizational commitment.[54] The second meta-analysis,[54] based on 13 longitudinal studies with a total of 62,916 participants, documented that baseline exposure to workplace bullying was significantly related to absenteeism and mental health problems at follow-up, which was usually conducted at 12 to 24 months.[54] Additionally, a significant inverted outcome was found between mental health problems at baseline and increased exposure to bullying at follow-up.[54]

Potential Perpetrators and Victims of Workplace Maltreatment

Bullying and other forms of victimization can reciprocally occur in the work environment among coworkers (lateral or horizontal mistreatment); between the employer or corporation, managers, supervisors, and employees (vertical victimization); or between a customer and an employee, provider, or establishment (Figure 12.1).

Maltreatment among Members of a Working Team

Victimization in the workplace can occur horizontally between coworkers, or vertically between subordinates and their superiors.

At least 14 studies[57-69,72] conducted in the last three decades have shown that, on the average, supervisors were identified considerably more frequently (73%) as the main perpetrators of workplace bullying than coworkers (44%). Yet, a few reports[71-73] have indicated that coworkers were, on the average, slightly more frequently (53%) recognized as bullies as compared to supervisors (49%), while in one Scandinavian study[74] supervisors and peers were equally identified as bullies, with a frequency of 54%. The participation of subordinates in bullying their superiors, as documented in all the studies just cited,[56-74] has been shown to happen at a low average frequency of 10%.

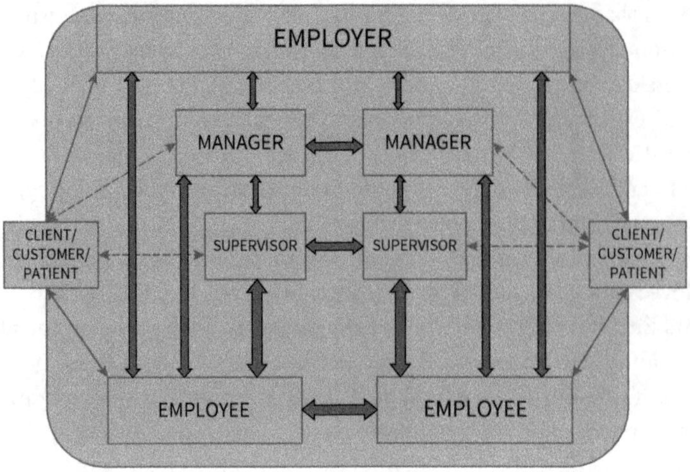

Figure 12.1. Potential perpetrators and victims of workplace maltreatment.

Corporate or Employer Victimization of Employees

Any employee can be victimized by the workplace organization, corporation, or employer through labor violations,[75,76] including employment discrimination, occupational safety and health violations, unfair labor practices, and wage theft. A 2008 survey[76] of more than 4,000 workers in low-wage industries in Chicago, Los Angeles, and New York City documented that almost 26% of the participants were paid below the minimal wage, and this violation occurred mostly among childcare workers (66%); beauty, dry cleaning, and general repair workers (50%); and sewing and garment workers (43%).[76] Of employees who worked overtime, 76% were exposed to overtime violations, by being paid regular rates rather than "time and a half," being paid less than regular rates, or not being paid for any overwork time.[76] The overtime violation rate was found to be the highest among childcare workers, with a frequency of 90% among those who worked more than 40 hours during the previous week.[76] Unauthorized foreign workers experience a higher frequency of violations of minimum wage (38%) as well as overtime (85%).

Maltreatment between Customers and Service Providers

Mistreatment by Customers, Clients, or Patients

In a study by Makarem et al.[56] of almost 450 Lebanese workers in central Beirut, 4% of the participants reported having been exposed to bullying by clients or students in the previous six months.

A survey[77] conducted in 2016 of 38,000 workers in 28 European countries showed that 16% of the respondents needed to deal with angry customers, clients, patients, or pupils 75% of the time or more. This is in contrast to Korean workers, among whom only 4% reported having to handle annoyed consumers at least 75% of the time.[78]

Many publications have examined mistreatment of service providers by their customers, as manifested by a wide range of behaviors, including bullying,[79-83] incivility,[84-98] harassment,[99-115] abuse,[116-121] aggression,[122-126] threats,[115,127-136] assault,[117,127,133,134,137-140] and/or violence.[120,129-132,141,142]

Bullying by Customers or Patients

Bishop and Hoel[81] conducted a systematic examination of the concept of "bullying by the customer" based on data drawn from semi-structured interviews of 38 employees dealing with the public ("frontliners") who worked in job centers that were part of the British Public Employment Service. The study[81] addressed the employees' perceptions of their job duties and the main purpose of their responsibility, the degree to which they liked or disliked their employment, their experience in interacting with customers, and the coping strategies that they used to deal with difficult interactions. Furthermore, the investigators also utilized a one-month direct observation, shadowing the frontliners, as well as interviews with some managers and union activists. The research[81] showed that the employees "frequently perceived customer behavior as extremely negative and unwanted," and mostly described the behavior as "offensive, terrible, personally insulting, degrading, abusive, and aggressive." The negative behaviors were reported to occur regularly and frequently with the same customers. Furthermore, the frontliners indicated that, regardless of how offensive a customer was to them, "they were still expected to be polite back and continue to give good customer service,"[81] a situation that demonstrated "a perceived imbalance of power tilted in favor of the customer."[81] Moreover, the customers' negative actions led to anxiety and frustration among the mistreated employees, who were also exposed to stigmatization by coworkers and managers, who often blamed them for their misfortune, judging them as having poor service customer skills or as lacking them. Additionally, the victimized frontliners (as well as managers and coworkers) did not recognize customers' negative actions as bullying, but rather explained them as "part of the job," and therefore expected the frontliners to accept the problem and move forward.

Ilse and Neilipovitz[82] highlighted the notion of bullying of health providers by patients, families, or their substitute decision makers (PFSDs) and defined this form of mistreatment "as occurring when PFSDs use offensive, intimidating, malicious or insulting behavior, along with misuse of power, to undermine, defame, or abuse the recipient, with the intention of forcing their will on the recipient." Their description of this type of bullying also indicated that it usually involves verbal abuse and different forms of "reputational intimidation," such as legal actions or grievances addressed to hospital leadership or management, media, or government officials, and more recently using social media or "online rating systems" to spread adverse remarks. The usual goals of bullying by patient and families recognized in this report[82] were those of wishing to obtain unnecessary medical care, treatment, or investigations, and/or to get preferential treatment or "expectation for service that is different from the standard of medical and hospital care."[82] Yet, the concept of bullying by patients and families requires differentiation from circumstances when PFSDs may behave in an atypical manner due to anger and frustration, leading to yelling or abuse.[82] Also, Ilse and Neilipovitz[82] addressed the legal and ethical obligations of health leaders in dealing with the problem of bullying behavior by patients and families, as well as the ethical obligations and duties of patients and their families to "avoid either uncivil behavior or needless waste."[143] Ultimately, the authors[82] emphasized the responsibilities of health organizations to tackle the issue of PFSD bullying by commitment of resources and senior management involvement, by the development of a formal multidisciplinary behavioral management team to support frontline caregivers in difficult situations, and by a change in the organizational culture around PFSD bullying that previously subtly suggested to the victimized providers to "let it go" rather than report it.

An initial study of the prevalence of patient bullying was conducted by Sansone et al.,[83] based on a survey of 61 primary care suburban physicians in a midwestern US city. The study aimed to assess the participants' experience in the previous 12 months of being exposed to different types of maltreatment by their patients. The majority (85%) of the respondents reported that patients cussed out their office staff, while 61% indicated that they were bullied by patients to write a prescription, and more than a third of the participants recounted attempts by patients to bully them by proxy (i.e., via an administrator; Table 12.3).

Incivility of Consumers

Uncivil behaviors have been characterized as "rude and discourteous, displaying a lack of regard for others."[84] Distinctive instances of uncivil behavior by customers may include carrying on with complaints despite efforts to help them, use of an inappropriate manner in addressing the service provider (e.g., "Hey you"), and making inappropriate gestures to get attention (e.g., snapping fingers; Table 12.4).

Sommovigo et al.[85] conducted a systematic review of research on customer incivility and verbal aggression based on 53 studies focusing on antecedents to customers' misbehavior, coping strategies used by service providers, effects of these forms of mistreatment on service providers' well-being, and practical implications for the manager. The review[85]

Table 12.3. Annual Prevalence of Patient Bullying by Types of Mistreatment[83]

Occurring > 30%	Occurring < 30%
The patient cussed out the office staff (85%).	The patient verbally bullied the physician to make a referral (26%).
The patient verbally bullied the physician to write a prescription (61%).	The physician is concerned about being followed home by an angry patient (26%).
The patient verbally bullied the physician to write a form (46%).	The patient verbally bullied the physician when being confronted by the provider (25%).
The patient verbally bullied the physician by proxy (i.e., via an administrator; 43%).	The patient assumed an intimidating posture to threaten the physician (20%).
The patient made a verbal threat to the office staff (43%).	The patient shook a fist at the office staff (15%).
The police or security was called to remove the patient from the office (41%).	The patient made a verbal threat against the physician (10%).
The patient assumed an intimidating posture to threaten the office staff (39%).	The patient shook a fist at the physician in anger (3%).
The patient walked out in anger before the appointment was finished (38%).	A physician's family member was threatened by a patient (3%).
The patient verbally bullied the physician when limits were set on the patient (34%).	The patient made a threat to physically harm the physician (2%).
The patient cussed out the physician (33%).	The physician had property damage by an angry patient (2%).

Table 12.4. Examples of Customers' Incivility (Wilson and Holmwall[84])

Continuing to complain despite efforts made by the service provider to help the customer.	Using inappropriate manner to address the service provider (i.e., "Hey you").
Making gestures to denote impatience (i.e., eye rolling, sighing).	Failing to acknowledge significant efforts made by the service provider to help.
Grumbling to service provider about slow service during busy times.	Complaining to the service provider that there are too few employees working.
Making negative remarks to service provider about the organization.	Complaining to the service provider about the value of goods and services.
Blaming the service provider for a problem not caused by the employee.	Making inappropriate gestures to get attention (i.e., snapping fingers)
Pestering the service provider to make exceptions to company's policy.	Being irritated with the service provider because the company is out of a product.

examined studies that focused on the psychological aspects of the customer, including anger or malicious traits,[85] psychological obstructionism,[144] or personal biases and prejudices,[86] as antecedents for uncivil or aggressive behavior. Furthermore, Sommovigo's study[85] looked at the research that focused on the customers' dissatisfaction with service[86] (e.g., problem with a product, being given scripted responses to a concern) or workplace characteristics[144] (inability to find wanted items, long queues, uncleanness, being exposed to other frustrated clients and noises) as potential causes for customers' uncivil behavior. Moreover, the review[85] comprehensively researched the studies that explored the range of employees' reactions to uncivil or verbally aggressive acts by customers, either by reciprocation and sabotage of customers[144-149] or by nonreciprocation and the use of coping strategies like serving customers with a smile (emotional labor),[150] pretending or faking positive emotions (surface acting),[151] modifying inner emotions to match expressed emotions with the demands of service rules (deep acting),[151] discussing problems with others (social sharing of negative events),[152] providing concessions and additional effort to meet customer demands,[153,154] or seeking assistance from a peer or support from a supervisor or manager.[153,154] Additionally, an examination of the research addressing the consequences of customer incivility and verbal aggression highlighted the development of employees' emotional dissonance,[155-159] emotional exhaustion,[87,160-161] impairment in working memory,[162] increased turnover intentions,[163,164] job dissatisfaction,[84,157,158] and tendency to mistreat their coworkers.[144,149]

Harassment by Customers or Patients

Most of the studies that examine the problem of harassment by customers or patients focus on sexual harassment,[99-101,104,105-107,111-115,165-167] while few reports focus on stalking.[102,103,168]

Vincent-Höper et al.[101] developed and validated a measure for assessing sexual harassment by patients or clients that was used in a study of 181 German healthcare employees. The study[101] found that more than 60% of the respondents observed some people unnecessarily exposing themselves in front of the respondents, received repeated requests for a date, were asked intrusive or personal questions by a client (e.g., sexual preference, relationships status, body measurements), or were hugged or touched in a way that made them feel uncomfortable. Furthermore, this research[101] documented that all forms of sexual harassment (nonverbal, verbal, or physical) are associated with emotional exhaustion, psychological strain, depressive symptoms, and psychosomatic complaints.

Stalking is a form of harassment described as "repeated and persistent attempts to impose unwanted contact and/or communication on another person."[169] McIvor et al.[168] investigated the frequency of patients' stalking of 198 psychiatrists working in a large mental health organization in London, England. The participants reported having been stalked by a patient in two or more circumstances (21%), and most of the psychiatrists (81%) experienced stalking at work. Close to 60% of the patients involved in stalking were males, and 39% of the stalkers had a personality disorder. The stalking actions were likely to be persistent, in some cases up to 16 years, while the average was 26 months.

A survey by Galeazzi et al.[170] of 361 mental health professionals working in Modena, Italy, showed that 11% of them were stalked by patients, with unwanted communications or repeated contacts occurring on more than 10 occasions, for a period of more than one month, causing anxiety.[170] Almost all of the stalkers (90%) were under the "direct care of the clinician."[170] Nearly 25% of the victimized clinicians received threats, 13% stated that their property was damaged, and 7% were physically attacked by the stalker.[170] With regard to the reason for the stalking, about half of the participants indicated that the motive could have been the patient's wish for more closeness, while 13% of the harassed clinicians considered that the stalking started as the patient's retaliation for perceived mistreatment by the provider (e.g., a refusal to certify a disability), and in less than 10% of the cases the "stalking campaign" began "after termination of the therapeutic relationship by the mental health professional."[170]

Abuse by Customers or Patients

In a study by Truman et al.[116] involving 162 pediatric nurses in the United States, verbal abuse by patient and families was found to occur very frequently. The study indicated that 82% of the participants reported having been verbally abused an average of four times per month. Almost half of the nurses continued to think about the episode for a few days or a week or more, feeling angry or powerless, and 14% of them thought of leaving their position.[116]

The incidence of abuse of medical practitioners by patients and families was studied by Miedema et al.[171] in a survey of 720 Canadian family physicians. The research[171] showed that almost a third of the participants were exposed to an abusive encounter in the previous month, involving a patient or a patient's relative. All the abused physicians experienced a minor event, such as being exposed to rudeness, disrespect, humiliation, loudness, anger, insult, or verbal threat,[171] while 26% of the participants suffered a major incident, in which the abuser threw an object, slammed a door, broke or smashed an object, or spoke, looked, or gestured in a manner perceived as an unwanted sexual advance. Only 8% of the victimized physicians were maltreated with physical aggression, sexual assault, or stalking.[171] It is of interest that 55% of the abused participants did not know of any policies to protect them, while 76% did not ask for help, and 64% did not report the abusive incident.[171]

An examination of patients' physical and emotional abuse of nurses working in Canadian hospitals or long-term facilities was conducted by Shield and Wilkins[172] using data from the 2005 National Survey of the Work and Health of Nurses,[173] and it determined that "34% of nurses reported physical assault by a patient in the previous year and 47% reported emotional abuse."[172] Both types of abuse were significantly associated with staffing resource inadequacy, unfavorable nurse–physician working relations, low support from supervisors, and little coworker backing.[172]

Bi et al.[174] investigated the effects on restaurant frontline employees caused by the actions of customers "who may behave improperly and disrupt service through verbal abuse, physical abuse, and/or sexual harassment"[175] (known as jay-customers[176]). The research was based on a survey of 302 workers who provided face-to-face restaurant services in several cities of South Korea. The study identified that the types of abuse by customers that may frequently affect restaurant frontline employees included demeaning, derogatory, or condescending remarks; physical damage; vandalism/theft; as well as offensive sexual comments or sexual molestation. All forms of abuse were found to influence job stress (i.e., exhaustion, burnout), with physical abuse having the strongest effect, followed by sexual harassment and verbal abuse.[174] One of the interesting findings of this study was the moderate effect that the employee's empowerment may have on the effects of verbal abuse and job stress.[174] Specifically, the study documented that verbal abuse positively increases job stress if the employees have less power/authority to correct the customer's abuse by themselves.[174] Yet, empowerment was found to have an insignificant effect in moderating the effects of physical abuse or sexual harassment on job stress, and high empowerment of employees did not reduce the contribution of verbal abuse to job anxiety.[174]

Physical Assault or Violence by Customers or Patients

The European Foundation's Fourth European Survey[42] showed that, in 2005, 4% of workers were subjected to physical violence by people outside their workplace. It also underscored that health professionals reported one of the highest levels of exposure to violence among all occupations.[42]

Li et al.[141] quantified pooled prevalence estimates of workplace physical violence against healthcare professionals by patients and visitors. Their research, which was based on systematic review and meta-analysis of 65 studies published between 2000 and 2018, reported one-year prevalence estimates for 61,800 healthcare professionals from 30 countries. They found an overall one-year prevalence of 19%, with the highest pooled prevalence registered in WHO Region European countries (26.4%) and the lowest occurrence recorded among WHO Region South-East Asia countries (5.6%).[141]

The risk of assaults on psychiatrists by their patients was highlighted in 1976 by Madden et al.[177] in a survey of 115 psychiatrists who held faculty appointments at the University of Maryland School of Medicine. Their study showed that 42% of the participants reported having been assaulted "during their career" in a variety of clinical and administrative positions.[177] Sixty percent of the assaulted psychiatrists were residents, 16% were in private practice, and 19% were in administrative positions.[177] The assaults most often occurred at the beginning of their careers while they were working in emergency rooms or prisons.[177]

The frequency and sequelae of patient attacks suffered or witnessed by psychotherapists was studied by Daniel and Anadria[178] through an online survey of 915 therapists in Germany, Austria, and Switzerland. The research documented that 51% of the respondents reported having been the victim of, or witness to, a physical assault by a patient or "imminent threat of injury or death."[178] After the physical assault, almost a third of the affected therapists experienced some symptoms of PTSD, lasting more than a month, while nearly 3% suffered manifestations of a full PTSD diagnosis.[178]

Mistreatment of Customers, Clients, or Patients

The notion of consumers (customers, clients, or patients) being mistreated by service providers or corporations has been examined in the areas of rudeness or disrespect, sabotage, misconduct, abuse, and/or fraud.

Rudeness, Incivility, or Disrespect toward Customers or Patients

The notion and relevance of "social regard" as experienced by consumers during their interaction with a service provider were highlighted by Butcher et al.[179] and were defined as "the genuine respect, deference, and interest shown to the customer by the service provider such that the customer feels valued or important in the social interaction."[179] A survey[179] of 406 customers who received services in different sectors (including hairdressing, café, or naturopath establishments) documented that social regard had a significant influence on customer satisfaction, but above all it was a more relevant predictor of all surveyed café customers' satisfaction than the sense of value for money or the perceived core service quality.[179]

Respectful interaction with consumers is particularly critical with individuals who are more vulnerable, like medical patients, given their dependence and anxiety about abandonment.[180]

The nature and significance of appropriate and respectful treatment of patients were carefully examined by Silverman et al.[180] from the perspective of "etiquette and manners." The research underscored the relevance of "bedside manner," including dressing appropriately, knocking on a patient's door before asking and waiting for permission to enter the room, positioning oneself so that one's eyes are level with or below the patient's eyes, being flexible with one's language, avoiding prognostication, keeping one's promises, and/or silencing one's pager before starting a conversation that will deliver bad news.[180] Above all, the research emphasized the significance of not only barring any rude, lewd, or crude behavior toward patients and their families, but also protecting them from witnessing rudeness between health professionals.[180]

The need to expand the culture of respect toward patients among all medical staff was emphasized by Walsh[181] in a paper about managing the practice-first impression at the front desk. Walsh recommended that medical practices "re-engineer" office procedures in order to provide patients "greater choice, control, autonomy, and service" and "to avoid destructive and disruptive behaviors and conditions, such as noise, interference, excessive repetition, long waits, appointment delays, and staff rudeness."[181] In the same context, Hills provided recommendations for practical procedures in the management of the medical practice telephone, including detailed advice on how "to take accurate and complete telephone messages without turning off callers or misleading them," as well as how to use, and not abuse, a hold button.[182]

Within the scope of disrespectful, abusive, or neglectful care of patients, several studies[183-186] provided evidence about the poor treatment given to women during childbirth around the world. Bohren et al.[187] undertook a systematic review of 65 studies from 34 countries, with the objective of developing an evidence typology of, identification criteria for, and operational definitions of the mistreatment of women during facility-based childbirth. Among different themes of mistreatment the review[187] identified were concerns about use of harsh or rude language; judgmental or accusatory comments; poor communication, including language and interpretation barriers; lack of supportive care; denial or lack of birth companions; lack of respect for women's preferred birth position; and lack of privacy.[187]

Sabotage of Consumers

The notion of "service sabotage" was explained by Harris and Ogbonna[188] as "organizational member behaviors that are intentionally designed to affect service." This concept was used in a field research study[188] based on 182 in-depth interviews with organizational members from four firms in the hospitality industry. The study aimed to explore, describe, and classify the types, antecedents, and consequences of service sabotage by frontline staff members. More than 90% of the respondents indicated that service sabotage was a daily occurrence in their organizations, with the behaviors occurring either covertly or openly as well as intermittently or regularly.[188] The most common type of service sabotage performed or witnessed by almost half of the respondents was the "customary public service sabotage" displayed in front of coworkers, such as affecting the speed of service contrary to the customer's wishes, patronizing or condescending to the customer, or purposely adhering to annoying rules to slow the service. In addition, 25% of the respondents participated in or witnessed "customary private service sabotage," involving covert, personalized antiservice action to obtain revenge for a perceived offense or snub caused by the consumer—examples were serving smaller portions of a requested meal or a "bad beer." "Sporadic public service sabotage," reported by 17% of the participants in the survey,[188] occurs sporadically in front others with an action that disrupts the service encounter by deliberately damaging property or even hurts the client, and then immediately apologizing for "accidental clumsiness." A minority of participants (11%) indicated that they had been involved in very occasional covert disruptive behavior without the customer's knowledge that was caused by either impulsivity or frustration. These behaviors usually involved hygienic issues, such as spitting in somebody's meal.

Abuse of Consumers

Almost all the published studies about abuse of consumers pertain to patients' being abused in the field of healthcare. Swanberg et al.[189-197] extensively studied the problem of abuse in the healthcare system (AHC) and defined it[189] as "acts by any healthcare personnel at any healthcare institution" that "might have been perceived as abusive from an emotional, physical or sexual aspect." The notion of AHC[190] was previously included as one of the maltreatment categories in the NorVold Abuse Questionnaire (NorAQ),[198] besides emotional, physical, and sexual abuse, with each category ranging in qualitative magnitude from mild to severe. Mild AHC was explained[190,198] as any feeling of offense, degradation, or being blackmailed or disrespected experienced during a healthcare visit and causing later disturbance or suffering. Moderate AHC has been described[198] as having "experienced that a 'normal' event, while visiting health services, suddenly became a really terrible and insulting experience" without the patient fully understanding how this could occur. Finally, severe AHC was defined[190] as "having felt purposely hurt physically or mentally or grossly violated, or as having felt that one's body was used to one's disadvantage for someone else's purpose." The lifetime prevalence of AHC and health problems associated with adult abuse in health care (AAHC) in Nordic gynecological patients was ascertained in a study[190] involving more than 3,600 women from Denmark, Finland, Iceland, Norway, and Sweden who were surveyed using the NorAQ.[198] This research[190] documented that the prevalence of any lifetime experience of AHC in the five Nordic countries varied from 13% in Norway to 25% in Finland,

and 8% to 20% of patients were still experiencing abuse at the time of the study. Women who were AAHC victims but without additional adult experience of emotional, physical, or sexual abuse had a significantly higher risk of suffering from physical complaints [adjusted odds ratio (AOR) = 2.5], posttraumatic stress symptoms (AOR = 3.8), or sleep problems (AO = 2.4).[190]

Mannava et al.[199] reviewed 81 studies to identify the attitudes and behaviors of maternal healthcare providers in low- and middle-income countries toward their patients. The review showed that 59 of the studies reported on only negative providers' attitudes, including verbal abuse, rudeness (e.g., ignoring or ridiculing patients), neglect, physical abuse, absenteeism, unavailability of providers, corruption, lack of regard for privacy, poor communication, or unwillingness to accommodate traditional practices.[199] Two-thirds of all the studies reported how the negative maternal healthcare providers' attitudes and behaviors affected maternal emotional well-being, patients' satisfaction with care, overall access to quality services, and maternal health outcomes.[199]

For the past three decades, many studies[200-212] have examined the mistreatment of patients by health professionals' sexual misconduct. The notion of sexual misconduct was first proposed in 1981 by Burgess,[200] in a study based on interviews of 16 patients who were examined by a gynecologist in a manner that they felt was "sexually abusive." The mistreatment, which led to patients' physical discomfort and sexual arousal, was characterized by either "lengthy examination" (20–30 minutes), "misuse of the physicians' hands" (being touched all over the perineum and genital area or having the clitoris touched and rubbed), absence of a nurse during the examination, or excessive use of lubricant.[200]

A nationwide survey of more than 1,300 US psychiatrists was conducted in 1985 by Gartrell et al.[202] to assess the participants' attitudes about sexual contact with patients and to ascertain the prevalence of sexual misconduct among the respondents. The participants were asked to limit their answers to adult patients, who were defined as "a person who has reached the legal age of consent for sexual relations."[202] In the context of this study,[202] sexual contact was defined as contact that "was intended to arouse or satisfy sexual desire in the patient, therapist, or both."[202] The survey documented that 6% of the participants indicated that they had sexual contact with their own patients.[202] Eighty-one percent of the perpetrators were male, and 2% of all the participants reported that they had been sexually involved with their own therapist. As for the reason for engaging in sexual contact, 73% of the offenders indicated that they were driven by "love" or "pleasure," while 19% "intended the contact to enhance the patient's self-esteem and/or to provide a restitutive emotional experience for the patient."[202] Yet, some participants gave different reasons for being involved with patients, including "loss of control," "exploitation," "judgment lapse," "impulsivity," "therapist enhancement," and "personal needs."[202]

From 2000 through 2009, 2 per 1000 Canadian physicians[213] were disciplined by their provincial licensing authorities because of sexual misconduct, while during the decade from 2003 to 2013, 1 per 1000 US physicians[214] had one or more licensure punitive actions due to sexual transgressions with their patients.

A comprehensive study of sexual misconduct by Australian health professionals was conducted by Bismarck et al.[212] based on a retrospective cohort analysis of national data of notifications to health regulators of this type of mistreatment. During the period of 2011–2016, Australian health practitioners received sexual misconduct notifications at the rate of 2 per 1,000. The highest risk for potential perpetration of sexual misconduct was found among males (AOR = 6.48), professionals between 46 and 55 years old (AOR = 2.74), and psychiatrists (AOR = 23.1) and psychologists (AOR = 13.4).

The notion of "treatment boundary violations" as warning signs in the development of therapist sexual misconduct[215] was thoroughly examined by Simon,[216] who put forward guidelines to ensure boundaries are maintained between the therapist and the patient, including, among others, the need to interact verbally and to minimize physical contact; the need to ensure no previous, present, or future relationship with the patient; maintenance of relative therapist neutrality; the need to foster psychological separateness from the patient; and provision of a consistent, private, and professional setting.[216]

Corporate Victimization of Consumers

Consumers can be victimized by corporate practices like consumer fraud, production and sale of faulty goods, and deceptive advertisement.[75]

Consumer fraud can be understood as "any fraudulent financial transactions in which individuals feel that they have been financially taken advantage of."[217] This notion can include "being sold unsuitable products, being a victim of misrepresentation of information (e.g., hidden fees or unclear transaction terms), but also experiencing misusage of money by third parties (e.g., embezzlement of investments)."[217] According to a survey conducted during 2011 by the US Federal Trade Commission,[218] almost 11% of US adults were victims of one or more consumer frauds. The most frequently reported scams were the purchase of fraudulent weight-loss products, prize promotions, or work-at-home programs, or being billed for a buyers' club membership or Internet services that one had not agreed to purchase.[218] Almost 33% of the victims learned about the products through the Internet, and 20% of targets received the fraudulent information though print media (direct mail solicitations, newspaper or magazine advertisements, and posters or flyers), while "telemarketing was the source of information in just under 10% of incidents."[218] Victims of fraud were more likely to be willing to take risks, to have limited numeric skills, and to have more debt than they could handle financially. It is relevant to note that individuals who had experienced serious negative life events in the previous two years (e.g., loss of a job, divorce, death of a family member or close friend, serious illness) "were more than two-and-a-half times as likely to have experienced fraud as were those who had not suffered such a negative event."[218]

Croall[219] published an article examining consumers' victimization through corporate crimes and identified a range of wrongdoings (Table 12.5), presented an outline of some of the transgressions, and reviewed characteristics of victims and offenders.

Croall's article[219] focused primarily on different forms of transgressions that may occur in the food industry, as well as wrongdoing in the consumer goods and services business. Among offenses committed in the food industry, failure to observe hygiene regulations that resulted in food poisoning was cited as "a major source of death and illness for consumers."[219] Other concerns related to "legalized adulteration,"[220] as in the case food being adulterated with water during processing without the added water being declared on the outer label. In the same context, concerns were raised about other food additives being used and not labeled, such as genetically modified (GM) ingredients or starch, hard fats, and hydrogenated oils.[220] Also, the consumer may be misled by labels indicating that the product is "low fat" or "nutritious" while it actually contains "high amount of salt, fat, or sugar."[221] Furthermore,

Table 12.5. Areas of Consumer Complaints about Corporate Abuse[219]

Automobile sales[224,225]	Food adulteration[219]	Home repair and maintenances[225]	Misleading indications[219]
Automotive repair and services[224,225]	Food contents[219]	Household goods[224]	Misleading pictures[219]
Collection and billing practices[224]	Food packaging[219]	Internet and ecommerce[224]	Real estate[224]
Cosmetics[219]	Food poisoning[219]	Marketing malpractice[224]	Telecommunications[224,225]
Credit and financial services[224,225]	Home improvements[224]	Misleading descriptions	Utilities[225]

the customer may be misled by the use of terms like *fresh*, *natural*, *traditional*, or *authentic*; deceptive images and/or food packaging; and a larger-than-required package that implies it contains a larger amount of product.[222]

Croall's study[219] also provided details on the potential risks facing customers of the cosmetics and toiletries industry, which uses thousands of products with unknown long-term effects. The study also highlighted the abuse that consumers of home and car repairs and service or maintenance may be exposed to.[219]

Strategies for the Prevention of Workplace Bullying

In 2017, Guillen et al.[223] suggested that there was a need for the development of "large, well-controlled trials" of workplace bullying prevention strategies effective on the levels of society/policy, organization/employer, job/task, and individual/job interface, employing "validated and reliable outcome measures of bullying and a minimum of six months follow-up."[223]

Future Directions

Future public health research related to workplace bullying and other forms of maltreatment may consider:

- Expanding the range of work milieu's stakeholders beyond employees, supervisors, and managers to include consumers and corporations/employers
- Widening the scope of workplace bullying by encompassing all forms of mistreatment, abuse, aggression, or neglect perpetrated by, or affecting, any work milieu's stakeholder
- Examining the morbidity, safety risks, and mortality associated with maltreatment in the workplace
- Developing large, well-controlled studies of workplace maltreatment prevention interventions, working on the levels of society/policy, organization/employer, job/task, and individual/job interface,[223] with the use of validated and reliable outcome measures

of victimization and related morbidity[223] as well as a meaningful follow-up of at least one year
- Implementing periodic national or regional surveys to ascertain the rate or prevalence of workplace maltreatment and associated health and well-being risks

Notes

1. Results of a search under the term *workplace bullying* as keyword in Elsevier, Scopus, interdisciplinary citation and abstract database covering more than 23,000 peer-reviewed journals, tracking cited and citing literature. https://www.elsevier.com/solutions/scopus. Accessed September 1, 2022.
2. Results of a search under the term *workplace bullying* as a MeSH major topic for PubMed search. http://www.ncbi.nlm.nih.gov/pubmed. Accessed September 2, 2022.
3. Alderman C. Bullying in the workplace: a survey. *Nurs Stand.* 1997;11(35):22–24..
4. Graveson G. Workplace bullying—the abuse of power. *Br J Theatre Nurs.* 1998;7(11):21–23.
5. Quine L. Workplace bullying in NHS Community Trust: staff questionnaire survey. *BMJ.* 1999;318(7178):228–232. Cited by Zapf et al.[61]
6. Rayner C. The incidence of workplace bullying. *J Community Appl Soc Psychol.* 1997;7(3):199–208..
7. Rayner C, Hoel H. A summary review of literature regarding workplace bullying. *J Community Appl Soc Psychol.* 1997;7(3):181–191.
8. Crawford N. Bullying at work: a psychoanalytic perspective *J Community Appl Soc Psychol.* 1997;7(3):219–225.
9. O'Moore M, Seigne E, McGuire L, Smith M. Victims of workplace bullying in Ireland. *Ir J Psychol.* 1998;19(2-3):345–357..
10. Tidwell A. The role of workplace conflict in occupational health and safety. *J Occup Health Safety Aust N Z.* 1998;14(6):587–592.
11. Einarsen S, Matthiesen S, Skogstad A. Bullying, burnout and well-being among assistant nurses. *J Occup Health Safety Aust N Z.* 1998;14(6):563–568.
12. Hirsh HL. Sexual harassment in the health care workplace. *Nurs Homes.* 1981;30(3):46–47..
13. Biles GE. A program guide for preventing sexual harassment in the workplace. *Pers Adm.* 1981;26(6):49–56.
14. Gosselin HL. Sexual harassment on the job: psychological, social, and economic repercussions. *Can Ment Health.* 1984;32(3):21–24, 32.
15. Mathews B, Bismark MM. Sexual harassment in the medical profession: legal and ethical responsibilities. *Med J Aust.* 2015;203(4):189–192.
16. Goerth CR. Violence in the workplace emerges as growing health and safety problem. *Occup Health Safety.* 1988;57(5):53.
17. Hales T, Seligman PJ, Newman SC, Timbrook CL. Occupational injuries due to violence. *J Occup Med.* 1988;30(6):483–487.
18. Zhao S, Liu H, Ma H, et al. Coping with workplace violence in healthcare settings: social support and strategies. *Int J Environ Res Public Health.* 2015;12(11):14429–14444.
19. Leymann H. Mobbing and psychological terror at workplaces. *Violence Vict.* 1990;5(2):119–126.

20. Sahin B, Cetin M, Cimen M, Yildiran N. Assessment of Turkish junior male physicians' exposure to mobbing behavior. *Croat Med J.* 2012;53(4):357–366.
21. Smith PK, Singer M, Hoel H, Cooper CL. Victimization in the school and the workplace: are there any links? *Br J Psychol.* 2003;94(Pt 2):175–188.
22. Leyman H. *Handanleitung für den LIPT-Fragebogen* [Leymann inventory of psychological terror]. Tübingen, Germany: Dgvt-Verlag; 1996. Cited in Niedhammer S, David S, Degioani S, et al. La version française du questionnaire de Leymann sur la violence psychologique au travail: le "Leymann Inventory of Psychological Terror" (LIPT). *J Epidemiology Public Health.* 2006 Jun 1;54(3):245–262.
23. Olweus D. *Bullying at School: What We Know and What We Can Do.* Oxford, England: Blackwell Publishers; 1993:9.
24. Einarsen S, Hoel H, Zapf D, Cooper C. The concept of bullying at work. In: Einarsen S, Hoel H, Zapf D, Cooper CL, eds. *Bullying and Emotional Abuse in the Workplace: International Perspectives in Research and Practice.* London, England: Taylor & Francis; 2003:15.
25. Leymann, H. (1990). *Handbok for anvandning av LIPT-formularetforkartlaggningavrisker for psykiskt vdld arbetsmiljon* [The LIPT questionnaire—a manual]. Stockholm, Sweden: Violen. Cited in Leymann (see Note 240).
26. Einarsen S, Hoel H, Notelaers G. Measuring exposure to bullying at work: validity, factor structure and psychometric properties of the Negative Acts Questionnaire–Revised. *Work Stress.* 2009;23(1):24–44.
27. Keashly L, Neuman J. Bullying in the workplace: its impact and management. *Empl Rights Empl Policy J.* 2004;8(2):335–373.
28. Kwan SS, Tuckey MR, Dollard MF. The Malaysian Workplace Bullying Index (MWBI): a new measure of workplace bullying in Eastern countries. *PLOS One.* 2020;15(1):e0223235.
29. Rhoads JM. Overwork. *JAMA.* 1977;237(24):2615–2618.
30. Netterstrøm B, Juel K. Impact of work-related and psychosocial factors on the development of ischemic heart disease among urban bus drivers in Denmark. *Scand J Work Environ Health.* 1988:231–238. Cited by Michie S, Cockcroft A. Overwork can kill: especially if combined with high demand, low control, and poor social support. *BMJ.* 1996;312(7036):921–923.
31. Hiyama T, Yoshihara M. New occupational threats to Japanese physicians: karoshi (death due to overwork) and karojisatsu (suicide due to overwork). *J Occup Environ Med.* 2008;65(6):428–429.
32. Kondo N, Oh J. Suicide and karoshi (death from overwork) during the recent economic crises in Japan: the impacts, mechanisms and political responses. *J Occup Environ Med.* 2010;64(8):649–650.
33. Ke DS. Overwork, stroke, and karoshi-death from overwork. *Acta Neurol Taiwan.* 2012;21(2):54–59.
34. Eguchi H, Wada K, Smith DR. Recognition, compensation, and prevention of karoshi, or death due to overwork. *J Occup Environ Med.* 2016;58(8): e313.
35. Wong CW, Chan YH, Cheng YH, Lam CS. Is overwork a precipitant factor of idiopathic ventricular fibrillation? *Int J Cardiol.* 2016;223:218–219.
36. Yamauchi T, Yoshikawa T, Takamoto M, et al. Overwork-related disorders in Japan: recent trends and development of a national policy to promote preventive measures. *Ind Health.* 2017;55(3):293–302.
37. Lin RT, Lin CK, Christiani DC, et al. The impact of the introduction of new recognition criteria for overwork-related cardiovascular and cerebrovascular diseases: a cross-country comparison. *Sci Rep.* 2017;7(1):167.

38. Shan HP, Yang XH, Zhan XL, et al. Overwork is a silent killer of Chinese doctors: a review of Karoshi in China 2013–2015. *Public Health.* 2017;147:98–100.
39. Otsui K, Yamamoto J, Inoue N. Overwork accelerates thrombotic reaction: implications for the pathogenesis of Karoshi. *J Thromb Thrombolysis.* 2018;45(2):222–224.
40. Bannai A, Tamakoshi A. The association between long working hours and health: a systematic review of epidemiological evidence. *Scand J Work Environ Health.* 2014:5-18.
41. Atroszko PA, Demetrovics Z, Griffiths MD. Work addiction, obsessive-compulsive personality disorder, burn-out, and global burden of disease: implications from the ICD-11. *Int J Environ Res Public Health.* 2020;17(2):660.
42. Parent-Thirion A, Fernández Macías E, Hurley J, Vermeylen G. Fourth European Working Conditions Survey, European Foundation for the Improvement of Living and Working Conditions, Annex 1, Survey Methodology. https://www.eurofound.europa.eu/sites/default/files/ef_files/pubdocs/2006/98/en/2/ef0698en.pdf. Accessed September 4, 2022.
43. Parent-Thirion A, Fernández Macías E, Hurley J, Vermeylen G. Fourth European Working Conditions Survey, European Foundation for the Improvement of Living and Working Conditions, Violence, Harassment and Discrimination at the Workplace. https://www.eurofound.europa.eu/sites/default/files/ef_files/pubdocs/2006/98/en/2/ef0698en.pdf. Accessed September 4, 2022.
44. Parent-Thirion A, Vermeylen G, van Houten G, Lyly-Yrjänäinen M, Biletta I, Cabrita J, with the assistance of Niedhammer I. *Eurofound Fifth European Working Conditions Survey.* Luxembourg: Publications Office of the European Union; 2012:57–58. https://www.eurofound.europa.eu/en/publications/2012/fifth-european-working-conditions-survey-overview-report. Accessed September 27, 2023.
45. Alterman T, Luckhaupt SE, Dahlhamer JM, Ward BW, Calvert GM. Job insecurity, work-family imbalance, and hostile work environment: prevalence data from the 2010 National Health Interview Survey. *Am J Ind Med.* 2013;56(6):660–669.
46. Lee RT, Brotheridge CM. When prey turns predatory: workplace bullying as a predictor of counter aggression/bullying, coping, and well-being. *Eur J Work Organ Psychol.* 2006;15(3):352–377..
47. Statistics Canada. Violence in the Workplace. https://www.statcan.gc.ca/pub/11-402-x/2008/2693/ceb2693_002-eng.htm. Accessed September 4, 2022.
48. Einarsen S. Harassment and bullying at work: a review of the Scandinavian approach. *Aggress Violent Behav.* 2000;5(4):379–401. Cited by Tsuno et al (see Note 49).
49. Tsuno K, Kawakami N, Inoue A, Abe K. Measuring workplace bullying: reliability and validity of the Japanese version of the Negative Acts Questionnaire. *J Occup Health.* 2010;52(4):216–226.
50. Leymann H. The content and development of mobbing at work. *Eur J Work Organ Psychol.* 1996;5(2):165–184. Cited by Tsuno et al.[49]
51. Petrović IB, Vukelić M, Čizmić S. Rocking at 81 and rolling at 34: ROC cut-off scores for the Negative Acts Questionnaire–Revised in Serbia. *Front Psychol.* 2017;7:2058.
52. Einarsen S, Hoel H, Notelaers G. Measuring exposure to bullying and harassment at work: validity, factor structure and psychometric properties of the Negative Acts Questionnaire–Revised. *Work Stress.* 2009;23(1):24–44. Cited by Tsuno et al.[49]
53. Bowling NA, Beehr TA. Workplace harassment from the victim's perspective: a theoretical model and meta-analysis. *J Appl Psychol.* 2006;91(5):998.
54. Nielsen MB, Einarsen S. Outcomes of exposure to workplace bullying: a meta-analytic review. *Work Stress.* 2012;26(4):309–332.

55. Wheeler AR, Halbesleben JR, Shanine K. Eating their cake and everyone else's cake, too: resources as the main ingredient to workplace bullying. *Business Horiz.* 2010;53(6):553–560. Cited by Kemp V. Antecedents, consequences, and interventions for workplace bullying. *Curr Opinion Psychiatry.* 2014;27(5):364–368.
56. Makarem NN, Tavitian-Elmadjian LR, Brome D, Hamadeh GN, Einarsen S. Assessment of workplace bullying: reliability and validity of an Arabic version of the Negative Acts Questionnaire-Revised (NAQ-R). *BMJ Open.* 2018;8(12):e024009.
57. Niedl K. *Mobbing/Bullying am Arbeitsplatz. Eine empirische Analyse zum Phänomen sowie zu personalwirtschaftlich relevanten Effekten von systematischen Feindseligkeiten.* [Mobbing at work. An empirical analysis of the phenomenon and the effect of systematic harassment on human resource management]. Munich, Germany: Hamp; 1995. Cited by Zapf D, Einarsen S, Hoel H, Vartia M. Empirical findings on bullying in the workplace. In: Einarsen S, Hoel H, Zapf D, Cooper CL, eds. *Bullying and Emotional Abuse in the Workplace: International Perspectives in Research and Practice.* London, England: Taylor & Francis; 2003:116–124.
58. Björkqvist K, Österman K, Hjelt-Bäck M. Aggression among university employees. Aggress Behav. 1994;20(3):173–184. Cited by Zapf et al.[57]
59. Zapf D. Mobbing in organisationen–Überblick zum Stand der Forschung. *Z Arb Organ.* 1999;43(1):1–25. Cited by Zapf et al.[57]
60. Mackensen von Astfeld S. *Das Sick-Building-Syndrom unter besonderer Berucksichtigung des Einflusses von Mobbing* [The sick building syndrome with special consideration of the effects of mobbing]. Hamburg, Germany: Verlag Dr Kovac; 2000. Cited by Zapf et al.[57]
61. Zapf D, Knorz C, Kulla M. On the relationship between mobbing factors, and job content, social work environment, and health outcomes. *Eur J Work Organ Psychol.* 1996;5(2):215–237. Cited by Zapf et al.[57]
62. zur Mühlen L, Normann G, Greif S. Stress and bullying in two organisations. Faculty of Psychology. University of Osnabrück. 2001 Cited by Zapf et al.[57]
63. O'Moore M. *Summary Report on the National Survey on Workplace Bullying in Ireland.* Dublin, Ireland: The Anti-Bullying Research Centre, Trinity College; 2000. Cited by Zapf et al.[57]
64. O'Moore M, Seigne E, McGuire L, Smith M. Victims of bullying at work in Ireland. *J Occup Health Safety Aust N Z.* 1998;14:569–574. Cited by Zapf et al.[57]
65. Ege H. *I Numeri del Mobbing: La Prima Ricerca Italiana* [The frequency of bullying. The first Italian research]. Bologne, Italy: Pitagora Editrice; 1998. Cited by Zapf et al.[57]
66. Holzen Beusch EV, Zapf D, Schallberger U. Warum Mobbingopfer ihre Arbeitsstelle nicht wechseln [Why the victims of bullying do not change their job]. *Z Personalforschung.* 1998. Cited by Zapf et al.[57]
67. Rayner C. The incidence of workplace bullying. *J Community Appl Soc Psychol.* 1997;7(3):199–208. Cited by Zapf et al.[57]
68. UNISON. *UNISON Members' Experience of Bullying at Work.* London, England: UNISON; 1997. Cited by Zapf et al.[57]
69. Hoel H, Cooper CL, Faragher B. The experience of bullying in Great Britain: the impact of organizational status. *Eur J Work Organ Psychol.* 2001;10(4):443–465. Cited by Zapf et al.[57]
70. Vartia M. Psychological harassment (bullying, mobbing) at work. In: Kaupinen-Toropainen K, ed. *OECD Panel Group on Women, Work, and Health.* Helsinki, Finland: Ministry of Social Affairs and Health; 1993:149–152. Cited by Zapf et al.[57]
71. Vartia M, Hyyti J. Gender differences in workplace bullying among prison officers. *Eur J Work Organ Psychol.* 2002;11(1):113–126. Cited by Zapf et al.[57]

72. Cowie H, Jennifer D, Neto C, et al. Comparing the nature of workplace bullying in two European countries: Portugal and the UK. In: *Transcending the Boundaries: Integrating People, Processes, and Systems. Proceedings of the 2000 Conference*. Brisbane, Australia: Griffith University; 2000:128-133. Cited by Zapf et al.[57]
73. Leymann H. *Mobbing-Psychoterror am Arbeitsplatz und Wie Man Sich Dagegen Wehren Kann* [Mobbing-Psychological Terror at Work, and How One Can Defend Oneself]. Reinbeck, Germany: Rowohlt; 2013. Cited by Zapf et al.[57]
74. Einarsen S, Skogstad A. Prevalence and risk groups of bullying and harassment at work. *Eur J Work Organ Psychol*. 1996;5(2):185–202. Cited by Zapf et al.[57]
75. Shichor D. Corporate deviance and corporate victimization: a review and some elaborations. *Int Rev Victimol*. 1989;1(1):67–88.
76. Bernhardt A, Milkman R, Theodore N, et al. Broken laws, unprotected workers: violations of employment and labor laws in America's cities. https://escholarship.org/uc/item/1vn389nh. Accessed September 5, 2022.
77. Eurofound. *Sixth European Working Conditions Survey – Overview Report* (2017 update). Luxembourg: Publications Office of the European Union; 2017. Cited by Eurofound and International Labour Organization (see Note 78).
78. Eurofound and International Labour Organization. *Working Conditions in a Global Perspective*. Luxembourg: Publications Office of the European Union; 2019:82–83. https://www.ilo.org/wcmsp5/groups/public/---dgreports/---dcomm/---publ/documents/publication/wcms_696174.pdf. Accessed September 4, 2022.
79. Mendonca A, D'Cruz P, Noronha E. Beauty service workers' encounters with abusive customers: furthering the concept of external bullying at work. *Indian Perspectives on Workplace Bullying: A Decade of Insights*. 2018:205–235.
80. Ram Y. Hostility or hospitality? A review on violence, bullying and sexual harassment in the tourism and hospitality industry. *Curr Issues Tourism*. 2018;21(7):760–774.
81. Bishop V, Hoel H. The customer is always right? Exploring the concept of customer bullying in the British Employment Service. *J Consumer Cult*. 2008;8(3):341–367.
82. Ilse R, Neilipovitz D. Addressing bullying behaviour by patients and families. *Healthc Manage Forum*. 2019;32(4):224–227.
83. Sansone RA, Sansone LA, Wiederman MW. Patient bullying: a survey of physicians in primary care. *Prim Care Companion J Clin Psychiatry*. 2007;9(1):56–58. Cited by Ilse and Neilipovitz.[82]
84. Wilson NL, Holmvall CM. The development and validation of the Incivility from Customers Scale. *J Occup Health Psychol*. 2013;18(3):310.
85. Sommovigo V, Setti I, Argentero P, O'Shea D. The impact of customer incivility and verbal aggression on service providers: a systematic review. *Work*. 2019;62(1):59–86..
86. Sliter M, Jones M. A qualitative and quantitative examination of the antecedents of customer incivility. *J Occup Health Psychol*. 2016;21(2):208. Cited by Sommovigo et al.[85]
87. Sliter M, Jex S, Wolford K, McInnerney J. How rude! Emotional labor as a mediator between customer incivility and employee outcomes. *J Occup Health Psychol*. 2010;15(4):468–481. Cited by Sommovigo et al.[85]
88. Harrison I, Trevethan CT, Pasciak F, Irwin A. Part and parcel: a qualitative interview study examining the experience of client rudeness by mental health workers. *Issues Ment Health Nurs*. 2020;41(2):122–131.
89. Bar-David S. What's in an eye roll? It is time we explore the role of workplace incivility in healthcare. *Isr J Health Policy Res*. 2018;7(1):1–3.

90. Walker DD, Van Jaarsveld DD, Skarlicki DP. Sticks and stones can break my bones but words can also hurt me: the relationship between customer verbal aggression and employee incivility. *J Appl Psychol.* 2017;102(2):163.
91. Walker DD, Van Jaarsveld DD, Skarlicki DP. Exploring the effects of individual customer incivility encounters on employee incivility: the moderating roles of entity (in)civility and negative affectivity. *J Appl Psychol.* 2014;99(1):151.
92. Kern JH, Grandey AA. Customer incivility as a social stressor: the role of race and racial identity for service employees. *J Occup Health Psychol.* 2009;14(1):46.
93. Walker DD, Van Jaarsveld DD, Skarlicki DP. Exploring the effects of individual customer incivility encounters on employee incivility: the moderating roles of entity (in)civility and negative affectivity. *J Appl Psychol.* 2014;99(1):151.
94. Alola UV, Olugbade OA, Avci T, Öztüren A. Customer incivility and employees' outcomes in the hotel: testing the mediating role of emotional exhaustion. *Tourism Manage Perspect.* 2019; 29:9–17.
95. Boukis A, Koritos C, Daunt KL, Papastathopoulos A. Effects of customer incivility on frontline employees and the moderating role of supervisor leadership style. *Tourism Manage.* 2020;77:103997.
96. Arnold KA, Walsh MM. Customer incivility and employee well-being: testing the moderating effects of meaning, perspective taking and transformational leadership. *Work Stress.* 2015;29(4):362–378.
97. Shin Y, Hur WM. When do service employees suffer more from job insecurity? The moderating role of coworker and customer incivility. *Int J Environ Res Public Health.* 2019;16(7):1298.
98. Vargas EA, Mahalingam R. Experiences of patient incivility: a qualitative study. *J Patient Exp.* 2020;7(4):615–620.
99. Gettman HJ, Gelfand MJ. When the customer shouldn't be king: antecedents and consequences of sexual harassment by clients and customers. *J Appl Psychol.* 2007;92(3):757.
100. Friborg MK, Hansen JV, Aldrich PT, et al. Workplace sexual harassment and depressive symptoms: a cross-sectional multilevel analysis comparing harassment from clients or customers to harassment from other employees amongst 7603 Danish employees from 1041 organizations. *BMC Public Health.* 2017;17(1):1–2.
101. Vincent-Höper S, Adler M, Stein M, Vaupel C, Nienhaus A. Sexually harassing behaviors from patients or clients and care workers' mental health: development and validation of a measure. *Int J Environ Res Public Health.* 2020;17(7):2570.
102. Kivisto AJ, Kivisto KL. Risk management with clients who stalk, threaten, and harass mental health professionals. *Am J Psychother.* 2018;71(3):110–120.
103. Sandberg DA, McNiel DE, Binder RL. Stalking, threatening, and harassing behavior by psychiatric patients toward clinicians. *J Am Acad Psychiatry Law Online.* 2002;30(2):221–229.
104. Notaro E, Pascoe V, Shinohara MM, DeNiro K. Sexual harassment from patient to provider. *Int J Womens Dermatol.* 2020;6(1):30.
105. Scholcoff C, Farkas A, Machen JL, et al. Sexual harassment of female providers by patients: a qualitative study. *J Gen Intern Med.* 2020;35(10):2963–2968.
106. Hemmat S, Khoong EC, Sharma AE, Sarkar U. Sharing stories, searching for solutions: sexual harassment of physicians by patients. *Am J Med.* 2019;132(10):e746.
107. Bratuskins PA, McGarry H, Wilkinson S. Sexual harassment of Australian female general practitioners by patients. *Med J Aust.* 2013;199(7):454.

108. Abrams KM, Robinson GE. Stalking by patients: doctors' experiences in a Canadian urban area. *J Nerv Ment Dis*. 2011;199(10):738–743.
109. Abrams KM, Robinson GE. Stalking by patients: doctors' experiences in a Canadian urban area (Part II)—physician responses. *J Nerv Ment Dis*. 2013;201(7):560–566.
110. Bird S. Strategies for managing and minimizing the impact of harassment and stalking by patients. *ANZ J Surg*. 2009;79(7-8):537–538.
111. Hibino Y, Hitomi Y, Kambayashi Y, Nakamura H. Exploring factors associated with the incidence of sexual harassment of hospital nurses by patients. *J Nurs Scholarsh*. 2009;41(2):124–131.
112. Hibino Y, Ogino K, Inagaki M. Sexual harassment of female nurses by patients in Japan. *J Nurs Scholarsh*. 2006;38(4):400–405.
113. Schneider M, Phillips SP. A qualitative study of sexual harassment of female doctors by patients. *Soc Sci Med*. 1997;45(5):669–676.
114. Kettl P, Siberski J, Hischmann C, Wood B. Sexual harassment of health care students by patients. *J Psychosoc Nurs Ment Health Serv*. 1993;31(7):11–13.
115. Chiodo GT, Tolle SW, Labby D. Sexual advances by patients in dental practice: implications for the dental and dental hygiene curricula. *J Dent Educ*. 1992;56(9):617–624.
116. Truman A, Goldman M, Lehna C, Berger J, Topp RV. Verbal abuse of pediatric nurses by patients and families. *Ky Nurse*. 2013;61(1):6–8.
117. Miedema BB, Hamilton R, Tatemichi S, et al. Monthly incidence rates of abusive encounters for Canadian family physicians by patients and their families. *Int J Fam Med*. 2010;2010:387202. doi:10.1155/2010/387202
118. Shields M, Wilkins K. Factors related to on-the-job abuse of nurses by patients. *Health Rep*. 2009;20(2):7.
119. Inoue M, Tsukano K, Muraoka M, Kaneko F, Okamura H. Psychological impact of verbal abuse and violence by patients on nurses working in psychiatric departments. *Psychiatry Clin Neurosci*. 2006 Feb;60(1):29–36
120. Lynch J, Appelboam R, McQuillan PJ. Survey of abuse and violence by patients and relatives towards intensive care staff. *Anaesthesia*. 2003;58(9):893–899.
121. Miedema B, Hamilton R, Lambert-Lanning A, et al. Prevalence of abusive encounters in the workplace of family physicians: a minor, major, or severe problem? *Can Fam Physician*. 2010;56(3):e101-e108.
122. Kind N, Eckert A, Steinlin C, Fegert JM, Schmid M. Verbal and physical client aggression—a longitudinal analysis of professional caregivers' psychophysiological stress response and burnout. *Psychoneuroendocrinology*. 2018; 94:11–16.
123. Gale C, Arroll B, Coverdale J. Aggressive acts by patients against general practitioners in New Zealand: one-year prevalence. *N Z Med J (Online)*. 2006;119(1237).
124. Saeki K, Okamoto N, Tomioka K, et al. Work-related aggression and violence committed by patients and its psychological influence on doctors. *J Occup Health*. 2011:1108050204.-
125. Gómez-Gutiérrez MM, Bernaldo-de-Quirós M, Piccini AT, Cerdeira JC. Posttraumatic stress symptomatology in pre-hospital emergency care professionals assaulted by patients and/or relatives: importance of severity and experience of the aggression. *J Interpers Violence*. 2016;31(2):339–354.
126. Rafaeli A, Erez A, Ravid S, Derfler-Rozin R, Treister DE, Scheyer R. When customers exhibit verbal aggression, employees pay cognitive costs. *J Appl Psychol*. 2012;97(5):931.

127. Faulkner LR, Grimm NR, McFarland BH, Bloom JD. Threats and assaults against psychiatrists. *J Am Acad Psychiatry Law Online*. 1990;18(1):37–46.
128. Acquadro Maran D, Varetto A, Zedda M, Franscini M. Health care professionals as victims of stalking: characteristics of the stalking campaign, consequences, and motivation in Italy. *J Interpers Violence*. 2017;32(17):2605–2625.
129. Edwards JA, Buckley P. Customer-perpetrated work-related violence: prevalence and trends in Britain. *Occup Med*. 2016;66(7):522–527.
130. Sanchez-Gallegos D, Viens DC. When the client is armed or dangerous: management of violent and difficult clients in primary care. *Nurse Pract*. 1995;20(6):26–32.
131. Zubairi AJ, Ali M, Sheikh S, Ahmad T. Workplace violence against doctors involved in clinical care at a tertiary care hospital in Pakistan. *Medicine*. 2019; 31:16–18.
132. Lewis ML, Dehn DS. Violence against nurses in outpatient mental health settings. *J Psychosoc Nurs Ment Health Serv*. 1999;37(6):28–33.
133. Dubin WR, Wilson SJ, Mercer C. Assaults against psychiatrists in outpatient settings. *J Clin Psychiatry*. 1988;49(9):338–345.
134. Dvir Y, Moniwa E, Crisp-Han H, Levy D, Coverdale JH. Survey of threats and assaults by patients on psychiatry residents. *Acad Psychiatry*. 2012;36(1):39–42.
135. McKenna BG, Poole SJ, Smith NA, Coverdale JH, Gale CK. A survey of threats and violent behaviour by patients against registered nurses in their first year of practice. *Int J Ment Health Nurs*. 2003;12(1):56–63.
136. Coverdale J, Gale C, Weeks S, Turbott S. A survey of threats and violent acts by patients against training physicians. *Med Educ*. 2001;35(2):154–159.
137. Stubbs B, Dickens G. Physical assault by patients against physiotherapists working in mental health settings. *Physiotherapy*. 2009;95(3):170–175.
138. Tattoli L, Bosco C, Grattagliano I, Di Vella G. The risk of assault against mental health professionals: a fatal case report and literature review. *Forensic Sci Med Pathol*. 2019;15(2):276–280.
139. Appelbaum PS, Dimieri RJ. Protecting staff from assaults by patients: OSHA steps in. *Psychiatr Serv*. 1995;46(4):333–334.
140. Madden DJ, Lion JR, Penna MW. Assaults on psychiatrists by patients. *Am J Psychiatry*. 1976;133(4):422–425.
141. Li YL, Li RQ, Qiu D, Xiao SY. Prevalence of workplace physical violence against health care professionals by patients and visitors: a systematic review and meta-analysis. *Int J Environ Res Public Health*. 2020;17(1):299.
142. Vanderslott J. A study of incidents of violence towards staff by patients in an NHS Trust hospital. *J Psychiatr Ment Health Nurs*. 1998;5(4):291–298.
143. Evans HM. Do patients have duties? *J Med Ethics*. 2007;33(12):689–694. Cited by Sansone et al.[83]
144. Van Jaarsveld DD, Walker DD, Skarlicki DP. The role of job demands and emotional exhaustion in the relationship between customer and employee incivility. *J Manage*. 2010;36(6):1486–1504. Cited by Sommovigo et al.[85]
145. Torres EN, van Niekerk M, Orlowski M. Customer and employee incivility and its causal effects in the hospitality industry. *J Hospitality Marketing Manage*. 2017;26(1):48–66. Cited by Sommovigo et al.[85]
146. Wang M, Liao H, Zhan Y, Shi J. Daily customer mistreatment and employee sabotage against customers: examining emotion and resource perspectives. *Acad Manage J*. 2011;54(2):312–334. Cited by Sommovigo et al.[85]

147. Skarlicki DP, Van Jaarsveld DD, Walker DD. Getting even for customer mistreatment: the role of moral identity in the relationship between customer interpersonal injustice and employee sabotage. *J Appl Psychol.* 2008;93(6):1335–1347. Cited by Sommovigo et al.[85]
148. Shao R, Skarlicki DP. Service employees' reactions to mistreatment by customers: a comparison between North America and East Asia. *Personnel Psychol.* 2014;67(1):23–59. Cited by Sommovigo et al.[85]
149. Walker DD, Van Jaarsveld DD, Skarlicki DP. Exploring the effects of individual customer incivility encounters on employee incivility: the moderating roles of entity (in) civility and negative affectivity. *J Appl Psychol.* 2014;99(1):151. Cited by Sommovigo et al.[85]
150. Grandey AA. Emotional regulation in the workplace: a new way to conceptualize emotional labor. *J Occup Health Psychol.* 2000;5(1):95. Cited by Sommovigo et al.[85]
151. Song G, Liu H. Customer-related social stressors, and emotional exhaustion: the mediating role of surface and deep acting. *Soc Behav Pers.* 2010;38(10):1359–1366. Cited by Sommovigo et al.[85]
152. Rose AJ. Co-rumination in the friendships of girls and boys. *Child Dev.* 2002;73(6):1830–1843. Cited by Sommovigo et al.[85]
153. Echeverri P, Salomonson N, Åberg A. Dealing with customer misbehavior: the role of practical judgement in service provision. InQUIS 11–Services Conference, June 11-14, 2009, Wolfsburg, Germany, 2009. Cited by Sommovigo et al.[85]
154. Fisk GM, Neville LB. Effects of customer entitlement on service workers' physical and psychological well-being: a study of waitstaff employees. *J Occup Health Psychol.* 2011;16(4):391. Cited by Sommovigo et al.[85]
155. Molino M, Emanuel F, Zito M, Ghislieri C, Colombo L, Cortese CG. Inbound call centers and emotional dissonance in the job demands–resources model. *Front Psychol.* 2016;7:1133. Cited by Sommovigo et al.[85]
156. Yoo JJ, Kim TT, Lee G. When customers complain: the value of customer orientation in service recovery. *Cornell Hospitality Q.* 2015;56(4):411–426. Cited by Sommovigo et al.[85]
157. Karatepe OM, Yorganci I, Haktanir M. Outcomes of customer verbal aggression among hotel employees. *Int J Contemp Hospitality Manage.* 2009;21(6):713–733. Cited by Sommovigo et al.[85]
158. Goussinsky R. Does customer aggression more strongly affect happy employees? The moderating role of positive affectivity and extraversion. *Motivation Emotion.* 2011;35(2):220–234. Cited by Sommovigo et al.[85]
159. Wegge J, Dick RV, Bernstorff CV. Emotional dissonance in call centre work. *J Manage Psychol.* 2010;25(6):596–619. Cited by Sommovigo et al.[85]
160. Karatepe OM, Nkendong RA. The relationship between customer-related social stressors and job outcomes: the mediating role of emotional exhaustion. *Econ Res.* 2014;27(1):414–426. Cited by Sommovigo et al.[85]
161. Kim TT, Paek S, Choi CH, Lee G. Frontline service employees' customer-related social stressors, emotional exhaustion, and service recovery performance: customer orientation as a moderator. *Serv Bus.* 2012;6(4):503–526. Cited by Sommovigo et al.[85]
162. Rafaeli A, Erez A, Ravid S, Derfler-Rozin R, Treister DE, Scheyer R. When customers exhibit verbal aggression, employees pay cognitive costs. *J Appl Psychol.* 2012;97(5):931–950. Cited by Sommovigo et al.[85]
163. Han SJ, Bonn MA, Cho M. The relationship between customer incivility, restaurant frontline service employee burnout and turnover intention. *Int J Hospitality Manage.* 2016;52:97–106. Cited by Sommovigo et al.[85]

164. Li X, Zhou E. Influence of customer verbal aggression on employee turnover intention. *Manage Decision*. 2013;51(4):890–912. Cited by Sommovigo et al.[85]
165. Gabay G, Shafran Tikva S. Sexual harassment of nurses by patients and missed nursing care—a hidden population study. *J Nurs Manage*. 2020;28(8):1881–1887.
166. Kagan I, Gaash T, Grigorash S, Sela M, Maximov Y, Cohen S. Sexual harassment by patients: the difference experience of female doctors, nurses, and nurse aids. *Med Law*. 2015;34:5.
167. Baker L. Sexual harassment by patients forces doctors to alter their practice. *BMJ*. 2014;348.
168. McIvor RJ, Potter L, Davies L. Stalking behaviour by patients towards psychiatrists in a large mental health organization. *Int J Soc Psychiatry*. 2008;54(4):350–357.
169. Mullen PE, Purcell R, Stuart GW. Study of stalkers. *Am J Psychiatry*. 1999;156(8):1244–1249. Cited by McIvor et al.[168]
170. Galeazzi GM, Elkins K, Curci P. Emergency psychiatry: the stalking of mental health professionals by patients. *Psychiatr Serv*. 2005;56(2):137–138.
171. Miedema BB, Hamilton R, Tatemichi S, et al. Monthly incidence rates of abusive encounters for Canadian family physicians by patients and their families. *Int J Fam Med*. 2010;2010:387202. doi:10.1155/2010/387202
172. Shields M, Wilkins K. Factors related to on-the-job abuse of nurses by patients. *Health Rep*. 2009;20(2):7.
173. Shields M, Wilkins K. *Findings from the 2005 National Survey of the Work and Health of Nurses*. Statistics Canada; Catalogue 83-003-XPE. Ottawa, Ontario: Minister of Industry, 2006 Cited by Shields and Wilkins.[172]
174. Bi Y, Choi S, Yin J, Kim I. Stress on frontline employees from customer aggression in the restaurant industry: the moderating effect of empowerment. *Sustainability*. 2021;13(3):1433.
175. Harris LC, Reynolds KL. Jaycustomer behavior: an exploration of types and motives in the hospitality industry. *J Serv Mark*. 2004;18:339–357. Cited by Bi et al.[174]
176. Lovelock CH. *Product Plus: How Product and Service Equals Competitive Advantage*. New York, NY: McGraw-Hill Companies; 1994. Cited by Bi et al.[174]
177. Madden DJ, Lion JR, Penna MW. Assaults on psychiatrists by patients. *Am J Psychiatry*. 1976;133(4):422–425.
178. Daniels JK, Anadria D. Experiencing and witnessing patient violence—an occupational risk for outpatient therapists? *Psychiatr Q*. 2019;90(3):533–541.
179. Butcher K, Sparks B, O'Callaghan F. Beyond core service. *Psychol Marketing*. 2003;20(3):187–208.
180. Silverman BC, Stern TW, Gross AF, Rosenstein DL, Stern TA. Lewd, crude, and rude behavior: the impact of manners and etiquette in the general hospital. *Psychosomatics*. 2012;53(1):13–20.
181. Walsh AL. Managing your practice's first impression: the process of front-desk reengineering. *J Med Pract Manage*. 2004;19(5):264–271.
182. Hills LS. Telephone techniques and etiquette: a medical practice staff training tool. *J Med Pract Manage*. 2007;23(3):166–170.
183. Bohren MA, Hunter EC, Munthe-Kaas HM, Souza JP, Vogel JP, Gülmezoglu AM. Facilitators and barriers to facility-based delivery in low-and middle-income countries: a qualitative evidence synthesis. *Reprod Health*. 2014;11(1):1–7. Cited by Bohren et al (see Note 187).
184. Chadwick RJ, Cooper D, Harries J. Narratives of distress about birth in South African public maternity settings: a qualitative study. *Midwifery*. 2014;30(7):862–868. Cited by Bohren et al (see Note 187).

185. D'Ambruoso L, Abbey M, Hussein J. Please understand when I cry out in pain: women's accounts of maternity services during labour and delivery in Ghana. *BMC Public Health.* 2005;5:140. Cited by Bohren et al (see Note 187).
186. Janevic T, Sripad P, Bradley E, Dimitrievska V. "There's no kind of respect here": a qualitative study of racism and access to maternal health care among Romani women in the Balkans. *Int J Equity Health.* 2011;10:53. Cited by Bohren et al (see Note 187).
187. Bohren MA, Vogel JP, Hunter EC, et al. The mistreatment of women during childbirth in health facilities globally: a mixed-methods systematic review. *PLOS Med.* 2015;12(6):e1001847.
188. Harris LC, Ogbonna E. Exploring service sabotage: the antecedents, types, and consequences of frontline, deviant, antiservice behaviors. *J Serv Res.* 2002;4(3):163–183.
189. Swahnberg K, Wijma B, Wingren G, Hilden M, Schei B. Women's perceived experiences of abuse in the health care system: their relationship to childhood abuse. *BJOG.* 2004;111(12):1429–1436.
190. Swahnberg K, Schei B, Hilden M, et al. Patients' experiences of abuse in health care: a Nordic study on prevalence and associated factors in gynecological patients. *Acta Obstet Gynecol Scand.* 2007;86(3):349–356.
191. Swahnberg K, Zbikowski A, Wijma B. Ethical lapses: staff's perception of abuse in health care. *J Psychosom Obstet Gynecol.* 2010;31(3):123–129.
192. Swahnberg K, Wijma B. Staff's perception of abuse in healthcare: a Swedish qualitative study. *BMJ Open.* 2012;2(5):e001111.
193. Swahnberg K, Hearn J, Wijma B. Prevalence of perceived experiences of emotional, physical, sexual, and health care abuse in a Swedish male patient sample. *Violence Vict.* 2009;24(2):265–279.
194. Swahnberg K, Thapar-Björkert S, Berterö C. Nullified: women's perceptions of being abused in health care. *J Psychosom Obstet Gynecol.* 2007;28(3):161–167.
195. Swahnberg K, Edholm S, Fredman K, Wijma B. Men's perceived experiences of abuse in health care: their relationship to childhood abuse. *Int J Mens Health.* 2012;11(2)
196. Swahnberg K, Wijma B, Hearn J, Thapar-Björkert S, Berterö C. Mentally pinioned: men's perceptions of being abused in health care. *Int J Mens Health.* 2009;8(1):60.
197. Swahnberg K, Davidsson-Simmons J, Hearn J, Wijma B. Men's experiences of emotional, physical, and sexual abuse and abuse in health care: a cross-sectional study of a Swedish random male population sample. *Scand J Public Health.* 2012;40(2):191–202.
198. Swahnberg IK, Wijma B. The NorVold Abuse Questionnaire (NorAQ): validation of new measures of emotional, physical, and sexual abuse, and abuse in the health care system among women. *Eur J Public Health.* 2003;13(4):361–366.
199. Mannava P, Durrant K, Fisher J, Chersich M, Luchters S. Attitudes and behaviours of maternal health care providers in interactions with clients: a systematic review. *Glob Health.* 2015;11(1):1–7.
200. Burgess AW. Physician sexual misconduct and patients' responses. *Am J Psychiatry.* 1981;138(10):1335–1342.
201. Shapiro ET, Morrow CK. Sex in the MD's office. *Hastings Cent Rep.* 1987;17(3):11–12.
202. Gartrell N, Herman J, Olarte S, Feldstein M, Localio R. Psychiatrist-patient sexual contact: results of a national survey. I: Prevalence. *Am J Psychiatry.* 1986;143(9):1126–1131.
203. Herman JL, Gartrell N, Olarte S, Feldstein M, Localio R. Psychiatrist-patient sexual contact: results of a national survey, II: Psychiatrists' attitudes. *Am J Psychiatry.* 1987;144(2):164–169.

204. Coverdale JH, Thomson AN, White GE. Social and sexual contact between general practitioners and patients in New Zealand: attitudes and prevalence. *Br J Gen Pract.* 1995;45(394):245–247.
205. Gallop R. Abuse of power in the nurse–client relationship. *Nurs Stand.* 1998;12(37):43.
206. Luepker ET. Effects of practitioners' sexual misconduct: a follow-up study. *J Am Acad Psychiatry Law Online.* 1999;27(1):51–63.
207. Zook R. Sexual misconduct by health care providers. *J Psychosoc Nurs Ment Health Serv.* 2001;39(6):40–47.
208. Campbell RJ, Yonge O, Austin W. Intimacy boundaries: between mental health nurses & psychiatric patients. *J Psychosoc Nurs Ment Health Serv.* 2016;43(5):32–39.
209. Elkin KJ, Spittal MJ, Elkin DJ, Studdert DM. Doctors disciplined for professional misconduct in Australia and New Zealand, 2000–2009. *Med J Aust.* 2011;194(9):452–456.
210. DuBois JM, Walsh HA, Chibnall JT, et al. Sexual violation of patients by physicians: a mixed-methods, exploratory analysis of 101 cases. *Sex Abuse.* 2019;31(5):503–523.
211. DuBois JM, Walsh HA, Chibnall JT, et al. Sexual violation of patients by physicians: a mixed-methods, exploratory analysis of 101 cases. *Sex Abuse.* 2019;31(5):503–523.
212. Bismark MM, Studdert DM, Morton K, Paterson R, Spittal MJ, Taouk Y. Sexual misconduct by health professionals in Australia, 2011–2016: a retrospective analysis of notifications to health regulators. *Med J Aust.* 2020;213(5):218–224.
213. Alam A, Klemensberg J, Griesman J, Bell CM. The characteristics of physicians disciplined by professional colleges in Canada. *Open Med.* 2011;5(4): e166–e172.
214. AbuDagga A, Wolfe SM, Carome M, Oshel RE. Cross-sectional analysis of the 1039 US physicians reported to the National Practitioner Data Bank for sexual misconduct, 2003–2013. *PLOS One.* 2016;11(2):e0147800.
215. Simon RI. The natural history of therapist sexual misconduct: identification and prevention. *Psychiatr Ann.* 1995;25(2):90–94. Cited by Simon (see Note 216).
216. Simon RI. Therapist–patient sex: from boundary violations to sexual misconduct. *Psychiatr Clin North Am.* 1999;22(1):31–47.
217. Brenner L, Meyll T, Stolper O, Walter A. Consumer fraud victimization and financial well-being. *J Econ Psychol.* 2020;76:102243.
218. Anderson KB. *Consumer Fraud in the United States, 2011: The Third FTC Survey.* Washington, DC: Federal Trade Commission; 2013. https://www.ftc.gov/sites/default/files/documents/reports/consumer-fraud-united-states-2011-third-ftc-survey/130419fraudsurvey_0.pdf. Accessed September 4, 2022.
219. Croall H. White collar crime, consumers and victimization. *Crime Law Soc Change.* 2009;51(1):127–146. https://hal.archives-ouvertes.fr/hal-00478394/document. Accessed September 4, 2022.
220. Lawrence F. *Not on the Label: What Really Goes into the Food on Your Plate.* London, England: Penguin Books; 2004. Cited by Croall.[219]
221. Which? Nutrition labelling. 2005. Cited by Croall.[219]
222. Clinard M, Yeager P. *Corporate Crime.* New York, NY: Free Press; 1980. Cited by Croall.[219]
223. Gillen PA, Sinclair M, Kernohan WG, Begley CM, Luyben AG. Interventions for prevention of bullying in the workplace. *Cochrane Database Syst Rev.* 2012;4.
224. Foley RJ. Consumer complaints soared in 2002. *Wall Street Journal.* 2003. Cited by Croall.[219]
225. Biswell K. Consumers and standards: increasing influence. *Consumer Policy Rev.* 2004;14(6):177–185. Cited by Croall.[219]

13
Victimization at Home

What Is Known?

This chapter examines the wide range of maltreatment that can occur in a home, afflicting any household[1,2] member, including a domestic employee.

Bullying among Siblings

Recognition of the occurrence of bullying among siblings and its association with peer victimization is growing, but this form of maltreatment is still largely unrecognized by professionals and society at large, where it is understood as "normal sibling rivalry." Clinical attention to this form of bullying needs to be considered within the larger picture of domestic victimization.

Since the initial study of bullying among siblings by Duncan[3] in 1999, a considerable number of studies[4,5,6-36] and reviews[12,37] have been published that exclusively[4-12,15-22,24,25,29-32,34-37] or partly[13,14,23,26-28,30,33] deal with this form of victimization.

Definition

The concept of bullying among siblings, as stated in the literature,[3-13,37] is based on the verbal, physical, and psychological types of victimization, which were first listed by Olweus[38] to define school bulling. Studies on the subject have also utilized other terms, such as *sibling aggression*, *sibling violence*, or *sibling abuse*, to describe aggressive sibling ineractions.[7,10,39] Wolke et al.[12] adapted the uniform definition of peer bullying[40] to define sibling bullying as:

> Any unwanted aggressive behavior(s) by a sibling that involves an observed or perceived power imbalance and is repeated multiple times or is highly likely to be repeated; bullying may inflict harm or distress on the targeted sibling, including physical, psychological, or social harm. It encompasses two modes of bullying (direct and indirect) as well as four types of bullying (physical, verbal, relational, and damage to property).[12]

The notion of sibling victimization was outlined by Tucker et al.[9] as being mistreated by a "juvenile sibling" and involving physical assault, with or without an object, or regardless of any ensuing injury; having a personal item forcibly taken away or stolen and never given back; having personal items broken or ruined purposely; or being made to feel "bad or scared" by being called names or being told mean things.[9]

Prevalence and Correlates

Tucker et al.[9] studied a nationally representative sample of more than 1,700 US children and adolescents and showed that almost 38% of the participants had been exposed to a type of sibling victimization in the previous year. The highest rates of victimization (45%) were experienced by children younger than 10 years old, with the frequency gradually diminishing through adolescence down to 28% among young people 14 to 17 years old. Physical aggression was found to be the most common form of maltreatment (32%), as compared to property damage or theft (5% to 6%) or psychological bullying (3%). Furthermore, sibling victimization was found to be "higher for males, whites, pre-adolescents, and those who were closer in age to their sibling."[9]

A survey[10] by Tippet and Wolke of more than 4,200 10- to 15-year-old adolescents living in the United Kingdom demonstrated that almost 45.8% of youths had been victims of sibling aggression, while 35.6% had been aggressive toward their siblings in the previous six months, with physical aggression, verbal maltreatment, and stealing being the most prevalent forms of victimization. The study[10] also showed a significant association between sibling victimization with having two or more siblings, being the eldest sibling, experiencing harsh parenting, living in poverty and/or with financial stress, and having poorer relationships with parents.

Being a victim of sibling aggression has been found[10] to be significantly associated with being a victim of school bullying [adjusted OR (AOR) = 1.69], while a more significant link has been established between perpetration of sibling aggression and being a bully toward peers [adjusted OR (AOR) = 2.63] or even further being involved in school bullying in the dual role of bully/victim [adjusted OR (AOR) = 3.44].

The prevalence of sibling bullying among children with and without autism spectrum disorder (ASD) was evaluated by Toseeb et al.[32] using data from a prospective population-based study comparing 475 11-year-old children with ASD and 13,702 age-matched children without ASD. The study showed that children with ASD were more likely to be bullied by their siblings [relative risk ratio (RRR) = 1.44 [0.98,3.13]] or to be both bully and victim (RRR = 1.49 [1.09,2.04]), as compared to children without ASD.

Sibling Bullying and Psychiatric Risks

As discussed in Chapter 4, Bowes et al.[8] showed that being bullied by a sibling is a risk factor for depression and self-harm in early adulthood. Their longitudinal study initially surveyed more than 6,900 12-year-old British children about sibling bullying and followed up 50% of them, at age 18, to ascertain depression, anxiety, and self-harm. Bowes et al. documented that children who reported being bullied by a sibling several times a week had twice the risk of depression and self-harm in young adulthood, as compared to those who were not bullied by their siblings, even after adjustment for confounding factors. Although a significant risk (OR = 1.83) was established for anxiety in young adulthood for children who were bullied by siblings, this association was weakened (OR = 1.51) after adjustment for individual and family characteristics.

Bar-Zomer and Brunstein Klomek[15] examined the moderating role of attachment on the association between sibling bullying and depression or suicidal ideation among 279 Israeli students age 10 to 17. Their study[15] showed that children and adolescents who participated in sibling bullying were 3.7 times more likely to experience clinical depression and 2.3 times more prone to suffer from suicidal ideation than children not involved in sibling bullying. Furthermore, Bar-Zomer and Brunstein Klomek found that a safe attachment to one's father (but not to one's mother) diminished the association between sibling bullying and depression/suicidal ideation. Yet, when suicidal ideation was assessed while excluding depression, attachment to one's father did not moderate the association between sibling bullying involvement and suicidal ideation, a finding indicating that depression plays a significant role in the association between sibling bullying and suicidal ideation.[15]

A study to ascertain the association between sibling bullying in middle childhood and psychotic disorder in early adulthood was conducted by Dantchev et al.,[31] based on the investigation of almost 4,000 participants from a UK community-based birth cohort, with sibling bullying being reported at 12 years and psychotic disorder being assessed at 18 years. The research showed that participants who were victimized by a sibling several times a week were almost three times at risk of experiencing psychotic disorder at 18 years (OR = 2.92), while those who bullied their siblings several times a week were almost 3.5 times at risk of developing a psychotic disorder (OR = 3.49). Another report,[34] based on the study by Dantchev et al.,[31] determined that frequent sibling bullying perpetration predicted antisocial behavior (OR = 1.74), while frequent sibling bullying victimization increased the risk of nicotine dependence (AOR = 2.87), even after adjustment for other forms of maltreatment.

An association between sibling bullying and psychotic-like experiences (i.e., magical thinking, delusional ideation, or hallucinatory experiences) was ascertained in a cross-sectional study by Liu et al.,[36] based on the investigation of more than 3,200 students from eight junior middle schools in three cities of Hunan Province, China.

Abuse among Siblings

Maltreatment among siblings has been examined under the concepts of abuse, violence, and victimization among siblings,[41-80] and several publications emphasized that this form of maltreatment is a far more common indication of family violence than is regularly recognized.[41-48,64,76] Some studies have focused their scope on distinct types of sibling abuse: physical,[9,60,73,74,78] sexual,[50,51,54,56,63,66] emotional/psychological,[9,28,60,68,73,74,78] and/or property related[9] abuse. Most aspects of what is defined as abuse among siblings have been dealt with in studies under the notion of bullying.

Physical Abuse or Violence among Siblings

The notion of physical abuse among siblings can be understood, based on a composite of previous definitions,[9,60,74,81,82] as an intentional violent physical act or behavior perpetrated by a juvenile sibling residing in the same household as the child or adolescent victim. These behaviors can include, but are not limited to, pinching, scratching, hair-pulling, shoving, kicking, slapping, hitting, biting, punching, or choking. They may or may not include the use of an instrument, such as a belt, broom handle, rubber hose, coat hunger, hairbrush, stick, bat, gun, rifle, broken glass, or knife, and may or may not result in injuries. A 2008 survey conducted by Tucker et al.[81] to establish the prevalence of sibling victimization in the United States documented that 32% of children and youth (ages 1 month to 17 years) from two-child families with a juvenile sibling in the home, had experienced physical assault perpetrated by the sibling in the previous year, while at least 4% were exposed to physical assault associated with a weapon or resulting in an injury.[81]

An examination by Krienert and Walsh[39] of more than 33,000 incidents of juvenile sibling violence reported to law enforcement agencies in the United States in the years 2000 to 2005 showed that 74% of the victims and 88% of the offenders were between 14 and 21 years old. Most of the offenders (73%) were males, while a majority (58%) of the victims were females.[39] The victim was younger than the offender in 61% of the incidents, while in 39% of the cases, the victim was of equal age or older than the perpetrator. The offender's hands or feet were used as a weapon in almost 70% of the incidents, while in 10% of the cases, guns, knives, and other objects were utilized. Minor injuries occurred in 52% of the assaults, while only 3% of the reported cases involved major injuries.[39]

Sibling Homicide

Sibling homicide has been examined by Peck and Heide[83] in a study based on national data from the US Uniform Crime Reports[84] pertaining to the arrests of youths (under age 18) for killing their siblings during the 32-year period from 1976 to 2007. During this period, 801 of the 44,147 juveniles arrested for homicide (1.8%) allegedly killed their siblings; 75% of the offenders were 14 years old or older, and 85% were males. Seventy percent of the juvenile siblicides were perpetrated against brothers, while the remaining 30% were committed against sisters, and most of the offenders were arrested in large cities. Most of the siblicides (63%) were committed with a gun, while 24% involved the use of a knife.

Sexual Abuse among Siblings

Sibling sexual abuse has been defined by Morill[85] as "sexual behavior between siblings that is not age appropriate, not transitory and not motivated by developmentally appropriate curiosity." This definition[85] includes as examples of sibling sexual abuse, "inappropriate fondling, touching, sexual contact, groping, indecent exposure, masturbation, exposure to pornography, oral sex, anal sex, digital penetration, and intercourse."[85] Normal common sexual behaviors in children 2 to 6 years old have been described as transient and responsive to parental distraction and redirection (e.g., touching/masturbating genitals in public/private, viewing/touching siblings' genitals, showing genitals to peers, standing or sitting too close, or trying to view peer/adult nudity).[85,86]

A study by Finkelhor,[87] based on the survey of almost 800 undergraduates at six New England colleges and universities, found that 15 females and 10 males reported a sibling sexual experience, and 40% reported they were less than 8 years old at the time of the experience, while 73% occurred when at least one of the partners was older than 8, and 35% occurred when one partner was older than 12. Because 23% of the occurrences took place between siblings who were 5 or more years apart in age, it raised the question of exploitation. Children 8 years old or younger were mostly involved in exhibiting, fondling, or touching genitals; while those age 9 or above were mostly engaged in fondling and touching, as in intercourse or attempted intercourse. Thirty percent of the activities happened only once, with no recurrence, but 27% of the episodes continued for over a year.[87]

Sibling incest has been reported to occur three to five times more frequently than parental incest,[41,88] yet its true prevalence remains unknown.[89] Krienert and Walsh[89] analyzed 13,013 incidents of sibling sexual abuse reported to law enforcement agencies in the United States during 2000 to 2007. Their study[89] documented that most of the victims were less than 13 years old, with a mean age of 8 years, and 71% of the victims were female. Among the offenders 92% were males with only 32% of them being 12 years or younger.[89] Eighty-four percent of the victims and offenders were white.[89] Most reported cases involved biologically related offenders and victims, yet 27% of the incidents involved step-siblings.[89] The victims were younger than the offenders in almost 95% of the incidents, and the age difference between victim and offender was 3 years or more in 82% of the incidents.[89] Forcible fondling was the most prevalent type of reported sibling sexual abuse (55%), followed by forcible rape (23%), forcible sodomy (17%), and sexual assault with an object (5%).[89] The majority of the incidents (89%) did not result in injuries.[89]

Psychological/Emotional Abuse among Siblings

Emotional abuse among siblings can be characterized as behaviors or attitudes (Table 13.1) perpetrated by one sibling against another and causing psychological distress. These behaviors have also been typified by recent studies as psychological or verbal bullying.

According to a 2008 survey conducted by Tucker et al.,[81] psychological victimization by siblings was reported by 2.7% of more than 1,500 participants 2 to 17 years old, with highest risk of victimization among those responders who were 2 to 5 years old (OR = 4.27) and 6 to 9 years old (OR = 3.32).[81]

Sibling Property Abuse

The notion of property victimization as a type of abuse among siblings was characterized by Tucker et al.[81] as either forcible theft/taking of a sibling's belongings or vandalism (breaking

Table 13.1. Examples of Sibling Psychological Abuse[58,68]

Being:		
Annoyed	Insulted	Scorned
Belittled	Intimidated	Shamed
Called names	Isolated	Teased
Frightened	Made fun of	Terrorized
Harassed	Provoked	Threatened
Humiliated	Rejected	Told lies about being adopted
Ignored	Ridiculed	Told mean things

or ruining a sibling's things on purpose). This form of victimization was found to be prevalent among 5% to 6% of juveniles surveyed by Tucker et al.[81] Forcible taking/theft of a sibling's belongings by another sibling was more prevalent among children age 2 to 5 (12.7%) than children age 6 to 9 (4.3%), while vandalism by siblings was more frequently experienced by children age 6 to 9 (10%) than by children age 2 to 5 (6.8%).[81]

Victimization among Parents

Definition

Victimization among parents encompasses all forms of physical, sexual, verbal, emotional, or relational abuse or maltreatment between a mother or father and their present or former married, common-law, or civil union spouse or domestic partner.

Studies exploring this key area of maltreatment can be found under the categories of domestic, marital, or spousal violence, aggression, or abuse, as well as intimate partner violence (IPV).

Flury et al.[90] provided examples of forms of domestic violence in a review of the subject that focused on Central European countries. In this study,[90] physical violence was understood as an intentional physical harm or threats to somebody's body, while sexual abuse was clinically understood as any form of unwanted sexual activity. Psychological or emotional violence was exemplified by negative verbal communication leading to outrage, offenses, humiliation, or exhaustion, as well as by exercising control of the other partner through social isolation, banning social contacts, confiscation of money, and forbidding or forcing the person to work.[90]

Prevalence and Correlates

A World Health Organization (WHO) study[91] of global and regional estimates of violence against women, based on data extracted from 79 countries and two territories, indicates that the global lifetime prevalence of IPV among ever-partnered women is 30%. This prevalence gradually rises from 29.4%, for women 15 to 19 years old, to its peak of 37.8% in the group 40 to 44 years old, and then gradually declines to 22.2% by age 65 to 69.[91]

There is a wide regional variation in the prevalence of ever-partnered women having experienced IPV, ranging from 65.6% in central sub-Saharan Africa, to the lowest prevalence, 16.3%, in East Asia.[91]

A survey[92] of almost 1,500 US women attending a family planning clinic in Iowa showed that women in urban areas and large rural towns reported the lowest prevalence (14% to 16%) of IPV, whereas women in small rural towns reported the highest prevalence (22.5%).[92]

The limited number of published studies[93-96] on female-to-male IPV includes a report by Mills et al.[96] documenting that among 282 heterosexual men surveyed in an emergency department, 29.3% had a positive history of IPV. In a study[97] based on a survey of 972 Swedish adults, all forms of IPV occurring in the previous year had similar prevalence in women and men. All forms of IPV were linked to limited social support, growing up with domestic violence, and being single, widowed, or divorced.

According to data from the National Crime Victimization Survey,[98] during the decade from 2003 to 2012, IPV accounted for 14.6% of all violent victimization in the United States, with current or former boyfriends/girlfriends representing the most frequent perpetrators (7.8%), followed by spouses (4.7%) and former spouses (2%). Females had a higher rate (6.2/1,000) of IPV than males (1.4/1,000), and individuals age 18 to 24 had the highest rate (8.7%) of IPV. Almost one in two incidents resulted in injuries, with 11% of them being serious, and 43% of incidents led to bruises or cuts. Almost 34% of the episodes required injury treatment, with half of them needing medical attention.

Spouse Abuse and Health Risks

Perinatal Risks

A WHO study led by Pallitto et al.,[99] based on a survey of more than 17,000 women in 10 countries, demonstrated that IPV is linked with significantly increased risk of unintended pregnancy (AOR = 1.69) and abortion (AOR = 2.68).[99]

Pavev et al.[100] conducted a study linking hospital records for infants born in the military health system in 2006–2007 to Family Advocacy Program-substantiated cases of IPV among military parents. The research showed that infants of mothers exposed to IPV were at higher risk for low birth weight (AOR = 1.52).[100]

Depression and Suicide

Devries et al.[101] conducted a systematic review of longitudinal studies intended to determine the extent to which IPV, in both men and women, was associated with incident depression and suicide attempts. The 16 studies they reviewed were published before 2013, and the authors noted the limitation of their review, which was based on studies that lacked an adjustment for common risk factors. Their analysis indicated that, among women, exposure to IPV intensified the risk of depressive symptoms and of suicide attempts, while at the same time depressive symptoms can increase the odds of IPV. Among men, there was some indication of a link between IPV and depressive symptoms, but no evidence of "an association between IPV and incident suicide attempts, or between depressive symptoms and incident IPV."[101]

Injuries

Fanslow and Robinson[102] conducted a survey of 2,855 adult New Zealand women to ascertain the degree of injuries resulting from IPV. Their study showed that 50% the women who experienced physical and/or sexual IPV in their lifetime were injured at least once as result of the violence. Among those who were injured by IPV, the most common injuries were abrasions or bruises, followed by cuts, punctures, bites, and injuries to eyes or ears. It is important to underline that approximately 14% of the women received care as needed on all occasions, but only half of them reported the reason for the injury to the health professional.[102]

Intimate Partner Homicide

Belfrage and Rying[103] investigated all cases of spouse homicide in Sweden between 1990 and 1999 (N = 164), using as a control all other cases of homicide (non-spouse violence) occurring in Sweden during the same period (N = 690). Their study[103] showed that the suicide rate among spousal homicide perpetrators (24%) was significantly higher than the suicide rate among perpetrators in the control group (4%). Almost 80% of the spousal homicide perpetrators received a forensic psychiatric examination, and almost all of them received one psychiatric diagnosis, while 34% were sentenced to forensic psychiatric treatment.

An examination of fatal violence among marriage partners in the United States during the decade of 1976-85 was conducted by Mercy and Saltzman[104] using data from the Federal Bureau of Investigation's Supplemental Homicide Reports. The investigation identified 16,595 spousal homicides, representing 8.8% of all homicides reported during that period, at a rate of 1.6 per 100,000 married persons.[104]

Maltreatment of Parents by Their Children

Maltreatment of parents by their children is an area of family or domestic abuse that has remained marginally studied[105-112] in comparison to the extensive research on child maltreatment.[113] The concept has been investigated and reported using varied terminology: "battered parents,"[105] "violence toward parents,"[106] "parent abuse,"[107,108,110] "child–parent violence,"[109,111] and "aggression to parents."[112]

Definition

The concept of maltreatment of parents by their children as understood in this chapter can be defined, based on an adapted description of "parent abuse,"[106,107] as any physical, verbal, relational, or psychological action or behavior of a child or adolescent that affects a parent with physical and/or emotional harm by being injured, threatened, intimidated, humiliated, manipulated, or controlled.

The notion of violence toward parents or parent abuse has been defined as "any act perpetrated by a child or adolescent that causes a parent to feel threatened, intimated, and controlled."[107,108] It includes physical abuse (e.g., hitting, spitting, punching holes in the walls, and throwing or breaking things), psychological victimization (e.g., intimidation or instilling fear), emotional maltreatment (e.g., making manipulative threats or making unrealistic demands), and financial mistreatment (e.g., stealing parents' money or belongings, destroying the home or the parents' belongings, incurring debts the parents must cover, or demanding that the parents buy certain things).[108,114]

Prevalence and Correlates

No published studies on prevalence of abuse toward parents by children or adolescents could be found at this time. Different studies have estimated that the rate of parental abuse ranges from 7% in two-parent families[115] to 29% in one-parent families.[116]

A review of research on adolescent-initiated parental abuse conducted by Hong et al.[110] underscored that this type of maltreatment is more often perpetrated by adolescents than by younger children; that males are more prone to assault parents than females; that assault of mothers is more likely to occur among white youth, while no racial differences have been reported for father abuse; and that "mothers are more likely to be abused than fathers."[110]

Walsh and Ktienert[117] examined data for almost 18,000 incidents of violence against parents reported to police agencies in the United States during 2002 and involving children and adolescents age 21 or younger. The research showed that 80% of the reports pertained to simple assaults of parents (the offender did not display a weapon and the victim did not suffer severe or aggravated bodily injuries), 12% of the incidents involved aggravated assault (the offender used a weapon or displayed it in a threatening manner, or the victim suffered severe injuries), and 8% of the cases involved parental intimidation.[117] Males accounted for 63% of the offenders, while 70% of the victims were mothers, with biological mothers the most common target (90.5%).[117] Most victims (45%) were 41 to 50 years old, and most offenders (60%) were 14 to 17 years old.[117] Major injuries (e.g., broken bones, loss of teeth, possible internal injury, severe laceration, or loss of consiousness[118]) occurred in 12% of aggravated assaults.[117]

No published studies have been found documenting emotional health risks affecting parents who are maltreated by their children.

Parricide

The magnitude and characteristics of incidents of killing of their parent(s) (parricide) by youth were examined by Walsh et al.[119] in a study based on almost 2,600 cases reported in the United States from 1976 to 2003, involving offenders 21 years old or younger. The research showed that males were more frequently perpetrators of parricide, exceeding females almost 7 to 1, with males being more prevalent among those 18 to 21 years old and females peaking in the 14- to 17-year-old group.[119] Most of parricide victims (75%) were fathers (patricide), and almost 80% of all victims were 31 to 50 years old.[119] Guns were the predominant weapon of choice for male offenders (67%) as well as females (60%), while a knife was used by more females (33%) than males (20%).[119]

Buyuk et al.[120] conducted a medico-legal evaluation of 39 Turkish adolescent (age 18 or younger) parricide offenders based on a retrospective analysis of forensic records of cases that occurred between 1994 and 2005. Almost 80% of the offenders were males, with a mean age of 15 years.[120] Biological fathers made up 69% of the victims. Weapons used were mostly firearms (54%) and cutting devices (26%), and 5% of offenders applied strangulation.[120] There was a history of physical abuse in 46% of the cases and sexual abuse in almost 8% of the incidents.[120] There was no psychiatric history found for almost 90% of the offenders, while schizophrenia and psychotic disorder (otherwise unclassified) were diagnosed in 10% of the perpetrators.[120]

Elder Abuse by Adult Offspring Living in the Same Household

According to a UN report on living arrangements of older persons[121] as of 2017, a global average of 55% of people age 60 or over resided in a household with their children, with estimates ranging from a low of 5.5% in the Netherlands to a high of 94.8% in Afghanistan.[121] More than half of older persons co-resided with their children in 93% of countries or areas in Asia, 77% in Latin America and the Caribbean, and 73% in Africa.

Pillemer and Finkelhor[122] investigated the prevalence and nature of maltreatment of the elderly based on a stratified random sample of 2,020 community-dwelling elderly persons (65 years or older) in the Boston metropolitan area. They found that 4.4% of the participants who lived with their children were exposed to diverse types of maltreatment, with 2.5% being physically abused, 1.8% being verbally mistreated, and 0.4% neglected. There were no significant differences in the rates of abuse in relation to race or age of the victims nor in relation to their religion and educational or economic background.[122]

Maltreatment of Custodial Grandparents by Their Grandchildren

Households where a grandparent is co-residing with grandchildren and none of the parents of the grandchildren is present, known as a skip-generation households, account, in most countries, for less than 5% of all family units.[123] Yet, skip-generation households are common in sub-Saharan Africa, the Caribbean, and Central America.[124]

In the more than 45 years since the problem of elder abuse was highlighted by the article titled "Granny Battering,"[125] there have been no studies conducted to ascertain the prevalence and correlates of victimization of custodial grandparents by their grandchildren, a form of maltreatment that has been characterized as a hidden phenomenon.[126] Nevertheless, some studies[126-128] have attempted to illustrate custodial grandparents' vulnerability to different forms of abuse through narratives that hint at maltreatment by custodial grandchildren, yet the episodes of abuse were not recognized as such by the grandparents and/or were not reported.

Child Abuse or Maltreatment

Child abuse has been the most studied[113] aspect of victimization at home since the public health relevance of maltreatment was brought to light with the landmark publication on the battered child syndrome.[129] The notion of child maltreatment has evolved in the last 60 years from its initial recognition as physical abuse[130] to encompass neglect as well as sexual and psychological abuse. This chapter also considers violent discipline as a form of mistreatment.

Definitions

Child Maltreatment

WHO defines child maltreatment as:

> the abuse and neglect that occurs to children under 18 years of age. It includes all types of physical and/or emotional ill-treatment, sexual abuse, neglect, negligence, and commercial or other exploitation, which results in actual or potential harm to the child's health, survival, development, or dignity in the context of a relationship of responsibility, trust, or power.[131]

In the United States, each jurisdiction (state, territory, or District of Columbia) has its own definition of child abuse and neglect, based on criteria established by the Child Abuse

Prevention and Treatment Act (CAPTA),[132] which characterizes child abuse and neglect, at a minimum, as "any recent act or failure to act on the part of a parent or caretaker which results in death, serious physical or emotional harm, sexual abuse or exploitation; or an act or failure to act, which presents an imminent risk of serious harm."[132] Amendments to CAPTA require that the definition of child abuse and neglect include sex trafficking victims, as well as that the states report "the infants identified by healthcare providers as being affected by substance abuse or withdrawal symptoms resulting from prenatal drug exposure, or [by] a fetal alcohol spectrum disorder."[132]

Physical Abuse

According to WHO, "physical abuse of a child is that which results in actual or potential physical harm from an interaction or lack of an interaction, which is reasonably within the control of a parent or person in a position of responsibility, power, or trust. There may be single or repeated incidents."[133]

Child Neglect

Child neglect has been defined as:

> the failure to provide for the development of the child in all spheres: health, education, emotional development, nutrition, shelter, and safe living conditions, in the context of resources reasonably available to the family or caretakers and causes or has a high probability of causing harm to the child's health or physical, mental, spiritual, moral,or social development. This includes the failure to properly supervise and protect children from harm as much as is feasible.[133]

Sexual Abuse

WHO describes child sexual abuse as

> the involvement of a child in sexual activity that he or she does not fully comprehend, is unable to give informed consent to, or for which the child is not developmentally prepared and cannot give consent, or that violates the laws or social taboos of society. Child sexual abuse is evidenced by this activity between a child and an adult or another child who by age or development is in a relationship of responsibility, trust, or power, the activity being intended to gratify or satisfy the needs of the other person. This may include, but is not limited to, inducement or coercion of a child to engage in any unlawful sexual activity; exploitative use of a child in prostitution or other unlawful sexual practices; exploitative use of children in pornographic performances and materials.[133]

Emotional Abuse

Child emotional abuse has been characterized as:

> the failure to provide a developmentally appropriate, supportive environment, including the availability of a primary attachment figure, so that the child can develop a stable and full range of emotional and social competencies commensurate with her or his personal potentials and in the context of the society in which the child dwells. There may also be acts toward the child that cause or have a high probability of causing harm to the child's health

or physical, mental, spiritual, moral, or social development. These acts must be reasonably within the control of the parent or person in a relationship of responsibility, trust, or power. Acts include restriction of movement, patterns of belittling, denigrating, scapegoating, threatening, scaring, discriminating, ridiculing or other non-physical forms of hostile or rejecting treatment.[133]

Violent Discipline

A recent UNICEF report on violence in the lives of children and adolescents[134] has defined violent discipline as any physical punishment or psychological aggression. In this context, physical punishment is explained as "shaking, hitting, or slapping a child on the hand/arm/leg, hitting on the bottom or elsewhere on the body with a hard object, spanking or hitting on the bottom with a bare hand, hitting or slapping on the face, head, or ears, and hitting or beating hard and repeatedly.[134] Severe physical punishment is characterized as "hitting or slapping a child on the face, head or ears, and hitting or beating a child hard and repeatedly."[134]

Psychological aggression is defined as "shouting, yelling, or screaming at a child, as well as calling a child offensive names, such as 'dumb' or 'lazy.' "[134]

Prevalence and Correlates

Maltreatment

From 2001 through 2015, Stoltenborgh et al. published[135-139] a series of meta-analyses, based on hundreds of studies, aiming to ascertain the global prevalence of sexual abuse,[135] emotional abuse,[136] neglect,[137] and physical abuse.[138] Across countries, sexual abuse was found to be self-reported by 127 per 1,000 children, with higher rates for females (180/1,000) than males (76/1,000).[135] Furthermore, the global prevalence, based on self-reports, of emotional abuse was 363/1,000[136]; physical neglect, 163/1,000[137]; emotional neglect, 184/1,000[138]; and physical abuse, 226/1,000.[139]

According to the US Child Maltreatment Report,[132] during 2019, 59.5 children and adolescents per 1,000 population were referred to Child Protective Services (CPS) for possible exposure to maltreatment. Subsequently, 80% of these referrals (47.2 children and adolescents per 1,000 population) received either an investigation[140] or an alternative response[141] from the local CPS. During that year, there were approximately 656,000 US children and adolescents for whom their state determined at least one maltreatment was substantiated or indicated. This equates to 8.9 victims of maltreatment per 1,000 children in the population.[132]

More than a quarter (28%) of the victims were 2 years old or younger, with 15% of all victims being less than 1 year old. The rate of victimization for females (9.4/1,000) was higher than for males (8.4/1,000).[132] "American-Indian or Alaska Native children had the highest rate of victimization, at 14.8 per 1,000 children in the population of the same race or ethnicity, while African American children had the second highest rate, at 13.8 per 1,000 children in the population of the same race or ethnicity."[132] Seventy-five percent of the victims were neglected, 18% were physically abused, and 9% were sexually victimized, with 15% of the victims experiencing two or more types of maltreatment.[132]

Risk factors among caregivers that may increase the likelihood of child maltreatment were found to be drug abuse (29%), domestic violence (29%), and having public assistance support (27%). Almost 40% of the victims were maltreated by their mothers acting alone, 23% were victimized by their fathers acting alone, and 21% were abused by both parents,[132] while 14% of victims were maltreated by a perpetrator who was not a parent (e.g., a relative, an unmarried partner of parent, an unrelated adult or child, a foster sibling, a babysitter, or household staff). Most of the perpetrators (83%) were 18 to 44 years old, and 53% were female.[132]

Challenges caused by the COVID-19 pandemic that influenced child maltreatment included job loss, income reduction, and parenting problems. These factors were investigated by Wong et al.[142] through a cross-sectional online survey of 600 randomly sampled parents, age 18 or older, who had lived with a child 10 years old or younger in Hong Kong between May 29 and June 16, 2020. Wong et al.[142] showed that income reduction was significantly associated with severe physical assault[143] (OR = 3.29) and very severe physical assaults[143] (OR = 7.69) against children. Job loss was also significantly associated with severe physical assaults[143] (OR = 3.68) and very severe physical assaults[144] (OR = 4.05) against children.[142]

Child Fatalities Linked to Abuse and Neglect

During the Federal Fiscal Year[145] of 2019, 2.5 per 100,000 children in the United States died from abuse and neglect, with "boys having a higher rate of child fatality (2.98/100,000 in the population) than girls (2.2/100,000 in the population)."[146] Of the children who died, 70% were less than 3 years old, with almost 50% of them being less than a year old, and they died at a rate of 22.94 per 100,000 population of infants, representing 3.3 times the mortality rate for children less than 1 year old (6.87 per 100,000 infants).[146]

Prevalence of Violent Discipline

The UNICEF report on violence in the lives of children and adolescents[134] documented that, worldwide, 75% of children age 2 to 4 years suffer from violent discipline by their caregivers on a regular basis, while 60% of children age 12 to 23 months are punished by physical means. Furthermore, the UNICEF report[134] indicates that almost 50% of 1-year-old children in 29 countries are exposed to shouting, yelling, or screaming as a form of discipline, while 30% are subjected to spanking.[134] "In most of the countries with data, children from wealthier households are equally likely to experience violent discipline as those from poorer households."[134]

Predictors of Physical Punishment

The use of physical punishment to deal with parent–child conflict has been related to parental cognition, affect, and history of physical punishment in childhood.[147] It has been documented that parental agreement with, or approval of, physical punishment is associated with its use.[148] Parents who think that children's misbehavior is "intentional and controllable"[147] are more likely to react with punishment,[149] and mothers who are angry or irritable when a conflict occurs are more likely to spank than a parent who is in a neutral or positive mood.[150] Furthermore, one's experience of physical punishment in childhood has been found to be associated with one's use of corporal punishment in adulthood.[151]

Wong et al.[142] documented, in their study about the impact of COVID-19 on child maltreatment, that parental confidence in discussing with their children issues related to COVID-19 and in implementing their children's health practices was significantly associated with less corporal punishment.[142]

Effects of Corporal Punishment

There is always the risk of injury in the use of physical punishment.[152] A review of physical abuse cases that occurred in Canada in 2003 showed that 75% of the incidents were intended by the parents to be corporal punishment.[153]

Cuartas et al.[154] conducted a study to examine whether 40 children (M_{age} = 11.60) who had been spanked a few or more times, but never physically or sexually abused, exhibited altered neural function in response to stimuli that suggested the presence of an environmental threat, as compared to 107 children who were never spanked, as well as 20 children with a history of physical and sexual abuse. The research documented that the children with a history of being spanked a few times or more frequently demonstrated, on functional magnetic resonance imaging (fMRI), greater activation in multiple regions of the medial and lateral prefrontal cortex when exposed to fearful relative to neutral faces, as compared to children who were never spanked. Yet, children who were spanked showed the same pattern of brain activation to fearful relative to neutral faces as children with history of abuse, suggesting that "spanking may alter neural responses to environmental threats in a manner similar to more severe forms of maltreatment."[154]

Liu and Wang[155] investigated the moderating role of HPA axis activity in the relationship between corporal punishment and child anxiety, through a cross-sectional study of 158 Chinese school-age children. The research[155] documented that corporal punishment was positively associated with child anxiety. Low morning basal cortisol exacerbated the relations between paternal corporal punishment and child anxiety, and flatter diurnal rhythm exacerbated the relations between both paternal and maternal corporal punishment and child anxiety.

The effects of corporal punishment on Chinese preschoolers' executive function and the moderating effects of cortisol stress reactivity were ascertained by Xing et al.[156] in a longitudinal study involving 152 Chinese preschoolers. The research demonstrated that both maternal and paternal corporal punishment were negatively correlated with children's executive functioning one year later.[156] Furthermore, children with low cortisol stress reactivity levels who experienced maternal corporal punishment in the previous year showed poorer global executive functioning and working memory than children with high cortisol stress reactivity.[156]

The association between corporal punishment and restricted development of cognitive ability was explored by Straus and Paschall[157] in a four-year longitudinal study of 806 children age 2 to 4 and 704 children age 5 to 9. Their results[157] demonstrated that, in both cohorts, children of mothers who used minimal or no corporal punishment at the start of the study gained cognitive ability faster, four years later, than those who were spanked.

It should be noted that a controversy about the significance of the association between corporal punishment and negative long-term outcomes has been underscored by meta-analyses of published research by Paolucci and Violato[158] in 2003, and by Ferguson[159] in 2013; both analyses indicated that corporal punishment has minimal behavioral, emotional, and cognitive effects.[158,159] Yet, on the other side of the controversy, in 2016, Gershoff and Grogan Kaylor[160] focused specifically on spanking and conducted a meta-analysis of a total of 111 unique effect sizes representing almost 161,000 children. Gershoff and Grogan Kaylor[160] found 13 of 17 mean effect sizes were significantly different from zero, indicating an association between spanking and increased risk for harmful child consequences, including low moral internalization, aggression, antisocial behavior, externalizing behavior problems, internalizing behavior problems, mental health problems, negative parent–child relationships, impaired cognitive ability, low self-esteem, and risk of physical abuse from parents.[160]

Maltreatment of Domestic Workers

It would be remiss not to consider a domestic worker as a member of a household who could potentially be exposed to domestic maltreatment.

A domestic worker is identified as any person involved, on a regular occupational basis, in work performed in, or for, a household or households.[161] At least 52.6 million men and women are employed as domestic workers across the world, and most (83%) are women.[162] These estimates "do not include children who have not yet reached working age, which in many countries is set at 15 or 16 years."[162] "There are an estimated 3.5 million children aged 5 to 11 years who work as domestic workers, and 3.8 million child domestic workers between the ages of 12 and 14 years."[162] Domestic work is strongly connected with international migration, because domestic workers not only look for work in their home countries, but also often move to other countries in search of better employment opportunities.[162]

Domestic workers are potentially exposed to victimization risks that are inherent in their dual role as employees and household members, which may subject them to workplace and/or domestic maltreatment.

Adverse Working Conditions Affecting Domestic Workers

Overwork

The International Labour Organization's Domestic Workers Convention of 2011, Chapter 10,[163] requires that each member state take measures to ensure

> equal treatment between domestic workers and workers generally in relation to normal hours of work, overtime compensation, periods of daily and weekly rest and paid annual leave in accordance with national laws, regulations, or collective agreements, taking into account the special characteristics of domestic work.[163]

It also requires that "rest should be at least 24 consecutive hours."[163]

Long working hours are especially common among live-in domestic workers, who usually work on a full-time basis but are frequently required to be always available.[164] It is noteworthy that almost 45% of domestic workers worldwide, most of them living in Asia and the Middle East, are not entitled to any weekly rest.[162]

Being Undervalued

According to a 2020 Economic Policy Institute report developed by Wolfe et al.,[165] domestic workers in the United States are paid, on average, just 74 cents for every dollar that their peers make, even when compared with demographically similar workers.[165] Also, US domestic workers are three times as likely to be living in poverty as other workers, and only one in five receives health insurance coverage through their job.[165] Worldwide, almost 36% of all domestic workers are not entitled to parental leave under national law, and this situation is more prevalent in the Middle East, Asia, and the Pacific.[165]

Failure to Receive Payment of Wages

Delayed payment or nonpayment of wages as an adverse work condition affecting foreign domestic workers has been noted by several Human Rights Watch reports.[166-168]

Other Adverse Circumstances

Malhotra et al.[169] conducted a systematic review of the scientific and gray literature to ascertain health issues among foreign domestic workers. The review identified as commonly perceived health risks: substandard sleeping accommodations, with lack of privacy or having their own room[166,170]; food deprivation (requiring permission to eat, being fed only once a day, or receiving inadequate food)[166,170]; denial of medical treatment[177]; confiscation of passport[170]; and restrictions of freedom of movement[170] or on communications with their family.[170]

Abuse and Harassment of Domestic Workers

In the last decade, many studies[166-192] have addressed domestic workers' risk of abuse or harassment, as well as the health correlates[171] associated with their maltreatment. There are at least nine published reports[166,167,174,178,180,189-192] documenting the extent of exposure to several types of abuse suffered by domestic workers, mostly migrants, in 10 countries (Table 13.2). All the surveys reflect a wide range of exposure to physical abuse experienced by domestic workers, ranging from as low as 2%[189] to 45%,[167] exposure to sexual abuse varies from 1%[189] to 17%,[178] and verbal/psychological maltreatment extends from 12%[187] to 88%[190] (Table 13.2).

A cross-sectional study by Bauleo et al.,[171] based on a survey of 201 domestic workers in Argentina, showed that 19% of them were exposed to physical or workplace violence, which was significantly associated with poor or fair self-reported general health (AOR = 7.3) as well as with symptoms of common mental disorders (AOR = 3.2).[171]

Future Directions

There is a need to foster, develop, and implement research efforts to enhance knowledge about the global prevalence, antecedents, correlates, and health consequences of:

- Bullying and other forms of mistreatment among siblings
- Victimization among parents
- Maltreatment of parents or custodial grandparents by their children or grandchildren
- Children's exposure to emotional abuse and violent discipline by their parents or custodians
- Victimization of domestic employees

Table 13.2. Frequency of Abuse Experienced by Domestic Workers in 10 Different Countries

Study/Report	Country	Sample Size	Physical abuse	Sexual abuse	Psychological/ Verbal Abuse
Hanley et al[189]	Canada	150	2%	1%	12%
Human Rights Watch[166]	Singapore	65	20%	9%	51%
Wong[190]	Singapore	58	24%	7%	88%
Human Rights Watch[167]	Kuwait	49	45%	14%	No frequency available
Human Rights Watch[191]	Saudi Arabia, Kuwait, Lebanon, United Arab Emirates	100	20%	13%	No frequency available
Human Rights Watch[192]	Malaysia	51	18%	14%	35%
Figueiredo et al[174]	Portugal	684	9.5%	No frequency available	46%
Ullah[178]	Hong Kong	215	18%	17%	19%
Cheung et al[180]	Hong Kong	105	20.5%	No frequency available	34%

Furthermore, future research should ascertain the frequency of co-occurrence of the distinct types of domestic maltreatment and their cumulative effect, as well as their association with different forms of victimization in other social settings, such as in school and the workplace.

Notes

1. United States Census Bureau, definition of household:

   > A household consists of all the people who occupy a housing unit. A house, an apartment or other group of rooms, or a single room is regarded as a housing unit when it is occupied or intended for occupancy as separate living quarters; that is, when the occupants do not live and eat with any other persons in the structure and there is direct access from the outside or through a common hall.

   https://www.census.gov/programs-surveys/cps/technical-documentation/subject-definitions.html#household. Accessed August 25, 2022.
2. "A household is defined as a group of persons who make common provision of food, shelter and other essentials for living." United Nations, Department of Economic and Social Affairs, Statistics Division. *Principles and Recommendations for Population and Housing Censuses,*

Revision 3. New York, NY: United Nations; 2017. ST/ESA/STAT/SER.M/67/Rev.3. Cited by United Nations, Department of Economic and Social Affairs, Population Division, 2019 (see Note 123).

3. Duncan RD. Peer and sibling aggression: an investigation of intra-and extra-familial bullying. *J Interpers Violence*. 1999;14(8):871–886.
4. Wolke D, Samara MM. Bullied by siblings: association with peer victimisation and behaviour problems in Israeli lower secondary school children. *J Child Psychol Psychiatry*. 2004;45(5):1015–1029.
5. Menesini E, Camodeca M, Nocentini A. Bullying among siblings: the role of personality and relational variables. *Br J Dev Psychol*. 2010;28(4):921–939.
6. Skinner JA, Kowalski RM. Profiles of sibling bullying. *J Interpers Violence*. 2013;28(8):1726–1736.
7. Tucker CJ, Finkelhor D, Turner H, Shattuck A. Association of sibling aggression with child and adolescent mental health. *Pediatrics*. 2013;132(1):79–84.
8. Bowes L, Wolke D, Joinson C, Lereya ST, Lewis G. Sibling bullying and risk of depression, anxiety, and self-harm: a prospective cohort study. *Pediatrics*. 2014;134(4):e1032–e1039.
9. Tucker CJ, Finkelhor D, Shattuck AM, Turner H. Prevalence and correlates of sibling victimization types. *Child Abuse Negl*. 2013;37(4):213–223.
10. Tippett N, Wolke D. Aggression between siblings: associations with the home environment and peer bullying. *Aggress Behav*. 2015;41(1):14–24.
11. Tanrikulu I, Campbell MA. Sibling bullying perpetration: associations with gender, grade, peer perpetration, trait anger, and moral disengagement. *J Interpers Violence*. 2015;30(6):1010–1024.
12. Wolke D, Tippett N, Dantchev S. Bullying in the family: sibling bullying. *Lancet Psychiatry*. 2015;2(10):917–929.
13. Coyle S, Demaray MK, Malecki CK, Tennant JE, Klossing J. The associations among sibling and peer-bullying, social support, and internalizing behaviors. *Child Youth Care Forum*. 2017;1–28.
14. Foody M, Samara M, O'Higgins Norman J. Bullying by siblings and peers: poly-setting victimization and the association with problem behaviours and depression. *Br J Educ Psychol*. 2020;90:138–157.
15. Bar-Zomer J, Brunstein Klomek A. Attachment to parents as a moderator in the association between sibling bullying and depression or suicidal ideation among children and adolescents. *Front Psychiatry*. 2018;9:72.
16. Ensor R, Marks A, Jacobs L, Hughes C. Trajectories of antisocial behaviour towards siblings predict antisocial behaviour towards peers. *J Child Psychol Psychiatry*. 2010;51(11):1208–1216.
17. Espelage DL, Low S, Rao MA, Hong JS, Little TD. Family violence, bullying, fighting, and substance use among adolescents: a longitudinal mediational model. *J Res Adolescence*. 2014;24(2):337–349.
18. Bouchard G, Plamondon A, Lachance-Grzela M. Parental intervention style and adult sibling conflicts: the mediating role of involvement in sibling bullying. *J Soc Pers Relat*. 2019;36(8):2585–2602.
19. Toseeb U, McChesney G, Dantchev S, Wolke D. Precursors of sibling bullying in middle childhood: evidence from a UK-based longitudinal cohort study. *Child Abuse Negl*. 2020;108:104633.

20. Toseeb U, McChesney G, Oldfield J, Wolke D. Sibling bullying in middle childhood is associated with psychosocial difficulties in early adolescence: the case of individuals with autism spectrum disorder. *J Autism Dev Disord.* 2020;50(5):1457–1469.
21. Dantchev S, Wolke D. Trouble in the nest: antecedents of sibling bullying victimization and perpetration. *Dev Psychol.* 2019;55(5):1059.
22. Plamondon A, Bouchard G, Lachance-Grzela M. Family dynamics and young adults' well-being: the mediating role of sibling bullying. *J Interpers Violence.* 2018:0886260518800313.
23. Morrill M, Bachman C, Polisuk B, Kostelyk K, Wilson S. An exploration of the relationship between experiences with sibling abuse and peer bullying: a pilot study. *J Child Adolesc Trauma.* 2018;11(1):113–120.
24. Naylor PB, Petch L, Williams JV. Sibling abuse and bullying in childhood and adolescence: knowns and unknowns. In: Barter, Christine, and David Berridge, eds. *Children Behaving Badly: Peer Violence between Children and Young People.* West Sussex, UK: John Wiley & Sons; 2011;31:47.
25. Taylor CB, Bryson S, Doyle AA, et al. The adverse effect of negative comments about weight and shape from family and siblings on women at high risk for eating disorders. *Pediatrics.* 2006;118(2):731–738.
26. Little L. Middle-class mothers' perceptions of peer and sibling victimization among children with Asperger's syndrome and nonverbal learning disorders. *Issues Compr Pediatr Nurs.* 2002;25(1):43–57.
27. Finkelhor D, Turner H, Ormrod R, Hamby SL. Trends in childhood violence and abuse exposure: evidence from 2 national surveys. *Arch Pediatrics Adolesc Med.* 2010;164(3):238–242.
28. Tucker CJ, Finkelhor D, Turner H, Shattuck AM. Sibling and peer victimization in childhood and adolescence. *Child Abuse Negl.* 2014;38(10):1599–1606.
29. Arseneault L. Sibling bullying is associated with anxiety, depression, and self-harm. *Evid-based Ment Health.* 2015;18(3):83.
30. Kim J, Kim E. Bullied by siblings and peers: the role of rejecting/neglecting parenting and friendship quality among Korean children. *J Interpers Violence.* 2019;34(11):2203–2226.
31. Dantchev S, Zammit S, Wolke D. Sibling bullying in middle childhood and psychotic disorder at 18 years: a prospective cohort study. *Psychol Med.* 2018;48(14):2321–2328.
32. Toseeb U, McChesney G, Wolke D. The prevalence and psychopathological correlates of sibling bullying in children with and without autism spectrum disorder. *J Autism Dev Disord.* 2018;48(7):2308–2318.
33. Dantchev S, Hickman M, Heron J, Zammit S, Wolke D. The independent and cumulative effects of sibling and peer bullying in childhood on depression, anxiety, suicidal ideation, and self-harm in adulthood. *Front Psychiatry.* 2019;10:651.
34. Dantchev S, Wolke D. Sibling bullying at 12 years and high-risk behavior in early adulthood: a prospective cohort study. *Aggress Behav.* 2019;45(1):18–32.
35. Liu X, Peng C, Yu Y, et al. Association between sub-types of sibling bullying and mental health distress among Chinese children and adolescents. *Front Psychiatry.* 2020;11.
36. Liu X, Wolloh MG II, Lin X, et al. The association between sibling bullying and psychotic-like experiences among children age 11–16 years in China. *J Affective Disord.* 2021;284:31–37.
37. Wolke D, Skew AJ. Bullying among siblings. *Int J Adolesc Med Health.* 2012;24(1):17–25.
38. Olweus D. *Bullying at School: What We Know and What We Can Do.* Oxford, England: Blackwell Publishers; 1993:9.

39. Krienert JL, Walsh JA. My brother's keeper: a contemporary examination of reported sibling violence using national level data, 2000–2005. *J Fam Violence*. 2011;26(5):331–342.
40. Gladden RM, Vivolo-Kantor AM, Hamburger ME, Lumpkin CD. *Bullying Surveillance Among Youths: Uniform Definitions for Public Health and Recommended Data Elements, Version 1.0*. Atlanta, GA: National Center for Injury Prevention and Control, Centers for Disease Control and Prevention, and U.S. Department of Education; 2014.
41. Caffaro JV, Conn-Caffaro A. Treating sibling abuse families. *Aggress Violent Behav*. 2005;10(5):604–623.
42. Kiselica MS, Morrill-Richards M. Sibling maltreatment: the forgotten abuse. *J Couns Dev*. 2007;85(2):148–160.
43. Rapoza KA, Cook K, Zaveri T, Malley-Morrison K. Ethnic perspectives on sibling abuse in the United States. *J Fam Issues*. 2010;31(6):808–829.
44. Mackey AL, Fromuth ME, Kelly DB. The association of sibling relationship and abuse with later psychological adjustment. *J Interpers Violence*. 2010;25(6):955–968.
45. Meyers A. A call to child welfare: protect children from sibling abuse. *Qual Soc Work*. 2014;13(5):654–670.
46. Button DM, Gealt R. High risk behaviors among victims of sibling violence. *J Fam Violence*. 2010;25(2):131–140.
47. Hoffman KL, Edwards JN. An integrated theoretical model of sibling violence and abuse. *J Fam Violence*. 2004;19(3):185–200.
48. Meyers A. Lifting the veil: the lived experience of sibling abuse. *Qual Soc Work*. 2017;16(3):333–350.
49. Rosenthal PA, Doherty MB. Serious sibling abuse by preschool children. *J Am Acad Child Psychiatry*. 1984;23(2):186–190.
50. Veigh MJ. 'But she didn't say no': an exploration of sibling sexual abuse. *Aust Soc Work*. 2003;56(2):116–126.
51. Bass LB, Taylor BA, Knudson-Martin C, Huenergardt D. Making sense of abuse: case studies in sibling incest. *Contemp Fam Ther*. 2006;28(1):87–109.
52. Simonelli CJ, Mullis T, Elliott AN, Pierce TW. Abuse by siblings and subsequent experiences of violence within the dating relationship. *J Interpers Violence*. 2002;17(2):103–121.
53. Caffaro J. Sibling abuse of other children. In: Geffner UR, Vieth V, Vaughan-Eden V, Rosenbaum A, Hamberger L, White J, eds. *Handbook of Interpersonal Violence Across the Lifespan*. Switzerland: Springer, Cham; 2020:1–28.
54. Yates P. Sibling sexual abuse: why don't we talk about it? *J Clin Nurs*. 2017;26(15-16):2482–2494.
55. Kominkiewicz FB. The relationship of child protection service caseworker discipline-specific education and definition of sibling abuse: an institutional hiring impact study. *J Hum Behav Soc Environ*. 2004;9(1-2):69–82.
56. Adler NA, Schutz J. Sibling incest offenders. *Child Abuse Negl*. 1995;19(7):811–819.
57. Witte S, Fegert JM, Walper S. Sibling relationship pattern in the context of abuse and neglect: results from a sample of adult siblings. *Child Abuse Negl*. 2020;106:104528.
58. McDonald C, Martinez K. Victim narratives of sibling emotional abuse. *Child Welfare*. 2019;97(2):1–21.
59. Tener D, Newman A, Yates P, Tarshish N. Child advocacy center intervention with sibling sexual abuse cases: cross-cultural comparison of professionals' perspectives and experiences. *Child Abuse Negl*. 2020;105:104259.
60. Perkins NH, Meyers A. The manifestation of physical and emotional sibling abuse across the lifespan and the need for social work intervention. *J Fam Soc Work*. 2020;23(4):338–356.

61. Relva IC, Fernandes OM, Mota CP. An exploration of sibling violence predictors. *J Aggress Conflict Peace Res.* 2013;5(1):47–61.
62. Eriksen S, Jensen V. All in the family? Family environment factors in sibling violence. *J Fam Violence.* 2006;21(8):497–507.
63. Tidefors I, Arvidsson H, Ingevaldson S, Larsson M. Sibling incest: a literature review and a clinical study. *J Sex Aggress.* 2010;16(3):347–360.
64. Meyers AB. Notes from the field: Understanding why sibling abuse remains under the radar and pathways to outing, professional development. *International J Soc Work Educ.* 2015;18(2):24–31. https://digitalcommons.molloy.edu/cgi/viewcontent.cgi?article=1001&context=swk_fac. Accessed September 28, 2023.
65. Alpert JL. Sibling child sexual abuse research review and clinical implications. *J Aggress Maltreat Trauma.* 1997;1(1):263–275.
66. Rayment-McHugh S, Nisbet I. Sibling incest offenders as a subset of adolescent sexual offenders. Paper presented at the Australian Institute of Criminology Child Sexual Abuse Conference. Adelaide, Australia, May 1–2, 2003. https://www.researchgate.net/profile/Ian-Nisbet-2/publication/45705705_Sibling_incest_offenders_as_a_subset_of_adolescent_sex_offenders/links/55a8253b08aea3d0867c39d3/Sibling-incest-offenders-as-a-subset-of-adolescent-sex-offenders.pdf. Accessed September 28, 2023.
67. Eriksen S, Jensen V. A push or a punch: distinguishing the severity of sibling violence. *J Interpers Violence.* 2009;24(1):183–208.
68. Whipple EE, Finton SE. Psychological maltreatment by siblings: an unrecognized form of abuse. *Child Adolesc Soc Work J.* 1995;12(2):135–146.
69. Stormshak EA, Bellanti CJ, Bierman KL. The quality of sibling relationships and the development of social competence and behavioral control in aggressive children. *Dev Psychol.* 1996;32(1):79.
70. Schulz-Heik RJ, Rhee SH, Silvern L, et al. Investigation of genetically mediated child effects on maltreatment. *Behav Genetics.* 2009;39(3):265–276.
71. Finkelhor D, Turner H, Ormrod R. Kid's stuff: The nature and impact of peer and sibling violence on younger and older children. *Child Abuse Negl.* 2006;30(12):1401–1421.
72. Lopes PP, Relva IC, Fernandes OM. Psychopathology and sibling violence in a sample of Portuguese adolescents. *J Child Adolesc Trauma.* 2019;12(1):11–21.
73. Perkins NH, O'Connor MK. Physical and emotional sibling violence: a necessary role for social work. *Soc Work.* 2015;61(1):91–93.
74. Perkins NH, Rai A, Grossman SF. Physical and emotional sibling violence in the time of COVID-19. *J Fam Violence.* 2021:1–8.
75. Kettrey HH, Emery BC. The discourse of sibling violence. *J Fam Violence.* 2006;21(6):407–416.
76. Khan R, Rogers P. The normalization of sibling violence: does gender and personal experience of violence influence perceptions of physical assault against siblings? *J Interpers Violence.* 2015;30(3):437–458.
77. Noland VJ, Liller KD, McDermott RJ, Coulter ML, Seraphine AE. Is adolescent sibling violence a precursor to college dating violence? Am J Health Behav. 2004;28(1): S13–S23.
78. Winters KE. Physical and emotional sibling violence and child welfare: a critical realist exploratory study [dissertation]. 2019. https://pdxscholar.library.pdx.edu/cgi/viewcontent.cgi?article=5880&context=open_access_etds. Accessed September 28, 2023.
79. Simonelli CJ, Mullis T, Elliott AN, Pierce TW. Abuse by siblings and subsequent experiences of violence within the dating relationship. *J Interpers Violence.* 2002;17(2):103–121.

80. Underwood RC, Patch PC. Siblicide: a descriptive analysis of sibling homicide. *Homicide Stud.* 1999;3(4):333–348.
81. Wiehe VR. *Sibling Abuse: Hidden Physical, Emotional, and Sexual Trauma.* Thousand Oaks, California: SAGE; 1997.
82. Caffaro J, Conn-Caffaro A. *Sibling Abuse Trauma.* New York, NY: Haworth Maltreatment & Trauma Press; 1998. Cited by Kiselica and Morrill-Richards.[42]
83. Peck JH, Heide KM. Juvenile involvement in fratricide and sororicide: an empirical analysis of 32 years of US arrest data. *J Fam Violence.* 2012;27(8):749–760.
84. Fox JA, Swatt ML. Uniform Crime Reports [United States]: Supplementary Homicide Reports with Multiple Imputation, Cumulative Files 1976-2007. Inter-university Consortium for Political and Social Research [distributor], 2009-02-24. https://doi.org/10.3886/ICPSR24801.v1. Accessed September 28, 2023. Cited by Peck and Heide.[83]
85. Morrill M. Sibling sexual abuse: an exploratory study of long-term consequences for self-esteem and counseling considerations. *J Fam Violence.* 2014;29(2):205–213.
86. Kellogg ND. Clinical report—the evaluation of sexual behaviors in children. *Pediatrics.* 2009;124(3):992–998.
87. Finkelhor D. Sex among siblings: a survey on prevalence, variety, and effects. *Arch Sex Behav.* 1980;9(3):171–194.
88. Smith H, Israel E. Sibling incest: a study of the dynamics of 25 cases. *Child Abuse Negl.* 1987;11(1):101–108. Cited by Krienert and Walsh (see Note 89).
89. Krienert JL, Walsh JA. Sibling sexual abuse: an empirical analysis of offender, victim, and event characteristics in National Incident-Based Reporting System (NIBRS) Data, 2000–2007. *J Child Sex Abuse.* 2011;20(4):353–372.
90. Flury M, Nyberg E, Riecher-Rossler A. Domestic violence against women: definitions, epidemiology, risk factors and consequences. *Swiss Med Wkly.* 2010;140(6):1–6. doi:10.4414/smw.2010.13099 https://smw.ch/index.php/smw/article/view/1179/1242. Accessed September 28, 2023.
91. García-Moreno C, Pallitto C, Devries K, Stöckl H, Watts C, Abrahams N. Global and regional estimates of violence against women: prevalence and health effects of intimate partner violence and non-partner sexual violence. World Health Organization; 2013. http://apps.who.int/iris/bitstream/10665/85239/1/9789241564625_eng.pdf. Accessed August 25, 2022.
92. Peek-Asa C, Wallis A, Harland K, Beyer K, Dickey P, Saftlas A. Rural disparity in domestic violence prevalence and access to resources. *J Womens Health.* 2011;20(11):1743–1749.
93. McCarthy SC. Men who sustain female-to-male partner violence: factors associated with where they seek help and how they rate those resources. *Violence Vict.* 2012;27(6):871.
94. Caetano R, Ramisetty-Mikler S, Harris TR. Neighborhood characteristics as predictors of male to female and female to male partner violence. *J Interpers Violence.* 2010;25(11):1986–2009.
95. Caetano R, McGrath C, Ramisetty-Mikler S, Field CA. Drinking, alcohol problems and the five-year recurrence and incidence of male to female and female to male partner violence. *Alcohol Clin Exp Res.* 2005;29(1):98–106.
96. Mills LD, Mills TJ, Taliaferro E, Zimbler A, Smith D. The prevalence of female-to-male intimate partner violence in an urban emergency department. *J Emerg Med.* 2003;25(2):215–218.
97. Nybergh L, Taft C, Enander V, Krantz G. Self-reported exposure to intimate partner violence among women and men in Sweden: results from a population-based survey. *BMC Public Health.* 2013;13(1):845.

98. Truman JL, Morgan RE. *Nonfatal Domestic Violence*. Washington, DC: US Department of Justice, Bureau of Justice Statistics; 2014. http://archive.mnadv.org/_mnadvWeb/wp-content/uploads/2011/07/BJS-Nonfatal-DV-2003-2012.pdf. Accessed August 25, 2022.
99. Pallitto CC, García-Moreno C, Jansen HA, Heise L, Ellsberg M, Watts C. Intimate partner violence, abortion, and unintended pregnancy: results from the WHO Multi-country Study on Women's Health and Domestic Violence. *Int J Gynecol Obstet*. 2013;120(1):3–9.
100. Pavey AR, Gorman GH, Kuehn D, Stokes TA, Hisle-Gorman E. Intimate partner violence increases adverse outcomes at birth and in early infancy. *J Pediatrics*. 2014;165(5):1034–1039.
101. Devries KM, Mak JY, Bacchus LJ, et al. Intimate partner violence and incident depressive symptoms and suicide attempts: a systematic review of longitudinal studies. *PLOS Med*. 2013;10(5):e1001439.
102. Fanslow JL, Robinson EM. Physical injuries resulting from intimate partner violence and disclosure to healthcare providers: results from a New Zealand population-based study. *Inj Prev*. 2011;17(1):37–42.
103. Belfrage H, Rying M. Characteristics of spousal homicide perpetrators: a study of all cases of spousal homicide in Sweden 1990–1999. *Crim Behav Ment Health*. 2004;14(2):121–133.
104. Mercy JA, Saltzman LE. Fatal violence among spouses in the United States, 1976–85. *Am J Public Health*. 1989;79(5):595–599.
105. Harbin HT, Madden DJ. Battered parents: a new syndrome. *Am J Psychiatry*. 1979;136(10):1288–1291.
106. Paterson R, Luntz H, Perlesz A, Cotton S. Adolescent violence towards parents: maintaining family connections when the going gets tough. *Aust N Z J Fam Ther*. 2002;23(2):90–100. Cited in Kennair and Mellor (see Note 31).
107. Cottrell B, Monk P. Adolescent-to-parent abuse: a qualitative overview of common themes. *J Fam Issues*. 2004;25(8):1072–1095.
108. Kennair N, Mellor D. Parent abuse: a review. *Child Psychiatry Hum Dev*. 2007;38(3):203–219.
109. Walsh JA, Krienert JL. A decade of child-initiated family violence: comparative analysis of child—parent violence and parricide examining offender, victim, and event characteristics in a national sample of reported incidents, 1995–2005. *J Interpers Violence*. 2009;24(9):1450–1477.
110. Hong JS, Kral MJ, Espelage DL, Allen-Meares P. The social ecology of adolescent-initiated parent abuse: a review of the literature. *Child Psychiatry Hum Dev*. 2012;43(3):431–454.
111. Calvete E, Orue I, Gámez-Guadix M. Child-to-parent violence: emotional and behavioral predictors. *J Interpers Violence*. 2013;28(4):755–772.
112. Margolin G, Baucom BR. Adolescents' aggression to parents: longitudinal links with parents' physical aggression. *J Adolesc Health*. 2014;55(5):645–651.
113. A PubMed search yielded more than 3,300 citations for studies including the term *child maltreatment* and more than 1,800 references for studies with this concept included in the title. https://www.ncbi.nlm.nih.gov/pubmed. Accessed August 25, 2022.
114. Cottrell B, Finlayson M. *Parent Abuse: The Abuse of Parents by Their Teenage Children*. Ottawa, Canada: Family Violence Prevention Unit, Health Canada; 2001. Cited by Kennair and Mellor.[108]
115. Peek CW, Fischer JL, Kidwell JS. Teenage violence toward parents: a neglected dimension of family violence. *J Marriage Fam*. 1985:1051–1058. Cited by Kennair and Mellor.[108]

116. Downey L. Adolescent violence: a systemic and feminist perspective. *Aust N Z J Fam Ther.* 1997;18(2):70–79. Cited by Kennair and Mellor.[108]

117. Walsh JA, Krienert JL. Child–parent violence: an empirical analysis of offender, victim, and event characteristics in a national sample of reported incidents. *J Fam Violence.* 2007;22(7):563–567.

118. Federal Bureau of Investigation. *Uniform Crime Reporting Guide: NIBRS Edition.* Washington, DC: US Department of Justice; 1992. Cited by Walsh and Krienert.[117]

119. Walsh JA, Krienert JL, Crowder D. Innocence lost: a gender-based study of parricide offender, victim, and incident characteristics in a national sample, 1976–2003. *J Aggress Maltreat Trauma.* 2008;16(2):202–227.

120. Buyuk Y, Kurnaz G, Eke SM, Ankarali HC, Oral G. Medico-legal evaluation of adolescent parricide offenders: thirty-nine cases from Turkey. *J Fam Violence.* 2011;26(1):1–7.

121. United Nations, Department of Economic and Social Affairs, Population Division. *Living Arrangements of Older Persons: A Report on an Expanded International Dataset.* New York, NY: United Nations; 2017:12. https://www.un.org/en/development/desa/population/publications/pdf/ageing/LivingArrangements.pdf. Accessed August 25, 2022.

122. Pillemer K, Finkelhor D. The prevalence of elder abuse: a random sample survey. *Gerontologist.* 1988;28(1):51–57.

123. United Nations, Department of Economic and Social Affairs, Population Division. *Patterns and Trends in Household Size and Composition: Evidence from a United Nations Dataset.* New York, NY: United Nations; 2019:29. https://www.un.org/en/development/desa/population/publications/pdf/ageing/household_size_and_composition_technical_report.pdf. Accessed August 25, 2022.

124. United Nations, Department of Economic and Social Affairs, Population Division. *Population Facts, April 2019.* New York, NY: Unied Nations; 2019:4. https://www.un.org/en/development/desa/population/publications/pdf/popfacts/PopFacts_2019-2.pdf. Accessed August 25, 2022.

125. Baker AA. Granny battering. *Modern Geriatr.* 1975;8:20–24. Cited by Kosberg and MacNeil (see Note 126).

126. Kosberg JI, MacNeil G. The elder abuse of custodial grandparents: a hidden phenomenon. *J Elder Abuse Negl.* 2003;15(3-4):33–53.

127. Bullock K, Thomas RL. The vulnerability for elder abuse among a sample of custodial grandfathers: an exploratory study. *J Elder Abuse Negl.* 2007;19(3-4):133–150.

128. Brownell P, Berman J, Nelson A, Fofana RC. Grandparents raising grandchildren: the risks of caregiving. *J Elder Abuse Negl.* 2003;15(3-4):5–31.

129. Kempe CH, Silverman FN, Steele BF, Droegemueller W, Silver HK. The battered-child syndrome. *JAMA.* 1962;181:17–24.

130. Fontana VJ, Donovan D, Wong RJ. The maltreatment syndrome in children. *N Engl J Med.* 1963;269(26):1389–1394.

131. Butchart A, Mikton C, Dahlberg LL, Krug EG. Global Status Report on Violence Prevention 2014, Part VII, Glossary. https://www.who.int/publications/i/item/9789241564793. Accessed August 25, 2022.

132. US Department of Health & Human Services, Children's Bureau. (2021). Child Maltreatment 2019. https://www.acf.hhs.gov/sites/default/files/documents/cb/cm2019.pdf. Accessed August 25, 2022.

133. World Health Organization. *Report of the Consultation on Child Abuse Prevention, 29–31 March 1999.* Geneva, Switzerland: WHO. http://apps.who.int/iris/handle/10665/65900. Accessed August 25, 2022.
134. United Nations Children's Fund. *A Familiar Face: Violence in the Lives of Children and Adolescents.* New York, NY: UNICEF; 2017. https://www.unicef.org/bulgaria/media/1511/file/BGR-violence-in-the-lives-of-children-and-adolescents-en.pdf. Accessed August 25, 2022.
135. Stoltenborgh M, Van Ijzendoorn MH, Euser EM, Bakermans-Kranenburg MJ. A global perspective on child sexual abuse: meta-analysis of prevalence around the world. *Child Maltreatment.* 2011;16(2):79–101.
136. Stoltenborgh M, Bakermans-Kranenburg MJ, Alink LR, van Ijzendoorn MH. The universality of childhood emotional abuse: a meta-analysis of worldwide prevalence. *J Aggress Maltreat Trauma.* 2012;21(8):870–890.
137. Stoltenborgh M, Bakermans-Kranenburg MJ, van Ijzendoorn MH. The neglect of child neglect: a meta-analytic review of the prevalence of neglect. *Soc Psychiatry Psychiatr Epidemiol.* 2013;48(3):345–355.
138. Stoltenborgh M, Bakermans-Kranenburg MJ, Ijzendoorn MH, Alink LR. Cultural–geographical differences in the occurrence of child physical abuse? A meta-analysis of global prevalence. *Int J Psychol.* 2013;48(2):81–94.
139. Stoltenborgh M, Bakermans-Kranenburg MJ, Alink LR, Ijzendoorn MH. The prevalence of child maltreatment across the globe: review of a series of meta-analyses. *Child Abuse Rev.* 2015;24(1):37–50.
140. Investigation of maltreatment reports in the United States: In most states, most maltreatment reports receive an investigation., which results in a determination (also known as a disposition), which can substantiate the allegation of maltreatment or conclude that there is not sufficient evidence under state law to conclude or suspect that the child was maltreated or is at risk of being maltreated.[132]
141. Alternative response to a maltreatment report in the United States:

    In some states, reports of maltreatment may not be investigated, but are instead assigned to an alternative track, called alternative response, family assessment response, or differential response. Cases receiving this response often include early determinations that the children have a low or moderate risk of maltreatment. According to states, alternative responses usually include the voluntary acceptance of CPS services and the agreement of family needs. These cases do not result in a formal determination regarding the maltreatment allegation or alleged perpetrator.[132]

142. Wong JY, Wai AK, Wang MP, et al. Impact of COVID-19 on child maltreatment: income instability and parenting issues. *Int J Environ Res Public Health.* 2021;18(4):1501.
143. Severe physical assault: Slapping somebody on the face, head, or ears; hitting on other parts of the body besides the bottom with a belt, hairbrush, stick, or other hard object; or throwing or knocking somebody down.[142]
144. Very severe physical assault: Beating somebody over and over as hard as one could, grabbing somebody by the neck and choking him/her, burning somebody on purpose, or threatening somebody with a gun.[142]

145. Federal Fiscal Year (FFY): The 12-month period from October 1 through September 30 used by the federal government. The fiscal year is designated by the calendar year in which it ends. https://budgetcounsel.com/cyclopedia-budgetica/cb-fiscal-year/#:~:text=The%20fiscal%20year%20is%20the,and%20ends%20September%2030%2C%202008. Accessed September 29, 2023.
146. US Department of Health & Human Services, Children's Bureau. Child Maltreatment 2019, Chapter 4, Fatalities. https://www.acf.hhs.gov/sites/default/files/documents/cb/cm2019.pdf. Accessed August 29, 2022.
147. Durrant JE, Broberg AG, Rose-Krasnor L. Predicting mother's use of physical punishment during mother–child conflicts in Sweden and Canada. *N Dir Child Adolesc Dev.* 1999;1999(86):25–41.
148. Corral-Verdugo V, Frias-Armenta M, Romero M, Munoz A. Validity of a scale measuring beliefs regarding the "positive" effects of punishing children: a study of Mexican mothers. *Child Abuse Negl.* 1995;19(6):669–679. Cited by Durrant et al.[147]
149. Dix T, Ruble DN, Zambarano RJ. Mothers' implicit theories of discipline: child effects, parent effects, and the attribution process. *Child Dev.* 1989:1373–1391. Cited by Durrant et al.[147]
150. Holden GW, Coleman SM, Schmidt KL. Why 3-year-old children get spanked: parent and child determinants as reported by college-educated mothers. *Merrill-Palmer Q.* 1995:431–452. Cited by Durrant et al.[147]
151. Simons R, Whitbeck L, Conger R, Chyi-In W. Intergenerational transmission of harsh parenting. *Dev Psychol.* 1991;27(1):159–171. Cited by Durrant et al.[147]
152. Gershoff ET. More harm than good: a summary of scientific research on the intended and unintended effects of corporal punishment on children. *Law Contemp Probs.* 2010;73:31.
153. Durrant JE, Trocmé N, Fallon B, Milne C, Black T, Knoke D. Punitive violence against children in Canada. *CECW Information Sheet E.* 2006;41. Cited by Gershoff.[152]
154. Cuartas J, Weissman DG, Sheridan MA, Lengua L, McLaughlin KA. Corporal punishment and elevated neural response to threat in children. *Child Dev.* 2021;92(3):821–832.
155. Liu L, Wang M. Parental corporal punishment, and child anxiety in China: the moderating role of HPA-axis activity. *J Affective Disord.* 2020;273:500–507.
156. Xing X, Yin T, Wang M. Cortisol stress reactivity moderates the effects of parental corporal punishment on Chinese preschoolers' executive function. *Child Abuse Negl.* 2019;88:288–297.
157. Straus MA, Paschall MJ. Corporal punishment by mothers and development of children's cognitive ability: a longitudinal study of two nationally representative age cohorts. *J Aggress Maltreat Trauma.* 2009;18(5):459–483.
158. Paolucci EO, Violato C. A meta-analysis of the published research on the affective, cognitive, and behavioral effects of corporal punishment. *J Psychol.* 2004;138(3):197–222.
159. Ferguson CJ. Spanking, corporal punishment and negative long-term outcomes: a meta-analytic review of longitudinal studies. *Clin Psychol Rev.* 2013;33(1):196–208.
160. Gershoff ET, Grogan-Kaylor A. Spanking and child outcomes: old controversies and new meta-analyses. *J Fam Psychol.* 2016;30(4):453.
161. International Labour Organization, C189—Domestic Workers Convention, 2011 (No. 189), Article 1. https://www.ilo.org/dyn/normlex/en/f?p=NORMLEXPUB:12100:0::NO::P12100_ILO_CODE:C189. Accessed September 29, 2023.
162. International Labour Organization. *Domestic Workers across the World: Global and Regional Statistics and the Extent of Legal Protection.* Geneva, Switzerland: International Labour

Office; 2013. https://www.ilo.org/wcmsp5/groups/public/---dgreports/---dcomm/---publ/documents/publication/wcms_173363.pdf. Accessed August 25, 2022.

163. International Labour Organization, C189—Domestic Workers Convention, 2011 (No. 189), Article 10. https://www.ilo.org/dyn/normlex/en/f?p=NORMLEXPUB:12100:0::NO::P12100_ILO_CODE:C189. Accessed September 29, 2023.
164. International Labour Organization. *Working Hours in Domestic Work.* Domestic Work Policy Brief No. 2. Geneva, Switzerland: International Labour Office; 2011. Cited by International Labour Office.[155] https://www.ilo.org/wcmsp5/groups/public/---dgreports/---dcomm/---publ/documents/publication/wcms_173363.pdf. Accessed August 25, 2022.
165. Wolfe J, Kandra J, Engdahl L, Shierholz H. *Domestic Worker Chartbook: A Comprehensive Look at the Demographics, Wages, Benefits, and Poverty Rates of the Professionals Who Care for Our Family Members and Clean Our Homes.* Washington DC, USA: Economic Policy Institute, 2020. https://files.epi.org/pdf/194214.pdf. Accessed August 25, 2022.
166. Human Rights Watch. *Maid to Order: Ending Abuses against Migrant Domestic Workers in Singapore.* New York, NY: Human Rights Watch; 2005. Cited by Malhotra et al (see Note 169).
167. Human Rights Watch. *Walls at Every Turn: Abuse of Migrant Domestic Workers through Kuwait's Sponsorship System.* New York, NY: Human Rights Watch; 2010. Cited by Malhotra et al (see Note 169).
168. Human Rights Watch. *Hidden in the Home: Abuse of Domestic Workers with Special Visas in the United States.* New York, NY: Human Rights Watch; 2001. Cited by Malhotra et al (see Note 169).
169. Malhotra R, Arambepola C, Tarun S, de Silva V, Kishore J, Østbye T. Health issues of female foreign domestic workers: a systematic review of the scientific and gray literature. *Int J Occup Environ Health.* 2013;19(4):261–277.
170. Jureidini R, Moukarbel N. Female Sri Lankan domestic workers in Lebanon: a case of 'contract slavery'? *J Ethnic Migrat Stud.* 2004;30(4):581–607. Cited by Malhotra et al.[169]
171. Bauleo MF, Van Dijk F, Radon K. One's workplace, other's home? Work and health of domestic workers in Argentina. *Ann Global Health.* 2018;84(3):450.
172. Ghaddar A, Khandaqji S, Ghattas J. Justifying abuse of women migrant domestic workers in Lebanon: the opinion of recruitment agencies. *Gac Sanit.* 2021;34:493–499.
173. DeSouza ER, Cerqueira E. From the kitchen to the bedroom: frequency rates and consequences of sexual harassment among female domestic workers in Brazil. *J Interpers Violence.* 2009;24(8):1264–1284.
174. Figueiredo MC, Suleman F, Botelho M. Workplace abuse and harassment: the vulnerability of informal and migrant domestic workers in Portugal. *Soc Policy Soc.* 2018;17(1):65–85.
175. Albin E, Mantouvalou V. The ILO convention on domestic workers: from the shadows to the light. *Ind Law J.* 2012;41(1):67–78.
176. Gilani I, Waqar S. Sexual harassment and coping strategies used by female domestic workers. *Pak J Psychol Res.* 2018:557–571.
177. Blackett A. Introduction: regulating decent work for domestic workers. *Can J Women Law.* 2011;23(1):1–46.
178. Ullah AA. Abuse and violence against foreign domestic workers: a case from Hong Kong. *Int J Area Stud.* 2015;10(2):221–238.
179. Huling A. Domestic workers in Malaysia: hidden victims of abuse and forced labor. *NYU J Int Law Polit.* 2011;44:629.

180. Cheung JT, Tsoi VW, Wong KH, Chung RY. Abuse and depression among Filipino foreign domestic helpers a cross-sectional survey in Hong Kong. *Public Health.* 2019;166:121–127.
181. Demetriou D. 'Tied visas' and inadequate labour protections: a formula for abuse and exploitation of migrant domestic workers in the United Kingdom. *Anti-Trafficking Rev.* 2015;29(5):1–10.
182. Jureidini R. The use and abuse of domestic workers: case studies in Lebanon and Egypt. In: Mary Romero, Valerie Preston, Wenona Giles, eds. *When Care Work Goes Global.* Oxfordshire, UK: Milton Park, Abingdon; 2016:95–113.
183. Pan SM, Yang JT. Outsiders in the family: abuse of migrant domestic workers in Taiwan. *Asian J Womens Stud.* 2012;18(1):87–117.
184. Huang S, Yeoh BS. Emotional labour and transnational domestic work: the moving geographies of 'maid abuse' in Singapore. *Mobilities.* 2007;2(2):195–217.
185. Murty OP. Maid abuse. *J Forensic Leg Med.* 2009;16(5):290–296.
186. Vandenberg ME, Bessell S. Diplomatic immunity and the abuse of domestic workers: criminal and civil remedies in the United States. *Duke J Comp Int Law.* 2015;26:595.
187. Vellos D. Immigrant Latina domestic workers and sexual harassment. *AMU J Gender Soc Policy Law.* 1996;5:407.
188. Lai Y, Fong E. Work-related aggression in home-based working environment: experiences of migrant domestic workers in Hong Kong. *Am Behav Scientist.* 2020;64(6):722–739.
189. Hanley J, Premji S, Messing K, Lippel K. Action research for the health and safety of domestic workers in Montreal: using numbers to tell stories and effect change. New Solut. 2011;20(4):421–439.) Cited by Malhotra et al.[169]
190. Wong A. *Identifying Work-Related Stressors and Abuses and Assessing Their Impact on the Health of Migrant Domestic Workers in Singapore.* Singapore: Humanitarian Organization for Migration Economics; 2010. Cited by Malhotra et al.[169]
191. Human Rights Watch. *Exported and Exposed: Abuses Against Sri Lankan Domestic Workers in Saudi Arabia, Kuwait, Lebanon, and the United Arab Emirates.* New York, NY: Human Rights Watch; 2007. Cited by Malhotra et al.[169]
192. Human Rights Watch. *Help Wanted: Abuses against Female Migrant Domestic Workers in Indonesia and Malaysia.* New York, NY: Human Rights Watch; 2004. Cited by Malhotra et al.[169]

14

Bullying and Other Forms of Maltreatment in Cyberspace

This chapter explores the diverse types of maltreatment that may affect people who interact in cyberspace, including cyberbullying and cybercrimes.

What Is Known?

The term *cyberspace* was coined by Gibson to describe a "graphic representation of data abstracted from banks of every computer in human system."[1] Cyberspace has been defined as a "complex environment resulting from the interaction of people, software, and services on the Internet by means of technology devices and networks connected to it, which does not exist in any physical form."[2] Cyberspace offers a new social place[3] that goes beyond geographical boundaries and transcends social milieus, therefore potentially widening the risk of exposure to victimization.

Cyberbullying

The topic of cyberbullying appeared in news reports[4] and peer-reviewed articles[5] as early as 2003. In the last two decades, there have been many published studies exploring its nature and concept,[6-18] prevalence,[19-29] correlates, predisposing factors,[30-64] ill effects,[65-91] and prevention.[92-103] Furthermore, cybervictimization has been comprehensively examined by several research-based books published in the last decade.[104-111]

The Definition and Nature of Cyberbullying

Patchin and Hinduja defined cyberbullying as "willful and repeated harm inflicted through the medium or electronic text."[112] In addition, cyberbullying can also mean electronic bullying, cybervictimization, cyberharassment, or cyberaggression.

Electronic bullying has been recognized in the uniform definition of bullying[113] as technology-based victimization that can be recognized by using the general definition of bullying.[114] In this context, cyberbullying contains four components: it is intentional, happens repeatedly, involves an imbalance of power, and occurs through electronic technologies. Furthermore, the potential anonymity[115] of the perpetrator is a unique characteristic of cyberbullying, as well the public aspects[116] of the victimization, due to a possibly vast audience.

A comprehensive review of cyberbullying research by Kowalki et al.[117] showed that published studies have defined cyberbullying by including behaviors that are common to

Table 14.1. Behaviors Occurring via Electronic Technologies

Being asked to do something sexual[118]	Exclusion[121]	Insulting[128]	Sending harmful, cruel text[132]
Blaming somebody for something that he/she has not done[9]	Flaming[121]	Leaving somebody out of things[119]	Sending mean notes[127]
Broadcasting[60]	Forgery[124]	Making fun of somebody[129]	Sending photos or videos of intimate scenes[133]
Calling someone hurtful names[119]	Forwarding a message without consent[125]	Masquerading[121]	Sending pornography[134]
Creating a mean webpage[120]	Happy slapping[126]	Name-calling[130]	Sharing photographs without permission[9]
Cyberstalking[121]	Harassment[14]	Outing[121]	Social exclusion[130]
Deception[60]	Hiding identity[124]	Receiving unwanted sexual text or photos[118]	Suggestive email[135]
Denigration[121]	Hostility[118]	Rumor spreading[130]	Telling lies[127]
Discrimination[122]	Humiliation[118]	Saying unwanted sexually related things to someone[119]	Threatening[135]
Embarrassment[123]	Ignoring[127]	Sending computer viruses on purpose[131]	Trickery[121]

bullying in any environment (e.g., insults, name-calling) and/or with actions unique to cyberbullying (Table 14.1)

The types of mistreatment that are unique to cyberbullying include:

- Broadcasting, defined as "making fun of someone by sending/posting stories/jokes or pictures about him/her"[60]
- Dissing, which is denigrating somebody online by "sending or posting gossip or rumors about a person to damage his or her reputation or friendships"[136]
- Flaming, which has been described as "sending or posting hostile, angry, or mischievous messages intended to inflame the emotions and sensibilities of others"[104]
- Hacking, defined as "knowingly accessing a computer system or network without authorization"[137]
- Happy slapping, which is an incident during which "an unsuspecting person is recorded being harassed or bullied in a way that usually involves some form of physical abuse," with the resulting photo or video sent around on cyberspace for public viewing[104]
- Identity theft, which is "knowingly electronically obtaining another person's credit card information without permission"[137]
- Impersonation, defined as "pretending to be someone else and sending or posting material to get that person in trouble or danger or to damage that person's reputation or friendships"[136]

- Outing, which means "sharing someone's secrets or embarrassing information or images online"[136]
- Trickery, which is the action of "talking someone into revealing secrets or embarrassing information, then sharing it online"[135]
- Virus writing, defined as "knowingly writing or using a program that would infect a computer or network"[137]

Prevalence

Canada

Data on the prevalence of Canadian adolescents' participation in cyberbullying has been documented in longitudinal research by Capadoccia et al.,[138] based on data from more than 1,700 students in grade 9 or higher who completed the Health Behavior in School-aged Children survey (HBSC) in Spring 2006 and Spring 2007. This investigation[138] documented that 6.5% of Canadian adolescents reported having been cyberbullied in the previous two months during 2006 and the frequency increased to 9.2% on the following year. Furthermore, data from the 2017–2018 HBSC[139] showed that an average of 13.16% of Canadian adolescents age 11 to 15 indicated that they had been exposed to cybervictimization in the previous couple of months.

United States

Prevalence of cyberbullying in the United States is discussed Chapter 2.

Europe and Asia

Review of data from the 2017–2018 HBSC[139] pertaining to adolescents (11 to 15 years old) in 40 European counties can be found in Chapter 2. A 2017–2019 large EU Kids Online[140] survey of children and adolescents 9 to 16 years old living in European countries showed that an average of 5% of youth were subject to cyberbullying at least every month in the previous year, and 9% were cyberbullied a few times during the previous 12 months[140] (Table 14.2). The same survey[140] also showed that an average of 17% of the participants reported that they had been exposed, at least every month or more often in the previous year, to hate messages that attacked certain individuals or groups. Also, an average of 7% of the respondents indicated that they experienced, almost every month during the prior year, some form of data misuse and privacy-related risks in the context of interpersonal, institutional, or business contacts.[140]

Chudal et al.[141] analyzed data from the Eurasian Child Mental Health Study,[142] which involves more than 21,000 adolescents (age 13 to 15) in 13 countries,[142] and documented that an average of 10.49% of the participants were exposed to cyberbullying only, or cyberbullying associated with traditional bullying, less than once a week or more frequently, in the previous six months.[141] The range of prevalence varied from 2.29% in Japan to as high as 21.17% in Russia (Table 14.3).[141]

Australia

Jadambaa et al.[143] conducted a systematic review and meta-analysis of 11 studies of cyberbullying prevalence in Australia conducted after 2006, and they found an estimated pooled prevalence of lifetime cyberbullying victimization of 7%.

Table 14.2. Frequency of Cyberbullying of Children[a] in the Previous Year, by Country (Adapted from EU Kids Online 2020[140])

Country	Frequent[b]	Occasional[c]	Country	Frequent[b]	Occasional[c]
Switzerland	5%	11%	Lithuania	4%	7%
Chechia	7%	8%	Malta	11%	10%
Greenland	3%	12%	Norway	3%	11%
Estonia	6%	11%	Poland	13%	13%
Spain	7%	9%	Portugal	6%	8%
France	2%	8%	Romania	7%	15%
Croatia	2%	4%	Serbia	6%	13%
Italy	2%	7%	Slovakia	4%	No data available

[a] All children 9 to 16 years old who use the Internet.
[b] At least every month.
[c] A few times.

Cyberbullying among Adults

A systematic review of 90 studies focused on cyberbullying among adults, conducted by Jenaro et al.,[144] indicated that almost 80% of the studies evaluated focused on college students, while 20% of the research reviewed explored college teachers, white collar workers, politicians, business and industrial personnel, and administrators. The prevalence rates of cyberbullying among "conservative studies requiring the occurrence of at least one negative act on a weekly basis over a six-month period to label the negative behavior as cyberbullying"[144] ranged from 2.8%[145] to 10.8%.[146]

Table 14.3. Six-Month Prevalence of Cyberbullying[a] in 13 European and Asian Countries, Calculated from Data Published by Chudal et al[141]

Country	Prevalence	Country	Prevalence
Russia	21.17%	Lithuania	11.21%
Indonesia	20.25%	China	8.94%
Israel	14.84%	Finland	8.68%
Iran	13.71%	Vietnam	7.54%
Singapore	12.91%	Greece	4.72%
Norway	12.31%	India	3.63%
		Japan	2.29%

[a] Cyberbullying only and cyberbullying associated with traditional bullying.

Wang et al.[147] examined the frequency of exposure to cyberbullying in a nationally representative sample of 20,848 adult New Zealanders who participated in the longitudinal New Zealand Attitudes and Value Study. Almost 15% of the participants indicated that they have been a target of cyberbullying in their lifetime, while 2.2% reported to have experienced cyberbullying in the previous month, during 2017.[147]

A 2020 nationally representative Pew Research Center survey[148] of more than 10,000 US adults showed that 41% of Americans have experienced some type of online harassment.[148] Furthermore, 25% of respondents indicated that they were subjected to more severe harassment.[148]

Correlates of Cyberbullying

Barlett and Gentile[149] developed a model drawn from learning-based theory that suggests that positive cyberbullying opinions predict later cyberbullying perpetration. Furthermore, it postulates that a "positive attitude towards cyberbullying" is developed by attitudes toward the strength and anonymity afforded by aggression against others in the mediated word.[149]

The empirical support of the Barlett and Gentile Cyberbullying Model was tested by a three-wave longitudinal study[34] of 161 participants age 18 to 24. The research documented that confidence in not being caught if engaging in mean online behavior (perceived anonymity), together with a strong belief that one can send mean messages to anybody regardless of one's own stature or muscularity (irrelevance of physical attributes), as ascertain at Wave 1, predicted 14 weeks later, at Wave 2, a positive cyberbullying attitude characterized by feelings that it is right "to bully others on line if they deserve it."[34] Subsequently, Wave 2 findings predicted cyberbullying perpetration three months later, at Wave 3.[34]

Sasson and Mesch[40] surveyed 495 students (10 to 18 years old) living in a large Israeli city and showed that the risk of online victimization was higher for females than for males, but not for younger or older adolescents.[40] Also, there was no significant association between time online and exposure to cybervictimization. Yet, risky behavior online, as manifested by disclosure of confidential information or sending frequent insults, was significantly associated with online victimization.[40] Parental guidance or nonintervention was not significantly associated with cyberbullying, but frequent parental control of their children's emails was linked to online victimization, a finding that leads to the authors' explanation that "perhaps parents who feel that something is bothering their children seek proof to confirm their suspicions."[40]

A cross-sectional study by Lam et al. (of 1,278 students in two main cities of Northeast China) aimed to determine a link between exposure to violent games and cyberbullying/victimization, and it documented that experience with moderately to severely aggressive online games was significantly linked with being both a perpetrator and a victim, as well as being a perpetrator only, of cyberbullying.[58] However, there was no evidence of a significant association between exposure to severe game violence and being a victim of cyberbullying.[58]

The effect of adolescents' exposure to media depicting antisocial and risky behavior on cyberbullying was investigated by den Hamer and Konijn[49] through a one-academic-year longitudinal study of 1,005 adolescents age 11 to 17. The research showed "that higher levels of exposure to media with antisocial and risk behavior content significantly contributed to higher initial rates of cyberbullying"[49] and that a surge in contact with antisocial media subjects was significantly associated with a rise of cyberbullying over time.[49]

Ill Effects of Cyberbullying

The association of cyberbullying victimization with self-reported health effects and substance abuse was examined by Kin et al.[65] in a study based on a second analysis of the 2014 Canadian General Social Survey on Victimization, which involved 31,907 participants age 15 or older living in the 10 provinces and territories. The results indicated that exposure to cybervictimization in the preceding 5 years was significantly associated with poor mental health [adjusted OR (AOR) = 4.26], binge drinking (AOR = 2.90), and drug use (AOR = 3.35).[65]

Fahy et al.[71] examined the association between involvement in cyberbullying and adolescent mental health in longitudinal research on 2,480 teenagers taking part in the Olympic Regeneration in East London study, which was developed to assess the impact of urban regeneration associated with the 2012 Olympic Games. The investigation documented that cybervictims and cyberbully-victims were significantly more likely than uninvolved adolescents to experience, at one-year follow-up, symptoms of depression (cybervictims, AOR = 1.44; cyberbully-victims, AOR = 1.54) and social anxiety (cybervictims, AOR = 1.52; cyberbully-victims, AOR = 1.44).[71]

A cross-sectional study by Sourander et al.[150] studied the link between cyberbullying and psychiatric/psychosomatic problems among 2,215 Finnish adolescents age 11 to 16 years. The analysis showed that cybervictims, as compared to noninvolved peers, were at higher risk of suffering from headaches (AOR = 3.1) or abdominal pain (AOR = 2.6) at least once a week or more frequently, as well as problems with falling asleep every, or almost every, night (AOR = 3.1).[150] Cyberbullies and cyberbully-victims were at higher risk of using alcohol once a week or more frequently (AOR = 6.1 and 6.3, respectively) as well as smoking weekly or daily (AOR = 2.9 and 2.7, respectively).[150]

Psychopathologic symptoms among participants of cyberbullying were investigated by Jung et al.[84] in a survey of 4,531 Korean youths (11 to 14 years old); the results showed that depressive and anxiety symptoms were significantly associated with cybervictims (AOR = 4.20), while aggressive behaviors were significantly associated with cyberbullies and cyberbully-victims (AOR = 2.9).[84]

Fu et al.[82] conducted an ecological study of 24 European countries to explore the relationship between cyberbullying and unnatural child death (accident, suicide, or assault), documenting that "countries with higher rates of cyberbullying were more likely to have a higher incidence of unnatural child death," without the "confounding effect of the national prevalence of depressive symptoms or traditional bullying."[82]

Prevention of Cyberbullying

As discussed in Chapter 7, among the few reported strategies to prevent cyberbullying are:

- Media Heroes,[151] a German cyberbullying prevention strategy that can be included in the regular school curriculum. The strategy is aimed at reducing cyberbullying by providing psychoeducation and social skills training through raising students' awareness about the nature and consequences of cyberbullying, fostering social responsibility, and enhancing the class climate, while also helping students to gain experience in self-protection.[151]

- The Cyber Friendly Schools (CFS) program, an Australian whole-school approach based on a "social-ecological conceptual framework"[98] intended to reduce cyberbullying by way of focusing on the online environments where students spent time, addressing the students' social competence in making positive cyber relationships, adopting Internet privacy and protection, promoting conduct and online skills, and promoting social responsibility, as well as raising awareness of legal issues while fostering reporting online.[98]
- The ConRed Program, a Spanish cyberbullying intervention initiative. ConRed is the abbreviation for the Spanish *Conocer, Construir and Convivir en la Red,* which translates as "The Knowing, Building and Living Together on the Internet Program."[152] ConRed utilizes a whole-school approach with a curriculum geared to foster empathy and sessions to raise awareness on Internet safety and to promote bullying prevention.[152]
- The KiVA program,[153] which is also used for prevention of traditional bullying, involves student lessons to raise awareness about the responsibility that the group has in preserving bullying or not and to foster empathy and support for the victim. The program also offers general guidance to parents.[153]

Cybercrime

Definition of Cybercrime

Gordon and Ford[154] defined cybercrime as "any crime that is facilitated or committed using a computer, network, or hardware device." This succinct but general definition takes into consideration the evolving range of computer-related crimes by providing a description that can be adapted to incorporate any future criminal variations in cyberoffending.[154] In the meantime, the characterization of cybercrime will vary according to international, national, or regional/ local legal recognition of any of the presently known forms of victimization associated with cyberspace.

Under the Council of Europe's Cybercrime Treaty of 2001,[155] each of the members of the Council of Europe formally agreed to adopt domestic legislation establishing as criminal offenses conduct pertaining to violations of the confidentiality, integrity, and availability of computer data and systems; computer-related transgressions; content-related offenses; and criminal infractions of copyright and related rights (Table14.4)

In the United States, the Computer Fraud and Abuse Act (CFAA), 18 U.S.C. 1030,[156] prohibits a range of behaviors, which were summarized by Doyle[157] as:

- Trespassing in a government computer
- Trespassing resulting in exposure of certain governmental, credit, financial, or commercial information
- Damaging a government computer, a bank computer, or a computer used in, or affecting, interstate or foreign commerce

Table 14.4. Types of Cyberoffenses Established by The Council of Europe's Cybercrime Treaty of 2001[155]

Illegal access[a]—Intentional access to the whole or any part of a computer system without right, by infringing security measures, with the intent of obtaining computer data or other dishonest intent, or in relation to a computer system that is connected to another computer system.	Computer-related forgery[b]—Intentionally and without right causing input, alteration, deletion, or suppression of computer data, resulting in inauthentic data with the intent that it be considered or acted on as if it were authentic, regardless of whether the data is directly readable and intelligible.
Illegal interception[a]—Intentional interception without right, made by technical means, of nonpublic transmissions of computer data to, from, or within a computer system, including electromagnetic emissions from a computer system carrying such computer data.	Computer-related fraud[b]—Intentionally causing the loss of property to another person by (a) any input, alteration, deletion, or suppression of computer data; (b) any interference with the functioning of a computer system, with fraudulent or dishonest intent of procuring, without right, an economic benefit for oneself or for another person.
Data interference[a]—Intentional damage, deletion, deterioration, alteration, or suppression of computer data without right.	Offenses related to child pornography[c]—Intentional commitment without right through a computer system of production, offer, distribution, or possession of child pornography.
System interference[a]—Intentional serious hindering without right of the functioning of a computer system by inputting, transmitting, damaging, deleting, deteriorating, altering, or suppressing computer data.	Offenses related to infringements of copyright and related rights.

[a] Offenses against the confidentiality, integrity, and availability of computer data and systems.

[b] Computer-related offenses.

[c] Content-related offenses.

- Committing fraud, an integral part of which involves unauthorized access to a government computer, a bank computer, or a computer used in, or affecting, interstate or foreign commerce
- Threatening to damage a government computer, a bank computer, or a computer used in, or affecting, interstate or foreign commerce
- Trafficking in passwords for a government computer, or when the trafficking affects interstate or foreign commerce
- Accessing a computer to commit espionage

Broadhurst[158] developed a broad typology of cybercrimes, with six categories:

- Interference with a lawful use of a computer (e.g., cybervandalism and terrorism, denial of service, or insertion of viruses, worms, and other malicious codes)[158]
- Dissemination of offensive materials (e.g., pornography/child pornography, racist content, treasonous or sacrilegious content)[158]
- Threatening communications (e.g., extortion, cyberstalking)[158]
- Forgery/counterfeiting (e.g., ID theft; IP offenses; software, CD, or DVD piracy; copyright breaches)[158]

- Fraud (e.g., payment card fraud, efunds transfer fraud, theft of Internet and telephone services, auction house and catalog fraud, consumer fraud, online securities fraud)[158]
- Other (such as illegal interception of communications, commercial/corporate espionage, communications in furtherance of criminal conspiracies, electronic money laundering)[158]

Prevalence of Cybercrime

The Federal Bureau of Investigation (FBI) 2020 Internet Crime Report[159] showed that, during the year 2020, the Internet Crime Complaint Center (IC3) received complaints about cybercrime perpetrated in the United States affecting 465,177 victims.

Fifty percent of the victims were, at least, exposed to either phishing,[160] vishing,[161] smishing,[162] or pharming[163] (and pharming includes "the use of unsolicited email, text messages, and telephone calls purportedly from a legitimate company requesting personal, financial, and/or login credentials").[159] Furthermore, not less than 23% of the victims were subjected to nonpayment for goods or services delivered or nondelivery of goods or services for which payment was made, while 16% of the victims were put at risk by extortion, 10% were endangered by a personal data breach, and 9% suffered from identity theft. Moreover, approximately 5% of the 2020 cybercrime victims in the United States suffered from either spoofing,[164] misrepresentation,[165] confidence fraud/romance,[166] harassment/threat of violence, business or personal email compromise, credit card fraud, government impersonation, crimes against children,[167] ransomware demands,[168] and/or malware/scareware/virus.[169]

The FBI 2020 Internet Crime Report also documented 707,217 victims of cybercrime in 21 countries, with almost 66% of the victims (465,177) having made reports in the United States, representing a rate of 1,400 victims per one million Internet users.[170] The US reporting rate was second only to the national frequency in the United Kingdom, where, in 2020, the estimated rate was 3,333 reported cybercrime victims per one million Internet users[170] (Table 14.5).

Correlates of Cybercrime

Srivastava et al.[171] investigated the factors affecting the cybercrime originating in a country by analyzing the data from 124 countries in relation to economic capital,[172] technological capital,[173] and cybersecurity preparedness.[174] This study demonstrated that "the economic capital and technological capital of a country are the primary factors that influence the frequency of cybercrime originating within it."[171] Also, the technological capital partially facilitates the link between economic capital of a country with its cybercrime frequency. Moreover, "the cybersecurity preparedness of a nation negatively moderates the relationship between technological capital and frequency of cybercrime originating within it."[171]

De Kimpe et al.[175] studied the relationship between Internet users' perceived knowledge about cybercrime and their trust about the Internet with their motivation for cybercrime prevention. This research,[175] based on a survey of 937 adult Belgian Internet users, showed that the participants who felt knowledgeable about online safety felt less vulnerable to cybercrime and were less likely to take protection actions. While feeling informed was linked with being more persuaded about the dangerousness of cybercrime, having high levels of

Table 14.5. Reported Number of Cybercrime Victims and Rates of Reported Cybercrime Victims in Top 21 International Victim Countries[159] for 2020

Country	Cybercrime Victims (N)[a]	Rate of Cybercrime Victims (Number per One Million Internet Users[b])	Country	Cybercrime Victims (N)[a]	Rate of Cybercrime Victims (Number per One Million Internet Users[b])
United Kingdom	216,633	3,333	Canada	5,399	15
United States	465,177	1,400	Italy	728	15
Belgium	1,023	98	Spain	618	15
Australia	1,807	81	Mexico	1,164	13
Hong Kong	407	60	Philippines	898	12
South Africa	1,754	48	Colombia	418	12
Greece	2,314	28	Brazil	951	6
France	1,640	28	Pakistan	443	6
Netherlands	450	25	Nigeria	443	5
Germany	1,578	20	India	2,930	4
			China	442	0.5

[a] Reported number of cybercrime victims for 2020, according to Federal Bureau of Investigation, Internet Crime Complaint Center, Internet Crime Report, 2020.[159]

[b] Estimated based on the number cybercrime victims[159] and the number of Internet users[170] for a given country for year 2000.

confidence in the safety of the Internet was linked to the feeling of being less vulnerable to cybercrime, and the perception that cybercrime is not a severe threat.[175] This study[175] also showed that Internet users with a higher level of education trusted the Internet less and were less convinced that they have the skills necessary to implement safety measures.[175]

Abdelhamid[176] investigated the effect of personality-based factors, such as health concerns, disposition to trust, and risk-taking, on phishing susceptibility in healthcare-related attacks. This study,[176] based on 200 adult participants residing in the United States, documented that health concerns led to higher phishing susceptibility; yet there was a larger influence of disposition to trust than of health concerns on phishing predisposition, and, above all, risk-taking propensity yields the highest phishing liability.[176] Male participants were found to have a lower phishing susceptibility than females.[176]

Impact of Cybercrime

Cheng et al.[177] investigated the effect of cybercrime victimization on self-perception of interpersonal relations, perceived control, perceived fairness, and subjective well-being through a population-based telephone survey of 1,018 Hong Kong participants, who were asked whether they experienced, in the previous year, any of the 10 most common types of cybercrime according to the Cyber Security and Technology Crime Bureau of the Hong Kong Police Force. The cybercrimes included online game-related crime, Internet/email account abuse, email scams, hacking, online shopping fraud, other online fraud, credit card misuse, online child pornography, social media deception, and naked chats. The findings[177] indicated that victims of cybercrime were significantly less trusting only of people online, but no significant relationship was found between cybercrime victimization and trust of all other members of offline social networks, including people met for the first time. Cybercrime victimization was also inversely related to perceived control, perceived fairness, and subjective well-being (i.e., the cognitive component of life satisfaction and affective component of happiness).[177]

Cybercrime during the COVID-19 Pandemic

The increase in cybercrime during the first half of 2020, coinciding with the beginning of the COVID-19 pandemic,[178-180] was highlighted by Monteith et a.[181]

A joint alert[178] from the United States Cybersecurity and Infrastructure Security Agency (CISA) and the United Kingdom's National Cyber Security Centre (NCSC) raised awareness about a "growing use of COVID-19-related themes by malicious cyber actors,"[178] which coincided with the surge of teleworking leading to the "increment in the use of potentially vulnerable services, such as virtual private networks (VPNs)."[178] This warning[178] specified that advanced persistent threat groups and cybercriminals were exploiting COVID-19 as a lure for phishing and for malware distribution. They were also registering new domain names containing wording related to coronavirus or COVID-19 and attacking newly deployed remote access and teleworking infrastructure.[178] The FBI indicated that, during the first five months of 2020, the IC3 received 320,000 complaints, almost the same number that they had received during the entire 12 months of 2019 (~ 400,000).

Monteith et al.[181] discussed the psychological implications of the increase in cybercrime coinciding with the COVID-19 pandemic.[178-180] They pointed out the psychological impact on victims of online fraud,[182] while also considering that mental illness may increase vulnerability to cybercrime. In support of the emotional risk affecting victims of cybercrime, the Monteith article[181] cited research by Golladay and Holtfreter[182] that ascertained the emotional and physical health impact of identity theft, which showed that recent (previous 12 months) identity theft victimization was very significantly associated with levels of emotional distress (anxiety, anger, depression) and physical consequences (headaches, high blood pressure, backaches). This association remained significant even after adjustment for previous victimization. The argument by Monteith et al.[181] that mental illness may increase vulnerability to cybercrime was partly derived from a 2012 study by Lichtenberg et al.[183] that used longitudinal data from the Health and Retirement Study.[184] The date indicated that having more depressive symptoms, as measured by the eight-item version of the CES-D,[185] significantly predicted new cases of fraud. The proposal by Monteith et al.[181] also originated from the results of a study by Claycomb et al.[186] that documented that at least 75% of a sample of 122 participants receiving psychiatric treatment who also received Social Security disability payment had experienced financial victimization in the previous month.[186] It should also be noted that this victimization occurred more frequently among participants who were younger, had more frequent psychiatric hospitalizations, used more alcohol in the previous 28 days, or had problems in managing their money.[186]

Future Directions

Future research to determine cross-country comparisons of youth prevalence of cyberbullying and its health correlates would benefit from having access to the national data collected by countries or territories in the GSHS.[187-189] Such a methodological approach would follow in the steps of the study by Nguyen et al.,[190] who applied GSHS data regarding the frequency of cyberbullying among adolescents in Vietnam. The GSHS[187-189] was developed by the World Health Organization (WHO) in collaboration with United Nations' UNICEF, UNESCO, and UNAIDS, and with technical assistance from the US Centers for Disease Control and Prevention, to generate data on health and social behavior among adolescents. It is a collaborative surveillance project designed to help countries measure and assess the behavioral risk factors and protective factors in 10 key areas among young people 13 to 17 years old. As of December 2013, representatives from more than 120 countries had been trained, and 94 countries had completed a GSHS. The GSHS data are owned by the official country-level agency[191] (e.g., Ministry of Health) that conducted or sponsored the survey. The GSHS questionnaires developed since 2017[192,193] include questions about exposure to cyberbullying in the previous year, providing cross-national data for comparison of prevalence of cyberbullying as well as associated health risks in more than 90 countries and territories, beyond the scope of nations already being regularly surveyed by the HBSC.[139]

There is also a need for cross-sectional studies, based on national representative samples, to establish cross-country comparisons of the prevalence of cyberbullying among adults. In this context, it would be advisable to utilize a uniform cybervictimization definition that is specific and inclusive of the forms of maltreatment in cyberspace, by incorporating not only typical bullying behaviors (e.g., being made fun of or called names, being harassed, having rumors spread about one), but also behaviors typical of cyberbullying (e.g., broadcasting, dissing, flaming) as well as cybercrimes (e.g., insertion of viruses, worms, and other malicious codes; ID theft).

The development of longitudinal studies is critical to understanding the antecedents and health consequence of exposure to cyberbullying across the life span, as well as its association with other forms of victimization.

Notes

1. Gibson W. *Neuromancer*. New York, NY: Ace Books, 1984. Cited by Strate L. The varieties of cyberspace: problems in definition and delimitation. *West J Commun*. 1999;63(3):382–412.
2. Hogan MD, Newton EM. *Supplemental Information for the Interagency Report on Strategic US Government Engagement in International Standardization to Achieve US Objectives for Cybersecurity*, Annex A, Terms and Definitions, page 41, NISTIR 8074, Volume 2. https://nvlpubs.nist.gov/nistpubs/ir/2015/NIST.IR.8074v2.pdf. Accessed June 2, 2021.
3. Morley D, Robins K. *Spaces of Identity: Global Media, Electronic Landscapes, and Cultural Boundaries*. London, England: Routledge; 1995.. Cited by Kitchin RM. Towards geographies of cyberspace. *Prog Hum Geogr*. 1998;22(3):385–406. http://mural.maynoothuniversity.ie/3919/1/RK_cyberspace.pdf. Accessed August 22, 2022.

4. Paulson A. Internet bullying. *The Christian Science Monitor.* December 30, 2003. https://www.csmonitor.com/2003/1230/p11s01-legn.html. Accessed August 22, 2022.
5. Servance RL. Cyberbullying, cyber-harassment, and the conflict between schools and the first amendment. *Wis Law Rev*. 2003:1213.
6. Moreno MA, Suthamjariya N, Selkie E. Stakeholder perceptions of cyberbullying cases: application of the uniform definition of bullying. *J Adolesc Health*. 2018;62(4):444–449.
7. Englander E, Donnerstein E, Kowalski R, Lin CA, Parti K. Defining cyberbullying. *Pediatrics.* 2017;140(suppl 2):S148–S151.
8. Runions KC, Bak M, Shaw T. Disentangling functions of online aggression: The Cyber-Aggression Typology Questionnaire (CATQ). *Aggress Behav*. 2017;43(1):74–84.
9. Betts LR, Spenser KA. Developing the cyber victimization experiences and cyberbullying behaviors scales. *J Genet Psychol*. 2017;178(3):147–164.
10. Hutson E. Cyberbullying in adolescence: a concept analysis. *Adv Nurs Sci*. 2016;39(1):60–70.
11. Alipan A, Skues J, Theiler S, Wise L. Defining cyberbullying: a multiple perspectives approach. *Annual Review of Cybertherapy and Telemedicine 2015: Virtual Reality in Healthcare: Medical Simulation and Experiential Interface*. 2016;219:9.
12. Carter JM, Wilson FL. Cyberbullying: a 21st century health care phenomenon. *Pediatr Nurs.* 2015;41(3):115.
13. Wright MF, Li Y. Normative beliefs about aggression and cyber aggression among young adults: a longitudinal investigation. *Aggress Behav*. 2013;39(3):161–170.
14. Menesini E, Nocentini A, Palladino BE, et al. Cyberbullying definition among adolescents: a comparison across six European countries. *Cyberpsychol Behav Soc Netw*. 2012;15(9):455–463.
15. Ybarra ML, Boyd D, Korchmaros JD, Oppenheim JK. Defining and measuring cyberbullying within the larger context of bullying victimization. *J Adolesc Health*. 2012;51(1):53–58.
16. Langos C. Cyberbullying: the challenge to define. *Cyberpsychol Behav Soc Netw.* 2012;15(6):285–289.
17. Vandebosch H, Van Cleemput K. Defining cyberbullying: a qualitative research into the perceptions of youngsters. *Cyberpsychol Behav*. 2008;11(4):499–503.
18. Slonje R, Smith PK. Cyberbullying: another main type of bullying? *Scand J Psychol*. 2008 Apr 1;49(2):147–154.
19. Ruiz-Maza JC, Sanchez-Salvatierra JM, Moreno-Arteaga CM. Cyberbullying in Peruvian schoolchildren and associated factors: analysis of a national survey. *Medwave.* 2017;17(7):e7015.
20. Rao J, Wang H, Pang M, et al. Cyberbullying perpetration and victimization among junior and senior high school students in Guangzhou, China. *Inj Prev*. 2019;25(1):13–19.
21. Gkiomisi A, Gkrizioti M, Gkiomisi A, Anastasilakis DA, Kardaras P. Cyberbullying among Greek high school adolescents. *Indian J Pediatrics*. 2017;84(5):364–368.
22. Brochado S, Soares S, Fraga S. A scoping review on studies of cyberbullying prevalence among adolescents. *Trauma Violence Abuse*. 2017;18(5):523–531.
23. Selkie EM, Fales JL, Moreno MA. Cyberbullying prevalence among US middle and high school–aged adolescents: a systematic review and quality assessment. *J Adolesc Health.* 2016;58(2):125–133.
24. Kessel Schneider S, O'Donnell L, Smith E. Trends in cyberbullying and school bullying victimization in a regional census of high school students, 2006–2012. *J Sch Health.* 2015;85(9):611–620.

25. Hamm MP, Newton AS, Chisholm A, et al. Prevalence and effect of cyberbullying on children and young people: a scoping review of social media studies. *JAMA Pediatrics*. 2015;169(8):770–777.
26. Gan SS, Zhong C, Das S, Gan JS, Willis S, Tully E. The prevalence of bullying and cyberbullying in high school: a 2011 survey. *Int J Adolesc Med Health*. 2014;26(1):27–31.
27. Lindfors PL, Kaltiala-Heino R, Rimpelä AH. Cyberbullying among Finnish adolescents—a population-based study. *BMC Public Health*. 2012;12(1):1027.
28. Arslan S, Savaser S, Hallett V, Balci S. Cyberbullying among primary school students in Turkey: self-reported prevalence and associations with home and school life. *Cyberpsychol Behav Soc Netw*. 2012;15(10):527–533.
29. Aricak T, Siyahhan S, Uzunhasanoglu A, et al. Cyberbullying among Turkish adolescents. *Cyberpsychol Behav*. 2008;11(3):253–261.
30. Garaigordobil M, Machimbarrena JM. Stress, competence, and parental educational styles in victims and aggressors of bullying and cyberbullying. *Psicothema*. 2017;29(3):335–340.
31. Wachs S, Whittle HC, Hamilton-Giachritsis C, Wolf KD, Vazsonyi AT, Junger M. Correlates of mono-and dual-victims of cybergrooming and cyberbullying: evidence from four countries. *Cyberpsychol Behav Soc Netw.* 2018;21(2):91–98.
32. Pfetsch JS. Empathic skills and cyberbullying: relationship of different measures of empathy to cyberbullying in comparison to offline bullying among young adults. *J Genet Psychol.* 2017;178(1):58–72.
33. Lee JY, Kwon Y, Yang S, Park S, Kim EM, Na EY. Differences in friendship networks and experiences of cyberbullying among Korean and Australian adolescents. *J Genet Psychol.* 2017;178(1):44–57.
34. Barlett C, Chamberlin K, Witkower Z. Predicting cyberbullying perpetration in emerging adults: a theoretical test of the Barlett Gentile Cyberbullying Model. *Aggress Behav.* 2017;43(2):147–154.
35. Fan CY, Chu XW, Zhang M, Zhou ZK. Are narcissists more likely to be involved in cyberbullying? Examining the mediating role of self-esteem. *J Interpers Violence*. 2016:0886260516666531.
36. Hong JS, Lee J, Espelage DL, Hunter SC, Patton DU, Rivers T. Understanding the correlates of face-to-face and cyberbullying victimization among US adolescents: a social-ecological analysis. *Violence Vict*. 2016;31(4):638.
37. Festl R, Quandt T. The role of online communication in long-term cyberbullying involvement among girls and boys. *J Youth Adolescence*. 2016;45(9):1931–1945.
38. Khoury-Kassabri M, Mishna F, Massarwi AA. Cyberbullying perpetration by Arab youth: the direct and interactive role of individual, family, and neighborhood characteristics. *J Interpers Violence*. 2019;34(12):2498–2524.
39. Orue I, Calvete E. Psychopathic traits and moral disengagement interact to predict bullying and cyberbullying among adolescents. *J Interpers Violence*. 2016:0886260516660302.
40. Sasson H, Mesch G. The role of parental mediation and peer norms on the likelihood of cyberbullying. *J Genet Psychol*. 2017;178(1):15–27.
41. Olenik-Shemesh D, Heiman T. Cyberbullying victimization in adolescents as related to body esteem, social support, and social self-efficacy. J Genet Psychol. 2017;178(1):28–43.
42. Sampasa-Kanyinga H, Hamilton HA. Use of social networking sites and risk of cyberbullying victimization: a population-level study of adolescents. *Cyberpsychol Behav Soc Netw.* 2015;18(12):704–710.

43. Meter DJ, Bauman S. When sharing is a bad idea: the effects of online social network engagement and sharing passwords with friends on cyberbullying involvement. *Cyberpsychol Behav Soc Netw*. 2015;18(8):437–442.
44. Runions KC, Bak M. Online moral disengagement, cyberbullying, and cyber-aggression. *Cyberpsychol Behav Soc Netw*. 2015;18(7):400–405.
45. Shin N, Ahn H. Factors affecting adolescents' involvement in cyberbullying: what divides the 20% from the 80%? *Cyberpsychol Behav Soc Netw*. 2015;18(7):393–399.
46. Van Ouytsel J, Walrave M, Vandebosch H. Correlates of cyberbullying and how school nurses can respond. *NASN Sch Nurse*. 2015;30(3):162–170.
47. Barlińska J, Szuster A, Winiewski M. The role of short- and long-term cognitive empathy activation in preventing cyberbystander reinforcing cyberbullying behavior. *Cyberpsychol Behav Soc Netw*. 2015;18(4):241–244.
48. Chang FC, Chiu CH, Miao NF, et al. Online gaming and risks predict cyberbullying perpetration and victimization in adolescents. *Int J Public Health*. 2015;60(2):257–266.
49. den Hamer AH, Konijn EA. Adolescents' media exposure may increase their cyberbullying behavior: a longitudinal study. *J Adolesc Health*. 2015;56(2):203–208.
50. Hemphill SA, Heerde JA. Adolescent predictors of young adult cyberbullying perpetration and victimization among Australian youth. *J Adolesc Health*. 2014;55(4):580–587.
51. Van Cleemput K, Vandebosch H, Pabian S. Personal characteristics, and contextual factors that determine "helping," "joining in," and "doing nothing" when witnessing cyberbullying. *Aggress Behav*. 2014;40(5):383–396.
52. Ciucci E, Baroncelli A. Emotion-related personality traits and peer social standing: unique and interactive effects in cyberbullying behaviors. *Cyberpsychol Behav Soc Netw*. 2014;17(9):584–590.
53. Chng GS, Liau A, Khoo A, Li D. Parental mediation and cyberbullying—a longitudinal study. *Stud Health Technol Inform*. 2014;199:98–102.
54. Floros GD, Siomos KE, Fisoun V, Dafouli E, Geroukalis D. Adolescent online cyberbullying in Greece: the impact of parental online security practices, bonding, and online impulsiveness. *J Sch Health*. 2013;83(6):445–453.
55. Shapka JD, Law DM. Does one size fit all? Ethnic differences in parenting behaviors and motivations for adolescent engagement in cyberbullying. *J Youth Adolescence*. 2013;42(5):723–738.
56. Elledge LC, Williford A, Boulton AJ, DePaolis KJ, Little TD, Salmivalli C. Individual, and contextual predictors of cyberbullying: the influence of children's provictim attitudes and teachers' ability to intervene. J *Youth Adolescence*. 2013;42(5):698–710.
57. Hinduja S, Patchin JW. Social influences on cyberbullying behaviors among middle and high school students. *J Youth Adolescence*. 2013;42(5):711–722.
58. Lam LT, Cheng Z, Liu X. Violent online games exposure and cyberbullying/victimization among adolescents. *Cyberpsychol Behav Soc Netw*. 2013;16(3):159–165.
59. Wachs S, D Wolf K, Pan CC. Cybergrooming: risk factors, coping strategies and associations with cyberbullying. *Psicothema*. 2012;24(4).
60. Ang RP, Goh DH. Cyberbullying among adolescents: the role of affective and cognitive empathy, and gender. *Child Psychiatry Hum Dev*. 2010;41(4):387–397.. Cited by Kowalski et al (see Note 117).
61. Wright MF. The role of technologies, behaviors, gender, and gender stereotype traits in adolescents' cyber aggression. *J Interpers Violence*. 2017:0886260517696858.

62. Wright MF. Predictors of anonymous cyber aggression: the role of adolescents' beliefs about anonymity, aggression, and the permanency of digital content. *Cyberpsychol Behav Soc Netw*. 2014;17(7):431–438.
63. Wright MF. The relationship between young adults' beliefs about anonymity and subsequent cyber aggression. *Cyberpsychol Behav Soc Netw*. 2013;16(12):858–862.
64. Modecki KL, Barber BL, Vernon L. Mapping developmental precursors of cyber-aggression: trajectories of risk predict perpetration and victimization. *J Youth Adolescence*. 2013;42(5):651–661.
65. Kim S, Boyle MH, Georgiades K. Cyberbullying victimization and its association with health across the life course: a Canadian population study. *Can J Public Health*. 2018;108(5-6):468–474.
66. Erreygers S, Vandebosch H, Vranjes I, Baillien E, De Witte H. The longitudinal association between poor sleep quality and cyberbullying, mediated by anger. *Health Commun*. 2018:1–7.
67. Ramos Salazar L. Cyberbullying victimization as a predictor of cyberbullying perpetration, body image dissatisfaction, healthy eating and dieting behaviors, and life satisfaction. *J Interpers Violence*. 2017:0886260517725737.
68. Kenny U, Sullivan L, Callaghan M, Molcho M, Kelly C. The relationship between cyberbullying and friendship dynamics on adolescent body dissatisfaction: a cross-sectional study. *J Health Psychol*. 2017:1359105316684939.
69. Kritsotakis G, Papanikolaou M, Androulakis E, Philalithis AE. Associations of bullying and cyberbullying with substance use and sexual risk taking in young adults. *J Nurs Scholarsh*. 2017;49(4):360–370.
70. Sampasa-Kanyinga H. Co-occurring cyberbullying and school bullying victimization and associations with mental health problems among Canadian middle and high school students. *Violence Vict*. 2017;32(4):671–687.
71. Fahy AE, Stansfeld SA, Smuk M, Smith NR, Cummins S, Clark C. Longitudinal associations between cyberbullying involvement and adolescent mental health. *J Adolesc Health*. 2016;59(5):502–509.
72. Tural Hesapcioglu S, Ercan F. Traditional and cyberbullying co-occurrence, and its relationship to psychiatric symptoms. *Pediatrics Int*. 2017;59(1):16–22.
73. Hébert M, Cénat JM, Blais M, Lavoie F, Guerrier M. Child sexual abuse, bullying, cyberbullying, and mental health problems among high schools students: a moderated mediated model. *Depress Anxiety*. 2016;33(7):623–629.
74. Ranney ML, Patena JV, Nugent N, et al. PTSD, cyberbullying, and peer violence: prevalence and correlates among adolescent emergency department patients. *Gen Hosp Psychiatry*. 2016;39:32–38.
75. Bottino SM, Bottino C, Regina CG, Correia AV, Ribeiro WS. Cyberbullying and adolescent mental health: systematic review. *Cad Saude Publica*. 2015;31:463–475.
76. Selkie EM, Kota R, Chan YF, Moreno M. Cyberbullying, depression, and problem alcohol use in female college students: a multisite study. *Cyberpsychol Behav Soc Netw*. 2015;18(2):79–86.
77. Spears BA, Taddeo CM, Daly AL, Stretton A, Karklins LT. Cyberbullying, help-seeking and mental health in young Australians: implications for public health. *Int J Public Health*. 2015;60(2):219–226.
78. Cénat JM, Hébert M, Blais M, Lavoie F, Guerrier M, Derivois D. Cyberbullying, psychological distress, and self-esteem among youth in Quebec schools. *J Affective Disord*. 2014;169:7–9.

79. Gini G, Espelage DL. Peer victimization, cyberbullying, and suicide risk in children and adolescents. *JAMA*. 2014;312(5):545–546.
80. Nixon CL. Current perspectives: the impact of cyberbullying on adolescent health. *Adolesc Health Med Ther*. 2014;5:143.
81. Sampasa-Kanyinga H, Roumeliotis P, Farrow CV, Shi YF. Breakfast skipping is associated with cyberbullying and school bullying victimization: a school-based cross-sectional study. *Appetite*. 2014;79:76–82.
82. Fu KW, Chan CH, Ip P. Exploring the relationship between cyberbullying and unnatural child death: an ecological study of twenty-four European countries. *BMC Pediatrics*. 2014;14(1):195.
83. Messias E, Kindrick K, Castro J. School bullying, cyberbullying, or both: correlates of teen suicidality in the 2011 CDC Youth Risk Behavior Survey. *Compr Psychiatry*. 2014;55(5):1063–1068.
84. Jung YE, Leventhal B, Kim YS, et al. Cyberbullying, problematic internet use, and psychopathologic symptoms among Korean youth. *Yonsei Med J*. 2014;55(3):826–830.
85. Magaud E, Nyman K, Addington J. Cyberbullying in those at clinical high risk for psychosis. *Early Intervent Psychiatry*. 2013;7(4):427–430.
86. Gámez-Guadix M, Orue I, Smith PK, Calvete E. Longitudinal and reciprocal relations of cyberbullying with depression, substance use, and problematic internet use among adolescents. *J Adolesc Health*. 2013;53(4):446–452.
87. Ortega R, Elipe P, Mora-Merchán JA, et al. The emotional impact of bullying and cyberbullying on victims: a European cross-national study. *Aggress Behav*. 2012;38(5):342–356.
88. Goebert D, Else I, Matsu C, Chung-Do J, Chang JY. The impact of cyberbullying on substance use and mental health in a multiethnic sample. *Matern Child Health J*. 2011;15(8):1282–1286.
89. Rose CA, Tynes BM. Longitudinal associations between cybervictimization and mental health among US adolescents. *J Adolesc Health*. 2015;57(3):305–312.
90. Vieno A, Gini G, Lenzi M, Pozzoli T, Canale N, Santinello M. Cybervictimization and somatic and psychological symptoms among Italian middle school students. *Eur J Public Health*. 2014;25(3):433–437.
91. Fridh M, Lindström M, Rosvall M. Subjective health complaints in adolescent victims of cyber harassment: moderation through support from parents/friends—a Swedish population-based study. *BMC Public Health*. 2015;15(1):949.
92. Roberto AJ, Eden J, Deiss DM, Savage MW, Ramos-Salazar L. The short-term effects of a cyberbullying prevention intervention for parents of middle school students. *Int J Environ Res Public Health*. 2017;14(9):1038.
93. Espelage DL, Hong JS. Cyberbullying prevention and intervention efforts: current knowledge and future directions. *Can J Psychiatry*. 2017;62(6):374–380.
94. Savage MW, Deiss DM Jr, Roberto AJ, Aboujaoude E. Theory-based formative research on an anti-cyberbullying victimization intervention message. *J Health Commun*. 2017;22(2):124–134.
95. Palladino BE, Nocentini A, Menesini E. Evidence-based intervention against bullying and cyberbullying: evaluation of the NoTrap! program in two independent trials. *Aggress Behav*. 2016;42(2):194–206.
96. Gradinger P, Yanagida T, Strohmeier D, Spiel C. Effectiveness, and sustainability of the ViSC Social Competence Program to prevent cyberbullying and cyber-victimization: class and individual level moderators. *Aggress Behav*. 2016;42(2):181–193.

97. Chaux E, Velásquez AM, Schultze-Krumbholz A, Scheithauer H. Effects of the cyberbullying prevention program media heroes (Medienhelden) on traditional bullying. *Aggress Behav*. 2016;42(2):157–165.
98. Cross D, Shaw T, Hadwen K, et al. Longitudinal impact of the Cyber Friendly Schools program on adolescents' cyberbullying behavior. *Aggress Behav*. 2016;42(2):166–180.
99. Barkoukis V, Lazuras L, Ourda D, Tsorbatzoudis H. Tackling psychosocial risk factors for adolescent cyberbullying: evidence from a school-based intervention. *Aggress Behav*. 2016;42(2):114–122.
100. Garaigordobil M, Martínez-Valderrey V. Effects of Cyberprogram 2.0 on "face-to-face" bullying, cyberbullying, and empathy. *Psicothema*. 2015;27(1).
101. Jacobs NC, Völlink T, Dehue F, Lechner L. Online Pestkoppenstoppen: systematic and theory-based development of a web-based tailored intervention for adolescent cyberbully victims to combat and prevent cyberbullying. *BMC Public Health*. 2014;14(1):396.
102. Roberto AJ, Eden J, Savage MW, Ramos-Salazar L, Deiss DM. Outcome evaluation results of school-based cybersafety promotion and cyberbullying prevention intervention for middle school students. *Health Commun*. 2014;29(10):1029–1042.
103. Williford A, Elledge LC, Boulton AJ, DePaolis KJ, Little TD, Salmivalli C. Effects of the KiVa Antibullying Program on cyberbullying and cybervictimization frequency among Finnish youth. *J Clin Child Adolesc Psychol*. 2013;42(6):820–833.
104. Hinduja S, Patchin JW. *Bullying Beyond the Schoolyard: Preventing and Responding to Cyberbullying*. Thousand Oaks, California, US: Corwin Press; 2009.
105. Kowalski RM, Limber SP, Agatston PW. *Cyberbullying: Bullying in the Digital Age*. Hoboken, New Jersey, USA: John Wiley & Sons; 2012.
106. Li Q, Cross D, Smith PK, eds. *Cyberbullying in the Global Playground: Research from International Perspectives*. John Wiley & Sons; 2012.
107. Patchin JW, Hinduja S, eds. *Cyberbullying Prevention and Response: Expert Perspectives*. Milton Park, Abingdon, Oxfordshire, UK: Routledge; 2012..
108. Hinduja S, Patchin JW. *School Climate 2.0: Preventing Cyberbullying and Sexting One Classroom at a Time*. Hoboken, New Jersey, USA: Corwin Press; 2012..
109. Patchin JW, Hinduja S. *Words Wound: Delete Cyberbullying and Make Kindness Go Viral*. Minneapolis, MN: Free Spirit Publishing; 2013..
110. Smith PK, Steffgen G. *Cyberbullying through the New Media: Findings from an International Network*. New York, NY, USA: Psychology Press; 2013..
111. Patchin JW, Hinduja S. *Bullying Today: Bullet Points and Best Practices*. Thousand Oaks, CA, USA: Corwin Press; 2016.
112. Patchin JW, Hinduja S. Bullies move beyond the schoolyard: a preliminary look at cyberbullying. *Youth Violence Juv Just*. 2006;4(2):148–169..
113. Gladden RM, Vivolo-Kantor AM, Hamburger ME, Lumpkin CD. *Bullying Surveillance Among Youths: Uniform Definitions for Public Health and Recommended Data Elements*, Version 1.0. Atlanta, GA; Centers for Disease Control and Prevention; 2014:7.. http://www.cdc.gov/violenceprevention/pdf/bullying-definitions-final-a.pdf. Accessed August 22, 2022.
114. According to the uniform definition, "Bullying is any unwanted aggressive behavior(s) by another youth or group of youths who are not siblings or current dating partners that involves an observed or perceived power imbalance and is repeated multiple times or is highly likely to be repeated. Bullying may inflict harm or distress on the targeted youth including physical, psychological, social, or educational harm."

115. Spears B, Slee P, Owens L, Johnson B. Behind the scenes and screens: insights into the human dimension of covert and cyberbullying. *Z Psychol.* 2009;217(4):189–196. Cited by Menesini et al.[14]
116. Nocentini A, Calmaestra J, Schultze-Krumbholz A, Scheithauer H, Ortega R, Menesini E. Cyberbullying: labels, behaviours, and definition in three European countries. *J Psychol Couns Sch.* 2010;20(2):129–142. Cited by Menesini et al.[14]
117. Kowalski RM, Giumetti GW, Schroeder AN, Lattanner MR. Bullying in the digital age: a critical review and meta-analysis of cyberbullying research among youth. *Psychol Bull.* 2014;140(4):1073.
118. Mishna F, Khoury-Kassabri M, Gadalla T, Daciuk J. Risk factors for involvement in cyber bullying: victims, bullies and bully-victims. *Child Youth Serv Rev.* 2012;34(1):63–70.. Cited by Kowalski et al.[117]
119. Hinduja S, Patchin JW. Cyberbullying: an exploratory analysis of factors related to offending and victimization. *Deviant Behav.* 2008;29(2):129–156. Cited by Kowalski et al.[117]
120. Yilmaz H. Cyberbullying in Turkish middle schools: an exploratory study. *Sch Psychol Int.* 2011;32(6):645–654. Cited by Kowalski et al.[117]
121. Akbulut Y, Eristi B. Cyberbullying and victimisation among Turkish university students. *Australas J Educ Technol.* 2011;27(7):1155–1170. Cited by Kowalski et al.[117]
122. Tynes BM, Rose CA, Williams DR. The development and validation of the online victimization scale for adolescents. *Cyberpsychology.* 2010;4(2). Cited by Kowalski et al.[117]
123. Goebert D, Else I, Matsu C, Chung-Do J, Chang JY. The impact of cyberbullying on substance use and mental health in a multiethnic sample. *Matern Child Health J.* 2011;15(8):1282–1286. Cited by Kowalski et al.[117]
124. Çetin B, Yaman E, Peker A. Cyber Victim and Bullying Scale: a study of validity and reliability. *Comput Educ.* 2011;57(4):2261–2271.. Cited by Kowalski et al.[117]
125. Palasinski M. Turning assault into a "harmless prank"—teenage perspectives on happy slapping. *J Interpers Violence.* 2013;28(9):1909–1923.
126. Lenhart A. Cyberbullying. Pew Internet & American Life Project. Retrieved from http://www.pewinternet.org/2007/06/27/cyberbullying/. Last updated August 22, 2022.
127. Beran T, Li Q. Cyber-harassment: A study of a new method for an old behavior. *J Educ Comput Res.* 2005;32(3):265–277. Cited by Kowalski et al.[117]
128. Gradinger P, Strohmeier D, Spiel C. Motives for bullying others in cyberspace. *Cyberbullying Glob Playground.* 2011:263. Cited by Kowalski et al.[117]
129. Patchin JW, Hinduja S. Cyberbullying and self-esteem. *J Sch Health.* 2010;80(12):614–621. Cited by Kowalski et al.[117]
130. Aoyama I, Barnard-Brak L, Talbert TL. Cyberbullying among high school students: cluster analysis of sex and age differences and the level of parental monitoring. *Int J Cyber Behav Psychol Learning.* 2011;1(1):25–35. Cited by Kowalski et al.[117]
131. Hunt C, Peters L, Rapee RM. Development of a measure of the experience of being bullied in youth. *Psychol Assess.* 2012;24(1):156–165. Cited by Kowalski et al.[117]
132. MacDonald CD, Roberts-Pittman B. Cyberbullying among college students: prevalence and demographic differences. Procedia Soc. 2010;9:2003–2009. Cited by Kowalski et al.[117]
133. Menesini E, Calussi P, Nocentini A. Cyberbullying, and traditional bullying: unique, additive, and synergistic effects on psychological health symptoms. In: Li Q, Cross D, Smith PK, eds. *Cyberbullying in the Global Playground: Research from International Perspectives.* Malden, MA: Blackwell; 2012:245–262. Cited by Kowalski et al.[117]

134. Finn J. A survey of online harassment at a university campus. *J Interpers Violence*. 2004;19(4):468–483. Cited by Kowalski et al.[117]

135. Berson IR, Berson MJ, Ferron JM. Emerging risks of violence in the digital age: lessons for educators from an online study of adolescent girls in the United States. *J Sch Violence*. 2002;1(2):51–71. Cited by Kowalski et al.[117]

136. Willard N. *Educator's Guide to Cyberbullying and Cyber-threats*. Center for Safe and Responsible Use of the Internet. https://education.ohio.gov/getattachment/Topics/Other-Resources/School-Safety/Safe-and-Supportive-Learning/Anti-Harassment-Intimidation-and-Bullying-Resource/Educator-s-Guide-Cyber-Safety.pdf.aspx. Accessed August 22, 2022.

137. Seigfried-Spellar KC, Treadway KN. Differentiating hackers, identity thieves, cyber-bullies, and virus writers by college major and individual differences. *Deviant Behav*. 2014;35(10):782–803.

138. Cappadocia MC, Craig WM, Pepler D. Cyberbullying: prevalence, stability, and risk factors during adolescence. *Can J Sch Psychol*. 2013;28(2):171–192.

139. Inchley J, Currie D, Budisavljevic S, et al, eds. *Spotlight on Adolescent Health and Well-being. Findings from the 2017/2018 Health Behaviour in School-aged Children (HBSC) Survey in Europe and Canada*. International Report. Volume 2. Copenhagen: WHO Regional Office for Europe; 2020:98–99. https://apps.who.int/iris/handle/10665/332104. Accessed August 22, 2022.

140. Smahel D, Machackova H, Mascheroni G, et al. (2020). EU Kids Online 2020: Survey Results from 19 Countries. https://www.lse.ac.uk/media-and-communications/assets/documents/research/eu-kids-online/reports/EU-Kids-Online-2020-March2020.pdf. Accessed August 20, 2022.

141. Calculated from Table 2 in Chudal R, Tiiri E, Klomek AB, et al. Victimization by traditional bullying and cyberbullying and the combination of these among adolescents in 13 European and Asian countries. *Eur Child Adolesc Psychiatry*. 2021:1–4.

142. The Eurasian Child Mental Health Study includes China, Finland, Greece, India, Indonesia, Iran, Israel, Japan, Lithuania, Norway, Russia, Singapore, and Vietnam. The group involves child and adolescent mental health experts in the participating countries to conduct cross-cultural, multisite research on the well-being and mental health of children and adolescents.[141]

143. Jadambaa A, Thomas HJ, Scott JG, Graves N, Brain D, Pacella R. Prevalence of traditional bullying and cyberbullying among children and adolescents in Australia: a systematic review and meta-analysis. *Aust N Z J Psychiatry*. 2019;53(9):878–888.

144. Jenaro C, Flores N, Frías CP. Systematic review of empirical studies on cyberbullying in adults: what we know and what we should investigate. *Aggress Violent Behav*. 2018;38:113–122.

145. Gardner D, O'Driscoll M, Cooper-Thomas HD, et al. Predictors of workplace bullying and cyber-bullying in New Zealand. *Int J Environ Res Public Health*. 2016;13(5):448. Cited by Jenaro et al.[144]

146. Privitera C, Campbell MA. Cyberbullying: the new face of workplace bullying? *Cyberpsychol Behav*. 2009;12(4):395–400. Cited by Jenaro et al.[144]

147. Wang MJ, Yogeeswaran K, Andrews NP, Hawi DR, Sibley CG. How common is cyberbullying among adults? Exploring gender, ethnic, and age differences in the prevalence of cyberbullying. *Cyberpsychol Behav Soc Netw*. 2019;22(11):736–741.

148. Pew Research Center. The State of Online Harassment. January 2021. https://www.pewresearch.org/internet/2021/01/13/the-state-of-online-harassment/. Accessed August 22, 2022.

149. Barlett CP, Gentile DA. Attacking others online: the formation of cyberbullying in late adolescence. *Psychol Popular Media Cult.* 2012;1(2):123.
150. Sourander A, Klomek AB, Ikonen M, et al. Psychosocial risk factors associated with cyberbullying among adolescents: a population-based study. *Arch Gen Psychiatry.* 2010;67(7):720–728.
151. Wölfer R, Schultze-Krumbholz A, Zagorscak P, Jäkel A, Göbel K, Scheithauer H. Prevention 2.0: Targeting cyberbullying@ school. *Prev Sci.* 2014;15(6):879–887.
152. Del Rey R, Casas JA, Ortega R. Impact of the ConRed program on different cyberbulling roles. *Aggress Behav.* 2016;42(2):123–135.
153. Kärnä A, Voeten M, Little TD, Poskiparta E, Kaljonen A, Salmivalli C. A large-scale evaluation of the KiVa Antibullying Program: grades 4–6. *Child Dev.* 2011;82(1):311–330.
154. Gordon S, Ford R. On the definition and classification of cybercrime. *J Comput Virol.* 2006;2(1):13–20.
155. Council of Europe, Convention on Cybercrime, Budapest, 23.XI.2001. https://rm.coe.int/1680081561. Accessed August 22, 2022.
156. Fraud and Related Activity in Connection with Computers. USC §1030. https://law.justia.com/codes/us/1994/title18/parti/chap47/sec1030. Accessed September 29, 2023.
157. Doyle C. *Cybercrime: A Sketch of 18 USC 1030 and Related Federal Criminal Laws.* Congressional Research Service; 2014. https://crsreports.congress.gov/product/pdf/RL/97-1025. Accessed September 29, 2023.
158. Broadhurst R. Developments in the global law enforcement of cyber-crime. *Policing.* 2006;29(3):408–433.
159. Federal Bureau of Investigation, Internet Crime Complaint Center. *Internet Crime Report, 2020.* https://www.ic3.gov/Media/PDF/AnnualReport/2020_IC3Report.pdf. Accessed August 22, 2020.
160. Phishing.org defines phishing as "a cybercrime in which a target or targets are contacted by email, telephone or text message by someone posing as a legitimate institution to lure individuals into providing sensitive data such as personally identifiable information, banking and credit card details, and passwords." https://www.phishing.org/what-is-phishing. Accessed August 22, 2022.
161. TrendMicro defines vishing as "phishing attacks that involve the use of voice calls, using either conventional phone systems or Voice over Internet Procotol (VoIP) systems." https://www.trendmicro.com/vinfo/us/security/definition/vishing. Accessed August 22, 2022.
162. According to TrendMicro, "Smishing (sometimes stylized as SMiShing) refers to phishing attacks that involve the use of messages sent using SMS (Short Message Service). False text messages are received by would-be victims, who in turn either reply directly or visit a phishing web site." https://www.trendmicro.com/vinfo/us/security/definition/smishing. Accessed August 22, 2022.
163. According to TrendMicro, "Pharming sets up a website that contains copies of pages from a legitimate website in order to capture confidential information from users, such as credit card, bank account, social security numbers and other sensitive personal information. Users are automatically redirected to malicious URLs when hackers hack into DNS servers and change IP addresses." https://www.trendmicro.com/vinfo/us/security/definition/pharming. Accessed August 22, 2022.
164. Spoofing occurs when "contact information (phone number, email, and website) is deliberately falsified to mislead and appear to be from a legitimate source. For example, spoofed

phone numbers making mass robocalls; spoofed emails sending mass spam; forged websites used to mislead and gather personal information. Often used in connection with other crime types."[159]

165. Misrepresentation occurs when "Merchandise or services were purchased or contracted by individuals online for which the purchasers provided payment. The goods or services received were of a measurably lesser quality or quantity than was described by the seller."[159]
166. Confidence/Romance Fraud is an individual's belief that "they are in a relationship (family, friendly, or romantic) and are tricked into sending money, personal and financial information, or items of value to the perpetrator or to launder money or items to assist the perpetrator. This includes the Grandparent's Scheme and any scheme in which the perpetrator preys on the complainant's heartstrings."[159]
167. Crimes against children encompass "anything related to the exploitation of children, including child abuse."[159]
168. Ransomware is "a type of malicious software designed to block access to a computer system until money is paid."[159]
169. Malware/scareware/virus is defined as "software or code intended to damage, disable, or capable of copying itself onto a computer and/or computer systems to have a detrimental effect or destroy data."[159]
170. DataReportal. Digital 2020, Complete Report Library, Search by Country. https://datareportal.com/library. Accessed August 22, 2022.
171. Srivastava SK, Das S, Udo GJ, Bagchi K. Determinants of cybercrime originating within a nation: a cross-country study. *J Glob Info Technol Manage.* 2020;23(2):112–137.
172. Economic capital is "a three-component latent variable composed of GDP per capita, trade freedom index, and education level of the nation's population."[171] Also, "education level of a nation is defined by two components, namely, average education in years and expected average education in years."[171]
173. Technological capital "has four components, i.e., (i) the percentage of individuals using the Internet, (ii) mobile-cellular telephone subscriptions per 100 inhabitants, (iii) fixed (wired) broadband subscriptions per 100 inhabitants, and (iv) wireless broadband subscriptions per 100 inhabitants."[171]
174. Cybersecurity preparedness of any country involves the "legal, technical, organizational, capability building, and cooperation measures"[171] to deal with cybercrime.
175. De Kimpe L, Walrave M, Verdegem P, Ponnet K. What we think we know about cybersecurity: an investigation of the relationship between perceived knowledge, internet trust, and protection motivation in a cybercrime context. *Behav Info Technol.* 2021:1–3.
176. Abdelhamid M. The role of health concerns in phishing susceptibility: survey design study. *J Med Internet Res.* 2020;22(5):e18394.
177. Cheng C, Chan L, Chau CL. Individual differences in susceptibility to cybercrime victimization and its psychological aftermath. *Comput Hum Behav.* 2020;108:106311.
178. Cybersecurity and Infrastructure Security Agency (CISA). Alert (AA20-099A): COVID-19 exploited by malicious cyber actors. April 8, 2020. https://us-cert.cisa.gov/ncas/alerts/aa20-099a. Accessed August 22, 2022. Cited by Monteith et al (see Note 181).
179. Interpol. *Cybercrime: Covid-19 Impact.* August 2020. https://www.interpol.int/en/News-and-Events/News/2020/INTERPOL-report-shows-alarming-rate-of-cyberattacks-during-COVID-19. Accessed August 22, 2022. Cited by Monteith et al (see Note 181).

180. *COVID-19 Fraud: Law Enforcement's Response to Those Exploiting the Pandemic. Hearing Before the Senate Judiciary Committee.* June 9, 2020 (statement of CA Shivers). https://www.fbi.gov/news/testimony/covid-19-fraud-law-enforcements-response-to-those-exploiting-the-pandemic. Accessed August 22, 2022. Cited by Monteith et al (see Note 181).

181. Monteith S, Bauer M, Alda M, Geddes J, Whybrow PC, Glenn T. Increasing cybercrime since the pandemic: concerns for psychiatry. *Curr Psychiatry Rep.* 2021;23(4):1–9.

182. Golladay K, Holtfreter K. The consequences of identity theft victimization: an examination of emotional and physical health outcomes. *Vict Offenders.* 2017;12(5):741–760.. Cited by Monteith et al.[181]

183. Lichtenberg PA, Sugarman MA, Paulson D, Ficker LJ, Rahman-Filipiak A. Psychological and functional vulnerability predicts fraud cases in older adults: results of a longitudinal study. *Clin Gerontol.* 2016;39(1):48–63.. Cited by Monteith et al.[181]

184. Health and Retirement Study. The Health and Retirement Study is a longitudinal project sponsored by the National Institute on Aging (NIA U01AG009740) and the Social Security Administration. https://hrs.isr.umich.edu/welcome-health-and-retirement-study. Accessed August 22, 2022.

185. Radloff LS. The CES-D Scale: a self-report depression scale for research in the general population. *Appl Psychol Meas.* 1977;1(3):385–340.. Cited by Lichtenberg et al.[183]

186. Claycomb M, Black AC, Wilber C, Brocke S, Lazar CM, Rosen MI. Financial victimization of adults with severe mental illness. *Psychiatr Serv.* 2013;64(9):918–920.. Cited by Monteith et al.[181]

187. World Health Organization. Global School-based Student Health Survey. https://www.who.int/teams/noncommunicable-diseases/surveillance/systems-tools/global-school-based-student-health-survey. Accessed August 22, 2022.

188. Centers for Disease Control and Prevention. Global School-based Student Health Survey, Background. https://www.cdc.gov/gshs/background/index.htm. Accessed August 22, 2022.

189. Centers for Disease Control and Prevention. Global School-based Student Health Survey, Overview. https://www.cdc.gov/gshs/pdf/GSHSOVerview.pdf. Accessed August 22, 2022.

190. Nguyen HT, Nakamura K, Seino K. Relationships among cyberbullying, parental attitudes, self-harm, and suicidal behavior among adolescents: results from a school-based survey in Vietnam. *BMC Public Health.* 2020;20(1):1–9.

191. Global School-based Student Health Survey (GSHS). Contact list of country representatives who have completed a GSHS survey implementation workshop. https://www.cdc.gov/gshs/pdf/web_master_coordinators_contact_list.pdf. Accessed August 22, 2022.

192. Global School-based Student Health Survey (GSHS). Core expanded questions for the Violence and Unintentional Injury Module. Question 21. *Manual for Conducting the Global School-based Student Health Survey.* Last updated October 13, 2017. https://cdn.who.int/media/docs/default-source/ncds/ncd-surveillance/gshs/2018-gshs-core-expanded-english.pdf?sfvrsn = c1c184b_2. Accessed August 22, 2022.

193. Global School-based Student Health Survey (GSHS). Core expanded questions 2021 Version. Question 24. https://cdn.who.int/media/docs/default-source/ncds/ncd-surveillance/gshs/2018-gshs-core-expanded-english.pdf?sfvrsn = c1c184b_2. Accessed August 22, 2022.

15
Maltreatment in the Neighborhood

What Is Known?

The notion of maltreatment in the neighborhood includes all forms of physical, sexual, verbal, psychological, or relational victimization or mistreatment experienced or witnessed by a person of any age and occurring in open public places of the local area where the person lives, studies, works, shops, plays, walks, runs, or drives through. Neighborhood victimization includes all acts of bullying, aggression, violence, intimidation, harassment, annoyance, incivility, disrespect, disregard, or exclusion of a person perpetrated by one or more people living (or not living) in that neighborhood. The maltreatment may affect the victim's physical or emotional well-being, reputation, property, belongings, or assets, and/or it may cause death.

Bullying in the Neighborhood

One of the very few studies addressing the nature and prevalence of neighborhood bullying, within the definition of bullying outlined by Olweus,[1] was undertaken by Percy-Smith and Mathews[2] and was based on semi-structured interviews of 181 young people, age 10 to 15, living in either the inner city (65%) or a suburban area (35%) of a large East Midland town in the United Kingdom. The research[2] showed that 46% of the participants living in the inner city and 27% of those residing in the suburban area reported having experienced bullying in their neighborhood. This mistreatment in public outdoor places was usually perpetrated by older adolescents, who moved into younger children's games, aiming to disrupt or take over ("barging in"); who used extortion or threats to make others participate in antisocial behavior; or who intimidated others through taunts, insults, threats, pushing and/or name-calling.[2]

A household survey conducted by Costa et al.[3] of almost 600 Brazilian adolescents age 14 to 17 living in Belo Horizonte documented that 26% of the adolescents surveyed were exposed to bullying, and almost one-third of the victims (7% of the total number of adolescents) experienced the bullying in the streets.[3]

Andershed et al.[4] conducted a survey of 2,912 Swedish eighth graders to ascertain whether adolescents who bully others in school are more violent in the streets at night than those who did not bully in schools. The research[4] showed that bullying behavior in school was significantly linked to engagement in street violence (e.g., unprovoked assault or threatening or forcing others to do something) or carrying a weapon while out in the streets. This association remained significant even after controlling for loitering and nights spent away from home.[4]

Aggression/Violence in the Streets

Youth Participation in Street Fights

At present there are no data available from national representative samples that document the prevalence of youth participation in street fights. Yet, based upon an analysis[5] of the US Health Behavior in School-aged Children (HBSC) survey conducted in 2009–2010,[6] it can be established that almost 4% of US adolescents in grades 5 to 10 reported having been involved in one or more physical fights with a "stranger" in the previous 12 months, while 25% of them (1% of US adolescents) were involved in four or more fights with a stranger each year. Although the HBSC data[6] do not provide information indicating in what environment the fights took place, it is possible that, given that the fights involved a stranger, they may have occurred in the street or neighborhood. Still, we cannot establish the prevalence of youth street fights between friends or people who know each other. Overall, the HBSC data[6] indicate that almost 15% of US adolescents were involved in one or more fights in the previous year, with a friend or somebody they knew, yet an unknown fraction of the physical fights occurred in the streets.

Victimization by Strangers

According to the US Department of Justice,[7] 37% of the violent victimizations committed by strangers during the period from 2005 to 2010 occurred in public places, including open areas, streets, public transportation, parking lots, or garages, while only 10% of violent victimizations perpetrated by an unknown person happened at the victim's home or at a friend's, neighbor's, or relative's residence. Based on the same statistics,[7] it is known that almost 80% of the violent victimization carried out by strangers involved simple or aggravated assault, while 24% of the crimes included rape or sexual assault.

During 2019, 8.1 per 1,000 persons (age 12 or older) living in the United States were violently victimized by a stranger, in contrast to 4.2 per 1,000 persons (age 12 or older) who were victims of domestic violence, or 2.5 per 1,000 persons (age 12 or older) who were victims of violence in intimate partner domestic relationships.[8]

Sampson[9] conducted a study to determine how individuals' characteristics and community circumstances concurrently increase or decrease the risk of personal stranger victimization. The research was conducted in 1982 and was based on a national survey of 10,905 individuals age 16 or older living in England and Wales. The study documented that "males suffer a risk of violent victimization by strangers over three times greater than females (3.6% of males vs. 1.1% of females),"[9] while single, divorced, or separated participants have 2.5 times more risk of being exposed to stranger violence than married people.[9] The risk of being exposed to stranger victimization was significantly higher for people who were out at night five to seven times a week (8.7%), as compared to participants who spent their evenings and nights in their home (2.3%). Furthermore, younger people (age 16 to 45) had 7.7 times higher risk of suffering stranger violence than people 48 years old or older. Moreover, Sampson's study showed that "residents of highly urbanized areas and areas of racial heterogeneity experience much higher risks of stranger theft than do residents of areas that are more racially homogeneous and lower in urbanization."[9]

Violence Linked to Street Gangs

Criminal street gangs have been defined as "ongoing groups, clubs, organizations, or associations of five or more individuals that have as one of their primary purposes the commission of one or more criminal offenses."[10] Gang activities include crimes like assault, drug trafficking, home invasion, homicide, intimidation, threats, carrying weapons, and sex trafficking.[11]

Miller[12] incorporated features of previous definitions of the term *youth gang* in defining it as a "a self-formed association of peers, united by mutual interests, with identifiable leadership and internal organization, who act collectively or as individuals to achieve specific purposes, including the conduct of illegal activity and control of a particular territory, facility, or enterprise."[12]

Pyrooz and Sweeten[13] investigated the frequency of youth gang membership in the United States and documented that approximately 2% of American youth self-reported active gang membership in 2011.[13] Interestingly, the investigation assessed the population exposure to local street gang densities in small areas by quantifying the density of street gang activity through the measurement of the number of "street gangs that exist[ed] within a 2-mile radius of each ZIP-code's population-weighted geographic centroid."[13]

Some researchers[14-16] have considered the use of the term *gang* to be problematic, given its highly sensitive and subjective nature[14] as well as the understanding that in reality "gangs are very complex social networks with unclear and constantly changing boundaries."[15] To circumvent these questions about interpretation, Sharpe et al.[16] used the term *delinquent youth group* to characterize "defined groups of young people who are involved in delinquent activities at a group level"—specifically, "young people who spend time in a group of three or more, including themselves; with the group, which has existed for more than three months, spending a lot of time in public places, engaged in delinquent or criminal behavior together in the previous year, and the group being characterized by a structural feature (name, area, leader or rules)."[16]

Gatti et al.[17] explored the link between deviant youth group membership and antisocial behavior through a large student survey involving more than 40,000 students in grades 7 to 9 who were attending different schools in 62 cities in 32 countries. A deviant youth group was defined as "any durable, street-oriented youth group whose own identity includes involvement in illegal activity."[17] Gatti et al. showed that 4.4% of the respondents identified themselves as members of a deviant youth group, with a range from 0.4% in Armenia to 16.8% in Ireland. Significantly more boys (5.9%) than girls (3%) were identified as member of such groups, as were second-generation migrants (5.8%) compared to not migrants (4%).[17] Members of a deviant youth group were significantly more at risk [adjusted odds ratio (AOR) = 9.1] than nonmembers of being involved in one or more delinquent activities (shoplifting; theft of a bicycle, moped, scooter, motorbike, or car; theft from a car; breaking into a building with intent to steal; and selling drugs). Also, members of a deviant youth group were more at risk (AOR = 7.12) of committing one or more violent offenses (assault, robbery, bag-snatching, vandalism, carrying a weapon, and group fighting) than students who did not identify themselves as members of a deviant youth group.[17]

People Living in the Streets

Unsheltered Homeless or People "Living Rough": Nature and Prevalence

The European Federation of National Organizations Working with the Homeless (FEANTSA)[18] has developed a typology of homelessness and housing exclusion, known as ETHOS,[19] which includes, among many other types of homelessness,[19] a category identified as people living rough, meaning people living in the streets or external public places "without a shelter that can be defined as living quarters."[19]

According to Our World in Data (a project of Global Data Change Lab[20-22]), the most common approach to determining the prevalence of homelessness is through so-called point-in-time[22] tallies of people who are sleeping in shelters or streets, to show the number of people "who are homeless on any given night."[22] Based on data from the US Department of Housing and Urban Development,[23] it is known that on one night in January 2019, there were approximately 568,000 people in the United States experiencing homelessness, with approximately 37% of them staying in "unsheltered locations, such as on the street, in abandoned buildings, or in other places not suitable for human habitation."[23] Of people staying in unsheltered locations (17,330), 8% were unaccompanied youth < 25 years old, and most of them (88%) were between 18 and 24 years old. It should be noted that 2.4% of the unsheltered unaccompanied youth in the United States were transgender individuals, in contrast to the estimated total population of transgender young adults, which is ~ 0.39 per 100 adults nationally.[24] Also, 4.6% the unsheltered were Native Americans (in contrast to their 1.3% share of the US population) and 1.7% were Pacific Islanders (in contrast to their 0.3% share of the total population).[25]

Of the people staying in an unsheltered location on one night of January 2019, almost 4% (7,811) were children and adolescents < 18 years old who were accompanied by an adult family member; they represented 1 per 10,000 US children and adolescents younger than 18.[25] Again, in the group of unsheltered accompanied youth, there was an overrepresentation of Native Americans (4.8%) and Pacific Islanders (12%).

In the streets of England, during one night of the autumn of 2016, there were 4,134 rough sleepers[26] counted/estimated, representing 7.4 per 100,000 people in England.[27] Almost 23% of the rough sleepers in the UK (940) were staying in unsheltered locations in London, meaning 10.7 of every 100,000 Londoners were rough sleepers,[28] and almost 60% of them were immigrants to the United Kingdom.[26]

Victimization of Unsheltered Adults

Ellsworth[29] investigated what is known about street crime victimization of adult homeless through an interdisciplinary systematic review of 33 peer-reviewed articles published from 1980 through 2017. The study[29] underscored the high rates of assault, robbery, and theft affecting the homeless,[30-36] as compared to victimization estimates in the general population.[37-39] The Ellsworth investigation[29] was based on the pooling[29] of quantitative findings from seven studies,[30-36] and it documented that almost 29% of homeless people have experienced physical attacks,[29] 24% "had their possessions forcibly taken from them,"[29] and 46% were victims of theft,[29] as compared to victimization estimations in the general population[37-39] indicating that 0.5% of people were robbed, 2.6% were victims of simple assault, 0.8% suffered aggravated assault, and 2.1% were exposed to theft.[29]

Homicide of Unsheltered Adults

A study conducted by Scott,[40] which reviewed data pertaining to 1,271 persons who died in King County in the State of Washington between 2009 and 2019 and who were presumed to be homeless at the time of death, showed that homicide accounted for 5.5% of the deaths among homeless people in King County, a rate that was 20 times higher than would have been expected for the general population of Washington.[40]

Street Children

The United Nations defines the term *street children* as "boys and girls for whom 'the street' (including unoccupied dwellings, wasteland, etc.) has become their home and/or source of livelihood."[41] The Consortium for Street Children[42] (CSC) defined the terms *street children* or *street-connected children* as young people who "depend on the streets to live and/or work, either on their own or with other children or family members, and have a strong connection to public places (e.g., streets, markets, parks, bus or train stations) and for whom the street plays a vital role in their everyday lives and identities."[43] Furthermore, "this wider group includes children who do not live or work on the street but regularly accompany other children or family members in the streets."[43]

UNICEF[44] described three categories of street children: children at risk (children of the urban poor, from whom street children surface), children on the street (who work in the streets to make an income but at night return to their homes), and children of the street (who live in the streets and have remote or infrequent contact with their homes).[45] The latter include orphans, refugees, runaways, and others "who have no contact with significant carers," and they "comprise only 5%–10% of street children."[46]

As of 2005, UNICEF[47] indicated that the number of street children was not clearly quantified, but it could be estimated to be in the tens of millions across the world.

Victimization of Street Children

In Toronto, Gaetz and O'Grady[48] studied 244 homeless youth (16 to 25 years old) who were interviewed in 2019 about life on the streets, including their experiences of criminal victimization. The research[48] documented that, in the previous 12 months, 48% of the youth were assaulted, 19% were sexually assaulted, and 33% were subjected to robbery, while 45% of these victims suffered physical injury and over 21% required attention in a hospital.[48]

Neighborhood Crime and Perception of Safety as Predictors of Vicarious Victimization

Neighborhood crime and perception or feeling of safety have been found to be significant predictors of vicarious victimization by exposure to violence in the neighborhood.[49]

Community Crime Victimization

According to the 2004–2005 International Crime Victims Survey[50] (ICVS), an average of 20% of individuals in 26 cities in developed countries[51] reported being victimized in the previous year by any of 10 "common crimes,"[52] while 28% of persons in five cities in developing countries[53] experienced being victimized in the previous year by one or more common crimes.[52] Property theft was the most frequent (5.4%) crime experienced in the previous year by people in cities of developed countries.[51] Persons in cities in developing countries[53] reported experiencing mostly burglary or pickpocketing (6.4%), as well as assault or robbery (6.1%),[50] in the previous year.

Duque et al.[54] interviewed a random sample of almost 2,100 non-institutionalized people age 12 to 60 years living in the city of Medellin, Colombia, to estimate the prevalence of witnesses and victims of different forms of interpersonal violence. The highest rates of violence witnessed over the life span were armed threats (41.4%) and robbery without weapon (25%), while 20% to 21% of people were direct victims of these forms of maltreatment in their lifetime.

A previous similar cross-sectional study by Duque et al.[55] of 3,007 adolescents and adults living in Bogota, Colombia, documented that 70% of the participants had witnessed assault with a weapon during their lifetime and 55% were direct victims of this type of violence.

Feeling of Safety

The 2004-2005 ICVS[50] indicated that 32% of people living in main cities in developed countries[5] felt unsafe or very unsafe walking alone in the streets after dark, while this sense of insecurity at night was reported by 61% of persons in cities of developing countries.[53]

According to the 2016 National Survey of Children's Health,[56] 6% of parents of children and adolescents living in the United States indicated that they "somewhat or definitely disagree that their children are safe in the neighborhood."[57] The perception of lack of safety varied between white-non-Hispanic parents (3.1%) and Hispanic parents (9.8%), black non-Hispanic parents (10.7%), Asian non-Hispanic parents (5.7%), and other non-Hispanic parents (7%).[58]

The Economist Intelligent Unit[59] studied the safety of 60 cities around the world using an array of indicators pertaining to several areas of urban well-being, including personal security. The "personal security index" was developed by considering "policies and decisions, such as level of police engagement, use of data-driven crime prevention, and the overall political stability of the country" where each city was located.[60] In addition, the index was based on "prevalence of petty and violent crime, safety perceptions, [and] assessment of the threat of civil unrest, military conflict, and terrorism."[60] While the average personal security score was 74.4 (for example, in Rome), the top 10 cities (scores from 94.94 to 87.42) were Singapore, Wellington, Osaka, Tokyo, Toronto, Taipei, Hong Kong, Melbourne, Stockholm, and Amsterdam, whereas the bottom 10 cities (scores from 59.24 to 31.85) were Jakarta, Teheran, Moscow, Johannesburg, Bogota, Quito, Yangon, Ho Chin Min City, Caracas, and Karachi.[61]

Neighborhood Fear of Crime

The relevance of individual and neighborhood factors in predicting neighborhood fear of crime was examined by McCrea et al.[62] in a study based on a survey of 1,610 adult residents of Brisbane, Australia. Over 30% of the respondents felt that it was not safe to walk in the streets after dark. The only four attributes found to be significantly predictive of fear of neighborhood crime were age, gender, neighborhood vandalism, and neighborhood cleanliness.[62]

Neighborhood Fear of Gangs

The question of whether the same or different individual or neighborhood factors predict neighborhood fear of crime versus fear of gangs was undertaken in research conducted by Katz et al.[63] Their study was based on a 2001 survey of 800 randomly selected participants, age 16 or older, who were residents of Mesa, Arizona, and who were drawn from a high- or low-gang area. The fear of crime was ascertained by asking the respondents whether they were worried about being the victim of a non-gang crime, being stopped by a stranger to ask for directions, the possibility that somebody might try to break into their home, and/or walking alone in the neighborhood because of non-gang-related concerns.[63] The fear of gangs was determined by asking the participants whether they worried about being the victim of a gang crime, that a gang member might hurt some member of their household, and/or that gangs were taking over their neighborhood.[63] The wide range of independent variables included individual demographic aspects (ethnicity, gender, age, education, income, and living or not living in a high-gang area); direct or vicarious victimization in the previous 12 months; residential stability, as measured by home ownership; perceptions of positive or negative changes in the neighborhood; and neighborhood cohesion, as determined by positive interaction of residents, such as helping neighbors out, interacting socially with neighbors, and/or watching neighbors' homes while they were on vacation.[63] Other independent variables pertained to subcultural diversity (concerns about racial and ethnic relations, foreign immigrants, and/or changing moral standards) and social disorder (teenagers hanging out in the streets; presence of drunks, prostitution, people fighting and arguing, and open drug dealing), as well as physical disorder (litter, abandoned cars, vacant houses, graffiti, vandalism, unmaintained property, and/or broken windows).[63] The study[63] found that fear of crime was significantly associated with all independent variables except race and indirect gang victimization. Fear of gangs was significantly related to all independent variables except gender.[63]

Neighborhood Impact of Mass Shootings

Lemieux et al.[64] assessed the incidence of mass shooting in the United States and Australia from 1981 to 2013. The study[64] defined a mass shooting as "an incident that resulted in the death by gunshot wound of four or more persons, and [that] was perpetrated by one or more offenders at the same site or at multiple sites as part of one related process."[64] It was understood that if the perpetrator was killed during or after the shooting, they were not included in the final victim count.[64] In the 33 years between 1981 and 2013, 13 mass shootings occurred in Australia, with the death of 104 people from gunshot wounds, corresponding to an average victimization rate of 0.41 per 100,000 population.[64] During the same time span, 73 mass shootings occurred in the United States, with 576 deaths, corresponding to a victimization rate of 1.81 per 100,000 population.[64] Thirty-eight percent of the Australian mass shootings and 25% the American mass killing incidents occurred in the community (streets, footpaths, and recreational sites).[64]

A study by Beard et al.[65] aimed at describing the prevalence of neighborhood mass shootings in Philadelphia from 2006 to 2015 and how these incidents were conveyed to the public through the news media. The investigation[65] identified 46 events, involving 212 victims. The investigators defined a mass shooting as a shooting in which four or more people were shot within 100 meters of each other during the period of one hour. The victims of neighborhood mass shootings, as compared to victims of other shootings, were likely to be younger, female, and non-white, and mass shootings were more likely than other shooting incidents to have fatalities.[65]

Interestingly, 15% of the mass shootings that occurred during 2006 to 2015 (at the frequency of one per year across Philadelphia in geographically diverse neighborhoods) did not receive any media coverage. The 39 mass shooting events that were covered in the media received 183 media reports, mostly (81%) in a feature or lead story, published in print (90%), and in the local/regional Philadelphia media (85%). In 99% of the reports, the headline did not describe the assailant (84%), did not provide the ages of victims (82%) or their gender (85%), and above all did not describe the event as a mass shooting.[65]

Lowe and Galea[66] conducted an examination of empirical investigations of the mental health consequences of mass shootings, based on 49 studies of 15 different mass shootings that occurred between 1984 and 2008. Posttraumatic stress symptoms were reported in 73% of the studies reviewed,[66] yet only 37% of the studies (based on 14 independent samples) documented a prevalence estimate of PTSD,[66] which varied from 3% among parents of children exposed to an elementary school shooting six to 14 months after the incident (using DSM-III-R criteria)[67] to 91% among the children in the same study (using proposed DSM-IV criteria).[68]

Major depression was the second most recognized psychiatric disorder assessed in a third of the studies reviewed,[66] with its prevalence estimated by only 16% of all studies using seven different samples.[66] The lowest prevalence of major depression was 4.9% among survivors of a cafeteria shooting in 1991 assessed one year after the incident (using DSM-III-R),[69] while the highest rate (71%) of major depression was documented among students two weeks after attacks on two university campuses.[70] The wide range of rates of mental disorders encountered in the review[66] was explained based on variation in sample characteristics, post-incident timing of the assessments, and different measures and diagnostic criteria.[66]

Neighborhood Fears of Terrorism

According to the 2019 wave of the Chapman University Survey of American Fears (CASF),[71] 51% of Americans were afraid, or very afraid, of a terrorist attack, a concern that was more prevalent in the community than being afraid of being murdered by a stranger (31%), being exposed to racial or hate crime (32%), gang violence (26%), or walking alone at night (23%).[72]

The differences between fear of terrorism and fear of violent crimes were explored by Onat et al.[73] in a study based on a comparative analysis of data from a nationally representative sample (N = 1,190) in the 2018 CASF.[74] The Onat study[73] attempted to ascertain whether the same factors that predict fear of crime could also explain fear of terrorism. The independent variables considered included demographic items (gender, race, education, age, employment, marital status, home ownership), political views, degree of religiosity, perceived risk of immigrant crime, and previous victimization in violent crime, as well as exposure to online or social media news.[73] Bivariate analyses showed that participants with higher levels of exposure to online news and news from social media reported higher levels of both fear of crime and fear of terrorism.[73] Also, participants who were female, non-white, and not married and who had a low level of education indicated higher levels of fear of both crime and terrorism.[73] At the same time, individuals who viewed immigrants as more apt to perpetrate crime, who were more politically moderate or conservative, and who considered themselves more religious were significantly likely to worry about terrorism.[73] Multivariate analysis indicated that older and religious respondents who consumed more news from online media had significantly higher levels of fear of terrorism than others.[73]

Neighborhood Safety and Its Health Impact

Psychological Symptoms

A study by Goldman-Mellor et al.[75] showed that adolescents who perceived their neighborhood to be unsafe were twice (OR = 2.4) as likely as those who perceived their neighborhood to be safe to report symptoms of depression and anxiety. However, those who lived in areas objectively distinguished by high levels of violent crime were no more likely (OR = 1.41) than their peers in safer areas to be psychologically afflicted.[75]

A cross-sectional survey by Polling et al.,[76] involving almost 1,700 adults living in two London neighborhoods, documented that those who somewhat or very seriously perceived neighborhood disorder (as characterized by vandalism, graffiti, crime, unsafety, and rubbish or litter) were more likely (OR = 2.12) to experience common mental illness than those who were directly affected by crime.[76]

Yimgang et al.[77] studied the impact of the civil unrest that occurred in April 2015 in the city of Baltimore on symptoms of depression suffered by mothers of young children living near the disturbance. The research[77] was based on cross-sectional surveys of almost 1,100 mothers of children mostly < 24 months old, from 17 months prior to the civil unrest through eight months after its occurrence. The study[77] used trend analysis and piecewise logistic regression to examine the effects of time as well as residential proximity moderation. After the unrest, prevalence of maternal depressive symptoms increased significantly in proximal, but not distal, neighborhoods, while the symptoms of depression returned to previous levels five months after the disturbance.[77]

Asthma

The association between exposure to community violence and asthma was studied by Sternthal et al.[78] in a longitudinal assessment of more than 2,000 children (from birth to 9 years old) living in Chicago. The study documented that violent crime was significantly associated with the frequency of asthma in a community, even after controlling for sociodemographic and individual characteristics.[78]

In a 26-week longitudinal study of almost 400 adults with moderate asthma aiming to ascertain the association of exposure to community violence and asthma-related outcomes, Apter et al.[79] showed that, over the study period, the participants who were exposed to violence had 2.27 times more asthma-related ED visits per month and 2.49 times more asthma-related hospitalizations per month than the adults not exposed to violence.[79]

Smoking

Shareck and Ellaway[80] found that adults who reside in areas of Scotland with high police-recorded crime rates or those who perceive high crime in their neighborhood are more likely to be current smokers, after controlling for individual characteristics, as compared to people living in low-crime areas.[80]

Weight Status

Forsyth et al.[81] surveyed more than 2,400 adolescents from 20 public schools in Minneapolis/St. Paul to examine the relationships of perceived and objective reports of neighborhood crime to adolescent physical activity and body mass index (BMI). The study determined that increased BMI among girls and boys was significantly associated with perceived crime and, among girls, with reported crime.[81] Yet, neither total reported crime nor perceived crime was significantly associated with physical activity, in either boys or girls.[81]

Cardiovascular Disease

A significant link between cardiovascular disease and neighborhood psychosocial hazards, such as violent crime, abandoned buildings, and signs of incivility, was established in a study by Augustin et al.[82] involving 140 adults, 50 to 70 years old, living in 65 contiguous neighborhoods in Baltimore, Maryland. The investigation showed, after adjustment for individual cardiac risk factors, that participants residing in areas with the highest level of psychosocial hazards had more than four times higher risk of a history of myocardial infarction, and more than three times higher chances of myocardial infarction, stroke, transient ischemic attack, or intermittent claudication than residents living in neighborhoods with the lowest degree of psychosocial danger.[82]

Sleep Disturbances

Bagley et al.[83] conducted a cross-sectional study of 252 adolescents living in the Southeast United States to explore the link between concerns about community violence and objective and subjective sleep parameters. The research documented that community violence was significantly associated with lower sleep efficiency, more long-wake episodes, and more sleep/wake problems and sleepiness, even after controlling for anxiety and demographic variables.[83]

Discrimination in the Streets

Over three decades ago, Feagin[84] conducted a study to investigate prevailing antiblack discrimination in public places, by obtaining data primarily through 37 in-depth interviews with black middle-class respondents in several cities of the United States. Despite its small sample size, the study showed that there were 28 discriminatory actions experienced in the streets, with 46% of them characterized as police threats or harassment, 18% as other threats or harassment, 25% as verbal epithets, and 7% as a feeling of avoidance.[84]

Perceived Discrimination

The term *perceived discrimination* has been defined as "a behavioral manifestation of a negative attitude, judgment or unfair treatment toward members of a group."[85] This perceptual dimension has been estimated through the use of the Every Day Discrimination Scale,[86] which consists of nine items and measures encounters pertaining to a sense of discrimination in the respondent's day-to-day life (e.g., being treated with less courtesy or less respect than other people are; people acting as if one is dishonest or not smart; people acting as if they are better than, or afraid of, oneself; being called names, insulted, threatened, or harassed; or receiving poorer services than other people at stores or restaurants).[86,87]

A national telephone/mail survey of more than 3,000 American adults, carried out in 1995–1996 by Kessler et al.,[88] documented that almost 61% of the adults reported exposure to any type of day-to-day discrimination. An average of 46% of them reported that people's behavior made them feel inferior or not smart or they were treated with less courtesy or respect than others.[88] Close to a third of respondents were threatened, harassed, insulted, or called names, and/or experienced that people were afraid of them or felt that they were dishonest.[88]

An average of 30% of respondents sensed that the reasons for perceived discrimination were race-ethnicity, gender, weight, and age, while around 5% understood that the reason for discrimination was religion; financial, occupational, or educational status; sexual orientation; physical disability; or other reasons.[88] Non-Hispanic blacks were significantly more at risk ($OR = 12.8$) than non-Hispanic whites for frequent day-to-day discrimination.[88]

Carlisle[89] conducted a comparative analysis to ascertain perceived discrimination among racial and ethnic subgroups in the United States, showing that Caribbean Americans (Haitians, Jamaicans, and Trinidadians) were the least likely (34.1%) to have never perceived discrimination as compared to Latino Americans (56.1%) or Asian Americans (57.6%).[89]

In 2008, Perez et al.[90] reported on the prevalence of perceived discrimination among a national sample of Latinos in the United States and documented that 30% of Latinos experienced daily discrimination, with those who were younger, male, and unmarried, and who had higher education and more income being more likely to report having felt discriminated against. Moreover, the discrimination was significantly more frequently experienced by those who were among the first generation born in the United States as well as those with a weak ethnic identity.[90]

Dulin-Keita et al.[91] studied 175 American children (age 7 to 12) to determine whether there were racial differences in the awareness of race as well as to determine their experience with racial discrimination. The investigation demonstrated that 75% of non-Hispanic black children were able to define race, as compared to 59% of Hispanic or non-Hispanic whites. Hispanic children had more everyday discrimination experiences, with 44% of them feeling that people thought that they were inferior.[91] Non-Hispanic black children reported a higher frequency (26.3%) of experiences of feeling that people were afraid of them, in comparison to 11.5% of Hispanics and 3% of non-Hispanic whites.[91]

A study by McLaughlin et al.,[92] based on an analysis of the United States 2004–2005 National Epidemiologic Survey on Alcohol and Related Conditions, with 34,653 respondents, revealed that perceived discrimination in public places in the previous 12 months was experienced by 18% of blacks, 9% of Hispanics, 14% of LGBT individuals, and 3% of women.[92] Blacks, Hispanics, and women who perceived discrimination were at significant risk of experiencing symptoms of generalized anxiety disorder (AOR = 2.3–2.8).

Street Harassment

Originally, street harassment was characterized by Di Leonardo[92] as an occurrence of one or more strange men accosting one or more women, "whom they perceive as heterosexual, in a public place [that] is not the woman's/women's worksite."[92] Bowman[93] defined street harassment as the "sexual harassment of women in public places by men who are strangers."[93]

In the process of exploring the terms and definitions of street harassment, Logan[94] emphasized the need for a definition that includes harassment directed not only at women but also at any group because of race, sexual orientation, age, size, ability, language, citizenship, religion, or ethnicity. Furthermore, Logan[94] endorsed the detailed definition advanced by Gardner,[95] which described street harassment as a "group of abuses, harrying, and annoyances characteristic of public places and uniquely facilitated by communication in public."[95]

Public harassment includes pinching, slapping, hitting, shouted remarks, vulgarity, insults, sly innuendo, ogling, and stalking. Public harassment is on a continuum of possible events, beginning when customary civility among strangers is abrogated and ending with the transition to violent crime (assault, rape, or murder).[95]

According to a 2019 National Study on Sexual Harassment and Assault,[96] based on a telephone survey of more than 2,000 adult women and men, 68% of female participants and

23% of males indicated that they have experienced sexual harassment in a public place (such as a street, park, beach, store, restaurant, mall, library, movie theater, museum, swimming pool, or gym) in their lifetime. The study also documented that 18% of women and 16% of men said the most recent experience occurred in the previous six months, while 45% of all respondents indicated that the most recent experience took place in the previous five years.[96]

Among women, the most common forms of sexual harassment included: being whistled or honked at, being stared at, being leered at aggressively, or being subjected to kissy noises or provocative sounds (like "pssst"). They were also be subjected to disrespectful or unwanted comments ("Hey baby," "Yo shorty," "Mami/Mamacita") and were called a sexist slur ("bitch," "ho," "slut").[96] Furthermore, comments were made about their body parts or they were asked inappropriate sexual questions.[96] Men were also subjected to whistling, honking, kissy noises, and "pssst" sounds; being leered at or stared at aggressively; or being exposed to homophobic or transphobic slurs.[96]

Among the adults who were sexually harassed, 30% of women and 18% of men experienced anxiety or depression, while 22% of women and 12% of men exposed to street harassment changed their route or regular routines.[96]

In a study by DelGreco and Christensen[97] that was based on a survey 252 female undergraduates of a Northeastern university, street harassment was positively related to anxiety and depression and negatively linked to sleep quality, while both anxiety and depression mediated the relationship between street harassment and sleep quality.[97]

Incivility in the Neighborhood

The notion of everyday incivility has been defined as "commonplace actions and interactions that are perceived to be rude or inconsiderate."[98] In 2000, Phillips and Smith[98] carried out a study to gather data on occurrences and views of incivility in public settings, utilizing semi-structured group techniques with 54 socially diverse adult residents of Melbourne, Australia. The research documented 294 episodes of incivilities in public places that were directly experienced or witnessed by the participants.[98] The majority of the incivilities (76%) were physical, with the most common examples recorded being road rage and aggressive and selfish driving (15%), followed by pushing and shoving (8%) and queue jumping (6%). Verbal incivilities accounted for 24% of the incivilities reported, with the most common (10%) being the use of inappropriate language (swearing, sexual remarks), followed by verbal aggression (4%). Of the reported physical incivilities, 4% or less were exemplified by spitting, littering, people walking into somebody or inconsiderate use of a footpath, aggressive use of a shopping cart, smoking, bad parenting, begging, and dirty looks.

A subsequent study on urban incivility, also by Phillips and Smith,[99] was based on a cross-sectional telephone survey of 1,621 adults throughout Australia and aimed to collect systematic narrative information on interpersonal encounters involving a rude stranger. The investigation showed that 61% of the uncivil encounters involved rude movements, with the most common instance (25%) being cutting somebody off or pushing in front of somebody, followed by cases of blocking somebody's way (10%), bumping into somebody (9%), invading somebody's space (6%), tailing somebody (4%), swerving in front of somebody (4%), or stopping abruptly in front of somebody (2%).[99] Of the other reported rudeness from a stranger, 11% concerned either bodily gestures (dirty or lewd looks, "the ups") or swearing, while 5% pertained to irritating sounds, such as a screaming, screeching, or shouting child or the beeping horn or revving engine of a motor vehicle.[99]

Dangerous Driving and Road Rage

Two decades ago, Dula and Geller[100] suggested that the concept of dangerous driving should encompass a spectrum of "driving behaviors that endanger or have the potential to endanger others."[100] The behaviors included: "a) intentional acts of aggression toward others; b) negative emotions experienced while driving, and c) risk taking."[100] Based on their review of previous literature,[101-107] they cited at least 24 examples of dangerous driving (Table 15.1)

The Dula Dangerous Driving Index[108] (DDDI) was developed to assess drivers' self-reported probability of driving hazardously. The DDDI encompasses 31 items pertaining to the categories of aggressive driving, negative emotions while driving, and risky driving[108] Its validity and reliability across cultures has been established, and it has been translated into Flemish, Chinese, Romanian, and French.[109-112]

The prevalence of road rage, defined as "a driver's uncontrolled aggressive behavior, apparently caused by the stresses of modern driving,"[113] was ascertained in a cross-sectional study of 131 current drivers who were patients waiting to be seen at an inner-London general practice clinic.[113] Fifty-three percent of them reported being exposed to a road rage incident in the previous five years, as a victim (29%), perpetrator (12%), or as both a victim and a perpetrator (11%).[30] Of the individuals involved in a road rage incident, 12% reported that an accident occurred immediately prior to the episode of road rage, 15% reported damage to a person or property during the incident, 32% indicated that either party got out of the car, and 7% required police involvement.[113]

Prevalence of road rage in Ontario was examined by Smart et al.[114] based on data from the 2001 Center for Addiction and Mental Health Monitor, a repeated cross-sectional telephone

Table 15.1. Examples of Dangerous Driving (Adapted from Dula and Geller[100])

Actual use of, or gesturing with, a gun	Cutting vehicles off	Glaring at another driver	Speeding 10–20 mph over the speed limit
Blocking an intersection or lane	Double parking	Intentionally braking suddenly	Tailgating
Cell phone usage	Failing to yield right of way	Passing on the shoulder	Thinking hostile thoughts about other drivers
Changing speed erratically	Failure to stop for pedestrians	Pulling into somebody else's parking space	Taking more than one parking space
Chasing other vehicles	Failure to use signals	Running a red light or stop sign	Using the vehicle as a battering object
Communicating threats or insults verbally, with gestures, or by horn-honking	Forcing one's way in front of a vehicle that has the right of way	Running vehicles off the road	Weaving in and out of traffic

survey of almost 1,400 adults. Nearly 50% of the respondents reported that they were shouted at, cursed at, or had rude gestures directed at them in the previous year, while 7% were threatened with damage to their vehicle or personal injury.

According to a 2014 report[115] prepared by the American Automobile Association Foundation for Traffic Safety, based on a nationally representative online survey of 2,705 licensed drivers age 16 and older, about 78% of the respondents indicated that they "engaged in at least one aggressive driving behavior at least once in the past year."[115] About half of the respondents had tailgated another vehicle, yelled at another driver, or honked their horn to show annoyance or anger; one-third of them had made an angry gesture at another driver; 24% had tried to block another driver from changing lanes; and 2% to 4% had intentionally cut off another vehicle, had exited their vehicle to confront another driver, or had bumped or rammed another vehicle on purpose.[115]

Incivility toward and among Cyclists

Car drivers' aggressive behavior toward cyclists was studied by Fruhen and Flin[116] through a 2013 online survey of 276 drivers age 18 or older. The study documented that aggressive warnings (cutting up, verbal abuse, sounding the horn, making a hand gesture, verbal threats, or flashing) were associated with younger age, being a male, having a negative attitude toward cyclists, having a negative attitude about risk taking, and subscribing to perceived social norms concerning aggressive warnings toward cyclists.[116]

An assessment of self-reported aggression among 623 Australian adult cyclists was conducted by Stephens et al.[117] using the Cyclist Anger Expression Inventory.[118] The results indicated that cyclists mostly dealt with their anger in an adaptive way (e.g., accepting there are frustrating situations, telling oneself to ignore it, or thinking of a positive solution). Yet, when cyclists were aggressive, they were most likely to convey their aggression by shouting or swearing aloud.[117] The physical expression of aggression was infrequent, and was more likely to be associated with crashes, as well as with younger male cyclists having a history of personal physical aggression, and was more likely to occur in "a group of riders who regularly ride on the road."[117]

Incivility and Pedestrian Safety

Recent research performed by Li et al.[119] examined the notion of raising incivility awareness to deter pedestrians from crossing red lights. The investigation[119] included three field experiments conducted at three busy, unpatrolled intersections, each in a different district of the city of Shanghai. The first experiment assessed the effectiveness of an incivility-awareness sign by assessing the frequency of crossing violations under the presence or absence of a warning sign. This trial showed a statistically significant difference in frequency of crossing violations: only 28% of infractions were committed by pedestrians who were exposed to a sign indicating that "Crossing at a red light is uncivil," in contrast to 33% of crossing transgressions made by pedestrians who were shown a no-crossing command sign, and 65% of violations among pedestrians who were not exposed to any sign.

The second experiment tested the efficacy of two civility-related signs as compared to two safety-related signs and showed that the lowest rate of violation (23%) was perpetrated by pedestrians who were exposed to a incivility-awareness sign, as compared to the 30% rate of infractions among individuals who saw a sign about civil awareness, 31% of crossing transgression among pedestrians exposed to a danger-awareness sign, 37% of infringements among people observing a safety-awareness sign, and 49% of violations when no sign was posted. The duration of the effectiveness of the incivility-awareness sign was tested in the third experiment, which showed that during the four weeks while the incivility sign was posted, the rate of violation remained below 37%, but it rebounded to 59% when the sign was removed.[119]

Dommes et al.[120] investigated human factors linked to red light violations, and more generally to safety-related behaviors at signalized crosswalks, in a study that linked the compilation of observational data with questionnaires answered by 422 French pedestrians. The results showed that running while crossing a street was more likely to happen if the pedestrian was younger, when traffic was heavy, and there were no reported crossing difficulties.[120] Also, the probability of a pedestrian's looking at the traffic while crossing was significantly associated with pedestrians crossing alone and with parked vehicles near the crosswalk, while looking at the pedestrian light while crossing "was significantly associated with heavy traffic and [was] observed among pedestrians reporting difficulty cross[ing] a road."[120]

Nuisance in the Neighborhood

The definition of *nuisance* is something "that is annoying, unpleasant or obnoxious"[121] and within a legal context as "something (as an act, object, or practice) that invades or interferes with another's rights or interests (as the use or enjoyment of property) by being offensive, annoying, dangerous, obstructive, or unhealthful."[122]

Paquin and Gambrill[123] explored the nature of annoyances between neighbors through a telephone survey of almost 200 adults living in Alameda County, California, in 1986. The study recorded that 90% of the respondents had experienced an average of almost three types of neighborhood nuisances in the preceding three years. Respondents reported that 43% of them were subjected to the annoyance of a neighbor's barking dog, and 33% were bothered by either the neighbor playing loud music, parking a car in the way, or having their dog mess in the respondent's yard.[123] Also, 25% of the participants were exposed to arguments with neighbors, and around 10% experienced their neighbor's child being noisy or damaging their property or their neighbors' being involved in criminal activity.[123] Verbal abuse by a neighbor was experienced by 6% of the respondents, while physical abuse by a neighbor was experienced by only 0.5%.[123]

Another assessment of frequency and type of nuisances experienced by neighbors was led by Adderley,[124] who conducted a survey, in 2006, of 414 adults living in New Providence, the Bahamas. A range of annoying circumstances were experienced by the neighbors at least once a week, with the most common (80%) being the barking of dogs at night and the noise of car systems, while the less frequently reported nuisance (26%) was the noise of air conditioning units (Table15.2).

An indication of the public health impact of neighborhood nuisance can be found in the results of a cross-sectional study by Agyemang et al.,[125] who investigated the associations

Table 15.2. Neighborhood Nuisances Experienced by Residents of the Island of New Providence, The Bahamas, during the Fall of 2006 (Adapted from Adderley[124])

Nuisance Experienced	Residents Responding (%) That the Nuisance Is Experienced Every Week or So	Nuisance Experienced	Residents Responding (%) That the Nuisance Is Experienced Every Week or So
Litter	84%	Beggars	48%
Car sound systems	82%	Dumping	44%
Dogs barking at night	80%	Neighbors' parties after midnight	43%
Car alarms	76%	Dogs barking during the day	42%
Unsupervised children	73%	Gangs	42%
Loud motorbikes (in convoy)	73%	Lawn mowing on Sunday mornings	40%
Domestic noises	67%	Abandoned cars	40%
Car horns	66%	Graffiti	40%
Noisy neighbors in the street	61%	Bonfires	40%
Bad parking	60%	Construction work/workers	35%
Unkempt yards/gardens	59%	Uninvited strangers calling at home	32%
Firecrackers	58%	Overflowing sewage	30%
Car pollution	55%	Noise from air conditioning units	26%

between neighborhood-level psychosocial stressors and self-rated health among more than 2,900 adults living in Amsterdam in 2003. The study showed that people experiencing high levels of neighborhood nuisance were at significant high risk (AOR = 1.99) of self-reporting fair to poor health, and this association was independent of individual-level demographic and socioeconomic factors.

Future Directions

Studies are needed to further the understanding of the nature, prevalence, and public health consequences of different forms of maltreatment occurring in the neighborhood. Advancing this line of research should bring the topic of neighborhood maltreatment to a level of development comparable to the degree achieved by studies of victimization in other milieus, such as the home, school, workplace, and cyberspace. Such knowledge will spur the inclusion of neighborhood victimization as a category in clinical detection tools and prevention strategies. In this context, there is a need to, at least, consider:

Table 15.3. Types of Maltreatment That Occur in a Neighborhood

Bullying	Incivility by, or toward, cyclists	Physical fights
Dangerous driving and road rage	Incivility by, or toward, pedestrians	Street harassment
Discrimination	Nuisance	Violent or property crimes

- Including questions pertaining to exposure to bullying and physical fights in the neighborhood in future versions of national[66,126] or multinational[65,67] health and behavioral risk surveys[65-67,126]
- Incorporating queries in future versions of national[127,128] or international victimization surveys[50,127,128] to ascertain exposure to different types of victimization or maltreatment in the neighborhood (Table 15.3) and their health impact (such as the feeling of safety as well as fear of crime, gangs, mass shootings, and terrorism)

Notes

1. Olweus D. *Bullying at School: What We Know and What We Can Do*. Oxford, England: Blackwell; 1993. Cited in Percy-Smith and Matthews (see Note 2).
2. Percy-Smith B, Matthews H. Tyrannical spaces: young people, bullying and urban neighborhoods. *Local Environ*. 2001;6(1):49–63.
3. Costa MR, Xavier CC, Andrade AC, Proietti FA, Caiaffa WT. Bullying among adolescents in a Brazilian urban center—"Health in Beagá" Study. *Rev Saude Publica*. 2015;49.
4. Andershed H, Kerr M, Stattin H. Bullying in school and violence on the streets: are the same people involved? *J Scand Stud Criminol Crime Prev*. 2001;2(1):31–49.
5. Second analysis of the HBSC conducted online, data not previously published. https://www.icpsr.umich.edu/web/NAHDAP/studies/34792. Accessed August 15, 2022.
6. Iannotti RJ. *Health Behavior in School-Aged Children (HBSC), 2009–2010*. Inter-university Consortium for Political and Social Research [distributor]; 2013.https://doi.org/10.3886/ICPSR34792.v1. Accessed August 15, 2022.
7. Harrell E. Violent victimization committed by strangers, 1993–2010. Bureau of Justice Statistics; 2012. https://bjs.ojp.gov/content/pub/pdf/vvcs9310.pdf. Accessed August 17, 2022.
8. Morgan RE, Kena G. Criminal victimization, 2018. Bureau of Justice Statistics; 2019:845..https://bjs.ojp.gov/content/pub/pdf/cv19.pdf. Accessed August 17, 2022.
9. Sampson RJ. Personal violence by strangers: an extension and test of the opportunity model of predatory victimization. *J Crim Law Criminol*. 1987;78:327.
10. Title 18 USC §521(a)(A). Cited by National Gang Intelligence Center, 2011 National Gang Threat Assessment. https://www.fbi.gov/stats-services/publications/2011-national-gang-threat-assessment. Accessed August 17, 2022.
11. National Gang Intelligence Center, National Gang Report, 2015. https://www.fbi.gov/file-repository/stats-services-publications-national-gang-report-2015.pdf/view. Accessed August 17, 2022.
12. Miller WB. *Crime by Youth Gangs and Groups in the United States*. Washington, DC: US Department of Justice, Office of Justice Programs, Office of Juvenile Justice and Delinquency

Prevention; 1992:21. https://www.bjs.gov/content/pub/pdf/cyggus.pdf. Last accessed August 26, 2021.

13. Pyrooz DC, Sweeten G. Gang membership between ages 5 and 17 years in the United States. *J Adolesc Health*. 2015;56(4):414–419.
14. Sullivan ML. Maybe we shouldn't study "gangs": does reification obscure youth violence? *J Contemp Crim Justice*. 2005;21(2):170–190. Cited by Sharp et al. (see Note 16).
15. Fleisher MS. Doing field research on diverse gangs: interpreting youth gangs as social networks. In: Huff R, ed. *Gangs in America III*. Thousand Oaks, CA: SAGE; 2002:199–218. Cited by Sharp et al. (see Note 16).
16. Sharp C, Aldridge J, Medina-Ariza J. *Delinquent Youth Groups and Offending Behavior: Findings from the 2004 Offending Crime and Justice Survey*. London, England: Home Office: 2006. https://www.research.manchester.ac.uk/portal/files/35506173/FULL_TEXT.PDF. Accessed August 17, 2022.
17. Gatti U, Haymoz S, Schadee HM. Deviant youth groups in 30 countries: results from the Second International Self-Report Delinquency Study. *Int Crim Justice Rev*. 2011;21(3):208–224.
18. European Federation of National Organizations Working with the Homeless (FEANTSA). https://www.feantsa.org/en/about-us/what-is-feantsa. Accessed August 17, 2022.
19. European Typology of Homelessness and Housing Exclusion (ETHOS). https://www.feantsa.org/download/ethos2484215748748239888.pdf. Accessed August 17, 2022.
20. Our World in Data, flagship project of Global Change Data Lab (see Note 21), which develops data and research to make progress with the world's largest problems. https://ourworldindata.org/about. Accessed August 17, 2022.
21. Global Change Data Lab, a nonprofit organization, chartered in England and Wales, whose purpose is to advance education in how global conditions and the Earth's environment are changing, through the production and maintenance of public online resources. https://global-change-data-lab.org/. Accessed August 17, 2022.
22. Ortiz-Ospina E, Roser M. Homelessness. Our World in Data; 2017. https://ourworldindata.org/homelessness?source = post_page. Accessed August 17, 2022.
23. Henry M, Watt R, Mahathey A, Oulette J, Sitller A. *The 2019 Annual Homeless Assessment Report (AHAR) to Congress, Part 1: Point-in-Time Estimates of Homelessness*. Washington, DC: US Department of Housing and Urban Development. https://www.huduser.gov/portal/sites/default/files/pdf/2019-AHAR-Part-1.pdf. Accessed August 17, 2022.
24. Meerwijk EL, Sevelius JM. Transgender population size in the United States: a meta-regression of population-based probability samples. *Am J Public Health*. 2017;107(2):e1–e8.
25. US Census Bureau. Quick Facts: United States, Population Estimates July 1, 2021. https://www.census.gov/quickfacts/fact/table/US/PST045219. Accessed August 17, 2022.
26. Department of Communities and Local Government, Housing and Statistical Release, Rough Sleeping Statistics, Autumn 2016, England. https://assets.publishing.service.gov.uk/government/uploads/system/uploads/attachment_data/file/585713/Rough_Sleeping_Autumn_2016_Statistical_Release.pdf. Accessed August 17, 2022.
27. Calculated on the basis of data from the Office for National Statistics, Population Estimates for the UK, England and Wales, Scotland and Northern Ireland: Mid 2016—Population of England Reaches 55 Million. https://www.ons.gov.uk/peoplepopulationandcommunity/populationandmigration/populationestimates/bulletins/annualmidyearpopulationestimates/mid2016#population-of-england-reaches-55-million. Accessed August 17, 2022.

28. Calculated on the basis of data from the Office for National Statistics, Subnational Population Projections for England 2016—London Is Projected To Be the Fastest Growing Region in England. https://www.ons.gov.uk/peoplepopulationandcommunity/populationandmigration/populationprojections/bulletins/subnationalpopulationprojectionsforengland/2016based#london-is-projected-to-be-the-fastest-growing-region-in-england. Accessed August 17, 2022.
29. Ellsworth JT. Street crime victimization among homeless adults: a review of the literature. *Vict Offenders*. 2019;14(1):96–118.
30. Huelsman M. Violence on Anchorage's 4th Avenue from the perspective of street people. *Alaska Med*. 1983;25(2):39–44. Cited by Ellsworth.[29]
31. Fischer PJ, Breakey WR. Homelessness and mental health: an overview. *Int J Ment Health*. 1985;14(4):6–41. Cited by Ellsworth.[29]
32. Padgett DK, Struening EL. Victimization, and traumatic injuries among the homeless: associations with alcohol, drug, and mental problems. *Am J Orthopsychiatry*. 1992;62(4):525–534. Cited by Ellsworth.[29]
33. Lam JA, Rosenheck R. The effect of victimization on clinical outcomes of homeless persons with serious mental illness. *Psychiatr Serv*. 1998;49(5):678–683. Cited by Ellsworth.[29]
34. Fitzpatrick KM, LaGory ME, Ritchey FJ. Dangerous places: exposure to violence and its mental health consequences for the homeless. *Am J Orthopsychiatry*. 1999;69(4):438–447. Cited by Ellsworth.[29]
35. Kushel MB, Evans JL, Perry S, Robertson MJ, Moss AR. No door to lock: victimization among homeless and marginally housed persons. *Arch Intern Med*. 2003;163(20):2492–2499. Cited by Ellsworth.[29]
36. Hudson AL, Wright K, Bhattacharya D, Sinha K, Nyamathi A, Marfisee M. Correlates of adult assault among homeless women. *J Health Care Poor Underserved*. 2010;21(4):1250–1262. Cited by Ellsworth.[29]
37. Bureau of Justice Statistics. *Criminal Victimization in the United States, 1983* (NCJ-96459). Washington, DC: US Department of Justice; 1985. Cited by Ellsworth.[29]
38. Bureau of Justice Statistics. *Criminal Victimization in the United States, 1986* (NCJ-106989). Washington, DC: US Department of Justice; 1987. Cited by Ellsworth.[29]
39. Bureau of Justice Statistics. *Criminal Victimization in the United States, 2015* (NCJ-250180). Washington, DC: US Department of Justice; 2016. Cited by Ellsworth.[29]
40. Scott RA. Without shelter, people die: disproportionate mortality rates among King County's homeless population, 2009–2019 (Order No. 28002474). Available from ProQuest Dissertations & Theses Global. (2437130095). Retrieved from https://gwlaw.idm.oclc.org/login?url=https://www.proquest.com/dissertations-theses/without-shelter-people-die-disproportionate/docview/2437130095/se-2
41. Volpi E. Street Children: Promising Practices and Approaches, page 2. World Bank Institute. Washington, DC, USA; 2002. https://documents1.worldbank.org/curated/en/344301468763803523/pdf/263880WBI0Street0children.pdf. Accessed October 12, 2023.
42. Consortium for Street Children. https://www.streetchildren.org/what-we-do/. Accessed August 17, 2022.
43. Consortium for Street Children. About Street Children. https://www.streetchildren.org/about-street-children/. Accessed August 17, 2022.
44. UNICEF. Latin American Seminar on Community Alternatives for Street Children. Brasilia, Brazil, 1984:12–15. Cited by Lalor (see Note 45).

45. Lalor KJ. Street children: a comparative perspective. *Child Abuse Negl.* 1999;23(8):759–770.
46. Taçon P. Marco and the malevolent monsters [Unpublished paper for presentation to the Organization of African Unity]; 1992. Cited by Lalor.[45]
47. UNICEF. *The State of the World's Children 2006: Excluded and Invisible.* UNICEF; 2005:40–41. https://www.unicef.org/reports/state-worlds-children-2006. Accessed October 1, 2023.
48. Gaetz S, O'Grady B, Buccieri K. *Surviving Crime and Violence: Street Youth and Victimization in Toronto.* Toronto, Ontario: JFCY & Homeless Hub; 2010. https://yorkspace.library.yorku.ca/xmlui/bitstream/handle/10315/29374/Surviving%20the%20Streets.JFCY_.September16.2010.pdf?sequence = 1. Accessed August 17, 2022.
49. Hartinger-Saunders RM, Rine CM, Nochajski T, Wieczorek W. Neighborhood crime and perception of safety as predictors of victimization and offending among youth: a call for macro-level prevention and intervention models. *Child Youth Serv Rev.* 2012;34(9):1966–1973.
50. Van Dijk J, Van Kesteren J, Smit P. Criminal victimisation in international perspective; 2007. https://repository.wodc.nl/bitstream/handle/20.500.12832/1204/ob257_full_text_tcm28-69406.pdf. Accessed October 12, 2023.
51. The 26 cities in developed countries included in the survey were: London (England), Tallinn (Estonia), Amsterdam (the Netherlands), Reykjavik (Iceland), Belfast (Northern Ireland), Dublin (Ireland), New York (United States), Copenhagen (Denmark), Stockholm (Sweden), Warsaw (Poland), Oslo (Norway), Helsinki (Finland), Zurich (Switzerland), Brussels (Belgium), Berlin (Germany), Istanbul (Turkey), Paris (France), Vienna (Austria), Edinburgh (Scotland), Rome (Italy), Sydney (Australia), Madrid (Spain), Athens (Greece), Budapest (Hungary), Lisbon (Portugal), and Hong Kong (SAR China). Cited by Van Dijk et al.[50]
52. Ten common crimes: Theft of a car; theft from a car; motorcycle theft; bicycle theft; burglary with entry; theft of personal property and pickpocketing; robbery; sexual offenses; assault and threats; consumer fraud. Cited by Van Dijk et al.[50]
53. The six cities in undeveloped countries included in the survey were: Phnom Penh (Cambodia), Maputo (Mozambique), Buenos Aires (Argentina), Johannesburg (South Africa), Sao Paulo (Brazil), and Rio de Janeiro (Brazil). Cited by Van Dijk et al.[50]
54. Duque LF, Montoya NE, Restrepo A. Violence witnessing, perpetrating and victimization in Medellin, Colombia: a random population survey. *BMC Public Health.* 2011;11(1):628.
55. Duque LF, Klevens J, Ramirez C. Cross sectional survey of perpetrators, victims, and witnesses of violence in Bogotá, Colombia. *J Epidemiol Community Health.* 2003;57(5):355–360.
56. Health Resources and Services Administration, Maternal and Child Health. 2016–17 National Survey of Children's Health, Fast Facts https://www.childhealthdata.org/docs/default-source/default-document-library/2016-17-nsch_fast-facts_final6fba3af3c0266255aab2ff00001023b1.pdf?sfvrsn = 569c5817_0. Accessed August 17, 2022.
57. Child and Adolescent Health Measurement Initiative. National Survey of Children's Health (2016-present). Data Resource Center for Child and Adolescent Health supported by the U.S Department of Health and Human Services, Health Resources and Services Administration (HRSA), Maternal and Child Health Bureau MCHB. Measures; State/Region: Nationwide; Topic: Neighborhood Safety and Support; Question: Indicator 7.2, Safe Neighborhood. https://www.childhealthdata.org/browse/survey. Accessed October 1, 2023.
58. Child and Adolescent Health Measurement Initiative. National Survey of Children's Health (2016-present). Data Resource Center for Child and Adolescent Health supported by the U.S Department of Health and Human Services, Health Resources and Services Administration (HRSA), Maternal and Child Health Bureau MCHB. Measures; State/Region: Nationwide;

Topic: Neighborhood Safety and Support; Question: Indicator 7.2, Safe Neighborhood; Sub-Group: Race/ethnicity—with Asian (National only). https://www.childhealthdata.org/browse/survey. Accessed October 1, 2023.

59. Economist Intelligent Unit, research division of The Economist Group. http://www.eiu.com/home.aspx. Accessed August 17, 2022.
60. The Economist Intelligence Unit. Safe Cities Index 2017, Security in a rapidly urbanizing world. Appendix 2: Index methodology, Index categories, Personal security, page 34. https://safecities.economist.com/safe-cities-index-2017/. Accessed October 1, 2023.
61. The Economist Intelligence Unit. Safe Cities Index 2017, Security in a rapidly urbanizing world. Category 4: Personal Security, page 2. https://safecities.economist.com/safe-cities-index-2017/. Accessed October 1, 2023.
62. McCrea R, Shyy TK, Western J, Stimson RJ. Fear of crime in Brisbane: individual, social and neighborhood factors in perspective. *J Sociol.* 2005;41(1):7–27.
63. Katz CM, Webb VJ, Armstrong TA. Fear of gangs: a test of alternative theoretical models. *Justice Q.* 2003;20(1):95–130.
64. Lemieux F, Bricknell S, Prenzler T. Mass shootings in Australia and the United States, 1981–2013. *J Criminol Res Policy Pract.* 2015;1(3):131–142.
65. Beard JH, Jacoby SF, James R, et al. Examining mass shootings from a neighborhood perspective: an analysis of multiple-casualty events and media reporting in Philadelphia, United States. *Prev Med.* 2019;129:105856..
66. Lowe SR, Galea S. The mental health consequences of mass shootings. *Trauma Violence Abuse.* 2017;18(1):62–82. Cited by Beard et al.[65]
67. Schwarz ED, Kowalski JM. Malignant memories: PTSD in children and adults after a school shooting. *J Am Acad Child Adolesc Psychiatry.* 1991;30(6):936–944. Cited by Lowe and Galea.[66]
68. Schwarz ED, Kowalski JM. Posttraumatic stress disorder after a school shooting: effects of symptom threshold selection and diagnosis by DSM-III, DSM-III-R, or proposed DSM-IV. *Am J Psychiatry.* 1991;148(5):592–597. Cited by Lowe and Galea.[66]
69. North CS, Smith EM, Spitznagel EL. One-year follow-up of survivors of a mass shooting. *Am J Psychiatry.* 1997;154(12):1696–1702. Cited by Lowe and Galea.[66]
70. Vicary AM, Fraley RC. Student reactions to the shootings at Virginia Tech and Northern Illinois University: does sharing grief and support over the Internet affect recovery? *Pers Soc Psychol Bull.* 2010;36(11):1555–1563. Cited by Lowe and Galea.[66]
71. Rapoport R, Berta K. *Methodology Report: American Fears Survey.* SSRS; 2019. https://www.chapman.edu/wilkinson/research-centers/babbie-center/_files/full-survey-methodology-2019.pdf. Accessed August 17, 2022.
72. Sheth S. *America's Top Fears 2019.* https://www.chapman.edu/wilkinson/research-centers/babbie-center/_files/americas-top-fears-2019.pdf. Accessed August 17, 2022.
73. Onat I, Guler A, Kula S, Bastug MF. Fear of terrorism and fear of violent crimes in the United States: a comparative analysis. *Crime Delinq.* 2021:00111287211036130.
74. Rapoport R, Berta K. *Methodology Report: American Fears Survey.* SSRS; 2018. https://www.chapman.edu/wilkinson/research-centers/babbie-center/_files/fear-2018/fear-V-methodology-report-ssrs.pdf. Accessed August 17, 2022. Cited by Onat et al.[73]
75. Goldman-Mellor S, Margerison-Zilko C, Allen K, Cerdá M. Perceived and objectively measured neighborhood violence, and adolescent psychological distress. *J Urban Health.* 2016;93(5):758–769.

76. Polling C, Khondoker M, Hatch SL, Hotopf M, SELCoH Study Team. Influence of perceived and actual neighborhood disorder on common mental illness. *Soc Psychiatry Psychiatr Epidemiol.* 2014;49(6):889–901.
77. Yimgang DP, Wang Y, Paik G, Hager ER, Black MM. Civil unrest in the context of chronic community violence: impact on maternal depressive symptoms. *Am J Public Health.* 2017;107(9):1455–1462.
78. Sternthal MJ, Jun HJ, Earls F, Wright RJ. Community violence and urban childhood asthma: a multilevel analysis. *Eur Resp J.* 2010;36(6):1400–1409.
79. Apter AJ, Garcia LA, Boyd RC, Wang X, Bogen DK, Ten Have T. Exposure to community violence is associated with asthma hospitalizations and emergency department visits. *J Allergy Clin Immunol.* 2010;126(3):552–557.
80. Shareck M, Ellaway A. Neighborhood crime and smoking: the role of objective and perceived crime measures. *BMC Public Health.* 2011;11(1):930.
81. Forsyth A, Wall M, Choo T, Larson N, Van Riper D, Neumark-Sztainer D. Perceived and police-reported neighborhood crime: linkages to adolescent activity behaviors and weight status. *J Adolesc Health.* 2015;57(2):222–228.
82. Augustin T, Glass TA, James BD, Schwartz BS. Neighborhood psychosocial hazards and cardiovascular disease: the Baltimore Memory Study. *Am J Public Health.* 2008;98(9):1664–1670.
83. Bagley EJ, Tu KM, Buckhalt JA, El-Sheikh M. Community violence concerns and adolescent sleep. *Sleep Health.* 2016;2(1):57–62.
84. Feagin JR. The continuing significance of race: antiblack discrimination in public places. *Am Sociol Rev.* 1991:101–116.
85. Pascoe EA, Smart Richman L. Perceived discrimination, and health: a meta-analytic review. *Psychol Bull.* 2009;135(4):531.
86. Williams DR, Yu Y, Jackson JS, Anderson NB. Racial differences in physical and mental health: socio-economic status, stress, and discrimination. *J Health Psychol.* 1997;2(3):335–351.
87. Banks KH, Kohn-Wood LP, Spencer M. An examination of the African American experience of everyday discrimination and symptoms of psychological distress. *Community Ment Health J.* 2006;42(6):555–570.
88. Kessler RC, Mickelson KD, Williams DR. The prevalence, distribution, and mental health correlates of perceived discrimination in the United States. *J Health Soc Behav.* 1999:208–230.
89. Carlisle SK. Perceived discrimination and chronic health in adults from nine ethnic subgroups in the USA. *Ethn Health.* 2015;20(3):309–326.
90. Pérez DJ, Fortuna L, Alegria M. Prevalence, and correlates of everyday discrimination among US Latinos. *J Community Psychol.* 2008;36(4):421–433.
91. Dulin-Keita A, Hannon Iii L, Fernandez JR, Cockerham WC. The defining moment: children's conceptualization of race and experiences with racial discrimination. *Ethn Racial Stud.* 2011;34(4):662–682.
92. di Leonardo M. Political economy of street harassment. *Aegis.* 1981; Summer. Cited by Logan (see Note 94).
93. Bowman CG. Street harassment and the informal ghettoization of women. Harvard Law Rev. 1993;106(3):517–580. Cited by Logan (see Note 94).
94. Logan LS. Street harassment: current and promising avenues for researchers and activists. *Sociol Compass.* 2015;9(3):196–211.
95. Gardner CB. *Passing By: Gender and Public Harassment.* Berkeley: University of California Press; 1995:4. Cited by Logan.[94]

96. *Measuring #MeToo: A National Study on Sexual Harassment and Assault.* UC San Diego Center on Gender Equity and Health: Stop Street Harassment; 2018. https://stopstreetharassment.org/wp-content/uploads/2012/08/2019-MeToo-National-Sexual-Harassment-and-Assault-Report.pdf. Accessed August 17, 2022.
97. DelGreco M, Christensen J. Effects of street harassment on anxiety, depression, and sleep quality of college women. *Sex Roles.* 2020;82(7):473–481.
98. Phillips T, Smith P. Everyday incivility: towards a benchmark. *Sociol Rev.* 2003;51(1):85–108.
99. Phillips T, Smith P. Rethinking urban incivility research: strangers, bodies, and circulations. *Urban Stud.* 2006;43(5-6):879–901.
100. Dula CS, Geller ES. Risky, aggressive, or emotional driving: addressing the need for consistent communication in research. *J Safety Res.* 2003;34(5):559–566.
101. James L, Nahl D. *Road Rage and Aggressive Driving: Steering Clear of Highway Warfare.* Amherst, NY: Prometheus Books; 2000. Cited by Dula and Geller.[100]
102. Lajunen T, Parker D, Stradling S. (1998). Dimensions of driver anger, aggressive, and highway code violations and their mediation by safety orientation in UK drivers. *Transp Res F Traffic Psychol Behav.* 1998;1:107–121. Cited by Dula and Geller.[100]
103. Parker, D., Lajunen, T., & Stradling, S. (1998). Attitudinal predictors of interpersonally aggressive violations on the road. *Transp Res F Traffic Psychol Behav.* 1998;1:11–24. Cited by Dula and Geller.[100]
104. Doob AN, Gross AE. (1968). Status of frustrator as an inhibitor of horn-honking responses. *J Soc Psychol.* 1968;76:213–218. Cited by Dula and Geller.[100]
105. Turner CW, Layton JF, Simons LS. Naturalistic studies of aggressive behavior: aggressive stimuli, victim visibility, and horn honking. *J Pers Soc Psychol.* 1975;31:1098–1107. Cited by Dula and Geller.[100]
106. Shinar D. Aggressive driving: the contribution of the drivers and the situation. *Transp Res F Traffic Psychol Behav.* 1998;1:137–160. Cited by Dula and Geller.[100]
107. Ellison-Potter P, Bell P, Deffenbacher J. The effects of trait driving anger, anonymity, and aggressive stimuli on aggressive driving behavior. *J Appl Soc Psychol.* 2001;31:431–443. Cited by Dula and Geller.[100]
108. Dula CS, Ballard ME. Development and evaluation of a measure of dangerous, aggressive, negative emotional, and risky driving. *J Appl Soc Psychol.* 2003 Feb 1;33(2):263–282.
109. Willemsen J, Dula CS, Declercq F, Verhaeghe P. The Dula Dangerous Driving Index: an investigation of reliability and validity across cultures. *Accid Anal Prev.* 2008;40(2):798–806.
110. Qu W, Ge Y, Jiang C, Du F, Zhang K. The Dula Dangerous Driving Index in China: an investigation of reliability and validity. *Accid Anal Prev.* 2014;64:62–68.
111. Iliescu D, Sârbescu P. The relationship of dangerous driving with traffic offenses: a study on an adapted measure of dangerous driving. *Accid Anal Prev.* 2013;51:33–41.
112. Richer I, Bergeron J. Differentiating risky and aggressive driving: further support of the internal validity of the Dula Dangerous Driving Index. *Accid Anal Prev.* 2012;45:620–627.
113. Fong G, Frost D, Stansfeld S. Road rage: a psychiatric phenomenon? *Soc Psychiatry Psychiatr Epidemiol.* 2001;36(6):277–286.
114. Smart RG, Mann RE, Stoduto G. The prevalence of road rage: estimates from Ontario. *Can J Public Health/Rev Can Santé Publique.* 2003;1:247–250.
115. AAA Foundation for Traffic Safety. Prevalence of Self-Reported Aggressive Driving Behavior: United States, 2014. https://aaafoundation.org/wp-content/uploads/2017/12/Prevalence-of-Aggressive-Drivig-2014.pdf. Accessed October 1, 2023.

116. Fruhen LS, Flin R. Car driver attitudes, perceptions of social norms and aggressive driving behavior towards cyclists. *Accid Anal Prev*. 2015;83:162–170.
117. Stephens AN, O'Hern S, Trawley S, Young KL, Koppel S. Self-reported aggression amongst active cyclists. *Accid Anal Prev*. 2019;128:46–52.
118. Møller M, Haustein S. Anger expression among Danish cyclists and drivers: a comparison based on mode specific anger expression inventories. *Accid Anal Prev*. 2017;108:354–360. Cited by Stephens et al.[117]
119. Li X, Hsee CK, Wang L. Incivility awareness could save lives. *Behav Sci Policy*. 2021;7(1):1–8. https://behavioralpolicy.org/articles/incivility-awareness-could-save-lives/. Accessed August 17, 2022.
120. Dommes A, Granié MA, Cloutier MS, Coquelet C, Huguenin-Richard F. Red light violations by adult pedestrians and other safety-related behaviors at signalized crosswalks. *Accid Anal Prev*. 2015;80:67–75.
121. *Merriam-Webster's Collegiate Dictionary*. 11th ed. Springfield, MA: Merriam-Webster; 2003:850. Cited by Adderley (see Note 124).
122. *Merriam-Webster's Dictionary of Law*. Springfield, MA: Merriam-Webster; 1996:333. Cited by Adderley (see Note 124).
123. Paquin GW, Gambrill E. The problem with neighbors. *J Community Psychol*. 1994;22(1):21–32. Cited by Adderley (see Note 124).
124. Adderley CR. Neighborhood nuisances in the Bahamas: the case of New Providence. *Int J Bahamian Stud*. 2008;14:4–12.
125. Agyemang C, van Hooijdonk C, Wendel-Vos W, Lindeman E, Stronks K, Droomers M. The association of neighborhood psychosocial stressors and self-rated health in Amsterdam, the Netherlands. *J Epidemiol Community Health*. 2007;61(12):1042–1049.
126. Statistics Canada, National Longitudinal Survey of Children and Adolescents, November 10, 2010. https://www23.statcan.gc.ca/imdb/p2SV.pl?Function=getSurvey&SDDS=4450. Accessed October 1, 2023.
127. Hamby SL, Finkelhor D, Ormrod RK, Turner HA. *The Juvenile Victimization Questionnaire (JVQ): Administration and Scoring Manual*. Durham, NH: Crimes Against Children Research Center; 2004. https://www.unh.edu/ccrc/sites/default/files/media/2022-02/the-juvenile-victimization-questionnaire-jvq-administration-scoring-manual.pdf. Accessed August 17, 2022.
128. US Department of Justice, Bureau of Justice Statistics. National Crime Victimization Survey (NCVS). https://bjs.ojp.gov/data-collection/ncvs#surveys-0. Accessed August 17, 2022.

16
Victimization in Adolescent Dating Relationships

What Is Known?

This chapter explores the nature, prevalence, and health effects of the different forms of victimization that can affect adolescents involved in a dating relationship, as well as the association with maltreatment in other social milieus.

Teen Dating Relationships: Concept and Prevalence

The notion of a dating relationship, also known as a romantic relationship, signifies "mutually acknowledged ongoing voluntary interactions"[1] that usually have "a distinctive intensity, commonly marked by expressions of affection and current or anticipated sexual behavior."[1] According to a study by Carver et al.,[2] based on national representative sample of more than 12,000 US adolescents in grades 7 to 12 who took part in the 1994–1995 National Longitudinal Study of Adolescent to Adult Health (Add Health), 55% of the participants engaged in a romantic relationship in the previous 18 months. A Pew Research Center Report[3] on a 2015 survey of a nationally representative sample of more than 1,000 US adolescents age 13 to 17 documented that 35% of the participants "ever dated, hooked up with, or [had] been otherwise romantically involved with another person,"[3] while 18% of the respondents were in a romantic relationship at the time of the survey.[3] The survey also found that 26% of all the adolescents met somebody for the first time in person (offline), while 8% of them had "dated or hooked up with someone they first met online."[3] Furthermore, 92% of teens who were in a dating relationship spent time with their significant others through messaging, while 86% to 87% of the dating adolescents spent time together in person or talking by phone. Around 70% of the adolescents involved in romantic relationships spent time together through social media or instant messaging; 55% indicated that they spent time with their partner through video chat, while 37% used email.

Victimization in a Dating Relationship

As adapted from the Centers for Disease Control (CDC) definition of intimate partner violence,[4] dating victimization can be defined as physical or sexual violence, stalking, or psychological aggression by a current or former intimate partner (boyfriend, girlfriend, dating or ongoing sexual partners) of the opposite or same sex, who may or not be cohabiting with the victim. This is differentiated from intimate partner violence among spouses (married, common-law, or civil union spouses or domestic partners).[4] The various aspects of dating victimization have been described[4] as follows:

- Physical violence "includes, but is not limited to, scratching, pushing, shoving, throwing, grabbing, biting, choking, shaking, hair-pulling, slapping, punching, hitting, burning, use of a weapon (gun, knife, or other object), and use of restraints or one's body, size, or strength against another person. Physical violence also includes coercing other people to commit any of the above acts."[4]
- Sexual violence is defined[4] as a "sexual act that is committed or attempted by another person without freely given consent of the victim or against someone who is unable to consent or refuse. It includes forced or alcohol/drug-facilitated penetration of a victim; forced or alcohol/drug-facilitated incidents in which the victim was made to penetrate a perpetrator or someone else; nonphysical pressured unwanted penetration; intentional sexual touching; or noncontact acts of a sexual nature. Sexual violence can also occur when a perpetrator forces or coerces a victim to engage in sexual acts with a third party."[4]
- Stalking is understood as a "pattern of repeated, unwanted attention and contact that causes fear or concern for one's own safety or the safety of someone else (e.g., family member, close friend)."[4] It can be exemplified, at least, by watching or following from a distance; leaving strange or potentially threatening items for the victim to find; repeated and unwanted phone calls, emails, or voice messages; spying with a listening device; sneaking into the victim's home or car; or approaching/showing up in place when the victim does not want to be seen.[4]
- Psychological aggression is explained[4] as use of verbal and nonverbal language with the purpose of harming somebody mentally or emotionally and/or exerting control over another person. It can be represented by name-calling; humiliation; degradation; coercive control; threats; exploitation of the victim's disability, sexual orientation, or immigration status; or exploitation of the perpetrator's real or perceived disability or immigration status.

Cyberdating Abuse

Zweig et al. defined the term *cyberdating abuse* as "the control, harassment, stalking, and abuse of one's dating partner via technology and social media."[5] Zweig et al.[5] provided examples of cyberdating victimization, such as being pressured or threatened by one's dating partner to send them a sexual or naked photo of oneself,[5] having embarrassing photos or images of oneself posted online by one's dating partner,[5] having rumors about oneself being spread in cyberspace by one's partner,[6] or feeling scared/unsafe because of chats or messages that were sent by one's dating partner.[5]

Prevalence of Adolescent Dating Victimization

Prevalence of Physical Dating Victimization

According to the Youth Risk Behavior Survey (YRBS),[7] 8.2% of US adolescents in grades 9 to 12 were physically hurt on purpose (hit, slammed into something, or injured with an object or weapon) by somebody they were dating or going out with, one or more times during the 12 months preceding the survey of 2019.[8] Female participants were significantly more likely than male respondents to have been subjected to physical dating violence (9.3% vs. 7.0%).[8] The frequency of physical dating violence was significantly higher among bisexual adolescents (13.6%) and those who were not sure of their sexual orientation (16.9%) than among heterosexual adolescents (7.2%).[8] No significant differences in the frequency of physical dating violence were found among US adolescents of different races as compared to whites, yet the prevalence of physical dating victimization among ninth graders (5.6%) was significantly lower than the frequency among tenth graders (8.1%), eleventh graders (8.7%), and twelfth graders (9.8%).[8]

Earlier studies[9-11] using the YRBS documented a 12-month prevalence of physical dating victimization among US adolescents that varied from 8%[10] to 10%.[10,11]

A 2000–2001 survey by Banyard and Cross,[12] involving more than 2,000 US adolescents in grades 7 to 10, found that almost 17% of the students were subjected to dating physical violence at one time in their life.[12]

Prevalence of Sexual Dating Victimization

As per the YRBS,[7] 9.7% of US adolescents in grades 9 to 12 were forced to do sexual things (kissing, touching, or having sexual intercourse) that they did not want to do by someone who they were dating or going out with, one or more times in the preceding 12 months of a 2021 survey.[13] Females were significantly more likely than males to have been subjected to sexual dating violence (15% vs. 4.00%).[13] The prevalence of sexual dating victimization among heterosexual adolescents (6.6%) was significantly lower than the prevalence among bisexual adolescents (20.8%) or those teens who were not sure of their sexual orientation (23.8%). No significant difference in the frequency of sexual dating victimization was found among US adolescents of different races as compared to whites, or among teens in different grades.

Earlier studies[10-12,14] using the YRBS found a life prevalence of sexual dating violence among US adolescents varying from 7.4%[14] to 13.2%.[12]

Prevalence of Psychological/Emotional Dating Violence and Abuse

A 2011–2012 study by Hébert et al.,[15] based on a sample of more than 3,400 adolescents in grades 10 to 12 living in Quebec, aimed at determining the prevalence of dating victimization, and it documented that 56.4% of the female respondents and 45.8% of the males experienced, in the previous 12 months, situations during an argument or conflict with a boyfriend or girlfriend when their dating partner said things that made them angry, being ridiculed or made fun of by their partner in front of others, or having their partner kept track of where they were and with whom. The high frequency of psychological dating victimization was also shown in cross-sectional surveys of adolescents conducted in 2013 by Fox et al.[16] in the United Kingdom, and by Zweig et al.[17] in the United States, documenting a one-year prevalence of 65.6%[16] and 47%,[17] respectively.

Prevalence of Cyberdating Abuse

In the fall of 2016, Smith et al.[18] surveyed almost 400 French-speaking high school students from Quebec (Canada), to determine the prevalence of cyberdating victimization (CDV). The survey showed that 17% of the participants reported having been cybervictimized by a romantic dating partner during the previous 12 months, with no significant difference in the rate of victimization by gender. The most frequent forms of CDV were online instances of insults, blackmail, being frightened, being threatened, or having rumors spread.

Similar findings of CDV were documented by Exner-Cortens et al.[19] in a study based on a representative sample of 3,711 Canadian adolescents (in grades 9 to 11). The study found that 17.5% of the teens reported having been victimized in cyberspace in the context of a dating relationship in the previous 12 months.[19]

In a longitudinal study of 1,042 Texan teen students, Temple et al.[20] documented that 24% of the participants reported having experienced one or more occurrences of CDV in the previous year.

Correlates of Adolescent Dating Victimization

Adolescent Dating Violence Victimization and Family Context

A multiwave longitudinal study by Foshee et al.,[21] based on surveys of 3,236 adolescents living in two rural counties of North Carolina, showed that low parent–adolescent closeness was significantly linked to elevated dating violence victimization (DVV) only in stable residential neighborhoods.[21] Also, family aggression was significantly linked to elevated DVV regardless of neighborhood stability. Yet, low parental monitoring and rule-setting were not significantly linked to DVV regardless of neighborhood characteristics and the only neighborhood characteristic significantly linked to DVV was ethnic heterogeneity.[21]

Adolescent DVV and Mental Health Risks

The association between teen DVV and multiple young adult health outcomes was investigated by Exner-Cortens et al.[22] through a longitudinal study based on a second analysis of three waves of the Add Health involving 5,681 adolescents (age 12 to 18), who reported heterosexual dating experiences at Wave 2 (1996). The study documented that female participants who experienced DVV at Wave 2 were at significantly higher risk of reporting heavy episodic drinking, depressive symptomatology, suicidal ideation, smoking, and intimate partner violence (IPV) at Wave 3 (at age 18 to 25) than female participants who did not experience adolescent DVV at Wave 2. Also, male participants experiencing DVV at Wave 2 were more at risk of reporting increased antisocial behaviors, suicidal ideation, marijuana use, and IPV at Wave 3 than males who did not experience DVV at Wave 2.

A study by Wolitzky-Taylor et al.,[23] which aimed at establishing the prevalence of correlates of dating violence in a sample of more than 3,600 US adolescents age 12 to 17, showed that "serious forms of dating violence" (i.e., sexual assault, physical assault, and/or drug/alcohol-facilitated rape perpetrated by a girlfriend, boyfriend, or other dating partner) are associated with posttraumatic stress disorder (OR = 3.58) and major depressive episode (OR = 3.68) "after controlling for significant demographics and other potentially traumatic and stressful events."[23]

Further evidence about the link between adolescents' DVV and their psychological well-being can be found in the results of a study by Callahan et al.,[24] based on a survey of 190 high school students living in southern Michigan. The research showed that adolescent females who were subjected to higher levels of DVV "were at significant risk of higher levels of post-traumatic stress and dissociation, even after controlling for demographic, family violence, and social desirability variable."[24] Among male students, "the levels of victimization were related to higher levels of anxiety, depression, and posttraumatic stress, even after controlling for other variables."[24]

Trauma symptoms associated with physical dating violence experienced by female adolescents have been found to function as a mediator of later revictimization in young adulthood, as shown in a 5-year longitudinal study led by Jouriles et al.[25]

A longitudinal study conducted by Forshee et al.[26] showed that psychological dating victimization predicted, in both males and females, increased alcohol use, while physical dating victimization predicted cigarette use. Increased marijuana use was associated with only physical dating victimization among females.

Suicide Risk

A significant association between DVV and suicidality has been highlighted by several studies[27-31] through cross-sectional[28,29,31] or longitudinal[27,30] investigations of US adolescents, who were surveyed through the YRBS,[28,29,31] the Healthy Teens Longitudinal Study,[27] or Add Health.[30] Among these studies,[27-31] we should underscore the work of Baiden et al.,[31] who examined the link between physical adolescent dating violence (ADV) and suicidal behaviors, using data derived from a cross-sectional survey more than 9,600 adolescents, while taking into account the exposure to other forms of victimization, such as bullying (in school or cyberspace) or experiencing forced sex, as part of the array of potential significant predictors of suicidality, which included being a sexual minority, experiencing depression, or binge drinking. The Baiden et al.[31] work showed that "adolescents who experienced physical [dating violence] were 1.92 times more likely to have experience suicidal ideation, 1.67 times more likely to have made a suicidal plan, and 2.42 times more likely to have attempted suicide during the past 12 months when compared with their counterparts who were dating but experienced no physical [dating violence]."[31]

Further, van Dulmen et al.[30] analyzed data from more than 4,600 individuals who were surveyed through different waves of a longitudinal study to determine the association of IPV and suicidality from adolescence into early adulthood. Their findings documented that "suicidality was associated with IPV victimization prospectively, but IPV victimization did not predict suicidality prospectively."[30]

Risk of Injuries

The prevalence of injuries from ADV was studied by Tharp et al.[32] using date from a longitudinal survey of 917 adolescents in grades 8 through 12 in a rural county of North Carolina. The investigation documented that 11.5% to 12.8% of the participants reported having been injured in the previous year due to physical/sexual dating victimization, with the likelihood of injuries decreasing significantly from eighth to twelfth grade. Furthermore, the risk of injuries due to exposure to three (psychological, sexual, and physical) forms of dating violence was significantly higher (AOR = 13.89) than the risk from exposure to one form of dating violence.[32]

According to Swahn et al.,[33] the frequency of injuries associated with reciprocal ADV is significantly greater than the occurrence of injuries associated with nonreciprocal ADV (10.1% vs 1.2%).[33]

ADV Victimization and Homicide

Adhia et al.[34] undertook an investigation to determine the proportion of adolescent homicides in the United States that were perpetrated by intimate partners. The study was based on analysis of data from the National Violent Death Reporting System from 2003 to 2016, and it showed that almost 7% of the adolescent homicides were committed by dating partners, with handguns being the most common mechanism of injury. Furthermore, 90% of the victims were female, with a mean age of 16.8 years.[34]

Association of ADV and Forms of Victimization

The co-occurrence of physical ADV with other forms of victimization was studied by Hamby et al.[35] using a telephone survey of 1,680 US adolescents who took part in the National Survey of Children's Exposure to Violence. The research showed that every victim of ADV gave an account of having been exposed to at least one other type of victimization. Specifically, a victim of ADV was found to be at significant risk of having been physically abused by a caregiver (AOR = 2.74), having been raped (AOR = 5.12), having been subjected to sexual harassment (AOR = 5.33), or having been exposed to polyvictimization (AOR = 5.40).[35]

The association of bullying victimization with physical and emotional ADV was explored by Debnam et al.[36] in a survey of 17,780 high school students in 12 Maryland counties. The research found that adolescents who were victims of physical, verbal, or relational bullying were more likely to have experienced physical or relational ADV.[36]

ADV Prevention Programs

Russell et al.[37] conducted a comprehensive review to identify relevant randomized controlled trials (RCTs) evaluating the effectiveness of ADV prevention programs in reducing the prevalence of ADV perpetration and/or victimization. The search, completed at the end of April

Table 16.1. Adolescent Dating Violence Prevention Programs, Randomized Controlled Trials, Examined by Russell et al.[37]

Safe Dates (Foshee et al.[38])	Building a Lasting Love (Langhinrichsen-Rohling and Turner[41])	It's Your Game (Peskin et al.[44])
JOVEN (Gonzalez-Guarda et al.[39])	Teen Choices (Levesque et al.[42])	Youth Relationships Project (Wolfe et al.[45])
Break the Cycle (Jaycox et al.[40])	Coaching Boys into Men (Miller et al.[43])	Fourth R (Wolfe et al.[46])

2019, led to a meta-analysis of nine RCTs[37-46] specifically measuring ADV perpetration and/or victimization as outcomes (Table 16.1) . All the programs[37-46] were found to significantly lower the perpetration of emotional and sexual ADV among adolescents in treatment groups as compared to youth in control groups.[37] Teen Choices[42] was the only individual ADV prevention program found to significantly reduce the risk of all types of ADV measured in the study.[37]

Future Directions

Looking ahead, research efforts should foster and facilitate the development and/or implementation of:

- National and regional assessments of the prevalence of adolescent dating victimization by including questions about this form of maltreatment in international surveys of adolescent health and well-being, such as the Health Behavior in School-aged Children (HBSC)[47] survey or the Global School-Based Student Health Survey (GSHS)[48]
- Longitudinal studies to explore the association of adolescent dating victimization with health and psychosocial risks, while accounting for other forms of victimization that could also predict similar risks
- Research-based evidence-supported programs for the prevention of adolescent dating violence
- Universal screening to ascertain exposure to victimization in dating relations and associated health problems among adolescents who are first seen in any clinical setting, as part of universal assessment to ascertain exposure to all forms of victimization
- Research-based therapeutic strategies to stop ongoing adolescent dating violence

Notes

1. Collins WA, Welsh DP, Furman W. Adolescent romantic relationships. *Annu Rev Psychol.* 2009;60:631–652.
2. Carver K, Joyner K, Udry JR. National estimates of adolescent romantic relationships. In: Florsheim P, ed. *Adolescent Romantic Relationships and Sexual Behavior: Theory, Research,*

and Practical Implications. New York, NY: Cambridge University Press; 2003:291–329. Cited by Collins et al.[1]

3. Lenhart A, Smith A, Anderson M. Teens, technology and romantic relationships. Pew Research Center, October 2015. https://www.pewresearch.org/internet/2015/10/01/teens-technology-and-romantic-relationships/. Accessed August 10, 2022.
4. Breiding MJ, Basile KC, Smith SG, Black MC, Mahendra RR. *Intimate Partner Violence Surveillance: Uniform Definitions and Recommended Data Elements, Version 2.0*. Atlanta, GA: National Center for Injury Prevention and Control; 2015. https://www.cdc.gov/violenceprevention/pdf/ipv/intimatepartnerviolence.pdf. Accessed August 10, 2022.
5. Zweig JM, Lachman P, Yahner J, Dank M. Correlates of cyber dating abuse among teens. *J Youth Adolescence*. 2014;43(8):1306–1321.
6. Picard P. *Tech Abuse in Teen Relationships*. Chicago, IL: Teen Research Unlimited; 2007. Cited by Zweig et al.[5]
7. Centers for Disease Control and Prevention (CDC), Youth Risk Behavior Surveillance System (YRBSS). https://www.cdc.gov/healthyyouth/data/yrbs/index.htm. Accessed August 12, 2022.
8. Basile KC, Clayton HB, DeGue S, Gilford JW, Vagi KJ, Suarez NA, ... Lowry R. Interpersonal violence victimization among high school students—youth risk behavior survey, United States, 2019. *MMWR Supplements*. 2020;69(1):28.
9. Coker AL, McKeown RE, Sanderson M, Davis KE, Valois RF, Huebner ES. Severe dating violence and quality of life among South Carolina high school students. *Am J Prev Med*. 2000;19(4):220–227. Cited by Stonard KE, Bowen E, Lawrence TR, Price SA. The relevance of technology to the nature, prevalence and impact of adolescent dating violence and abuse: a research synthesis. *Aggress Violent Behav*. 2014;19(4):390–417.
10. Eaton DK, Kann L, Kinchen S, et al. Youth risk behavior surveillance—United States, 2007. *MMWR Surveill Summ*. 2008;57(4):1–31. Cited by Stonard et al.[9]
11. Silverman JG, Raj A, Clements K. Dating violence and associated sexual risk and pregnancy among adolescent girls in the United States. *Pediatrics*. 2004;114(2):e220–e225. Cited by Stonard et al.[9]
12. Banyard VL, Cross C. Consequences of teen dating violence: understanding intervening variables in ecological context. *Violence Women*. 2008;14(9):998–1013. Cited by Stonard et al.[9]
13. Clayton HB, Kilmer G, DeGue S, Estefan LF, Le VD, Suarez NA, ... Thornton JE. Dating violence, sexual violence, and bullying victimization among high school students—youth risk behavior survey, United States, 2021. *MMWR Supplements*. 2023;72(1):66.
14. Eaton DK, Kann L, Kinchen S, et al. Youth risk behavior surveillance-United States, 2009. *MMWR Surveill Summ*. 2010;59(5):1–142. Cited by Stonard et al.[9]
15. Hébert M, Blais M, Lavoie F. Prevalence of teen dating victimization among a representative sample of high school students in Quebec. *Int J Clin Health Psychol*. 2017;17(3):225–233.
16. Fox CL, Corr ML, Gadd D, Butler I. Young teenagers' experiences of domestic abuse. *J Youth Stud*. 2013;17(4):510–526. Cited by Stonard et al.[9]
17. Zweig JM, Dank M, Lachman P, Yahner J. *Technology, Teen Dating Violence and Abuse, and Bullying*. Washington, DC: Urban Institute; 2013. Cited by Stonard et al.[9]
18. Smith K, Cénat JM, Lapierre A, Dion J, Hébert M, Côté K. Cyber dating violence: prevalence and correlates among high school students from small urban areas in Quebec. *J Affective Disord*. 2018;234:220–223
19. Exner-Cortens D, Baker E, Craig W. The national prevalence of adolescent dating violence in Canada. *J Adolesc Health*. 2021;69(3):495–502.

20. Temple JR, Choi HJ, Brem M, et al. The temporal association between traditional and cyber dating abuse among adolescents. *J Youth Adolescence*. 2016;45(2):340–349.
21. Foshee VA, Chang LY, Reyes HL, Chen MS, Ennett ST. The synergy of family and neighborhood on rural dating violence victimization. *Am J Prev Med*. 2015;49(3):483–491.
22. Exner-Cortens D, Eckenrode J, Rothman E. Longitudinal associations between teen dating violence victimization and adverse health outcomes. *Pediatrics*. 2013;131(1):71–78.
23. Wolitzky-Taylor KB, Ruggiero KJ, Danielson CK, et al. Prevalence and correlates of dating violence in a national sample of adolescents. *J Am Acad Child Adolesc Psychiatry*. 2008;47(7):755–762.
24. Callahan MR, Tolman RM, Saunders DG. Adolescent dating violence victimization and psychological well-being. *J Adolesc Res*. 2003;18(6):664–681.
25. Jouriles EN, Choi HJ, Rancher C, Temple JR. Teen dating violence victimization, trauma symptoms, and revictimization in early adulthood. *J Adolesc Health*. 2017;61(1):115–119.
26. Foshee VA, Reyes HL, Gottfredson NC, Chang LY, Ennett ST. A longitudinal examination of psychological, behavioral, academic, and relationship consequences of dating abuse victimization among a primarily rural sample of adolescents. *J Adolesc Health*. 2013;53(6):723–729.
27. Nahapetyan L, Orpinas P, Song X, Holland K. Longitudinal association of suicidal ideation and physical dating violence among high school students. *J Youth Adolescence*. 2014;43(4):629–640.
28. Belshaw SH, Siddique JA, Tanner J, Osho GS. The relationship between dating violence and suicidal behaviors in a national sample of adolescents. *Violence Vict*. 2012;27(4):580–591.
29. Olshen E, McVeigh KH, Wunsch-Hitzig RA, Rickert VI. Dating violence, sexual assault, and suicide attempts among urban teenagers. *Arch Pediatrics Adolesc Med*. 2007;161(6):539–545.
30. Van Dulmen MH, Klipfel KM, Mata AD, et al. Cross-lagged effects between intimate partner violence victimization and suicidality from adolescence into adulthood. *J Adolesc Health*. 2012;51(5):510–516.
31. Baiden P, Mengo C, Small E. History of physical teen dating violence and its association with suicidal behaviors among adolescent high school students: results from the 2015 Youth Risk Behavior Survey. *J Interpers Violence*. 2019:0886260519860087.
32. Tharp AT, McNaughton Reyes HL, Foshee V, Swahn MH, Hall JE, Logan J. Examining the prevalence and predictors of injury from adolescent dating violence. *J Aggress Maltreat Trauma*. 2017;26(5):445–461.
33. Swahn MH, Alemdar M, Whitaker DJ. Nonreciprocal and reciprocal dating violence and injury occurrence among urban youth. *West J Emerg Med*. 2010;11(3):264.
34. Adhia A, Kernic MA, Hemenway D, Vavilala MS, Rivara FP. Intimate partner homicide of adolescents. *JAMA Pediatrics*. 2019;173(6):571–577.
35. Hamby S, Finkelhor D, Turner H. Teen dating violence: co-occurrence with other victimizations in the National Survey of Children's Exposure to Violence (NatSCEV). *Psychol Violence*. 2012;2(2):111.
36. Debnam KJ, Waasdorp TE, Bradshaw CP. Examining the contemporaneous occurrence of bullying and teen dating violence victimization. *Sch Psychol Q*. 2016;31(1):76.
37. Russell KN, Voith LA, Lee H. Randomized controlled trials evaluating adolescent dating violence prevention programs with an outcome of reduced perpetration and/or victimization: a meta-analysis. *J Adolescence*. 2021;87:6–14.
38. Foshee VA, Bauman KE, Ennett ST, Suchindran C, Benefield T, Linder GF. Assessing the effects of the dating violence prevention program "Safe Dates" using random coefficient regression modeling. *Prev Sci*. 2005;6(3):245–258. Cited by Russell et al.[37]

39. Gonzalez-Guarda RM, Guerra JE, Cummings AA, Pino K, Becerra MM. Examining the preliminary efficacy of a dating violence prevention program for Hispanic adolescents. *J Sch Nurs*. 2015;31(6):411–421. Cited by Russell et al.[37]
40. Jaycox LH, McCaffrey D, Eiseman B, et al. Impact of a school-based dating violence prevention program among Latino teens: randomized controlled effectiveness trial. *J Adolesc Health*. 2006;39(5):694–704. Cited by Russell et al.[37]
41. Langhinrichsen-Rohling J, Turner LA. The efficacy of an intimate partner violence prevention program with high-risk adolescent girls: a preliminary test. *Prev Sci*. 2012;13(4):384–394. Cited by Russell et al.[37]
42. Levesque DA, Johnson JL, Welch CA, Prochaska JM, Paiva AL. Teen dating violence prevention: cluster-randomized trial of Teen Choices, an online, stage-based program for healthy, nonviolent relationships. *Psychol Violence*. 2016;6(3):421–432. Cited by Russell et al.[37]
43. Miller E, Tancredi DJ, McCauley HL, et al. "Coaching boys into men": A cluster-randomized controlled trial of a dating violence prevention program. *J Adolesc Health*. 2012;51(5):431–438. Cited by Russell et al.[37]
44. Peskin MF, Markham CM, Shegog R, et al. Effects of the It's Your Game .... Keep It Real program on dating violence in ethnic-minority middle school youths: a group randomized trial. *Am J Public Health*. 2014;104(8):1471–1477. Cited by Russell et al.[37]
45. Wolfe DA, Crooks C, Jaffe P, et al. A school-based program to prevent adolescent dating violence: A cluster randomized trial. *Arch Pediatrics Adolesc Med*. 2009;163(8):692–699. Cited by Russell et al.[37]
46. Wolfe DA, Wekerle C, Scott K, Straatman AL, Grasley C, Reitzel-Jaffe D. Dating violence prevention with at-risk youth: a controlled outcome evaluation. *J Consult Clin Psychol*. 2003;71(2):279. Cited by Russell et al.[37]
47. World Health Organization, Europe. Health Behavior in School-aged Children study. https://www.who.int/europe/initiatives/health-behaviour-in-school-aged-children-(hbsc)-study. Accessed August 12, 2022.
48. Global School-Based Student Health Survey, 2021 Version. https://cdn.who.int/media/docs/default-source/ncds/ncd-surveillance/gshs/gshs_core_module_questions_2021.pdf?sfvrsn=7d07af8_7. Accessed August 12, 2022.

17
Victimization in Competitive Sports

What Is Known?

In 2013, the notion of bullying in sports came to public attention via media reports about the alleged role of a US football player in harassing a teammate.[1-4] Yet the broad scope of victimization occurring in competitive games has been receiving news exposure for decades.[5-27] This chapter examines the different forms of victimization affecting players, coaches, managers, and fans participating in competitive sports. It could be argued that the spectrum of maltreatment discussed could have been reviewed under bullying in schools, in tertiary education, in the workplace, and in the community. Yet its occurrence transcends social milieus and justifies its receiving a separate chapter.

Victimization in sports

Definition

There is a lack of a standard research-based definition of victimization in sports,[28] yet a conceptual framework for future investigation has been developed by Stirling[29] based on various categories and constituents of harm or neglect that potentially can affect any participant in an athletic milieu. The notion of victimization discussed in this chapter follows Stirling's framework[29,30] and encompasses the wide range of abuse (physical, sexual, verbal, emotional) or neglect that can affect or be perpetrated by players, support staff, or spectators of organized competitive amateur or professional sports. Victimization can involve physical aggression (punching, beating, hitting, slapping); noncontact physical maltreatment (imposing physical exertion; denying access to needed water, sleep, food, or use of a toilet; unreasonable physical requirements as punishment), intentional or flagrant fouls that can caused physical harm; hazing; sexual assault or harassment; discrimination, exclusion, or rejection; verbal abuse (belittling, shouting, name-calling, degradation, intimidation, insults); and all forms of institutional or leadership neglect of the well-being of players, support staff, and spectators.

Prevalence

In 2018, Vveinhardt et al.[31] conducted a study to determine the prevalence of bullying behaviors and victimization among amateur athletes, based on a sample of 337 Lithuanian nonprofessional players involved in different sports. Their research documented that almost 36% of the respondents witnessed athletes being bullied by their team members, while 33% of the participants saw players being bullied by members of other teams. Furthermore, 16% of the players surveyed in the study[31] indicated that they bullied their team members, almost 13%

reported that they mistreated members of other teams, almost 20% acknowledged having been bullied by their teammates, and almost 18% indicated that they were bullied by members of other teams. Nearly 50% of the victims experienced verbal bullying, while 22% were subjected to physical victimization. Furthermore, the athletes surveyed reported that "5% of coaches bullied them daily, and 5.9% of coaches did that every week."[31]

Another report[32] of Vveinhardt's study[31] indicated that male athletes "are more aggressive physically, verbally, or nonverbally than women"[32] and that "persons who were bullied in the past also apply the same negative behavior themselves in sport activities later."[32]

Marracho et al.[33] explored the prevalence of bullying in sports in the regions of Portugal called Trás-os-Montes and Alto Douro, through a survey of 642 athletes (13 to 18 years old) involved in school and federated sports. The researchers found that 23.6% of students reported being involved in bullying during school sports, with 16.3% as bystanders, 4.9% as victims, and 2.3% as perpetrators. Almost 26% of participants reported involvement in bullying in the context of federated sports, with 5.9% as victims, 16.6% as bystanders, and 3.1% as perpetrators.[33]

The prevalence of sexual abuse in organized competitive sports was studied by Leahy et al.[34] using a survey of 370 Australian adults (from 18 to 60 years old) who had participated in organized athletic activities through a club system or through "elite level" programs organized by the Australian Institute of Sport (AIS). The survey found that 13.3% of athletes participating in elite sport activities were subjected to sexual abuse, as compared to 6.3% of those who participate in club sports. Also, 12.9% of female athletes reported sexual abuse, in contrast to 6.3% of their male counterparts.

In 2019, Herr et al.[35] conducted a study of exposure to maltreatment in sports among Canadian national team athletes. The research, developed on behalf of the University of Toronto with the support of Athletes CAN Safe Sport Committee, was based on a sample of 1,001 athletes, of whom 76% were at that time current athletes (mean age: 25.5 years) and 26% were retired players (mean age: 34.4 years) who had left their sport within 10 years before the survey. Neglect was the most frequent form of maltreatment, experienced by almost 67% of the current athletes and 76% of the retired players. The mistreatment included the experience of receiving "unequal treatment," "training while injured/exhausted," having to "sacrifice education/career," feeling "ignored," being "trained in unsafe conditions," being required to "try new skills before ready," being "left alone without care," or being "denied medical attention." Neglect was mostly experienced from coaches, followed by high-performance directors.

Emotional abuse was the second most common maltreatment, experienced by approximately 60% of the surveyed[35] Canadian athletes. The abuse was characterized as being shouted at in an angry or critical manner; being exposed to lies or rumors spread about oneself; being put down, embarrassed, or humiliated; being called names; or being ignored.[35] Only 4% to 5% of the athletes were exposed to physical abuse (excessive exercise; being forced to the ground; being hit, slapped, or punched) or sexual maltreatment.[35]

Physical Aggression in Sports

Physical Aggression Related to Foul Play

Players participating in some of the collision sports (ice hockey, rugby, American football) may experience different degrees of physical aggression that are "permissible" within the rules of the game and inherent in its strategies and tactics (e.g., tackling in rugby, blocking

Table 17.1. Examples of Physical Aggression That Is Considered Foul Play in Sports

Sport	Foul Play
American Football[37]	Clipping,[a] striking with fists, clubbing, kicking, or kneeing an opponent
Rugby[38]	Striking, tripping, kicking, or trampling on an opponent
Ice Hockey[39]	Attempt to injure, boarding,[b] butt-ending,[c] elbowing, or unnecessary roughness
Association Football (Soccer)[40]	Jumping or spitting at an opponent or kicking, charging, tripping, striking, pushing, holding, or tackling an opponent

[a] Clipping is blocking an opponent from behind below the waist, provided the opponent is not a runner.[41]

[b] Boarding is the action where a player pushes, trips or body checks an opponent causing them to go dangerously into the boards.[42]

[c] Butt-ending is the action whereby a player uses the shaft of the stick, above the upper hand to check an opposing player in any manner or attempts to jab an opposing player with his part of the stick.[43]

in American football, body checks in ice hockey).[36] Yet, it is incumbent on a referee's judgment to ascertain the legality of the aggressive act and decide, based on the rules of the sport, whether it constitutes an act of foul play, leading to restrictions or penalties. Still, the affected player may feel mistreated, with subsequent suffering of physical or emotional harm, whether or not the aggression has been deemed legitimate.

Organizations representing collision and contact sports (i.e., American football, rugby, ice hockey, soccer) have developed rules[44-47] to prevent players from committing serious aggressive actions that may cause injuries by considering them illegal or foul play (Table 17.1), and by prescribing significant penalties.

A study published in 1999 by Shields,[48] based on a survey of almost 150 high school athletic directors in the state of North Carolina, documented that at least 50% of the respondents agreed that player violence was in part attributable to local media hype, pep rallies, team cheers, and coaches' berating of players, while 29% indicated that athletes "accept violence between players as a part of the sport."[48]

A 1984 report by Watters et al.,[49] which was based on more than 2,700 sports injuries seen in an accident and emergency department in Edinburgh, showed that 24% of football (soccer) injuries were due to foul play, as compared to only 9% of the rugby injuries.[49]

Collins et al.[50] conducted an epidemiologic study to determine the frequency of injuries related to illegal activity or foul play in high school sports. Their study used data from the 2005–2006 and 2006–2007 National High School Sports-Related Injury Surveillance Study of young athletes who participated in nine sports (boy's football, soccer, basketball, wrestling and baseball, as well as girls' soccer, volleyball, basketball, and softball). Collins et al. showed that 6.4% of all high school sports-related injuries were associated with illegal activity, with the highest frequency encountered in girls' basketball (14%), girls' soccer (11.9%), and boys' soccer (11.4%).[50] A third of the injuries caused by foul play were to the head and face, and 25% resulted in concussions.[50]

Physical Aggression Related to Brawls

Physical fights or brawls occurring before, during, or after a sporting event, "among or between athletes and/or nonathlete participants (parents, coaches, referees, spectators, security personnel, etc.),"[50] have been in the spotlight for years,[6-14,26,44,51] and at times they have led to fatalities.[12,51]

In 2007, Fields et al.[45] commented that the publications considering brawling in sports focused on the fields of sociology and law, with very little literature on the subject coming from the public health field, and that has continued to be the case.[46-52]

Physical Violence against Sports Officials

A special report developed in 1998 by Cross[53] outlined incidents of physical aggression toward sports officials that were reported in the press[54-74] between 1995 and 1998; that were committed by players,[54-64,71-74] coaches,[65,66] or fans[67-70]; and that incurred reported injuries[54,57,58,60,61,65-67] and/or concusions.[55,59,62,66]

Fans and Physical Aggression in Sports

The attraction experienced by some spectators to physical violence among players has been studied mainly for hockey.[75-78] A study by Paul[75] to ascertain variations in game-to-game fans' attendance in the National Hockey League documented that "violence, specifically fighting, tends to attract fans in large numbers across the United States and Canada."[75]

A review of the problem of spectator violence in sports, published in 2000 by Roberts and Benjamin,[79] emphasized that this subject has been traditionally linked to professional football in Europe, with limited research having been done in North America.[80,81]

Smith[81] conducted a study of news coverage of collective violence related to sports occurring in North America based on reports published by the *Toronto Globe and Mail*, "Canada's most 'national' newspaper."[81] The study found that at least 39 cases of hockey-related collective violence or near violence, involving mainly spectators, occurred in North America between 1963 and 1973 and were featured in news reports by the Toronto newspaper.[81]

Lewis[82] researched American newspaper stories about sports violence occurring between 1960 and 1972 and found only 15 hockey-related episodes involving fan violence.

A wide range of media reports[83-122] published in the last decade, and mostly during 2021,[102-122] have underscored the occurrence and gravity of violence among sports fans occurring across the world, with some incidents resulting in injuries[96] or death.[85,95]

Spaaij[123] outlined seven categories of sport spectators' behaviors that can involve violence, including physical assault, fighting, verbal abuse, pitch invasion (unauthorized entry onto the playing field of sporting venues), discharge of missiles (throwing or kicking an object into the playing field or toward somebody), vandalism, and terrorism (politically driven act of violence to disrupt or intimidate).[123]

Football Hooliganism

The term *football hooliganism* was defined by Spaaij[124] as "the competitive violence of socially organized fan groups in football, principally directed against opposing fan groups." Although violence among football fans has been prevalent in the past, the phenomenon of "contemporary football hooliganism"[124] as an "organized" form of violence in sports, has been recognized as emerging in England in the 1960s.[124] At the beginning of the 21st century, some researchers[125,126] considered football hooliganism to be a universal occurrence, while Spaaij[124] argued that it has been primarily prevalent in Europe[127-141] and Latin America.[142-145]

Frosdick and Newton[146] studied the nature and extent of football hooliganism in England and Wales during the four football seasons from 1999–2000 to 2002–2003, based on data pertaining to football-related arrests, as available from the National Criminal Intelligence Service (NCIS) and the Home Office. The study results showed that, two decades ago, hooliganism was prevalent in 5% of the British football games and only one per 10,000 spectators was arrested for a football-related offense, mostly public disorder, sometimes for the use of missiles, and with one resulting injury for every 10 incidents.[146]

In Argentina, the murder of a football fan that occurred in November 1967[147,148] marked the "beginning of the institutionalization of football violence and the era of the *barra bravas*,"[149] which are well-organized groups of violent football fans with a "political element and a militant role in the electoral process."[149] Duke and Crolley[149] provided a comprehensive description of the barra bravas, whose members are between the ages of 20 and 25, while their leaders are over 30, with the "core" of the group being full-time professional militants, linked to a leader of the sports club, usually a "particular candidate for club president."[149] According to some news reports,[150,151] the members assemble during the week, they place projectiles in the ground a few days prior to a game, they go to the match as a group, they meet at half-time to discuss their plans, and they follow a structure that is "military in style."[149] They usually participate in some type of political activity, in exchange for funding for transportation to out-of-town matches and/or gifts of match tickets to be sold in the black market.[149] Between 1986 and 1993, the barra bravas were involved in 1,945 incidents, resulting in 3,148 injuries and 42 deaths.[152-155]

Sexual Violence in Sports

A systematic literature review on sexual violence against children in sports, conducted by Bjørnseth and Szabo,[156] led to a final qualitative synthesis of seven studies[157-163] that offers the most up-to-date information on the topic. The prevalence of this form of victimization was found[156] to have been examined in a retrospective study by Vertommen et al.,[159] based on the survey of more than 4,000 adults recruited from all regions in Flanders and the Netherlands. The research documented that 13% of the responding adults experienced being touched in a way that made them uneasy or being touched sexually against their will while they were involved in sports training during their childhood or adolescence.[159] It is of interest to note that the significant risk factors associated with sexual violence against children in sports include being female, being from an ethnic minority, having a disability, performing in competition at the international level, and being gay or bisexual.[159] In almost all the studies selected for review,[157,158,160-163] the coach was found to be the perpetrator, with male coaches more often being the offenders.

Leahy et al.[34] ascertained the prevalence of sexual abuse in organized competitive sport in Australia through a cross-sectional retrospective survey mailed to a sample of 370 of national elite athletes and local club players. The survey showed that the elite athletes reported higher levels (13.3%) of sexual abuse in sports than the local club players reported (6.3%). Females reported higher rates (12.0%) of sexual abuse in sports than did males (6.3%). Furthermore, national elite female participants experienced a higher rate (17.4%) of sexual abuse in sports than local club female players experienced (7.4%).

A call to sport health professionals to play a key role in the prevention and early detection of sexual harassment and abuse (SHA) in sport has been made by Marks et al.[164] in a prime article that provides a concise review of the nature and prevalence of sexual maltreatment in sport, the identity of the perpetrators, the risk factors, the physical and psychological consequences, and approaches for prevention. Marks et al.[164] delineated the range of "inappropriate sexual encounters" that can be experienced in sport, including sexual harassment, sexual abuse, gender harassment, hazing, and homophobia.[165-167] Furthermore, they highlighted that the diverse types of SHA can occur in all types of sports[168,169] and at all levels,[170-172] with the prevalence varying from 2% to 48%.[173-176] SHA in sports can also occur in a homosexual context.[177] Marks et al.[164] also emphasized that the perpetrators are not limited to those in a position of power, such as coaches,[178] but that athletes have also been found to harass their peers,[169] especially through hazing.[179,180] Marks et al.[164] brought to light the risk factors for SHA among athletes, including being a young woman, having a poor and distant relationships with parents, having low self-esteem, being a strong talent in one's sport, and having a strong dedication to one's sport.[164] Risk factors for SHA among coaches include being an older male, having a good reputation in the sport, and being trusted by the athlete's parents, while risks factors for SHA among sports' organizations include having many opportunities for trips away from home and/or having limited opportunities for reporting SHA.[164] Marks et al.[164] described the health and psychosocial problems linked to SHA in sports, including anxiety, eating disorders, depression, headaches, hypervigilance, nightmares, obsessive-compulsive behavior, hair-pulling, self-injury, substance abuse, and suicidal thoughts and/or attempts.[164] For prevention of SHA in sports, Marks et al.[164] advocated for the adoption of a prevention policy statement and efforts to raise awareness about SHA in sports, together with a clinical approach for disclosure of SHA in sports, accurate record completion, and mechanisms for reporting as well as providing support to stop the abuse.[164]

Emotional Abuse in Competitive Sports

Based on a review of the literature on emotional abuse of child elite athletes, Wilinsky and McCabe[181] described this type of maltreatment as "repeated screaming, shouting, humiliating, scapegoating, ignoring, belittling, rejecting, isolating, threatening, criticizing, using derogatory language and comments, denying attention and support, expressing intense anger, and/or committing aggressive acts, such as throwing equipment at, or in the presence of, the athlete."[181-186] Stirling and Kerr[185] defined emotional abuse in the athletic environment as:

> a pattern of deliberate noncontact behaviors by a person within a critical relationship role that has the potential to be harmful. Acts of emotional abuse include physical behaviors, verbal behaviors, and acts of denying attention and support. These acts have the potential to be spurning, terrorizing, isolating, exploiting/corrupting, or deny emotional

responsiveness, and may be harmful to an individual's affective, behavioral, cognitive, or physical well-being.[185]

A survey conducted by Alexander et al.[187] of more than 6,100 British students (age 18 to 22) investigated the range of maltreatment that the students experienced during their childhood and adolescence in sport settings. The survey documented that 70% of the athletes experienced, once or more frequently, emotional abuse, including being criticized about their performance, embarrassed, humiliated, teased, bullied, shouted at, sworn at, called names, ignored, or threatened.[187] Emotional abuse was more commonly experienced on a regular basis by those competing at an international echelon level (32%) rather than a recreational level (16%).[187] At the local/recreational level of sports competition, team members/peers were the most common perpetrators of emotional abuse (83%), while coaches/trainers were reported to be involved in 28% of the victimization experiences.[187] Yet, the rate of coaches/trainers as perpetrators of emotional abuse was much higher (56%) in international level sports competition.[187]

Body Shaming

Wilson and Kerr[188] characterized the experiences of body shaming encountered by athletes as a form of emotional abuse. Wilson and Kerr[188] conducted semi-structured interviews of eight retired female athletes in aesthetic sports who had been members of a Canadian national team, five of whom had competed in the Olympic Games. The athletes reported that they were exposed to negative comments about their physical appearance, body-weight monitoring, food and water restrictions, public criticism of their body, and punishment when body-related standards were not met.[188]As a result of this form of maltreatment, the athletes developed excessive control methods, developed eating disorders, experienced declining performance, and had decreased enjoyment in sports.[188]

Hazing in Sports

Crow and Macintosh[189] defined hazing in sports as "any potentially humiliating, degrading, abusive, or dangerous activity expected of a junior-ranking athlete by a more senior teammate, which does not contribute to either athlete's positive development, but is required to be accepted as part of a team, regardless of the junior-ranking athlete's willingness to participate."[189] This includes, but is "not limited to, any activity, no matter how traditional or seemingly benign, that sets apart or alienates any teammate based on class, number of years on the team, or athletic ability."[189]

A survey conducted by Waldron[190] of 232 student-athletes from seven high schools and three colleges/universities the United States showed that 42% of the respondents participated in at least one severe hazing activity, 50% participated in no less than one mild and one severe hazing episode, and 33% were involved in, at the minimum, one mild hazing incident. The most frequent severe hazing episodes consisted of being deprived of sleep, participating in drinking games, or acting as personal servant to others, while the most common mild hazing situations were having to associate with specific people and not others, being yelled at, cursed at, or sworn at, or being required to remain silent or being silenced.[190]

Discrimination in Sports

Three decades ago, a literature review of discrimination in professional sports, published by Kahn,[191] highlighted a history of racial discrimination by team owners,[192] coworkers,[193] and spectators.[194] The discrimination manifested as unequal pay, as was evident in significant basketball salary shortfalls for African American players in the 1980s[195-199], or salary discrimination (as suffered by French Canadian hockey defense players[200-202]). Several studies, published almost half a century ago or more, underlined the subject of positional segregation in sports, also known as "stacking," probably based on racial stereotypes. This type of discrimination has been demonstrated in studies showing that African American baseball players were found, in the past, to be underrepresented at pitcher and catcher positions[203,204] and in infield placement,[205,206] while they were overrepresented in the outfield[203,206] and at first base.[203] Also, Canadian Francophone hockey players were found, in the past, to be underrepresented in defense positions.[200]

Neglect in Sports

According to Nimal,[207] neglect is revealed in sports indirectly, making it difficult for the behavior to be identified. Yet, there are instances where coaches' behavior may represent negligence or a failure to recognize and attend to the physical, developmental, or psychological needs of the players,[208-214] such as when coaches hold unrealistic practice sessions.[215-223]

Two decades ago, the Committee on Sports Medicine and Fitness of the American Academy of Pediatrics issued a statement on intensive training and sports specialization in young athletes that emphasized the potential physical, developmental, and emotional risks associated with intensive youth sport training.[221] Furthermore, the committee recommended, among other things, that young people should not be pushed beyond their abilities and limits, that children should avoid specialization in a single sport before adolescence, and that coaches should have knowledge about "appropriate training techniques and equipment and the unique physical, physiologic, and emotional characteristic of young competitors."[221] It also recommended that coaches should know about, and avoid the risks of, heat injury, overtraining, poor nutritional intake, excessive physical stress, and overuse injuries.[221]

Stirling[29] highlighted that coaches have a critical responsibility for the physical, educational, emotional, and social well-being of young athletes, and that neglect by coaches can take many forms. Neglect can be exemplified by:

- refusing an athlete recovery time for an injury,
- disregarding or encouraging the use of enhancing drugs by an athlete,
- not allowing an athlete time to study,
- inadequate supervision of an athlete,
- not providing attention or performance feedback to a less successful athlete,

- chronic exclusion of an athlete from social events, or
- delaying psychological care of an athlete.[29]

Future Directions

There is a need to better understand the frequency of victimization in competitive sports, its association with health risks, and strategies for its prevention. Going forward, scholars and researchers need to promote and implement the development of:

- National cross-sectional studies to ascertain the prevalence of all forms of maltreatment affecting high school and college students participating in competitive sports, professional players/athletes, coaches, sports officials, and spectators
- Longitudinal research to determine the association of victimization in sports with psychosocial and health risks, while accounting for other forms of victimization that could also predict similar risks
- Evidence-based programs for the prevention of maltreatment in competitive sports
- Universal screening to ascertain exposure to victimization in competitive sports and associated health problems among patients who are first seen in any clinical setting, as part of a universal assessment to ascertain exposure to all forms of victimization (see Chapter 8)
- Research-based therapeutic strategies to stop ongoing victimization in competitive sports

Notes

1. Bell J. Martin situation in Miami brings bullying to forefront. *USA Today Sports*, November 3, 2013. https://www.usatoday.com/story/sports/nfl/2013/11/02/jonathan-martin-miami-dolphins-bullying-jarrett-bell-column/3393497/. Accessed August 8, 2022.
2. Associated Press. Richie Incognito bullying: Jonathan Martin could sue Dolphins under workplace laws, experts say. *The Oregonian*, November 14, 2013. http://www.oregonlive.com/nfl/index.ssf/2013/11/richie_incognito_bullying_jona.html. Accessed August 8, 2022.
3. Demby G. Dolphins' story is about race and bullying, but not the way you think. National Public Radio, November 7, 2013. https://www.npr.org/sections/codeswitch/2013/11/07/243728867/dolphins-story-is-about-race-and-bullying-but-not-the-way-you-think. Accessed August 8, 2022.
4. Branch J, Belson K. In bullying case, questions on N.F.L. culture. *New York Times*, November 4, 2013. http://www.nytimes.com/2013/11/05/sports/football/for-the-nfl-a-question-of-hazing-or-abuse.html?mtrref = www.google.com&gwh = 2EF5BF3C0EB9653F441581E02CB583C1&gwt = pay. Accessed August 8, 2022.
5. Daniel M, Ebbert S. Father banned in youth hockey incident. *Boston Globe*, January 7, 2005. http://archive.boston.com/news/local/massachusetts/articles/2005/01/07/father_banned_in_youth_hockey_incident/. Accessed August 8, 2022.
6. Italy to address violence at soccer games. *China Daily*, April 14, 2005. http://www.chinadaily.com.cn/english/doc/2005-04/14/content_434186.htm. Accessed August 8, 2022.

7. Johnson C. Parents turn violent during youth sports. CBC News, November 15, 2006. https://www.cbsnews.com/news/parents-turn-violent-during-youth-sports/. Accessed August 8, 2022.
8. Italian league halted by violence. *BBC Sport,* February 2, 2007. http://news.bbc.co.uk/sport2/hi/football/6326513.stm. Accessed August 8, 2022.
9. Germany gets serious about football violence. *Der Spiegel*, November 1, 2006. https://www.spiegel.de/international/rising-racism-in-stadiums-germany-gets-serious-about-football-violence-a-445903.html. Accessed August 8, 2022.
10. Smith T. Crowd violence flares at Open tennis. *Independent*, January 23, 2009. http://www.independent.co.uk/sport/tennis/crowd-violence-flares-at-open-tennis-1513647.html. Accessed August 8, 2022.
11. Stevens H. When football fans attack: how to fix the NFL's violence problem. *The Atlantic*, August 25, 2011. https://www.theatlantic.com/entertainment/archive/2011/08/when-football-fans-attack-how-to-fix-the-nfls-violence-problem/244095/. Accessed August 8, 2022.
12. Scores killed in Egypt football violence. *Aljazeera,* February 1, 2012. https://www.aljazeera.com/news/2012/2/1/scores-killed-in-egypt-football-violence. Accessed August 8, 2022.
13. Brocchetto M, Shoichet CE. Brazil: police fire tear gas as fierce fighting erupts in football stands. *CNN*, December 8, 2013. http://www.cnn.com/2013/12/08/sport/brazil-football-fight/index.html. Accessed August 8, 2022.
14. Duarte F, Wilson J, Walker S, Bandini P, Doyle P. Football violence: a view from around the world. *Guardian*, December 19, 2013. https://www.theguardian.com/football/2013/dec/19/football-violence-view-around-world. Accessed August 8, 2022.
15. Hobson W, and Rich S. 290 coaches, officials tied to U.S. Olympic groups have been accused of sexual misconduct since 1982, *Washington Post. Chicago Tribune*, November 18, 2017. http://www.chicagotribune.com/sports/ct-olympic-sexual-abuse-20171118-story.html. Accessed August 8, 2022.
16. Kaplan P. Tennessee football coach Butch Jones accused of "bullying and mental abuse" in Antone Davis resignation letter. *USA Today Network*—Tennessee, November 9, 2017. http://www.knoxnews.com/story/sports/college/university-of-tennessee/football/2017/11/09/antone-davis-resignation-letter-butch-jones-vol-for-life-tennnessee-football-vols-ut/848001001/. Accessed August 8, 2022.
17. Smith C. Former California prep baseball player sues coach for $150,000, claims benching was bullying. *USA Today High School Sports,* August 15, 2017. http://usatodayhss.com/2017/former-california-prep-baseball-player-sues-coach-for-150000-claims-benching-was-bullying. Accessed August 8, 2022.
18. Hope N, Keatings D. The climate of fear is real in British gymnastics. BBC Sport, November 13, 2017. https://www.bbc.com/sport/gymnastics/41976299. Accessed August 8, 2022.
19. Sargeant K. Amid bullying allegations, Rutgers coach fired for "Mike Rice tactics." NJ.com, November 16, 2017. http://www.nj.com/rutgersfootball/index.ssf/2017/11/rutgers_fires_swimming_coach_accused_of_mike_rice.html. Accessed August 8, 2022.
20. Kelner M. UK sport may hit British para-swimming in pocket over bullying crisis. *Guardian,* October 24, 2017. https://www.theguardian.com/sport/2017/oct/24/uk-sport-british-para-swimming-bullying-crisis-chris-furber. Accessed August 8, 2022.
21. Morse B, Davies A. FIFA fears recent abuse cases in women's football are just "tip of the iceberg." *CNN Action News Now,* October 18, 2021. https://www.cnn.com/2021/10/18/football/womens-football-abuse-fifa-cmd-spt-intl/index.html. Accessed August 8, 2022.

22. Associated Press. Jets' Harrison overcame years of bullying to achieve dreams. *USA Today*, December 1, 2018. https://www.usatoday.com/story/sports/nfl/2018/12/01/jets-harrison-overcame-years-of-bullying-to-achieve-dreams/38650735/. Accessed August 8, 2022.
23. Ramsay G. Violence and abuse are too often a part of the child athlete's experience in Japan—report. *CNN Sports*, July 20, 2020. https://www.cnn.com/2020/07/20/sport/japan-child-athletes-abuse-hurman-rights-watch-report-spt-intl/index.html. Accessed August 8, 2022.
24. The Athletic Staff. Coach shot in shoulder during Argentine football match amid fan violence. *The Athletic*, November 1, 2021. https://theathletic.com/news/coach-shot-in-shoulder-during-argentine-football-match-amid-fan-violence/HOvSew20SKj4/. Accessed August 8, 2022.
25. White M. Violence prompts Sto-Rox High to move home football game. *Pittsburgh Post-Gazette*, October 31, 2021. https://www.post-gazette.com/sports/high-school-football/2021/10/31/Sto-Rox-violence-home-football-games-WPIAL-playoffs/stories/202110310223. Accessed August 8, 2022.
26. Evans S. FIFA investigating "abhorrent" violence at Wembley. *The Star*, October 13, 2021. https://www.thestar.com.my/sport/football/2021/10/13/soccer-fifa-condemn-039abhorrent039-violence-at-wembley. Accessed October 2, 2023.
27. Associated Press. German gymnastics coach removed after bullying investigation. *ESPN*, May 4, 2021. https://www.espn.com/olympics/gymnastics/story/_/id/31388484/german-gymnastics-coach-removed-bullying-investigation. Accessed August 8, 2022.
28. Bachand CR. Bullying in sports: the definition depends on who you ask. *Sports Stud Sports Psychol.* 2017;9:1-4.
29. Stirling AE. Definition and constituents of maltreatment in sport: establishing a conceptual framework for research practitioners. *Br J Sports Med.* 2009;43(14):1091–1099.
30. Stirling AE, Bridges EJ, Cruz EL, Mountjoy ML. Canadian Academy of Sport and Exercise Medicine position paper: abuse, harassment, and bullying in sport. *Clin J Sport Med.* 2011;21(5):385–391.
31. Vveinhardt J, Fominiene VB, Jesevičiūtė-Ufartienė L. Prevalence of bullying and victimization in amateur sport: a case of Lithuania. In: Gómez Chova L, López Martínez A, Candel Torres I, eds. *ICERI 2018: 11th Annual International Conference of Education, Research, and Innovation.* IATED; 2018:8238–8244. https://library.iated.org/view/VVEINHARDT2018PRE. Accessed August 9, 2022.
32. Vveinhardt J, Fominienė VB. Gender, and age variables of bullying in organized sport: is bullying "grown out of"? *J Hum Sport Exerc.* 2020;15(4):747–761.
33. Marracho P, Coelho E, Pereira A, Nery M, Rosado A. Young people and bullying in sports—exploratory research in an inland northern region of Portugal. *J Phys Educ Sport.* 2021;21(4):1904–1912.
34. Leahy T, Pretty G, Tenenbaum G. Prevalence of sexual abuse in organised competitive sport in Australia. *J Sex Aggress.* 2002;8(2):16–36.
35. Kerr G, Willson E, Stirling A. Prevalence of maltreatment among current and former national team athletes. *Partnership with AthletesCAN*, 1–51. https://athletescan.ca/wp-content/uploads/2014/03/prevalence_of_maltreatment_reporteng.pdf. Accessed October 13, 2023.
36. Kerr JH. Issues in aggression and violence in sport: the ISSP position stand revisited. *Sport Psychol.* 2002;16(1):68–78.
37. 2021 Official Playing Rules of the National Football League, Rule 12, Player Conduct. Section 2, Personal Fouls, pages 48–53. https://operations.nfl.com/media/5427/2021-nfl-rulebook.pdf. Accessed August 8, 2022.

38. RFU Regulations, RFU Regulation 19-Discipline (Appendix 2). https://www.englandrugby.com/dxdam/e2/e2574ff9-fea3-4114-bba8-ca78694a05ea/Regulation%2019%20Appendix%202.pdf. Accessed August 8, 2022.
39. USA Hockey, 2021–25, Official Rules of Ice Hockey, Playing Rules, pages 61–67. https://cdn1.sportngin.com/attachments/document/603a-2502129/2021-25_USAH_Playing_Rules.pdf. Accessed August 8, 2022.
40. Fédération Internationale de Football Association (FIFA), Laws of the Game, 2015/2016, Law 12, Fouls and Misconduct, page 37. https://digitalhub.fifa.com/m/3f3e15cc1ab8977b/original/datdz0pms85gbnqy4j3k-pdf.pdf. Accessed August 8, 2022.
41. NFL Football Operations, Rule 3, Section 6, Clipping. https://operations.nfl.com/the-rules/nfl-video-rulebook/clipping/. Accessed August 9, 2022.
42. USA Hockey, Section Six, Playing Rules, Rule 603, Boarding. https://www.usahockeyrulebook.com/page/show/1084647-rule-603-boarding. Accessed August 9, 2022.
43. USA Hockey, Section Six, Playing Rules, Rule 606, Butt-Ending. https://www.usahockeyrulebook.com/page/show/1084650-rule-606-butt-ending. Accessed August 9, 2022.
44. Hagerty M. The punch: how an infamous moment in Houston sports changed basketball forever. National Public Radio, December 8, 2017. https://www.houstonpublicmedia.org/articles/news/2017/12/08/255471/the-punch-how-an-infamous-moment-in-houston-sports-changed-basketball/ Accessed August 8, 2022.
45. Fields SK, Collins CL, Comstock RD. Conflict on the courts: a review of sports-related violence literature. *Trauma Violence Abuse*. 2007;8(4):359–369.
46. Romanet I, Graillon N, Le Roux MK, et al. Hooliganism and maxillofacial trauma: the surgeon should be warned. *J Stomatol Oral Maxillofac Surg*. 2019;120(2):106–109.
47. Shepherd J. Football hooliganism, delinquency, and public health. *Medico-Legal J*. 1991;59(1):50–52.
48. Shields EW Jr. Intimidation and violence by males in high school athletics. *Adolescence*. 1999;34(135):503–521.
49. Watters DA, Brooks S, Elton RA, Little K. Sports injuries in an accident and emergency department. *Emerg Med J*. 1984;1(2):105–111.
50. Collins CL, Fields SK, Comstock RD. When the rules of the game are broken: what proportion of high school sports-related injuries are related to illegal activity? *Inj Prev*. 2008;14(1):34–38.
51. Gleeson S. Four dead as rival fans riot at Honduras soccer game. *USA Today,* August 19, 2019. https://www.usatoday.com/story/sports/soccer/2019/08/19/soccer-riots-four-dead-after-fight-breaks-out-game-honduras/2049092001/ Accessed August 8, 2022.
52. Sekulic M, Kühl S, Connert T, Krastl G, Filippi A. Dental, and jaw injuries sustained by hooligans. *Dent Traumatol*. 2015;31(6):477–481.
53. Cross T. Special report: assaults on sports officials. *Marq Sports L Rev*. 1997;8:429. https://scholarship.law.marquette.edu/cgi/viewcontent.cgi?referer=&httpsredir=1&article=1257&context=sportslaw. Accessed October 3, 2023.
54. Topp B. Incident in black and white. *Referee*. February, 1996:36. Cited by Cross.[53]
55. Prep wrestler punished for head-butting referee. *Referee*. June, 1996:19. Cited by Cross.[53]
56. N.J. teen sentenced in umpire assault. *Referee*. July, 1996:14. Cited by Cross.[53]
57. Umpire won't let attack intimidate him. *Referee*. November, 1996: 17. Cited by Cross.[53]
58. Football official rammed by player. *Referee*. November, 1996:18. Cited by Cross.[53]
59. Ref beaten; judge's sentence draws criticism. *Referee*. September, 1996:12. Cited by Cross.[53]

60. Ex-CFL player punches ref in touch football game. *Referee.* January,1997:16. Cited by Cross.[53]
61. High school player sentenced for ref assault. *Referee.* February, 1997:16. Cited by Cross.[53]
62. High school football ref knocked out. *Referee.* February,1997:14. Cited by Cross.[53]
63. Stock C. Attack on ref doesn't surprise Bears. *Edmonton Journal.* February 28, 1996:C3. Cited by Cross.[53]
64. Nelson P. Ellis issues apologies: Dragons' star awaits team, league sanctions. *Des Moines Register.* January 19, 1998:3. Cited by Cross.[53]
65. Radel C. Ref beatings in Ky. become spectator sport. *Cincinnati Enquirer.* February 9, 1996:B01. Cited by Cross.[53]
66. Basketball ref beaten; criminal, civil charges follow. *Referee.* June, 1996:18. Cited by Cross.[53]
67. Youth football official attacked, then charged with assault. *Referee.* January, 1997:15. Cited by Cross.[53]
68. Invasion of officials' locker room costs fan. *Referee.* July, 1996:7.
69. D.A. accused of accosting ref. *Referee.* May, 1996:14. Cited by Cross.[53]
70. Fan faces trial for punching football official. *Referee.* February, 1997:18. Cited by Cross.[53]
71. NBA refs accosted in separate incidents. *Referee.* June, 1996:15. Cited by Cross.[53]
72. Cohn L. NBA should take its cue from soccer. *Santa Rosa Press Democrat.* April 11, 1996:C1. Cited by Cross.[53]
73. MacMullan J. First Rodman, then Van Exel, now Magic: why all the official bashing? *Sports Illustrated.* 1996;(84)16:69. Cited by Cross.[53]
74. NBA suspends Barkley, Drexler: players also draw fines. *STAR-TRIB.* December 21, 1996:02C. Cited by Cross.[53]
75. Paul RJ. Variations in NHL attendance: the impact of violence, scoring, and regional rivalries. *Am J Econ Sociol.* 2003;62(2):345–364. Cited by Fields et al.[45]
76. Jones JC, Ferguson DG, Stewart KG. Blood sports and cherry pie: some economics of violence in the National Hockey League. *Am J Econ Sociol.* 1993;52(1):63–78. Cited by Paul.[75]
77. Jones JC, Nadeau S, Walsh WD. The wages of sin: employment and salary effects of violence in the national hockey league. *Atlantic Econ J.* 1997;25(2): 191–192. Cited by Paul.[75]
78. Jones JC, Stewart KG, Sunderman R. From the arena into the streets: hockey violence, economic incentives, and public policy. *Am J Econ Sociol.* 1996;55(2):231–243. Cited by Paul.[75]
79. Roberts J, Benjamin C. Spectator violence in sports: a North American perspective. *Eur J Crim Policy Res.* 2000;8(2):163–181.
80. Edwards H, Rackages V. The dynamics of violence in American sport: some promising structural and social considerations. *J Sport Soc Issues.* 1977;1(2):3–31. Cited by Roberts and Benjamin.[79]
81. Smith MD. Precipitants of crowd violence. *Sociol Inquiry.* 1978;48(2):121–131. Cited by Roberts and Benjamin.[79]
82. Lewis JM. Fan violence: an American social problem. In: Lewis M, ed. *Research in Social Problems and Public Policy*, Volume 2. Greenwich, CT: JAI Press; 1982:175–206. Cited by Roberts and Benjamin.[79]
83. Football violence: South America's interminable problem. France 24, December 22, 2018. https://www.france24.com/en/20181222-football-violence-south-americas-interminable-problem. Accessed August 8, 2022.
84. Barreiro R. Why is watching soccer so dangerous in Argentina? *El Pais*, May 2, 2017. https://english.elpais.com/elpais/2017/05/02/inenglish/1493718727_034529.html. Accessed August 8, 2022.

85. Barreiro R. Argentina soccer fan dies after being pushed off stands. *El Pais*, April 18, 2017. https://english.elpais.com/elpais/2017/04/17/inenglish/1492424704_367509.html. Accessed August 8, 2022.
86. Szlifman J. More football violence in Argentina and new tragedies in South America. *Play the Game*. 18.04.2013. https://www.playthegame.org/news/more-football-violence-in-argentina-and-new-tragedies-in-south-america/. Accessed August 8, 2022.
87. ESPN staff. Unruly Argentina fans set to be barred from World Cup. ESPN, May 9, 2018. https://www.espn.com/soccer/fifa-world-cup/story/3489770/unruly-argentina-fans-set-to-be-barred-from-world-cup. Accessed August 8, 2022.
88. Argentina's hooligans: the endless cycle of football violence. France 24, November 27, 2018. https://www.france24.com/en/20181127-argentinas-hooligans-endless-cycle-football-violence. Accessed August 8, 2022.
89. Parkin S. The rise of Russia's neo-Nazi football hooligans. *Guardian*, April 24, 2018. https://www.theguardian.com/news/2018/apr/24/russia-neo-nazi-football-hooligans-world-cup. Accessed August 8, 2022.
90. Petkova M. Russian football hooligans face a crackdown ahead of World Cup. *Aljazeera*, April 11, 2018. https://www.aljazeera.com/features/2018/4/11/russian-football-hooligans-face-a-crackdown-ahead-of-world-cup. Accessed August 8, 2022.
91. Mosko A. Soccer shame: 3 violent clashes involving Russian football fans. *Russia Beyond*, June 15, 2018. https://www.rbth.com/sport/2016/06/15/soccer-shame-3-violent-clashes-involving-russian-football-fans_603291. Accessed August 8, 2022.
92. Associated Press. FIFA calls fan violence in Brazil 'very sad.' *USA Today*, December 9, 2013. https://www.usatoday.com/story/sports/soccer/2013/12/09/fifa-calls-fan-violence-in-brazil-very-sad/3919881/. Accessed August 8, 2022.
93. Uribarri J. SEE IT: Brazilian soccer fans riot in the stands during Vasco da Gama-Paranaense game. *New York Daily News*, December 9, 2013. https://www.nydailynews.com/sports/soccer/soccer-riot-control-brazil-article-1.1541545. Accessed August 8, 2022.
94. Jenner F. Colombian football rivalry turns deadly after fight between fans. Colombia Focus, February 26, 2018. https://colombiafocus.com/colombian-football-rivalry-turns-deadly-after-fight-between-fans. Accessed August 8, 2022.
95. Fahmy MF, Lee I. Anger flares in Egypt after 79 die in soccer riot. CNN, February 2, 2012. https://www.cnn.com/2012/02/02/world/africa/egypt-soccer-deaths/index.html. Accessed August 8, 2022.
96. Southgate G. Czech Republic vs England: one football fan injured and 31 people detained for 'rioting' in Prague. *Independent*, October 11, 2019. https://www.independent.co.uk/sport/football/international/czech-republic-vs-england-31-fans-rioting-arrested-violence-euro-2020-qualifying-a9152871.html. Accessed August 8, 2022.
97. Thompson O. Mobs, violence, discrimination: the Italian ultra problem. *Sporting Ferret*, July 6, 2020. https://www.sportingferret.com/2020/07/06/mobs-violence-discrimination-the-italian-ultra-problem/. Accessed August 8, 2022.
98. Worst fan violence 'since 2000' after Danish cup final. *The Local DK*, May 26, 2017. https://www.thelocal.dk/20170526/worst-fan-violence-since-2000-after-danish-cup-final/. Accessed August 8, 2022.
99. Friend N. Fan violence, firebombs and teargas force Greek derby to be abandoned. CNN. March 18, 2019. https://www.cnn.com/2019/03/18/football/panathinaikos-olympiakos-fan-violence/index.html. Accessed August 8, 2022.

100. Greek football plagued by hooligans and violence. DW, March 21, 2019. https://www.dw.com/en/greek-football-plagued-by-hooligans-and-violence/a-48008499. Accessed August 8, 2022.
101. AFP. Turkey crackdown on football violence. *World Soccer Talk,* August 10, 2017. https://worldsoccertalk.com/2017/08/10/turkey-crackdown-on-football-violence/. Accessed August 9, 2022.
102. Reuters. Survival of French football at stake after latest fan violence, sports minister warns. ESPN, November 22, 2021. https://www.espn.com/soccer/french-ligue-1/story/4527200/survival-of-french-football-at-stake-after-latest-fan-violencesports-minister-warns. Accessed August 9, 2022.
103. Wright N, Bell J. The challenge of violence in sport. *The Williams Record,* December 1, 2021. https://williamsrecord.com/458653/opinions/the-challenge-of-violence-in-sport/. Accessed August 9, 2022.
104. Doyle P. Shocking rise of fan disorder leaves Ligue 1 facing an existential crisis. *Guardian,* November 27, 2021. https://www.theguardian.com/football/2021/nov/27/ligue-1-supporters-disorder-violence. Accessed August 9, 2022.
105. Schiller R. Clubs should sanction fans involved in violence before FAI Cup final, minister says. Independent.ie, November 29, 2021. https://www.independent.ie/news/clubs-should-sanction-fans-involved-in-violence-before-fai-cup-final-minister-says-41100073.html. Accessed August 9, 2022.
106. Associated Press. Euro 2020 final review shows England fans 'endangered lives.' Sports Illustrated. December 3, 2021. https://www.si.com/soccer/2021/12/03/england-fans-euro-2020-final-wembley-stadium-review. Accessed August 9, 2022.
107. Hill GA. Kept quiet for 15 months, sports fans are back at games. For better and worse. *Washington Post,* May 29, 2021. https://www.washingtonpost.com/sports/2021/05/29/unruly-sports-fan-history/. Accessed August 9, 2022.
108. Mansfield A. The 15 craziest fan brawls at sporting events. *Complex,* August 24, 2021. https://www.complex.com/sports/craziest-fan-brawls-sporting-events/. Accessed August 9, 2022.
109. Calhoun D. Galaxy, LAFC release joint statement regarding fan violence at games, Incidents following the Aug. 28 and Sunday's games are under investigation. *Los Angeles Daily News,* October 4, 2021. https://www.dailynews.com/2021/10/04/galaxy-and-lafc-release-joint-statement-regarding-fan-violence-at-games/. Accessed August 9, 2022.
110. Reuters, Coach shot in Argentine third-tier game amid fan violence. The Star, November 01, 2021. https://www.thestar.com.my/sport/football/2021/11/01/soccer-coach-shot-in-argentine-third-tier-game-amid-fan-violence. Accessed October 3, 2023.
111. Williams T. French football in crisis: missiles thrown, fans invading the pitch and matches abandoned. *The Athletic,* December 3, 2021. https://theathletic.com/2993808/2021/12/03/french-football-crisis-missiles-thrown-fans-invading-pitch-matches-abandoned/. Accessed August 9, 2022.
112. Bears vs. Rams: fans get in violent brawl...in bowels of SoFi stadium. *TMZ Sports,* September 13, 2021. https://www.tmz.com/2021/09/13/bears-rams-fans-brawl-nfl-los-angeles-sofi-stadium/. Accessed August 9, 2022.
113. Semini L. Albanian FA deplores fan violence, blames Polish supporters. AP News, October 14, 2021. https://apnews.com/article/soccer-sports-albania-world-cup-tirana-48adcdadbbc5d871ec0911106fb0f5f6. Accessed August 9, 2022.

114. Euros: Maguire's father hurt; UEFA investigate fan violence. Associated Press, July 13, 2021. https://apnews.com/article/euro-2020-sports-health-violence-europe-6aff3e0eae2c7ab4f3fef220f2a77848. Accessed August 9, 2022.

115. Contes B. Vikings fan gets decked twice by vicious blows to the head in violent brawl at Panthers stadium. Media ITE, October 18, 2021. https://www.mediaite.com/sports/vikings-fan-gets-decked-twice-by-vicious-blows-to-the-head-in-violent-brawl-at-panthers-stadium/. Accessed August 9, 2022.

116. United fan violence condemned by government and mayor. Reuters, March 5, 2021. https://www.eurosport.com/football/premier-league/2020-2021/football-news-manchester-united-fan-violence-condemned-by-government-and-mayor_sto8302362/story.shtml. Accessed August 9, 2022.

117. Evans S. FIFA investigating 'abhorrent' violence at Wembley. *The Star*, October 13, 2021. https://www.thestar.com.my/sport/football/2021/10/13/soccer-fifa-condemn-039abhorrent039-violence-at-wembley. Accessed October 3, 2023.

118. Nair S. WATCH: violence erupts in Argentina-Spain field hockey game on opening day of Tokyo Olympics 2020. *Essentially Sports,* July 23, 2021. https://www.essentiallysports.com/tokyo-olympics-news-watch-violence-erupts-in-argentina-spain-field-hockey-game-on-opening-day-of-tokyo-olympics-2020/. Accessed August 9, 2022.

119. JTA Staff. Argentine soccer fans chant about 'killing the Jews to make soap.' *Jerusalem Post,* March 26, 2021. https://www.jpost.com/diaspora/argentine-soccer-fans-chant-about-killing-the-jews-to-make-soap-663275. Accessed August 9, 2022.

120. Abu Much A. Israelis fed up with racist, anti-Muslim behavior of soccer fans. *Al-Monitor,* October 25, 2021. https://www.al-monitor.com/originals/2021/10/israelis-fed-racist-anti-muslim-behavior-soccer-fans. Accessed August 9, 2022.

121. Noryskiewicz A. Israeli soccer fans subjected to antisemitic abuse at 1st match in Berlin stadium built by the Nazis. CBS News, October 1, 2021. https://www.cbsnews.com/news/jewish-fans-antisemitic-abuse-berlin-maccabi-haifa-olympic-stadium-hitler-nazis/. Accessed August 9, 2022.

122. Wheeler C. Three Manchester United fans are hurt in Gdansk as a mob of Polish football hooligans dressed in black ambush the bar where they were drinking ahead of the Europa League final. MailOnline, May 26, 2021. https://www.dailymail.co.uk/sport/sportsnews/article-9620285/Manchester-United-fans-attacked-Gdansk.html. Accessed August 9, 2022.

123. Spaaij R. Sports crowd violence: an interdisciplinary synthesis. *Aggress Violent Behav.* 2014;19(2):146–155.

124. Spaaij R. *Understanding Football Hooliganism: A Comparison of Six Western European Football Clubs.* Amsterdam University Press; 2006.https://pure.uva.nl/ws/files/44222576/Thesis.pdf. Accessed October 3, 2023.

125. Dunning E, Murphy P, Waddington I, Astrinakis AE, eds. *Fighting Fans: Football Hooliganism as a World Phenomenon.* Dublin, Ireland: University College Dublin Press; 2002. Cited by Spaaij.[124]

126. Hua, T. Football "hooligans" and football supporters' culture in China. In: Manzenreiter W, Horne J, eds. *Football Goes East: Business, Culture and the People's Game in China, Japan and South Korea.* London, England: Routledge; 2004:87–101. Cited by Spaaij.[124]

127. Roversi A, Balestri C. Italian ultras today: change or decline? In: Dunning E, Murphy P, Waddington I, Astrinakis AE, eds. *Fighting Fans: Football Hooliganism as a World Phenomenon.* Dublin, Ireland: University College Dublin Press; 2002:131–142. Cited by Spaaij.[124]

128. Horak R. Things change: Trends in Austrian football hooliganism from 1977–1990. *Sociol Rev.* 1991;39(3):531–548. Cited by Spaaij.[124]
129. Piotrowski P. Soccer hooliganism in Poland: its extent, dynamism and psycho-social conditions. In: Jackson R, ed. *(Re)constructing Cultures of Violence and Peace.* Amsterdam: Rodopi; 2004. Cited by Spaaij.[124]
130. Pintér O, van Gestel J. Football's fighting fans: the Hungarian case. In: Dunning E, Murphy P, Waddington I, Astrinakis AE, eds. *Fighting Fans: Football Hooliganism as a World Phenomenon.* Dublin, Ireland: University College Dublin Press; 2002:106–117. Cited by Spaaij.[124]
131. Beiu A. Football related violence in Romania. In: Aquesolo Vegas J, ed. *Actas del X Congreso Internacional de Historia del Deporte.* Seville, Spain:CESH; 2005. Cited by Spaaij.[124]
132. Duke V, Slepička P. Bohemian rhapsody: football supporters in the Czech Republic. In: Dunning E, Murphy P, Waddington I, Astrinakis AE, eds. *Fighting Fans: Football Hooliganism as a World Phenomenon.* Dublin, Ireland: University College Dublin Press; 2002:49–61. Cited by Spaaij.[124]
133. Harsányi L. *Report on Hooliganism, Racism, Anti-Semitism and Intolerance in Slovak Football.* Bratislava, Yugoslavia: Ludia Proti Rasizm; 2005. Cited by Spaaij.[124]
134. Viñas C. *El Mundo Ultra: Los Radicales del Fútbol Español.* Madrid, Spain: Temas de Hoy; 2005. Cited by Spaaij.[124]
135. Mignon P. Le Francais feel-good factor. In: Perryman M, ed. *Hooligan Wars: Causes and Effects of Football Violence.* London, England: Mainstream; 2001:165–178. Cited by Spaaij.[124]
136. Courakis N. Football violence: not only a British problem. *Eur J Crim Policy Res.* 1998;6(2):293–302. Cited by Spaaij.[124]
137. Andersson T, Radmann A. Fans in Scandinavia. In: Brown A, ed. *Fanatics! Power, Identity and Fandom in Football.* London, England: Routledge; 1998:141–157. Cited by Spaaij.[124]
138. Spaaij RFJ. The prevention of football hooliganism: a transnational perspective. In: Aquesolo Vegas J, ed. *Actas del X Congreso Internacional de Historia del Deporte.* Seville, Spain:CESH; 2005:1–10. Cited by Spaaij.[124]
139. van Limbergen K, Walgrave L. *Sides, fans en hooligans: Voetbalvandalisme: feiten, achtergronden en aanpak.* Leuven en Amersfoort, the Netherlands: Acco; 1998. Cited by Spaaij.[124]
140. Giulianotti R. Hooligans and carnival fans: Scottish football supporter cultures. In: Armstrong G, Giulianotti R, eds. *Football Cultures and Identities.* London, England: Macmillan; 1999:29–40. Cited by Spaaij.[124]
141. Ek R. *Hooligans: Fakten, Hintergründe.* Analysen, Worms: Cicero Verlag, Munich, Germany; 1996. Cited by Spaaij.[124]
142. Archetti EP, Romero AG. Death and violence in Argentinian football. In: Giulianotti R, Bonney N, Hepworth M, eds. *Football, Violence and Social Identity.* London, England: Routledge; 1994:37–72. Cited by Spaaij.[124]
143. Alabarces P. "Aguante" and repression: football, politics and violence in Argentina. In: Dunning E, Murphy P, Waddington I, Astrinakis AE, eds. *Fighting Fans: Football Hooliganism as a World Phenomenon.* Dublin, Ireland: University College Dublin Press; 2002:23–36. Cited by Spaaij.[124]
144. de Toledo LH. Transgressão e violência entre torcedores de futebol. *Revista USP.* 1994;22:92–101. Cited by Spaaij.[124]
145. Panfichi A, Thieroldt J. Barras bravas: representation and crowd violence in Peruvian football. In: Dunning E, Murphy P, Waddington I, Astrinakis AE, eds. *Fighting Fans: Football*

Hooliganism as a World Phenomenon. Dublin, Ireland: University College Dublin Press; 2002:143–157. Cited by Spaaij.[124]
146. Frosdick S, Newton R. The nature and extent of football hooliganism in England and Wales. *Soccer Soc*. 2006;7(4):403–422.
147. Romero A. *Muerte En La Cancha*. Buenos Aires, Argentina: Nueva America; 1986. Cited by Duke and Crolley.[149]
148. Scher A, Palomino H. *Futbol: Pasion De Multitudes Y De Elites*. Buenos Aires, Argentina: CISEA; 1988. Cited by Duke and Crolley.[149]
149. Duke V, Crolley L. Football spectator behaviour in Argentina: a case of separate evolution. *Sociol Rev*. 1996;44(2):272–293.
150. Las barras bravas (informe especial). *El Grafico*, June 7, 1983. Cited by Duke and Crolley.[149]
151. Las barras bravas (informe especial). *Somos*, August 12, 1983. Cited by Duke and Crolley.[149]
152. La violencia disminuyo pero en las estadisticas. *Ambito*, December 27, 1993. Cited by Duke and Crolley.[149]
153. La ley del mas fuerte. *El Cronista*, May 18, 1992. Cited by Duke and Crolley.[149]
154. Futbol: se sextuplico la violencia. *La Razon*, April 20, 1989. Cited by Duke and Crolley.[149]
155. Futbol: donde esta la falla? *La Razon*, April 25, 1989. Cited by Duke and Crolley.[149]
156. Bjørnseth I, Szabo A. Sexual violence against children in sports and exercise: a systematic literature review. *J Child Sex Abuse*. 2018;27(4):365–385.
157. Vertommen T, Kampen J, Schipper-Van Veldhoven N, Wouters K, Uzieblo K, Van Den Eede F. Profiling perpetrators of interpersonal violence against children in sport based on a victim survey. *Child Abuse Negl*. 2017;63:172–182. Cited by Bjørnseth and Szabo.[156]
158. Parent S, Lavoie F, Thibodeau M-È, Hébert M, Blais M, Team PAJ2. Sexual violence experienced in the sport context by a representative sample of Quebec adolescents. 2016;31(16):2666–2686. Cited by Bjørnseth and Szabo.[156]
159. Vertommen T, Schipper-Van Veldhoven N, Wouters K, et al. Interpersonal violence against children in sport in the Netherlands and Belgium. *Child Abuse Negl*. 2016;51:223–236. Cited by Bjørnseth and Szabo.[156]
160. Fasting K, Sand TS. Narratives of sexual harassment experiences in sport. *Qual Res Sport Exerc Health*. 2015:1–16. Cited by Bjørnseth and Szabo.[156]
161. Hartill M. Exploring narratives of boyhood sexual subjection in male-sport. *Sociol Sport J*. 2014;31(1):23–43. Cited by Bjørnseth and Szabo.[156]
162. Fasting K, Brackenridge CH, Kjølberg G. Using court reports to enhance knowledge of sexual abuse in sport: a Norwegian case study. *Scand Sport Stud Forum*. 2013;4:49–67. http://dspace.brunel.ac.uk/bitstream/2438/7434/2/Fulltext.pdf. Cited by Bjørnseth and Szabo.[156]
163. Nielsen JT. The forbidden zone: intimacy, sexual relations, and misconduct in the relationship between coaches and athletes. *Int Rev Sociol Sport*. 2001;36(2):165–182. Cited by Bjørnseth and Szabo.[156]
164. Marks S, Mountjoy M, Marcus M. Sexual harassment, and abuse in sport: the role of the team doctor. *Br J Sports Med*. 2012;46(13):905–908.
165. Brackenridge CH. "He owned me basically . . . " Women's experience of sexual abuse in sport. *Int Rev Sociol Sport*. 1997;32:115–130. Cited by Marks et al.[164]
166. International Olympic Committee. Consensus Statement on Sexual Harassment & Abuse in Sport. 2007. Cited by Marks et al.[164]
167. Hoover NC. National Survey: Initiation Rites and Athletics for NCAA Sports Teams. Alfred University, 1999. Cited by Marks et al.[164] https://www.alfred.edu/about/news/studies/_docs/hazing.pdf. Accessed October 3, 2023.

168. Fasting K, Brackenridge CH, Sundgot-Borgen J. Prevalence of sexual harassment among Norwegian female elite athletes in relation to sport type. *Int Rev Sociol Sport.* 2004;39:373–386. Cited by Marks et al.[164]
169. Fasting K, Brackenridge CH, Sundgot-Borgen J. Experiences of sexual harassment and abuse amongst Norwegian elite female athletes and non-athletes. *Res Q Exerc Sport.* 2003;74:84–97. Cited by Marks et al.[164]
170. Brackenridge CH. Fair play or fair game: child sexual abuse in sport. *Int Rev Sociol Sport.* 1994;29:287–299. Cited by Marks et al.[164]
171. Vanden Auweele Y, Openacker J, Vertommen T, et al. Unwanted sexual experiences in sport: perceptions and reported prevalence among Flemish female student-athletes. *Int J Sport Exerc Psychol.* 2008; 6:354–365. Cited by Marks et al.[164]
172. Fasting K, Brackenridge CH, Miller KE, et al. Participation in college sports and protection from sexual victimization. *Int J Sport Exerc Psychol.* 2008;16:427–441. Cited by Marks et al.[164]
173. Fasting K, Brackenridge CH, Sundgot-Borgen J. *Females, Elite Sports, and Sexual Harassment: The Norwegian Women Project 2000.* Oslo, Norway: Norwegian Olympic Committee; 2000. Cited by Marks et al.[164]
174. Kirby S, Greaves L, Hankivsky O. *The Dome of Silence: Sexual Harassment and Abuse in Sport.* London, England: Zed Books; 2000. Cited by Marks et al.[164]
175. Tomlinson A, Yorganci I. Male coach/female athlete relations: gender and power relations in competitive sport. *J Sport Soc.* 1997;21:134–155. Cited by Marks et al.[164]
176. Volkwein K, Schnell F, Sherwood D, et al. Sexual harassment in sport: perceptions and experiences of American female student-athletes. *Int Rev Sociol Sport.* 1997;32:283–295. Cited by Marks et al.[164]
177. Brackenridge CH, Bishopp D, Moussali S, et al. The characteristics of sexual abuse in sport: a multidimensional scaling analysis of events described in media reports. *Int J Sport Exerc Psychol.* 2008;16:385–406. Cited by Marks et al.[164]
178. Volkwein-Caplan K, Schnell F, Devlin S, et al. Sexual harassment of women in athletics vs academia. *J Sex Aggress.* 2002;8:69–82. Cited by Marks et al.[164]
179. Kirby SL, Wintrup G. Hazing and initiation: sexual harassment and abuse issues. *J Sex Aggress.* 2002;8:41–60. Cited by Marks et al.[164]
180. Waldron J, Lynn Q, Krane V. Duct tape, Icy Hot & paddles: narratives of initiation onto US male sport teams. *Sport Educ Soc.* 2011;16:111–125. Cited by Marks et al.[164]
181. Wilinsky CL, McCabe A. A review of emotional and sexual abuse of elite child athletes by their coaches. *Sports Coach Rev.* 2020:1–.6.
182. Gervis M, Dunn N. The emotional abuse of elite child athletes by their coaches. *Child Abuse Rev.* 2004;13(3):215–223. Cited by Wilinsky and McCabe.[181]
183. Kavanagh E, Brown L, Jones I. Elite athletes' experience of coping with emotional abuse in the coach–athlete relationship. *J Appl Sport Psychol.* 2017;29(4): 402–417. Cited by Wilinsky and McCabe.[181]
184. Stirling AE, Kerr GA. Elite female swimmers' experiences of emotional abuse across time. *J Emot Abuse.* 2007;7(4):89–113. Cited by Wilinsky and McCabe.[181]
185. Stirling AE, Kerr GA. Defining and categorizing emotional abuse in sport. *Eur J Sport Sci.* 2008;8(4):173–181. Cited by Wilinsky and McCabe.[181]
186. Stirling AE, Kerr GA. Initiating and sustaining emotional abuse in the coach–athlete relationship: an ecological transactional model of vulnerability. *J Aggress Maltreat Trauma.* 2014;23(2):116–135. Cited by Wilinsky and McCabe.[181]

187. Alexander K, Stafford A, Lewis R. *The Experiences of Children Participating in Organised Sport in the UK*. London, England: NSPCC; 2011. https://www.pure.ed.ac.uk/ws/portalfiles/portal/7971883/experiences_children_sport_main_report_wdf85014.pdf. Accessed August 9, 2021.
188. Willson E, Kerr G. Body shaming as a form of emotional abuse in sport. *Int J Sport Exerc Psychol*. 2021:1–9.
189. Crow RB, Macintosh EW. Conceptualizing a meaningful definition of hazing in sport. *Eur Sport Manage Q*. 2009:433–451. Cited by Waldron (see Note 190).
190. Waldron JJ. Predictors of mild hazing, severe hazing, and positive initiation rituals in sport. *Int J Sports Sci Coach*. 2015;10(6):1089–1101.
191. Kahn LM. Discrimination in professional sports: a survey of the literature. *ILR Rev*. 1991;44(3):395–418.
192. Okrent D, Wulf S. *Baseball Anecdotes*. New York, NY: Oxford University Press; 1989. Cited by Kahn.[191]
193. Becker G. *The Economics of Discrimination*. 2nd ed. Chicago, IL: University of Chicago Press; 1971. Cited by Kahn.[191]
194. Bradley B. *Life on the Run*. New York, NY: Quadrangle/New York Times Books; 1976. Cited by Kahn.[191]
195. Tygiel J. *Baseball's Great Experiment*. New York, NY: Oxford University Press; 1983. Cited by Kahn.[191]
196. Brown E, Spiro R, Keenan D. Wage and nonwage discrimination in professional basketball [Mimeo]. Pomona College, 1988. Cited by Kahn.[191]
197. Kahn LM, Sherer PD. Racial differences in professional basketball players' compensation. *J Labor Econ*. 1988;6(1):40–61. Cited by Kahn.[191]
198. Koch JV, Vander Hill CW. Is there discrimination in the "black man's game"? *Soc Sci Q*. 1988;69(1):83–94. Cited by Kahn.[191]
199. Wallace M. Labor market structure and salary determination among professional basketball players. *Work Occup*. 1988;15(3):294–312. Cited by Kahn.[191]
200. Grenier G, Lavoie M. Francophones in the National Hockey League: test of entry and salary discrimination [Mimeo]. University of Ottawa, 1988. Cited by Kahn.[191]
201. Jones JCH, Walsh WD. Salary determination in the National Hockey League: the effects of skills, franchise characteristics, and discrimination. *Ind Labor Relat Rev*. 1988;41(4):592–604. Cited by Kahn.[191]
202. Lavoie M. Stacking, performance differentials, and salary discrimination in professional ice hockey: a survey of the evidence. *Sociol Sport J*. 1989;6(1):17–35. Cited by Kahn.[191]
203. Pascal AH, Rapping LA. The economics of racial discrimination in organized baseball. In: Pascal AH, ed. *Racial Discrimination in Economic Life*. Lexington, MA: D. C. Heath; 1972:119–156. Cited by Kahn.[191]
204. Hill JR, Spellman W. Fay discrimination in baseball: data from the Seventies. *Ind Relat*. 1984;23(1):103–112. Cited by Kahn.[191]
205. Scully GW. Economic discrimination in professional sports. *Law Contemp Prob*. 1973;38(1):67–84. 1974a. "Discrimination: The Case of Baseball." In R. Noll, ed., Government, and the Sports Business. Washington, D.C: Brookings, pp. 221–73 Cited by Kahn.[191]
206. Christiano K. Salaries and race in professional baseball: discrimination 10 years later. *Sociol Sport J*. 1988;5(2):136–149. Cited by Kahn.[191]

207. Nirmal R. *Coaches' Perceived Impact of the Respect in Sport (RiS) Program on Bullying, Abuse, Neglect, and Harassment in Sports* [dissertation]. Vancouver: University of British Columbia. https://open.library.ubc.ca/soa/cIRcle/collections/ubctheses/24/items/1.0054461. Accessed August 9, 2022.
208. Mitten MJ. The coach and the safety of athletes: ethical and legal issues. In: Simon RL, ed. *The Ethics of Coaching Sports*. Routledge; 2013. Forthcoming, Marquette Law School Legal Studies Paper N0. 12–13. 2012. https://papers.ssrn.com/sol3/papers.cfm?abstract_id=2088091. Accessed October 4, 2023.
209. Anderson MK. *Fundamentals of Sports Injury Management*. Baltimore, MD: Lippincott Williams & Wilkins; 2003.
210. Statum C. Yes, it is your fault: cracking down on college coaches and administrators who ignore abuse. *U Ill L Rev*. 2020:1571.
211. Mirsafian H. Legal duties and legal liabilities of coaches toward athletes. *Phys Cult Sport*. 2016;69(1):5. https://sciendo.com/pdf/10.1515/pcssr-2016-0002. Accessed August 9, 2022.
212. Hekmat RR. Malpractice during practice: should NCAA coaches be liable for negligence. *Loy LA Ent L Rev*. 2001;22:613 https://digitalcommons.lmu.edu/cgi/viewcontent.cgi?referer=&httpsredir=1&article=1446&context=elr. Accessed October 4, 2023.
213. Partington N. Sports coaching and the law of negligence: implications for coaching practice. *Sports Coach Rev*. 2017;6(1):36–56. https://pureadmin.qub.ac.uk/ws/portalfiles/portal/60471213/Sports_coaching_and_the_law_of_negligence_implications_for_coaching_practice.pdf. Accessed August 9, 2022.
214. Herbert R. More isn't better: overtraining as a cause of action for coach negligence. *Cap U L Rev*. 2019;47:125.
215. Winsley R, Matos N. Overtraining and elite young athletes. In: Armstrong N, McManus AM, eds. *The Elite Young Athlete*. New York, NY: Karger; 2011:97–105.
216. DiFiori JP, Benjamin HJ, Brenner JS, et al. Overuse injuries and burnout in youth sports: a position statement from the American Medical Society for Sports Medicine. *Br J Sports Med*. 2014;48(4):287–288.
217. Stricker PR. Sports training issues for the pediatric athlete. *Pediatr Clin*. 2002;49(4):793–802.
218. Bergeron MF. The young athlete: challenges of growth, development, and society. *Curr Sports Med Rep*. 2010;9(6):356–358.
219. Podlog L, Eklund RC. Professional coaches' perspectives on the return to sport following serious injury. *J Appl Sport Psychol*. 2007;19(2):207–225.
220. Raedeke TD, Lunney K, Venables K. Understanding athlete burnout: coach perspectives. *J Sport Behav*. 2002;25(2).
221. Committee on Sports Medicine and Fitness. Intensive training and sports specialization in young athletes. *Pediatrics*. 2000;106(1):154–157.
222. Lloyd RS, Faigenbaum AD, Stone MH, et al. Position statement on youth resistance training: the 2014 International Consensus. *Br J Sports Med*. 2014;48(7):498–505.https://bjsm.bmj.com/content/48/7/498. Accessed October 4, 2023.
223. Normand JM, Wolfe A, Peak K. A review of early sport specialization in relation to the development of a young athlete. *Int J Kinesiol Sports Sci*. 2017;5(2):37–42.

18
Bullying and Other Forms of Victimization in Tertiary Education

What Is Known?

There is documented evidence supporting the continuity of being a bully, victim, or bully-victim from elementary school through college,[1] and it has been established that bullying experiences in childhood and adolescence relate to difficulties in psychological adjustment in young adulthood.[2]

This chapter reviews the maltreatment experiences prevalent in tertiary education, also known as postsecondary or higher education. It includes an examination of all facets of victimization, including bullying, hazing, incivility, sexual harassment, intimidation, and stalking, affecting students or trainees, teachers/instructors, and academic officials studying/working in undergraduate, graduate, and postgraduate education, including military training. As previously discussed (see Chapter 11), the tertiary education milieu is a place of work, where all its stakeholders can be affected by workplace bullying and other forms of victimization.

Bullying in Postsecondary Education

Bullying among College/University Students

Wensley and Campbell[3] explored the frequency of participation in traditional bullying and cyberbullying among 528 Australian first-year college students and found that almost 21% of the participants reported being a victim and 5% reported being a perpetrator of traditional bullying in the previous 12 months.[3] For cyberbullying, almost 12% of participants were victims, and 4% were perpetrators in the previous year. Nonheterosexual students reported a higher frequency of participation in traditional bullying, both as victims and perpetrators, while cyberbullying prevalence was found to be similar for heterosexual and nonheterosexual participants.[3]

Witnessing bullying in college was studied by Chapell et al.[4] in a survey of 1,025 undergraduate university students at a public university in the northeast of the United States. Almost 60% of the participants witnessed a student being bullied by another student, once or more frequently.[4] Furthermore, 44% of the students surveyed reported having witnessed a teacher bullying a student in college, once or more frequently.[4] In this survey[4] as well as in a report by Marraccini et al.,[5] 18% of college students indicated that a professor or instructor had bullied them.

An investigation focused on bullying at a Finnish university was conducted in May 2010 by Sinkkonen et al.[6] via a survey of 2,805 students (mean age 27 years and 72% female). The study showed that 5% of the participants reported having been bullied while studying or in the university milieu, with 2% being victimized daily or a couple of times a month. In half of the incidents, the perpetrator was another student, but nearly as frequently (44%), the perpetrator was a faculty member, or occasionally (6%) the victimizer was an administrative employee.[6] Furthermore, 11% of students indicated that they witnessed bullying on campus, but only 3% tried to intervene. Regarding the types of bullying identified in the study,[6] 65% of students who were bullied experienced indirect public or individual victimization through age discrimination, exclusion from a group, unfair or unequal treatment, getting inappropriate assignments, being treated disrespectfully or belittled, or being given ambiguous advice on purpose. Moreover, one-third of respondents who were bullied were affected by direct verbal mistreatment, such as being called names, picked on, reprimanded, or exposed to public ridicule.[6]

Bullying among Healthcare Students and Professional Trainees

Data on prevalence of bullying and other forms of maltreatment among US medical students can be found in a survey[7] of 1,630 graduates of 145 medical schools (who graduated in the academic year 2019–2020). The study found that 40% of graduates were embarrassed in public and 22% were publicly humiliated during medical school by other students, faculty, nurses, residents/interns, or other institution employees or staff.[7] Furthermore, 15% were subjected to offensive sexist remarks or names, while 5% to 7% were subjected to racially or ethnically offensive remarks or names, were required to perform personal services, were subjected to unwanted sexual advances, were denied opportunities for training or rewards based on gender, received lower evaluations or grades solely based on gender rather than performance, or were exposed to offensive behaviors based on personal beliefs or characteristics other than gender, race/ethnicity, or sexual orientation. A small segment (1%–3%) experienced offensive remarks/names related to sexual orientation, received lower evaluations or grades solely based on gender orientation rather than performance, or were physically harmed or threatened with physical harm.[7]

Ahmer et al.[8] led an effort to document the prevalence of bullying among medical students in Pakistan via a cross-sectional investigation of 342 medical students who were in their final year at six Pakistani medical colleges. Over half of the students (52%) indicated that they were bullied in medical college, with 16% being victimized at least once a month.[8] Among those who were bullied, almost 57% suffered verbal abuse, 16% felt deliberately ignored, 11% experienced exclusion, 5% were physically abused, and 2.5% were subjects of written abuse.[8] Most of the students who were bullied (73%) were subjected to maltreatment by a consultant (attending physician) or by a resident medical officer, while 18% were bullied by a peer or a nurse, and 9% by patients.[8]

A survey conducted by Gágyor et al.[9] to ascertain "negative experiences" among 400 students at a medical university in Germany documented that 56% felt "insufficiently appreciated," 45% felt ignored, 34% suffered verbal abuse, and 23% experienced humiliation. Furthermore, less than 10% reported sexual harassment, discrimination on other grounds, or physical abuse, while a small number (2%) felt discriminated against on ethnic or racial grounds.

A significant exposure to bullying in nursing school was documented by Karatas et al.[10] in a study based on 202 undergraduate nursing students enrolled at a university in southeastern

Turkey during the 2013–2014 academic year. More than three-quarters (78%) reported mistreatment in the previous six months, with approximately 50% to 60% being verbally abused, being exposed to rumors or gossip, being subjected to homework and job rotation as form of punishment in lieu of training, being ignored or excluded, being assigned impossible workloads, or being insulted with sarcastic, ironic, or offensive speech.[10] Only 24% of the students were victimized by peers, while the rest reported having been mistreated by clinical nurses, scholars, and other university employees.[10]

The extent to which undergraduate medical and nursing students experienced bullying and harassment during the first year on full-time placement was studied by Timm[11] through an online survey of 309 UK students. The study showed that nursing students were more likely (27%) to report having witnessed or experienced incidents of bullying or harassment of themselves or other people during their last seven months of full-time clinical placement, as compared to 18% of the medical students.[11]

Bullying among University Academic or Administrative Staff

Meriläinen and Kõiv[12] created an instrument for determining the level and nature of workplace bullying among faculty members based on the Negative Acts Questionnaire-Revised (NAQ-R)[13] and additional items dealing with sexual harassment, cyberbullying, and work-related mismanagement or dereliction. This research led to the development of the Academic Bullying Inventory (ABI-10),[12] based on a model of five representative types of workplace bullying and inappropriate behaviors in Estonian universities, including personal insults, work-related blame, professional misunderstanding, unreasonable work-related demands, and work-related malpractice (Table 18.1).

Table 18.1. Dimensions of the Academic Bullying Inventory (ABI-10) Based on 10 Items of the NAQ-R22

Dimensions of the of the ABI-10[12]	Items of the NAQ-R22[13]
Person-related insulting[12]	Repeated reminders of one's errors or mistakes[12,13]
	Being ignored or facing a hostile reaction when one approaches others[12,13]
Work-related blaming[12]	Being humiliated or ridiculed in connection with one's work[12,13]
	Having one's work being excessively monitored[12,13]
Professional understanding[12]	Being ordered to do work above one's level of competence[12,13]
	Having key areas of responsibility removed or replaced with more trivial or unpleasant tasks[12,13]
Unreasonable work-related demands[12]	Being given unreasonable tasks[12,13]
	Being exposed to an unmanageable workload[12,13]
Work-related malpractices[12]	Recognizing that somebody is purposefully wasting resources[12,13]
	Finding out that somebody is purposefully wasting resources[12,13]

Meriläinen et al.[14] investigated the prevalence, nature, and manifestations of academic bullying among university personnel based on a survey of 864 Estonian and 327 Finnish faculty employees, showing that 27% of the Estonian faculty experienced bullying in the previous six months, mostly once a month or less frequently, while almost 17% of the Finnish participants experienced bullying in the preceding half year, mostly once a month or less frequently, while this form victimization was not found to be related to the type of job.[14] In Finland, bullying was more frequently experienced during research-related work, while Estonian participants were more frequently bullied during personnel meetings.[14]

The most common (above 40%) form of maltreatment experienced by Estonian and Finnish faculty personnel was characterized by being subjected to personal insults, negative work-related remarks, ostracism, and professional demotion.[14] Thirty-two percent of Finnish participants and 17% of Estonian respondents reported having been exposed to overwork and other forms of abuse in work-related tasks (e.g., perpetrators engaged in impeding flow of necessary information, plagiarism, deception, and conscious distortion of subjects and track records).[14] Approximately one-quarter of respondents in both nations indicated that they were humiliated or ridiculed, were shouted at, and were the target of spontaneous anger or allegations, negative comments, name-calling, or threats of violence.[12] Sexual harassment was experienced by 1% of Finnish faculty and 3% of Estonian personnel, while cyberbullying was reported by 1% of Finnish personnel and 6% of Estonian academic staff.[14]

Finnish academic personnel were mostly (20%) mistreated through professional demotion, slander, and ostracism. The second most frequent form of bullying experienced by both the Estonian and Finnish participants was in the form of negligence related to work tasks, as manifested by deliberating causing harm, impeding flow of necessary information, or delaying official management tasks, as well as overwork (among the Estonian faculty) or conscious distortion of subjects and track records, plagiarism, deception, and conscious aggravation among the Finnish group.[14]

Zabrodska and Kveton[15] determined the prevalence of workplace bullying among 1,553 university employees in the Czech Republic, through a survey based on the NAQ-R22.[13] Most of the academic workers surveyed (82%) were involved in research and teaching (including PhD candidates), while the rest worked in administration, finance, and services.[15] The study demonstrated that almost 8% of the respondents had been bullied in the previous 12 months, at least occasionally, according to a definition of bullying as a "situation where one or several individuals persistently over a period of time perceive themselves to be on the receiving end of negative actions from one or several persons, in a situation where the target of bullying has difficulty in defending him- or herself against these actions."[15] When the participants were administered the NAQ-R22,[13] almost 14% of them reported that they had been exposed to at least one negative act, at best once a week, during the previous year.[15]

Keashly[16] developed an in-depth review of the extant global research on bullying in academia, focusing on the experiences of faculty as victims, perpetrators, and witnesses of workplace bullying. The review examined 70 studies conducted in 20 countries around the world, from 1990 through 2018, and documented that approximately 25% of faculty had been bullied in the previous 12 months, while 50% to 75% had witnessed bullying in the previous year.

Bullying in Military Training

There are some studies on bullying during military training,[17-23] as well as worldwide news reports on the subject.[24-35]

A survey conducted in 2002 by Magerøy et al.[17] of 1,604 military and civilian employees serving in the Royal Norwegian Navy documented that 2.5% of employees experienced bullying and almost 10% witnessed its occurrence. The highest frequencies were found among the most junior ranks (enlisted, petty officer, and ensign), with 3.6% of them being bullied and 14.5% witnessing.[17] Lack of fair leadership and unequal treatment were significantly associated with bullying.[17]

Vaara et al.[18] led a study of 328 Finnish female volunteer military personnel that showed that being bullied because of physical fitness was experienced by 12% of the participants.[18]

Kirke[19] defined bullying in the British military context as:

> actions and practices that are directed against one or more soldiers, that may be carried out deliberately or unconsciously, but cause humiliation, offense, and distress, and cannot be justified as aimed at achieving operationally advantageous results. Such actions may interfere with job performance and/or cause an unpleasant working and living environment.

Furthermore, Kirke[19] discussed the notion of "oppressive coercive behavior" that could be predictable in a relationship between senior and junior military personnel for "positive military ends" (i.e., the enforcement of formal discipline and the implementation of military training for combat). Yet, this needs to be differentiated from "toxic leadership" or negative oppressive behavior, which is a form of workplace bullying that exploits "the rank and authority structure for personal satisfaction."[19]

The British House of Commons Defence Committee's report on duty of care,[20] which ensures that the mental and physical well-being of military personnel are protected, has underlined that "incidents of bullying of recruits and trainees are probably the most evident form of duty of care failure."[20] The 2021 Armed Forces Continuous Attitude Survey,[21] based on a sample of more than 10,000 trained UK Regular Armed Forces, has documented that 11% of the respondents reported having been subject to bullying, discrimination, or harassment in the previous 12 months, while 89% of them did not make a complaint to the ombudsman, "either because they did not believe anything would be done if they [made] a complaint and/or they believe[d] a complaint could affect their career."[21]

Bullying within the United States Armed Forces has been characterized[22] as an "act of aggression" that "may involve the singling out of an individual from his or her coworkers, or unit, for ridicule because he or she is considered different or weak." It may encompass some of the following acts "when performed without military or governmental purpose": physically striking or threatening; intimidating, teasing, or taunting; berating; playing abusive or malicious tricks; subjecting someone to excessive or abusive use of water; forcing someone to consume food, alcohol, or drugs; and degrading or damaging someone's property or reputation.[22]

A study to ascertain the awareness of bullying behaviors among United States military was conducted in 2015 by the Defense Equal Opportunity Management Institute,[23] through a survey of about 620,000 active-duty personnel of all branches, excluding members of the

Coast Guard, Reserve, and National Guard. The study showed that 12% of the respondents, regardless of gender, perceived that, in their units, bullying was occurring, as manifested by excessive teasing of certain members to the point that they were unable to defend themselves, purposeful exclusion of certain members from social activities, and/or certain members' being frequently reminded of small errors or mistakes they have made, to belittle them.[23] Nonwhite/black service members perceived bullying slightly more frequently in their units (13%) than white/Caucasian service members (10%), while the perception of bullying in the units was more frequently experienced by junior enlisted members (15%) than by senior enlisted members (4.5%).[23]

Other Forms of Victimization in Postsecondary Education

In addition to the bullying affecting young adults in postsecondary education or training, there is a wide range of other maltreatment that may be experienced by postsecondary students and trainees, including hazing, incivility, harassment, intimidation, stalking, discrimination, and violence.

Hazing among University Students

A comprehensive insight into the nature and dimensions of hazing in US colleges is provided by the initial findings of the National Study of Student Hazing,[36,37] which is based on "the analysis of 11,482 survey responses from undergraduate students enrolled at 53 colleges and universities and more than 300 interviews with students and campus personnel at 18 of those institutions."[36] The study[36] describes the notion of hazing as "any activity expected of someone joining or participating in a group that humiliates, degrades, abuses, or endangers them regardless of a person's willingness to participate."[36] Its preliminary findings (2008) documented that more than half of the college population (55%) engaged in hazing, with common practices being participating in drinking games, humiliation, isolation, sleep deprivation, and sex acts, with incidents frequently posted on Web sites.[36] It is important to highlight that 90% of "students who experienced hazing did not consider themselves to have been hazed."[36]

Further findings of the National Study of Student Hazing,[38] based on a 2013 survey of almost 5,000 students in seven universities located in different regions of the United States, have documented that 26% of the respondents reported that "they experienced at least one behavior meeting the definition of hazing in order to join or maintain membership in their group, team or organization," with most frequent activity being participation in a drinking game.[38] The majority (73%) of the respondents indicated that they have knowledge of other groups' engaging in hazing behaviors, while more than half of the survey participants reported that hazing was most likely to occur off campus.[38]

The term *ragging*, as it is known in South Asian countries, applies to a form of hazing or initiation ritual perpetrated by senior university students on undergraduates new to the institution, involving months of physical, mental, and sexual torment.[39-41]

The report of a death linked to ragging[42] brought this serious form of maltreatment into public attention and led to a judicial review by the Supreme Court of India.[43]

Hazing among Military Trainees

A debate about what constitutes hazing in the US military and what the US military leadership should do to prevent it was triggered by news of a US Marine's suicide following alleged hazing.[44] An independent report by the US Government Accountability Office (GAO)[45] has indicated that, until 2015, the US Department of Defense identified the concept of hazing "as any conduct whereby a military member or members, regardless of service or rank, without proper authority causes another military member or members, regardless of service or rank, to suffer or be exposed to any activity which is cruel, abusive, humiliating, oppressive, demeaning, or harmful."[46] Furthermore, the GAO report clarified that "soliciting or coercing another to perpetrate any such activity was also considered hazing, and the actions could be verbal or psychological in nature."[46] Moreover, "actual or implied consent did not eliminate the culpability of the perpetrator."[46] Subsequent to the GAO report,[45] the US Department of Defense updated the hazing definition by specifying that "hazing involves bringing people into a group or new status, whereas bullying may involve the singling out of an individual for being different or weak."[47]

The GAO report has advised, among other recommendations, that the US Department of Defense and the US Coast Guard "regularly monitor policy implementation, issue guidance on the collection and tracking of hazing incident data and evaluate the prevalence of hazing."[47]

During the period of April 2016 to September 2017, more than 700 US military service members, from all Armed Forces, reported having been exposed to incidents of hazing, which were mostly (55%) of physical nature, followed by verbal hazing (28%), with the majority of the incidents (97%) affecting enlisted personnel, mostly (89%) males and usually (89%) occurring while personnel were on duty inside a military base.[48]

Pershing[38] reviewed data from a 1990 survey administered by the US General Accounting Office (GAO)[49] to a stratified sample of 527 cadet officers at the US Naval Academy (midshipmen) covering a range of areas pertaining to the treatment of military students. In this context, Pershing[38] underscored that more than 70% of the midshipmen, of both genders, reported having experienced hazing at least twice a month or more frequently, during their freshman year as "plebes," manifested by being screamed in face by an upperclassman or being required to memorize trivia and to recite it to upperclassmen, while half of the respondents indicated that they had to "brace" for an extended period of time or endure verbal harassment, insult, or ridicule.[38]

The GAO[49] has also ascertained the extent of hazing occurrences among freshmen cadets of the US Air Force Academy and US Military Academy, documenting a similar frequency of experiences as those reported by the US Naval Academy freshmen.[38] Furthermore, the GAO survey of US cadets and midshipmen[49] showed that "greater exposure to hazing-type activities was associated with higher levels of physical and psychological stress,"[49] as well as a high level of attrition and or deterrence to further a military career.[49]

Incivility

The notion of incivility as a form of maltreatment may overlap in part with the concept of bullying. Adapting from Cortina et al.,[50] as they applied the term *incivility* to its occurrence at the workplace, incivility relates to perceptions of lack of interpersonally fair or respectful treatment linked to personal experience of rudeness and insulting or unfriendly behavior.[50] It may include perceptions of being treated in a condescending manner, experiencing that one's opinion or statements are paid little attention or interest, being addressed improperly, being exposed to derogatory or demeaning remarks about oneself, being ignored or excluded from camaraderie, or being unwillingly drawn into a discussion of personal matters.[50]

A study by Lasiter et al.,[51] based on narratives of 152 senior baccalaureate nursing students from two US universities in the Midwest, showed that 24.5% of the students felt mistreated "in front of others," being criticized, being yelled at, being laughed at, being threatened, being belittled, or being cut off, and 6.4% experienced feeling that faculty members were uncivil by talking to others about them, by criticizing them, or by divulging information to others, thereby compromising student–faculty trust.[51] Furthermore, 30.8% experienced that the faculty made comments that made them feel incompetent, incapable, or stupid.[51] Moreover, 54.4% felt "belittled or unimportant when faculty members lost their assignments, threatened low grades, did not reply to emails, laughed at or mimicked them, interrupted them, talked down to them, seemed uncaring, did not listen or ignored them, or suggested a different career."[51]

Students' perception of classroom incivility was studied by Bjorklund and Rehling[52] through a survey of more than 3,600 undergraduate and graduate students at a public university of the Midwestern United States. The survey's participants listed the most uncivil classroom behaviors as instances of students' "continuing to talk after being asked to stop," "coming to class under the influence of alcohol or drugs," "allowing a cellphone to ring," and "conversing loudly with others."[52] The uncivil behaviors most recently observed in the classroom were cases of "text messaging" and "packing up books before class is over," while the least observed were the occurrences of "continuing to talk after being asked to stop" and "coming to class under the influence of alcohol or drugs."[52]

Connelly[53] highlighted a range of students' "more serious"[53] behaviors that have been perceived by faculty members as examples of student incivility, according to a 2000 survey conducted by the Center for Survey Research at Indiana University.[54] The range of behaviors that were "always"[54] considered by 50% or more of the surveyed[54] faculty as examples of "more serious"[53] incivility, extended from students' sarcastic remarks or gestures to students' not paying attention in class (Table 18.2).

Table 18.2. University Students' Behaviors Considered "More Serious" Examples of Incivility by Surveyed Faculty Members[53,54]

Making sarcastic remarks or gestures	Harassing comments directed at faculty member	Inappropriate email sent to faculty member
Threats of physical harm to faculty member	Hostile verbal attacks or challenges directed at faculty member	Cellphones or pager disruptions during class
Students taunting or belittling other students	Cheating on exams or quizzes	Use of computer for purpose not related to class
Vulgarity directed at faculty member	Conversation distracting other students or faculty member	Not paying attention in class

Harassment and Discrimination in Colleges or Universities

A systematic review by Fnais et al.[55] of 57 cross-sectional and two cohort studies demonstrated that 59.6% of medical students had faced at least one form of harassment or discrimination during their training, with verbal harassment being the most common (68.8%) form.[55] Among medical residents, 63.4% experienced harassment and discrimination during residency training, with gender discrimination being the most common (66.6%) form of mistreatment, followed by verbal harassment (58.2%), while racial prejudice was the least common (26.3%) type of discrimination.[55]

Cleary et al.[56] examined students' perceptions of sexual harassment by faculty members, based on a survey of 292 undergraduate and graduate students documenting that 8% of the respondents reported that they experienced physical advances, explicit sexual propositions, and sexual bribery as forms of harassment.[56]

Sexual harassment among a sample of 859 Chinese students at a local university of Hong Kong was studied by Tang et al.,[57] who showed that the most frequent (11%–12%) forms of sexual harassment by faculty members directed at female students included "unwanted leaning or cornering," having their hands being held, having arms put around their shoulders against their wishes, or having faculty talking or joking about the student's gender.[57] Among male students, 3% to 5% "reported receiving sexist remarks or sexually suggestive looks from their teachers, while 2% reported experiencing teachers' unwanted physical contacts as in leaning over, cornering, putting arms around shoulders, etc."[57] In reference to peer sexual harassment, twice as many female students as male students reported being sexually harassed.[57] An average of 23% of women experienced physically seductive behaviors and gender harassment by peers and around 10% experienced pressure for dates and sexual looks or gestures.[57]

A systematic review of studies published after 2000 conducted by Klein and Martin[58] found several reports[59-64] documenting a wide span of prevalence of sexual harassment occurring in college/university campuses, after matriculation or during study, ranging from 9%[59] to 80%,[64] with an average of 36%. The types of sexual harassment described included being exposed to inappropriate comments, jokes, or remarks about one's body, appearance, or sexual behavior; receiving unwanted sexual photos or videos; being flashed or unwillingly exposed to someone's genitals; or being subjected to sexual coercion. Perpetrators were more likely to be male[61] and a peer known to the victim,[61] while undergraduate women had been mainly sexually harassed by an undergraduate or graduate student, whereas female graduates were generally sexually harassed by a faculty member.[62]

The prevalence of stalking among college students have been studied by McNamara and Marsil,[65] based on an online stalking survey, conducted in 2007, of 1,773 university students (70% females) who attended a public university in the southeast of the United States. The research[65] revealed that 42.5% of students met the research definition for stalking victimization based on having been subjected to at least one of several stalking behaviors, including unwanted calls or calls with hang-ups; unwanted messages; unwanted gifts or emails; somebody waiting a considerable amount of time to see them; being followed or having someone suddenly show up; being watched, spied upon, or threatened; having personal property vandalized or destroyed; phone calls being monitored; and having private information about oneself being obtained through different unauthorized means.[65] It is noteworthy that 75% of stalking victims did not regard their incident as stalking.[65]

Harassment in Military Training

Rosenstein et al.[66] examined some published reports[67,68] documenting the rates of sexual harassment in the US military service academies during the academic years of 2006 to 2016. In this context, the research of Van Winkle et al.[67] showed that, in 2016, almost 50% of women and 12% of men in military service academies reported having been sexually harassed in the academic year prior to being surveyed.[67] Also, the research of Cook et al.[68] documented that, during the academic years of 2006 to 2016, the most common (49%) forms of sexist behavior experienced by cadets or midshipmen were being exposed to offensive sexual stories or jokes, receiving comments about one's sexual life, or being exposed to embarrassing gestures.[68] Of the surveyed military trainees, 17% reported having been subjected to unwanted sexual attention, as attempts to establish a sexual relationship, while 6% experienced sexual coercion.[68]

Estrada and Berggren[69] studied the incidence and nature of sexual harassment of female officers and cadets in the Swedish military, through a survey of 324 participants, showing that 97% of the cadets reported having experienced at least one sexually harassing episode in the previous 24 months.[69] The most common (97%) type of harassment was crude/offensive behavior (i.e., being told offensive jokes, being whistled at or called in a sexual way, being exposed to offensive sexual remarks, or being stared at in a manner that elicits discomfort).[69] Of the cadet participants, 79% indicated that they experienced sexist behaviors (being treated differently or in a condescending manner because of gender), while 59% reported having been the object of unwanted sexual attention (i.e., being subject to unwanted attempts to establish a romantic relationship).[69]

Violence in Colleges and Universities

A systematic review of 34 studies published since 2000, conducted by Fedina et al.,[70] indicated that unwanted sexual contact seems to be the most frequent type of sexual assault on campuses (including sexual coercion), followed by incapacitated rape and completed or attempted forcible rape. "Unwanted sexual contact" has been characterized[70] as "attempted or completed unwanted kissing, fondling, petting, or other sexual touching using physical force, threat of physical force, verbal coercion or a combination of these but excluding vaginal, anal, or oral intercourse." At least seven studies[71-77] have shown that more than 20% of college women were exposed to unwanted sexual contact after entering college.[70] "Incapacitated rape,"[70] defined as "completed vaginal, anal, or oral intercourse while intoxicated or while on drugs," is a form of sexual violence, documented by at least six studies[78-83] as having endangered a range of 3%[78] to 13%[82] of college women and 0.7%[83] of college men. Furthermore, nine studies[74,79-86] reviewed by Fedima et al.[70] have shown that 0.5%[83] to 8%[79] of college women and 0.5%[83] to 0.6%[81] of college men were subjected to "completed rape,"[70] described as "forcible vaginal, oral, or anal intercourse using physical force or threat of force."[70]

Rothman et al.[87] conducted a study to compare the rates of aggressive victimization among autistic versus non-autistic US college students, using the secondary analysis of de-identified and publicly available data from the college Healthy Minds Study (HMS),[88] which collects self-reported mental health data from US college students. The research,[87] based on the survey of 1,411 autistic and 218,430 non-autistic students from 78 colleges, showed that autistic students were almost twice as likely as non-autistic students to report emotional aggressive victimization in the previous year (44% vs. 26%%, $P < .001$).[87] Furthermore, autistic college students were more likely than non-autistic peers to report past year physical victimization (8.4% vs. 5.7%, $P < .001$).[87] Yet, autistic and non-autistic students reported similar one-year prevalence of sexual assault (9.3% and 9.0%, respectively).[87]

Sexual Victimization in Military Training

Snyder et al.[89] investigated the extent of sexual victimization at the three US military academies. Their study,[89] which was based on self-report data from more than 5,000 cadets and midshipmen who participated in the 2005 Service Academy Sexual Assault Survey, documented that 60% of the participants stated that they had been exposed to at least one type of sexual victimization in the previous year, with the most common type of victimization being sexual harassment (56%), followed by unwanted sexual attention (23%), unwanted sexual contact (16%), sexual coercion (8%), and rape (3%).[89] Close to 42% of males and just above 85% of females were exposed to at least one form of sexual victimization.[89] Of military trainees experiencing victimization, 25% were exposed to two or more types of maltreatment, with females experiencing polyvictimization at a significantly greater frequency than males (45% vs. 12%, respectively).[89]

Exposure to sexual violence in the US military was examined by Kimerling et al.,[90] based on outpatient data of 3,062,621 veterans (4.45% females) who were screened for military sexual trauma while treated in Veteran Health Administration clinics during 2003. The study documented that 21.4% of women and 1.08% of men reported that, while in the military, they received uninvited sexual attention (verbal remarks, being touched, being pressured for sexual favors) or someone used force or threat of force to have sexual contact with them against their will.[90]

A review of the literature on sexual assault in the US Armed Forces, conducted by Turchik and Wilson,[91] documented that between 9.5% and 33% of women reported having been exposed to an attempted or completed rape while serving in the military.[92-97]

Health Impact of Victimization in Postsecondary Education or Military Training

A survey study at two points in time from a sample of 2,118 freshmen from eight colleges and universities in the Midwestern United States, led by Rospenda et al.,[98] showed that bullying at college/university "consistently predicted alcohol consumption and problematic drinking, controlling for baseline drinking and other school and work stressors."[98]

A significant association between exposure to, or participation in, cyberbullying and depression and alcohol abuse was documented by Selkie et al.,[99] through a cross-sectional study of 235 undergraduate students from four universities in the United States. This study showed that students who cyberbullied others and were also cyberbullied had three times higher risk of depression [adjusted OR (AOR) = 3.2] as compared to those who were not exposed or participated in cyberbullying.[99] Those who only cyberbullied others had 4.5 times higher risk of depression (AOR = 4.5) as compared to those with no cyberbullying experience. There was no evidence of a significant link between being a victim of cyberbullying and depression.[99]

Participation in cyberbullying as a bully was significantly associated (AOR = 4.7) with problem alcohol use, defined as a frequency of drinking alcohol, frequency of binge drinking, and/or negative consequences associated with alcohol use.[99]

Sodl et al.[100] reported a case of a college student who developed myositis ossificans traumatica after a fraternity hazing, which consisting in being struck repeatedly on both of his thighs while standing at attention, with subsequent bilateral thigh pain and stiffness 6 weeks after the incident.[100]

At least four cases of death related to college hazing were reported in the United States during 2017.[101-104]

It has been documented that experiencing or witnessing incivility and hostility on a college campus mediates the relationship between sexual minority status and problematic drinking.[105] A survey by Woodford et al.[105] of 2,500 of undergraduate and graduate students showed that the significant risk of sexual minority college students' having alcohol problems is 20% as explained by exposure to personal incivility (e.g., seeing somebody being stared at, given dirty looks, being ignored or left out, and being "put down") and 14% as explained by ambient hostility (e.g., seeing someone being bullied or threatened, knowing someone who was followed in a threatening manner).[105]

Blanco et al.[106] investigated the link between exposure to sexual victimization among female university students and mental health problems, through a cross-sectional study of 871 Spanish university students, and documented that victims of sexual violence in the previous year, as compared to nonvictim students, were at significantly higher risk of suffering from depression (AOR = 1.69), anxiety (AOR = 1.95), eating disorders (AOR = 1.60), substance abuse (AOR = 1.99), and risk of suicide (AOR = 1.65) but were not at significant risk of suicide attempt (AOR = 1.01).

Strauss et al.[107] explored the association between stalking victimization and alcohol/drug abuse. Based on a cross-sectional study of 357 male and female undergraduates in current dating relationships, they showed that "stalking victimization from a dating partner was related to alcohol and drug use, even after controlling for age, gender, length of dating relationship, and physical aggression victimization."[107]

Future Directions

Research is needed to identify the frequency of different forms of maltreatment occurring in postsecondary education and training, their link to health risks, and strategies for their prevention. Therefore, there is a need to advance and implement:

- National cross-sectional studies to ascertain the prevalence of all forms of maltreatment affecting students or trainees, teachers/instructors, and academic officials studying/

working in undergraduate, graduate, and postgraduate education, including military training

- Longitudinal research to determine the association of victimization in postsecondary education and training with psychosocial and health risks
- Evidence-based programs for the prevention of maltreatment in postsecondary education and training
- Universal screening to identify victimization and associated health problems occurring in postsecondary education and training, among patients who are seen in any clinical setting, as part of a universal assessment to ascertain exposure to all forms of victimization (see Chapter 8)
- Research-based strategies for stopping ongoing victimization in postsecondary education and training

Notes

1. Chapell MS, Hasselman SL, Kitchin T, Lomon SN, MacIver KW, Sarullo P. Bullying in elementary school, high school, and college. *Adolescence.* 2006;41(164):633–648..
2. Sesar K, Barišić M, Pandža M, Dodaj A. The relationship between difficulties in psychological adjustment in young adulthood and exposure to bullying behaviour in childhood and adolescence. *Acta Med Acad.* 2012;41(2):131–144..
3. Wensley K, Campbell M. Heterosexual and non-heterosexual young university students' involvement in traditional and cyber forms of bullying. *Cyberpsychol Behav Soc Netw.* 2012;15(12):649–654.
4. Chapell M, Casey D, De la Cruz C, et al. Bullying in college by students and teachers. *Adolescence.* 2004;39(153):53–64.
5. Marraccini ME, Weyandt LL, Rossi JS. College students' perceptions of professor/instructor bullying: questionnaire development and psychometric properties. *J Am Coll Health.* 2015;63(8):563–572.
6. Sinkkonen HM, Puhakka H, Meriläinen M. Bullying at a university: students' experiences of bullying. *Stud Higher Educ.* 2014;39(1):153–165.
7. Association of American Medical Colleges. *Medical School Graduation Questionnaire, 2020 All Schools Summary Report*, pages 35–38, Behaviors experienced during medical school. https://www.aamc.org/media/46851/download. Accessed August 3, 2022.
8. Ahmer S, Yousafzai AW, Bhutto N, Alam S, Sarangzai AK, Iqbal A. Bullying of medical students in Pakistan: a cross-sectional questionnaire survey. *PLOS One.* 2008;3(12):e3889.
9. Gágyor I, Hilbert N, Chenot JF, et al. Frequency and perceived severity of negative experiences during medical education in Germany—results of an online survey of medical students. *GMS Z Med Ausbildung.* 2012;29(4).
10. Karatas H, Ozturk C, Bektas M. A study of bullying against nursing students. *J Nurs Res.* 2017;25(3):198–202.
11. Timm A. 'It would not be tolerated in any other profession except medicine': survey reporting on undergraduates' exposure to bullying and harassment in their first placement year. *BMJ Open.* 2014;4(7):e005140.
12. Meriläinen M, Kõiv K. Theoretical dimensions of bullying and inappropriate behavior among faculty members. *Scand J Educ Res.* 2019;63(3):378–392.

13. Einarsen S, Hoel H, Notelaers G. Measuring exposure to bullying and harassment at work: validity, factor structure and psychometric properties of the Negative Acts Questionnaire-Revised. *Work Stress*. 2009;23(1):24–44. Cited by Meriläinen and Kõiv.[12]
14. Meriläinen M, Käyhkö K, Kõiv K, Sinkkonen HM. Academic bullying among faculty personnel in Estonia and Finland. *J Higher Educ Policy Manage*. 2019;41(3):241–261.
15. Zabrodska K, Kveton P. Prevalence and forms of workplace bullying among university employees. *Empl Responsib Rights J*. 2013;25(2):89–108.
16. Keashly L. Workplace bullying, mobbing and harassment in academe: faculty experience. In: D'Cruz P, Noronha E, Keashly L, Tye-Williams S, eds. Special Topics and Particular Occupations, Professions, and Sectors. Handbooks of Workplace Bullying, Emotional Abuse and Harassment. Vol 4. Springer; 2019.
17. Magerøy N, Lau B, Riise T, Moen BE. Association of psychosocial factors and bullying at individual and department levels among naval military personnel. *J Psychosomat Res*. 2009;66(4):343–351.
18. Vaara JP, Viskari J, Kyröläinen H, Santtila M. Perceptions and attitudes of female soldiers toward physical performance and fitness standards in soldiers. *Milit Med*. 2016;181(10):1218–1223.
19. THE SHRIVENHAM PAPERS—Number 4 August 2007, Defence Academy of the United Kingdom, Shrivenham, Wiltshire, SN6 8LA, United Kingdom. https://publications.parliament.uk/pa/cm200405/cmselect/cmdfence/63/63.pdf. Accessed August 3, 2022.
20. House of Commons, Defence Committee. Duty of Care, Third Report of Session 2004-5, Volume I, Report, together with formal minutes, Ordered by The House of Commons to be printed March 3, 2005. https://publications.parliament.uk/pa/cm200405/cmselect/cmdfence/63/63.pdf. Accessed August 3, 2022.
21. UK Ministry of Defence. UK Regular Armed Forces Continuous Attitude Survey Results 2021. Published May 20, 2021, United Kingdom. https://assets.publishing.service.gov.uk/government/uploads/system/uploads/attachment_data/file/987969/Armed_Forces_Continuous_Attitude_Survey_2021_Main_Reportedited.pdf. Accessed August 3, 2022.
22. US Department of Defense. 2017 Annual Report on Hazing Prevention and Response in the Armed Forces, Appendix A, A-10. https://www.defenseculture.mil/Portals/90/Documents/Toolkit/RPT-2017_Annual_Hazing_Report_to_Congress-20200109.pdf?ver = 2020-01-09-123931-860. Accessed August 3, 2022.
23. Defense Equal Opportunity Management Institute, Directorate of Research, Development and Strategic Initiatives. Perceptions of Hazing and Bullying among U.S Military Service Members. Technical Report #18-16. October 18, 2016. https://www.defenseculture.mil/Portals/90/Documents/Research/Publications/TECR_18-16_Perceptions_of_Hazing_and_Bullying_Among_US_Military-20191202.pdf. Accessed August 3, 2022.
24. Soldiers jailed over South Korea bullying death. BBC News, October 30, 2014. http://www.bbc.com/news/world-asia-29828761. Accessed August 3, 2022.
25. Sang-Hun C. Outrage builds in South Korea in deadly abuse of a soldier. *New York Times*. August 6, 2014. https://www.nytimes.com/2014/08/07/world/asia/outrage-builds-in-south-korea-over-military-abuse.html. Accessed August 3, 2022.
26. Hajela D. Asian American soldier's suicide called a 'wake-up call' for the military. *Washington Post*. February 21, 2012. https://www.washingtonpost.com/politics/asian-american-soldiers-suicide-called-a-wake-up-call-for-the-military/2012/02/19/gIQA7Ke4QR_story.html?utm_term=.1f5567113260. Accessed August 3, 2022.

27. Sengupta K. Army training instructors suspended after bullying exposé. *Independent.* September 18, 2008. http://www.independent.co.uk/news/uk/home-news/army-training-instructors-suspended-after-bullying-expos-935413.html. Accessed August 3, 2022.
28. Norton-Taylor R. Army bullying, harassment and discrimination complaints rise sharply. *Guardian.* March 27, 2014. https://www.theguardian.com/uk-news/2014/mar/27/army-bullying-harassment-discrimination-complaints-rise. Accessed August 3, 2022.
29. Cox M. After Marine photo scandal, services issue social media guidelines. Military.com. March 20, 2017. https://www.military.com/daily-news/2017/03/20/marine-photo-scandal-services-issue-social-media-guidelines.html. Accessed August 3, 2022.
30. Owen J, Johnson A. One in 10 Army recruits "bullied and intimidated." *Independent.* November 16, 2008. https://www.independent.co.uk/news/uk/home-news/one-in-10-army-recruits-bullied-and-intimidated-1020494.html. Accessed August 3, 2022.
31. Myers M. Navy targets sailor bullies as hazing reports drop. *Navy Times.* August 28, 2016. https://www.navytimes.com/pay-benefits/military-benefits/2016/08/28/navy-targets-sailor-bullies-as-hazing-reports-drop/. Accessed August 3, 2022.
32. 8 US soldiers charged in bullying suicide. CBS. December 21, 2011. https://www.cbsnews.com/news/8-us-troops-charged-in-fellow-soldiers-death/. Accessed August 3, 2022.
33. Bullying in armed forces on rise, MoD figures reveal. *Guardian.* February 1, 2014. https://www.theguardian.com/uk-news/2014/feb/01/bullying-on-rise-armed-forces. Accessed August 3, 2022.
34. Army trainers "bullied recruits." BBC News. September 18, 2018. http://news.bbc.co.uk/2/hi/uk_news/7623567.stm. Accessed August 3, 2022.
35. Schreck C. Is the Russian army bullying soldiers to death? *Time.* June 21, 2010. http://content.time.com/time/world/article/0,8599,1998445,00.html. Accessed August 3, 2022.
36. Allan EJ, Madden M. Hazing in view: initial findings of the National Study of Student Hazing. The University of Maine, Orono, ME. March 11, 2008. https://www.stophazing.org/wp-content/uploads/2014/06/hazing_in_view_web1.pdf. Accessed August 3, 2022.
37. Allan EJ, Madden M. The nature and extent of college student hazing. *Int J Adolesc Med Health.* 2012;24(1):83–90.
38. Pershing JL. Men and women's experiences with hazing in a male-dominated elite military institution. *Men Masc.* 2006;8(4):470–492.
39. Pai SA, Chandra PS. Ragging: human rights abuse tolerated by the authorities. *Indian J Med Ethics.* 2009;6(2):60–61.
40. Garg R. Ragging: a public health problem in India. *Indian J Med Sci.* 2009;63(6):263.
41. Lekamwasam S, Rodrigo M, Wickramathilake M, et al. Preventing ragging: outcome of an integrated programme in a medical faculty in Sri Lanka. *Indian J Med Ethics.* 2015;12(4):227–230.
42. Sharma NK, Bodh A. Medical student killed in ragging. The Times of India. March 10, 2009. https://timesofindia.indiatimes.com/india/medical-student-killed-in-ragging/articleshow/4247603.cms. Accessed October 4, 2023.
43. The Honorable Supreme Court of India. Summary of the judgment of the Hon Supreme Court, delivered on the 8th of May 2009. https://www.nitt.edu/home/students/Supreme_Court_Judgment.pdf. Accessed August 3, 2022.
44. Associated Press. 3 face hazing charges after Marine commits suicide. Fox News. September 8, 2011. http://www.foxnews.com/us/2011/09/08/3-face-hazing-charges-after-marine-commits-suicide.html. Accessed August 3, 2022.

45. US Government Accountability Office (GAO). Report to Congressional Committees. DOD and Coast Guard: actions needed to increase oversight and management information on hazing incidents involving servicemembers. GAO-16-226. February 9, 2016. https://www.gao.gov/assets/680/675040.pdf. Accessed August 3, 2022.
46. Secretary of Defense memorandum. *Hazing*. August 28, 1997. Cited in US Government Accountability Office (GAO) report.[45]
47. Deputy Secretary of Defense memorandum. *Hazing and Bullying Prevention and Response in the Armed Forces*. December 23, 2015. Cited in US Government Accountability Office (GAO) report.[45]
48. US Department of Defense. 2017 Annual Report on Hazing Prevention and Response in the Armed Forces, DOD Hazing Data Analysis Summary, pages 22–25. https://www.defenseculture.mil/Portals/90/Documents/Toolkit/RPT-2017_Annual_Hazing_Report_to_Congress-20200109.pdf?ver = 2020-01-09-123931-860. Accessed August 3, 2022.
49. US General Accounting Office. *DOD Service Academies: More Changes Needed to Eliminate Hazing*. Document #GAO/NSIAD-93-36. Washington, DC: US General Accounting Office; 1992. Cited by Pershing.[38]
50. Cortina LM, Magley VJ, Williams JH, Langhout RD. Incivility in the workplace: incidence and impact. *J Occup Health Psychol*. 2001;6(1):64–80.
51. Lasiter S, Marchiondo L, Marchiondo K. Student narratives of faculty incivility. *Nurs Outlook*. 2012;60(3):121–126..
52. Bjorklund WL, Rehling DL. Student perceptions of classroom incivility. *Coll Teach*. 2009;58(1):15–18.
53. Connelly RJ. Introducing a culture of civility in first-year college classes. *J Gen Educ*. 2009;58(1):47–64.
54. Center for Survey Research. *A Survey on Academic Incivility at Indiana University: Preliminary Report*. University of Indiana, Bloomington; 2000. Cited by Connelly.[53]
55. Fnais N, Soobiah C, Chen MH, et al. Harassment and discrimination in medical training: a systematic review and meta-analysis. *Acad Med*. 2014;89(5):817–827.
56. Cleary JS, Schmieler CR, Parascenzo LC, Ambrosio N. Sexual harassment of college students: implications for campus health promotion. *J Am Coll Health*. 1994;43(1):3–10.
57. Tang CS, Yik MS, Cheung FM, Choi PK, Au KC. Sexual harassment of Chinese college students. *Arch Sex Behav*. 1996;25(2):201–215.
58. Klein LB, Martin SL. Sexual harassment of college and university students: a systematic review. *Trauma Violence Abuse*. 2021;22(4):777–792.
59. Campbell JC, Sabri B, Budhathoki C, Kaufman MR, Alhusen J, Decker MR. Unwanted sexual acts among university students: correlates of victimization and perpetration. *J Interpers Violence*. 2021;36(1–2):NP504–NP526. Cited by Klein and Martin.[58]
60. Cantor D, Fisher B, Chibnall S, et al. *Report on the AAU Campus Climate Survey on Sexual Assault and Sexual Misconduct*. Rockville, MD: Westat; 2015. Cited by Klein and Martin.[58]
61. Clodfelter TA, Turner MG, Hartman JL, Kuhns JB. Sexual harassment victimization during emerging adulthood: a test of routine activities theory and a general theory of crime. *Crime Delinq*. 2010;56:455–481. Cited by Klein and Martin.[58]
62. Kelley ML, Parsons B. Sexual harassment in the 1990s: a university-wide survey of female faculty, administrators, staff, and students. *J Higher Educ*. 2000;71:548–568. Cited by Klein and Martin.[58]

63. Hill C, Silva E. *Drawing the Line: Sexual Harassment on Campus*. Washington, DC: American Association of University Women Educational Foundation, 2005. Cited by Klein and Martin.[58]
64. Kearney LK, Gilbert LA. The role of ethnicity in Mexican American and Non-Hispanic White students' experience of sexual harassment. *Hisp J Behav Sci*. 2012;34:507–524. Cited by Klein and Martin.[58]
65. McNamara CL, Marsil DF. The prevalence of stalking among college students: the disparity between researcher- and self-identified victimization. *J Am Coll Health*. 2012;60(2):168–174.
66. Rosenstein JE, Angelis KD, McCone DR, Carroll MH. Sexual assault and sexual harassment at the US military service academies. *Milit Psychol*. 2018;30(3):206–218.
67. Van Winkle E, Hurley M, Creel A, et al. *2016 Service Academy Gender Relations Survey Overview Report*. OPA Report No. 2016-043. Alexandria, VA: Office of People Analytics, 2017. Cited by Rosenstein et al.[66]
68. Cook PJ, Van Winkle EP, Namrow N, et al. *2014 Service Academy Gender Relations Survey Overview Report*. DMDC Report No. 2014-016. Alexandria, VA: Defense Manpower Data Center, 2015. Cited by Rosenstein et al.[66]
69. Estrada AX, Berggren AW. Sexual harassment and its impact for women officers and cadets in the Swedish Armed Forces. *Milit Psychol*. 2009;21(2):162–185.
70. Fedina L, Holmes JL, Backes BL. Campus sexual assault: a systematic review of prevalence research from 2000 to 2015. *Trauma Violence Abuse*. 2018;19(1):76–93.
71. Andar S. *The Prevalence of College Sexual Assault among Women in the Digital Media Era: An Online Investigation of Potential Impacts from Social Networking, Pornography, Cyberbullying, and Sexting* [dissertation]. 2014. ProQuest Dissertations and Theses, AAT 3621761. Cited by Fedina et al.[70]
72. Flack WF, Caron ML, Leinen SJ, et al. Red zone: temporal risk for unwanted sex among college students. *J Interpers Violence*. 2008;23:(11). Cited by Fedina et al.[70]
73. Meyerson LA. *A Prospective Analysis of Sexual Assault and Alcohol Use among College Women* [dissertation]. 2002. ProQuest Dissertations and Theses, AAT 3080539. Cited by Fedina et al.[70]
74. Orchowski LM, Creech SK, Reddy MK, Capezza NM, Ratcliff T. College women's perceived risk to experience sexual victimization: A prospective analysis. *Violence Vict*. 2012;27:194–214.) Cited by Fedina et al.[70]
75. Palmer RS, McMahon TJ, Rounsaville BJ, Ball SA. Coercive sexual experiences, protective behavioral strategies, alcohol expectancies and consumption among male and female college students. *J Interpers Violence*. 2010;25: 1563–1578. Cited by Fedina et al.[70]
76. Walsh WA, Banyard VL, Moynihan MM, Ward S, Cohn ES. Disclosure and service use on a college campus after an unwanted sexual experience. *J Trauma Dissoc*. 2010;11:134–151. Cited by Fedina et al.[70]
77. Wiscombe, K. An exploratory analysis of sexual violence and rape myth acceptance at a small liberal arts university (Doctoral dissertation, University of Kansas). 2012. Cited by Fedina et al.[70]
78. Mohler-Kuo M, Dowdall GW, Koss MP. Correlates of rape while intoxicated in a national sample of college women. *J Stud Alcohol*. 2004;65:37–45. Cited by Fedina et al.[70]
79. McCauley JL, Ruggiero KJ, Resnick HS, Conoscenti LM, Kilpatrick DG. Forcible, drug-facilitated, and incapacitated rape in relation to substance use problems: results from a national sample of college women. *Addict Behav*. 2009;34:458–462. Cited by Fedina et al.[70]

80. Krebs CP, Lindquist CH, Barrick K. The Historically Black College and University Campus Sexual Assault (HBCU-CSA) study. Research Triangle Park, NC: US Department of Justice; 2011. Cited by Fedina et al.[70]
81. Krebs CP, Lindquist CH, Warner TD, Fisher BS, Martin SL. The campus sexual assault (CSA) study: Final report. Washington, DC: National Institute of Justice, US Department of Justice. 2007. Cited by Fedina et al.[70]
82. Kalof L. Vulnerability to sexual coercion among college women: a longitudinal study. *Gender Issues*. 2000;18:47–58. Cited by Fedina et al.[70]
83. Hines DA, Armstrong JL, Reed KP, Cameron AY. Gender differences in sexual assault victimization among college students. *Violence Vict.* 2012;27:922–940. Cited by Fedina et al.[70]
84. Fisher BS, Cullen FT, Turner MG. The sexual victimization of college women. December 2000 U.S. Department of Justice, Office of Justice Programs, National Institute of Justice, Washington, DC NCJ 182369. 2000. Cited by Fedina et al.[70] https://www.ojp.gov/pdffiles1/nij/182369.pdf. Accessed October 4, 2023.
85. Gidycz CA, Orchowski LM, King CR, Rich CL. Sexual victimization and health-risk behaviors: a prospective analysis of college women. *J Interpers Violence.* 2008;23:744–763. Cited by Fedina et al.[70]
86. Humphrey JA, White JW. Women's vulnerability to sexual assault from adolescence to young adulthood. *J Adolesc Health.* 2000;27:419–424. Cited by Fedina et al.[70]
87. Rothman EF, Heller S, Graham Holmes L. Sexual, physical, and emotional aggression, experienced by autistic vs. non-autistic US college students. *J Am Coll Health.* 2021:1–9.
88. The Healthy Minds Network. The Healthy Minds Study—Student Survey. https://healthymindsnetwork.org/hms/. Accessed August 3, 2022.
89. Snyder JA, Fisher BS, Scherer HL, Daigle LE. Unsafe in the camouflage tower: sexual victimization and perceptions of military academy leadership. *J Interpers Violence.* 2012;27(16):3171–3194.
90. Kimerling R, Gima K, Smith MW, Street A, Frayne S. The Veterans Health Administration and military sexual trauma. *Am J Public Health.* 2007;97(12):2160–2166.
91. Turchik JA, Wilson SM. Sexual assault in the US military: a review of the literature and recommendations for the future. *Aggress Violent Behav.* 2010;15(4):267–277.
92. Bostock DJ, Daley G. Lifetime and current sexual assault and harassment victimization rates of active-duty United States Air Force women. *Violence Against Women.* 2007;13:927–944. Cited by Turchik and Wilson.[91]
93. Coyle BS, Wolan DL, Van Horn AS. The prevalence of physical and sexual abuse in women veterans seeking care at a Veterans Affairs medical center. *Milit Med.* 1996;161:588–593. Cited by Turchik and Wilson.[91]
94. Murdoch M, Pryor JB, Polusny MA, Gackstetter GD. Functioning and psychiatric symptoms among military men and women exposed to sexual stressors. *Milit Med.* 2007;172:718–725. Cited by Turchik and Wilson.[91]
95. Sadler AG, Booth BM, Nielson B, Doebbeling BN. Health-related consequences of physical and sexual violence: women in the military. *Obstet Gynecol.* 2000;96:480–493. Cited by Turchik and Wilson.[91]
96. Skinner KM, Kressin N, Frayne S, et al. The prevalence of military sexual assault among female Veterans' Administration outpatients. *J Interpers Violence.* 2000;15:291–310. Cited by Turchik and Wilson.[91]

97. Surís A, Lind L, Kashner TM, Borman PD. Mental health, quality of life, and health functioning in women veterans: differential outcomes associated with military and civilian sexual assault. *J Interpers Violence.* 2007;22:179–197. Cited by Turchik and Wilson.[91]
98. Rospenda KM, Richman JA, Wolff JM, Burke LA. Bullying victimization among college students: negative consequences for alcohol use. *J Addict Dis.* 2013;32(4):325–342.
99. Selkie EM, Kota R, Chan YF, Moreno M. Cyberbullying, depression, and problem alcohol use in female college students: a multisite study. *Cyberpsychol Behav Soc Netw.* 2015;18(2):79–86.
100. Sodl JF, Bassora R, Huffman GR, Keenan MA. Case report. *Clin Orthop Related Res.* 2008;466(1):225–230.
101. Deak M. Penn State frat members gave pledge 18 drinks in less than 90 minutes, video shows. (Bridgewater, NJ) *Courier News.* November 13, 2017. https://www.usatoday.com/story/news/nation-now/2017/11/13/penn-state-frat-charges/859524001/. Accessed January 25, 2022.
102. Rossman S. LSU student dies following hazing ritual, 10 charged. USA Today Network, October 12, 2017. https://www.usatoday.com/story/news/nation-now/2017/10/12/10-charged-lsu-students-hazing-death/757063001/. Accessed October 4, 2023.
103. Associated Press. Nine face hazing charges in death of Florida State pledge Andrew Coffey. NBC News, January 17, 2018. https://www.nbcnews.com/storyline/hazing-in-america/nine-face-hazing-charges-death-florida-state-pledge-andrew-coffey-n838301. Accessed August 3, 2022.
104. Texas State University suspends all Greek activities following death of 20-year-old fraternity pledge. ABC News, November 14, 2017. https://abcnews.go.com/US/texas-state-university-suspends-greek-activities-death-20/story?id=51150380. Accessed October 4, 2023.
105. Woodford MR, Krentzman AR, Gattis MN. Alcohol and drug use among sexual minority college students and their heterosexual counterparts: the effects of experiencing and witnessing incivility and hostility on campus. *Subst Abuse Rehabil.* 2012;3:11.
106. Blanco V, López L, Otero P, Torres ÁJ, Ferraces MJ, Vázquez FL. Sexual victimization and mental health in female university students. *J Interpers Violence.* 2021:08862605211005148.
107. Strauss CV, Haynes EE, Cornelius TL, Shorey RC. Stalking victimization and substance use in college dating relationships: an exploratory analysis. *J Interpers Violence.* 2016:0886260516663899.

19

Bullying and Other Forms of Maltreatment in Prisons

What Is Known?

This chapter explores what is known about the nature, prevalence, and consequences of bullying and other forms of victimization affecting people living and working in prisons. Furthermore, the chapter considers the notion of the prison environment as a workplace milieu, a view already considered in the Swedish Work Environment Act[1] and the Finnish Occupational Safety and Health Act,[2] which regard as employees either "persons in institutional care performing work that they have been assigned"[1] or "work done by persons serving a court sentence."[2] In this context, the concept of workplace maltreatment can be applied to some forms of mistreatment affecting prison staff and inmates in a similar way.

Bullying among Prison Inmates

For the past two decades there have been a growing number of published reports highlighting the concept, frequency, and correlates of bullying among people in confinement.[3-19] Most of these studies are based on young and adult inmates confined in prisons in the United Kingdom and Ireland.

The Conceptual Framework

Jane Ireland, leading researcher in the field of bullying behaviors in the prison environment, developed a working definition stating that:

> An individual is being bullied when he or she is the victim of direct and/or indirect aggression happening on a weekly basis, by the same or different perpetrator(s). Single incidences of aggression can also be viewed as bullying, particularly those that are severe and where the individual either believes or fears that he or she is at risk of future victimization by the same perpetrator or others.[3]

This definition adapts to the culture of the prison milieu and departs from the traditional research notion of school bullying by not requiring the elements of repetitive pattern, imbalance of power, and intentionality as conceptual constraints.[6]

To determine the occurrence of bullying behaviors in prisons, in 1988 Ireland developed the Direct and Indirect Prisoner behavior Checklist (DIPC),[4,8] subsequently modified in 2002 as DIPC-R©.[5] This research instrument[8] contains items that imply direct bullying (physical, psychological, verbal, or sexual mistreatment or theft), indirect victimization (gossiping and spreading rumors), and coercion, signifying "aggression in which the perpetrator interacts directly with the victim in order to force them to engage in a specific behavior."[8] Among the examples of prison's coercion, the DIPC[8] includes being forced to buy or give one's canteen to or for someone else, being forced to ask one's family to send money for another prisoner, being coerced to carry drugs for another prisoner, being forced to do other chores or jobs that pertain to other prisoners, lying for someone, or being forced to clean another prisoner's cell.

Ireland and Ireland[9] developed a study to explore how offenders define bullying, based on a survey of 332 UK young and adult male inmates; they showed that many definitions given by the participants pertained to physical and verbal aggression, with almost all centering on "taking things" as a type of bullying. Seven percent of respondents alluded to "indirect forms of bullying"[9] and 11% of the surveyed inmates explained bullying by the effects it caused on the victim, primarily feelings of fear. Most of the participants (77%) did not regard bullying as a repetitive type of aggression and therefore a single act of hostility could be sufficient to be interpreted as bullying. Likewise, almost half of the adult inmates considered that bullying could occur accidentally, and therefore intentionality was not a conceptual requisite for bullying.[9] Almost half of the adult participants did not feel that *bullying* was a good term to be used in a prison milieu, suggesting other terms instead, such as *victimizing, abusing, intimidating, taxing, baroning, rail-roading, hassling*, or *cockroaching*.[9]

Prevalence of Bullying among Inmates

A survey led by Ireland[10] of 309 British young and adult inmates of all genders, utilizing the DIPC,[11] documented that almost 52% of the participants reported having been exposed in the previous week to at least one form of interaction defined by the researcher as being victimized. Of those who were victimized, 42% experienced indirect bullying, while 33% were exposed to direct bullying, mostly psychological and verbal (23%), followed by physical (16%), theft-related (10%), and sexual (2.3%).

The prevalence of bullying in Irish prisons was assessed by Leddy and O'Connell[12] through the interview of 232 prisoners; 57% of the participants indicated that they participated in bullying as victims and or as bullies. Forty-seven percent indicated that they were bullied, and 25% reported bullying others.[12] Thirty percent of the victims suffered verbal and emotional abuse, 16% suffered assault without a weapon, 7% were assaulted with a weapon, and almost 5% were exposed to taunting, physical abuse, or robbery, while only 2% experienced exploitation.

The frequency of bullying among young inmates in the province of British Columbia, Canada, was examined by Viljoen et al.,[13] in a 2000 study based on a sample of 244 male and female offenders, age 13 to 19, from nine youth custody facilities in that province.

Seventy-seven percent of the participants identified themselves as bullies and or victims, with 37% reporting having been involved as both perpetrators and victims; 32% participated only as bullies, while only 8% indicated that they were only victims of bullying.[13] Significantly more females than males were bullied by "being touched or grabbed in a sexual way" (26% vs.

14%) or experienced "unwanted sexual comments or jokes" (22% vs. 5%).[13] Approximately 40% of the inmates were subjected to mean and unpleasant words and around 30% received threats or intimidation. Almost 24% of males and 11% of females reported being punched, hit, or beaten up.[13]

A 1995 survey by Power et al.[14] of more than 700 inmates from all Scottish Young Offenders Institutions established that 76% of the participants had seen bullying being perpetrated during their present sentence at their current prison.[14] Furthermore, 29% of the respondents indicated that they had been bullied by other inmates, with more than a third of them being bullied almost every day; 16% reported that they bullied other prisoners, and 33% indicated that they were bullied by staff during that sentence and at that prison.[14] Being threatened was the most frequent (75%) of the forms of bullying experienced by the victims, followed by exposure to untrue rumors (39%), name-calling (28%), and physical assault (20%).[14]

A descriptive analysis, directed by Ireland,[16] of 107 bullying incidents recorded by staff in one male young offender institution over a period of 14 months, showed that psychological and verbal bullying were the most frequent (72%) forms of maltreatment reported, followed by physical bullying (32%) and theft-related incidents (23%), with no sexual bullying reported.[16]

The prevalence of bullying in a high-security hospital was studied by Ireland,[15] through a semi-structured interview of 30 patients who were detained with the legal classification of psychopathic disorder[15] or with the diagnosis of at least one personality disorder, and who were housed in units of 15 to 20 patients. Thirty staff members working in those units were also interviewed. Among patients and staff, 20% reported having witnessed a patient being bullied in the previous week, and 23% of the participating patients reported having been bullied in the previous week. Most frequently (average 14%), victims experienced theft-related victimization; verbal abuse, or being made to do tasks/chores. Less frequently (7% or less), victims were exposed to physical or sexual assaults, intimidation, ostracism, or having their property damaged.[15]

Bullying among Inmates and Health Risks

The association between psychological health and bullying behavior among juvenile offenders was explored by Ireland[17] through a survey of 202 offenders, age 15 through 21. The study[17] documented that those respondents who reported they were bullied as well as those who were both bullied and bullied others, reported more symptoms related to "somatic concerns, severe depression, anxiety, and insomnia" than those who bullied others or those not involved in bullying.[17]

Blaauw et al.[18] examined the link between bullying in prisons and suicide risk in a study based on the review of files of 95 suicide victims in Dutch jails and prisons and the interview of 221 nonsuicidal jail inmates and 53 suicidal jail inmates. The research[18] showed that 34% of the prisoners who committed suicide felt bullied prior to their death, while 22% of the completed suicides were preceded by serious incidents of bullying that made the suicide victims fear for their life or the life of a family member.[18] Among inmates who were interviewed, those with a high suicide risk "more often reported being victims of bullying than did the comparison group of nonsuicidal inmates (66% vs. 34%)."[18]

Bullying among Prison Officers

The prevalence of workplace bullying in prisons was studied by Vartia and Hyyti,[19] through a survey of almost 900 Finish prison officers, showing that 20% of the participants reported having been bullied by one or more coworkers or supervisors in the previous six months. For this study,[19] bullying was defined as a situation "when somebody is a target of enduring and repetitive negative acts, scorn, or oppressing or devaluating behavior."[19] No significant differences in exposure to workplace bullying were found between male and female officers, with the exception of the younger group of officers (< 35 years old), where female officers reported having been more frequently bullied (25%) than their male colleagues (15%).[19] "Twenty-one percent of the female victims and 12% of the male victims were bullied daily or almost daily."[19] The most common forms of bullying experienced by both male and female officers were derogatory comments behind the victim's back, spreading of negative rumors, criticism, and/or the devaluation of the officer's job or contribution.[19] Female officers experienced significantly more frequent sexual harassment than male counterparts. Male officers were equally bullied by other officers as well as by supervisors, while female officers were mostly (75%) bullied by peers.[19]

Sexual Abuse in Prisons

A National Inmate Survey[20] implemented by the US Bureau of Justice Statistics between February 2011 and May 2012, based on a study of more than 94,000 inmates, documented that 1.8% of juvenile inmates (ages 16 to 17) held in adult prisons and jails reported sexual victimization by other inmates in the previous 12 months, while a similar prevalence (2%) was reported by adult inmates.[20] Approximately 3.2% of juvenile inmates held in adult prisons and jails reported having experienced staff sexual misconduct, a rate that was not significantly different from 2.4% of adults in prisons and 1.8% of adults in jails.[20] Sexual victimization, as defined in this survey,[20] implied any unwanted sexual contact with another inmate or any unwilling or willing sexual contact with a staff involving oral, anal, or vaginal penetration; "hand jobs"; or touching of the inmate's buttocks, thigh, penis, breasts, or vagina in a sexual way.[20]

A study of prevalence of sexual victimization in Spanish prisons conducted by Caravaca-Sanchez and Wolff,[21] based on a survey of 2,709 adult male and female inmates, showed that 12% of female inmates reported having been subjected to sexual victimization in the previous six months, as compared to 6% of male inmates.[21]

Wolff et al.[22] investigated the rates of sexual victimization among prison inmates with and without mental disorders, through a survey of more than 7,500 adult inmates housed in 13 state prisons within a single mid-Atlantic state prison system in the United States. The researchers reported that 8% of the male participants who indicated that they have been treated for a mental disorder (i.e., depression, schizophrenia, posttraumatic stress disorder, bipolar disorder, and/or an anxiety disorder) had been exposed to sexual victimization in the previous six months, as compared to 3% of the participants with no history of mental disorder.[22] Furthermore, 23% of females with any mental disorder reported having been exposed to sexual victimization in the previous 6 months, as compared to 8% of female inmates without a mental disorder.[22]

An analysis by Wolff and Shi[23] of 200 incidents of sexual victimization reported by a random sample of almost 7,000 adult male inmates indicated that 13% of those who were victimized by another inmate and 28% of those who were assaulted by a staff member were required to perform sexual acts to protect themselves from future acts.[23] About 50% of the inmates sexually victimized by other inmates reported having suffered fear, anxiety, insomnia, flashbacks, depression, and/or nightmares, while 68% experienced anger.[23] Furthermore, 53% of the victims suffered one or more physical injuries—primarily injuries to their anus or throat (20%), bruises, cuts, or scratches (27%), or being knocked unconscious (14%)—with approximately one-third requiring medical attention.[23]

According to the 2018 National Survey of Youth in Custody,[24] based on report from more than 6,000 confined youth (< 18 years old) housed in 327 facilities across the United States, 6% of imprisoned adolescent males and almost 3% of incarcerated adolescent females reported having been subjected during the previous year to sexual misconduct perpetrated by a staff member, involving any sexual act regardless of coercion, force, or consent.[24] Youth-on-youth sexual victimization in the previous 12 months was reported by almost 4.7% of adolescent confined females, as compared to 1.6% of imprisoned adolescent males.[24] Adolescent inmates who identified themselves as gay, lesbian, or bisexual reported higher rates (12%) of sexual victimization in the previous year by other inmates or staff, as compared to 6% of heterosexual young inmates. The difference in the reported rates of sexual victimization were more striking between the youth who identified with a different gender than assigned at birth (19%), as compared to 6.8% of young, confined inmates who identified with their assigned gender.[24]

Walsh et al.[25] examined the association between childhood maltreatment experiences (sexual, physical, or emotional abuse; physical or emotional neglect; or combination of these experiences) and inmate-perpetrated sexual victimizations, through a survey of 168 female inmates recruited from a state correctional facility in the Midwest of the United States. The study[25] demonstrated that each form of childhood maltreatment was associated with experiencing prison sexual coercion, as manifested by being verbally pressured into engaging in sexual touching or oral, vaginal, or anal sex.[25] Yet, fewer associations were encountered between different forms of childhood maltreatment and forced prison sexual experiences.[25] Furthermore, emotional dysregulation, as assessed by the Difficulties in Emotion Regulation Scale (DERS),[26] mediated links between childhood maltreatment, mostly concurrent victimizations, and verbal sexual coercion in prison; however, it was not linked to physically forced prison sexual incidents.[25]

Physical Aggression in Prisons

The frequency of physical victimization in prisons was studied by Wolff et al.,[27] based on a survey of almost 7,800 adult male and female inmates held in different prisons in a single mid-Atlantic state prison system in the United States.[27] The investigation[27] established that 21% of males and females reported having been physically victimized by another inmate in the previous six months, while almost 25% of male inmates and 8% of female prisoners reported having experienced physical victimization by a staff member in the previous six months. The survey[27] exemplified physical victimization as episodes of drowning attempts and being slapped, hit, kicked, bitten, choked, beaten up, or threatened/harmed with a knife or a shank.

The work of Wolff and Shi[23] showed that being threatened or harmed with a knife or shank was the most frequent form of physical assault among 39% those attacked by another inmate and among 25% of those assaulted by staff.[23] The second most common form of physical assault to an inmate was being slapped, hit, kicked, or bitten, occurring among 16% of those assaulted by another inmate and among 20% of those prisoners attacked by staff.[23] Bruises, cuts, and scratches were the most frequent injuries suffered by one-third of inmates attacked by either another inmate or a staff member, followed by stab wounds, which occurred in 10% of inmates attacked by another inmate, and being knocked unconscious, which occurred in 10% of prisoners assaulted by a staff.[23] Among the inmates physically assaulted by another inmate or staff, anger was the most frequent emotional reaction, experienced by about 70% of victims, while approximately one-third suffered from depression, difficulties in sleeping, and fear.[23]

Inmate-on-Staff Assaults

Sorensen et al.[28] conducted a study to describe the patterns associated with "serious inmate-on-staff assaults," defined as "resulting in injury requiring treatment beyond first aid."[28] This study,[28] based on the examination of 79 assaults perpetrated during 2007–2008 by 96 inmates confined in the facilities of the Texas Department of Criminal Justice, revealed that the assaults were uncommon (53 per 100,000 inmates annually) but were even more sporadic (2.2 per 100,000 inmates) as the seriousness of the injuries worsened to require hospitalization or reconstructive surgery.[28]

Overall Victimization in Prisons

Polyvictimization

The notion of exposure to polyvictimization in prisons was highlighted by Listwan et al.[29] in a 2006–2007 cross-sectional study that examined 1,642 individuals who had just been released from the Ohio Department of Rehabilitation and Corrections and placed in halfway house locations across the state. The study[29] examined whether the participants witnessed somebody being victimized and/or whether they were directly victimized during the previous 12 months in prison with one or more forms of victimization, including thefts, fighting, emotional abuse, or sexual assault.[29] Most frequently, the former inmates reported having experienced three or four types of victimization, with about 27% of the participants in the study indicating that they had been victimized in three or four different ways. Witnessing victimization occurred more frequently than being directly victimized, as exemplified by 92% of previous inmates having witnessedg fighting and 29% having experienced fighting or 95% having witnessed emotional abuse and only 40% having experienced this form of maltreatment. The study[29] also showed, through a multivariate regression model, that some variables, such as the inmate's perception of the prison environment and correctional officers or having been diagnosed with a mental illness, were factors that significantly predicted a risk for polyvictimization in prison.[29]

Additional understanding about the occurrence of polyvictimization in prisons emerged from a study led by Caravaca-Sánchez and Wolff that was based on a randomly selected sample of almost 2,500 male inmates held at eight Spanish adult prisons. The investigation[30] showed that almost one-third of the inmates reported having experienced two or three type of victimization (emotional, physical, or sexual) during a six-month period, with 22.2% reporting two forms of maltreatment and 5.6% of the respondents recounting exposure to three types of victimization.[30] Multivariate regression analysis showed that having experienced childhood and adulthood sexual victimization as well as adulthood physical victimization in the community "was associated with a 0.813 increase in the number of different types of victimization experienced in a six-month period of incarceration."[30]

Predictors of Prison Victimization

Steiner et al.[31] conducted a systematic review of evidence published between 1980 and 2014 regarding the causes and correlates of prisoner victimization, showing that the inmate's variables more likely to be linked to violent victimization included being of young age; being a security risk; being introverted; having been employed prior to incarceration, and or physically/sexually abused before confinement. Also, this study[31] has documented several inmates' routines and experiences in prison found to be associated with violent victimizations, including being an inmate not housed with the general population; being involved in recreation activities; having a significant history of misconduct; perceiving the prison not to be safe and or having less favorable views of staff.[31] In addition, there were several prison characteristics, found to be predictors of a higher rate of violent victimization, as being a maximum-security facility; having a linear architectural design; housing a large population; and being a prison where officers perceived the rules being underenforced.[31]

Fear of Victimization in Prisons

The role of fear of victimization in prisons as a predictor of general well being was investigated by McCorkle[32] through a study of 300 inmates housed at the Tennessee State Prison, whose psychological well-being was assessed with the General Well-Being Scale (GWB),[33] an 18-item scale intended to measure depression, anxiety, and various psychophysiological symptoms. The fear of victimization was quantified by summing answers to questions about how safe one feels in prison; how much one worries about being attacked during the prison sentence and how one estimates the risk of being attacked during the prison sentence.[32] Furthermore, the participants were assessed with an index of their victimization experiences during that prison sentence. as well as with a measurement of other prison stresses such as missing family and friends; missing freedom; missing a specific object or activity; regrets about the past; concerns about the future; boredom; lack of privacy and inadequacies of facilities.[32] The strength of the association between fear of victimization and GWB was found to be significant ($P < .001$).

Mistreatment of Inmates by the Prison System

The prison system can mistreat the inmates through either the development and implementation of policies that allow for abuse, discrimination, or disrespect of the prisoners or through the neglect in advancing and executing procedures to foster the physical and emotional well-being and safety of the convicts.

The United Nations Standard Minimum Rules for the Treatment of Prisoners (SMRs),[34] initially adopted by the UN Congress on the Prevention of Crime and the Treatment of Offenders in 1955, and its latest revision, known as the Nelson Mandela Rules,[35] provide guidelines for a comprehensive model system of penal institutions intended for what is "generally accepted as being good principles and practice in the treatment of prisoners and prison management."[35] In this context the Nelson Mandela Rules[35] cover a wide range of recommended prison guidelines that are intended to curb the implementation of procedures that afflict, discriminate against, or disrespect inmates. These guidelines[35] were also envisioned to promote and sustain the prisoners' safety, well-being, security, and rehabilitation.

In the rest of this chapter, I will postulate, based on the review of these guidelines,[35] potential areas of abuse or neglect of inmates, by the prison system, due to failure to observe the Nelson Mandela Rules.[35]

Abuse of Inmates by the Prison System

Inmates can be abused by a penal system that allows the application of cruel, inhuman, or degrading treatment or punishment such as torture; corporal or collective punishment; indefinite or prolonged isolation; placement in a dark or constantly lit cell; prohibition of family contact; use of any instrument of restraint for reprimand or reduction of prisoner's diet or drinking water, regardless of any circumstances that could be invoked as a justification for a penalty.[36] Also, the penal system could mistreat convicts though harassment, intimidation, or disrespect of inherent human dignity and privacy, in the conduct of intrusive searches, including strip and body cavity searches and searches of cells, which are undertaken without an unequivocal need.[37]

Furthermore, prisoners could be abused by the prison because of being required to perform work that is afflictive; in slavery or servitude; for the personal or private benefit of a prison staff; without equitable remuneration and/or required to work beyond the maximum daily and weekly working hours as fixed by law or by administrative regulation, taking into account local rules or custom in regard to the employment of free employees.[38]

Torture of Inmates

The concept of torture as defined in the United Nations 1984 Convention against torture and other cruel, inhuman, or degrading treatment or punishment, signifies "any act by which severe pain or suffering, whether physical or mental, is intentionally inflicted on a person for such purposes as obtaining from him or a third person information or a confession, punishing him for an act he or a third person has committed or is suspected of having committed, or intimidating or coercing him or a third person, or for any reason based on discrimination of any kind, when such pain or suffering is inflicted by or at the instigation of or with the consent or acquiescence of a public official or other person acting in an official capacity. It does not include pain or suffering arising only from, inherent in or incidental to lawful sanctions."[39]

Between January 2009 and May 2013, Amnesty International received reports of torture from 141 countries, even though 165 nations were parties to the UN Convention against Torture.[40]

Modvig and Jaranson[41] have exemplified the wide range of known methods of physical torture as beatings; mutilations; amputations; near drowning or emotional torment such as threats of rape, death, or torture to victim and/or family; mock execution; experiencing the torture of others.[41]

According to the International Rehabilitation Council for Torture Victims (IRCT),[42] more than 60,000 survivors of torture from around the world, were provided rehabilitation and support for justice during the year 2021.[43] Almost 70% of torture survivors were care for in countries from the Pacific; North Africa, Middle East, and sub-Sahara areas, 20% in Europe and Asia and 11% in the Americas.[43] Of survivors treated by IRCT's members, 48% were living in poverty, according to the criteria in their respective countries, as compared to a "global average of roughly 20% living below the internationally recognized medium poverty line."[43]

Kalt et al.[44] conducted a systematic review of 23 studies, published between 2000 and 2011, to ascertain evidence of exposure to violence and associated health problems among adults seeking asylum in high income host counties. This review[44] has documented that the prevalence of torture was above 30% across all studies and the history of torture, in those survivors seen in clinics, was correlated with PTSD.[45]

Prison Solitary Confinement

Solitary confinement has been characterized as a physical isolation of inmates in which they are confined in their cells, separated from other prisoners, for approximately 23 hours each day (usually 22 to 24 hours).[46,47] The use of solitary confinement still takes place in Western penal systems as a method to preserve prison lawfulness; as a punitive or corrective strategy or as an administrative policy for inmates who are considered an "escape risk or a risk to themselves or to prison order in general." Some inmates, like sex offenders, may want voluntary isolation to evade harassment from other prisoners, and solitary confinement is sometimes used to prevent to stop pre-trial detainees from influencing witnesses or 'to force out a confession."[46]

In the last three decades many jurisdictions in the United States have developed or modernized correctional facilities or units, known as "Supermax," characterized as a "highly restrictive, high-custody housing unit within a secure facility, or an entire secure facility, that isolates inmates from the general prison population and from each other due to grievous crimes, repetitive assaultive or violent institutional behavior, the threat of escape or actual escape from high-custody facility(s), or inciting or threatening to incite disturbances in a correctional institution."[48]

The prevalence of symptoms associated with prison solitary confinement have been investigated by Haney[49] in a study based on face-to face interviews of 100 randomly selected prisoners confined to a "supermax prison" that housed the prisoners in virtual isolation with almost complete idleness for extremely long period of time."[49] More than 80% of the inmates interviewed were suffering from anxiety; headaches; lethargy, and trouble in sleeping, while more than half to two-thirds of them experienced nightmares; dizziness; loss of appetite and heart palpitations.[49] Also, more than 70% of the prisoners participating in this evaluation, experienced ruminations; oversensitivity to stimuli; confused thought processes; social withdrawal and chronic depression, while more than 40% suffered from hallucinations and perceptual distortions and almost one third had suicidal thoughts.[49]

Neglect of Inmates by the Prison System

Inmates can be mistreated by the prison system through neglect in developing or implementing policies, projects, programs, or procedures to foster and preserve the prisoners' physical and emotional well-being and safety. Negligence by the penal system in providing to the needs of the inmates, as recommended by the guidelines provided by the UN SMRs,[34] could be categorized into at least five areas such as preserving safety; maintaining physical and emotional health and well-being of inmates; providing prisoners rehabilitation and after-release care and support for administrative assistance and legal rights.

Neglect in Preserving Inmates' Safety

Neglect in preserving the security of inmates can be evidenced by the penal system's failure to keep different categories of prisoners in separate institutions or parts of an institution "according to their sex, age, criminal record, the legal reason for their detention and the necessities of their treatment."[50] Also, lack of care by the prisons, could be shown by allowing overcrowding[51]; failure to safeguard inmates' personal property[52] or lack of staff's training in early detection of inmates' mental health issues; management of violent inmates through appropriate use of force or restraints and by implementation of defusing techniques such as negotiation and mediation while avoiding inhuman or degrading treatment or punishment.[53]

Overcrowding of Prisons

According to the World Prison Brief,[54] during 2021, 119 countries and territories had a prison occupancy level above 100% of official capacity while 22 countries had above 200% occupancy level.[55]

Ross et al.[56] have recently conducted a narrative review of studies, published between 2000 and 2022, focusing on the effects of overcrowding in high security environments, highlighting research which documented a link between prison overcapacity and inmates' mortality[57] and suicide risk.[58]

Rabe[57] explored the impact or prison density(overcrowding) on prison mortality in a study based on supranational data from the Council of Europe Annual Penal Statistics from 1997 to 2008. This research[57] through a multiple regression analysis has shown that, in the European Union, mortality rate in prison is only influenced by prison density (as a marker of overcrowding).[57]

Wolff et al.[58] examined the association between overcrowding and prisoner acts of self-harm and self-strangulation hanging events, based on a cross-sectional study at a pretrial prison in Geneva, Switzerland between 2006 and 2014. Information of overcrowding was obtained from annual prison records and data of self-harm requiring medical attention, as documented by registered nurses immediately after its occurrence, was found in protected computerized files. This research[58] indicated that overcrowding in more than 200%, prevalent in the period of 2011-2014, was significantly ($P < .001$) associated with an increment in the rate of self-strangulation/hangings, but not with all self-harm events. It is of note that there was no change, between 2006 and 2014 of any demographics that could have impacted in self-harm such as gender, area of origin, foreign residency, religion, or psychiatric treatment.[58]

Neglect in Protecting Inmates' Physical and Mental Health and Well-Being

Neglect in protecting inmates' physical and mental health and well-being could be shown by the failure of the disciplinary facility in providing all appropriate accommodations to ensure that prisoners with physical or mental disabilities have complete and suitable access to all aspects of prison life.[59] Also lack of attention by the prison to the prisoners' health and well-being could be exemplified by the negligence in securing appropriate natural and/or artificial light and ventilation[60]; providing adequate sanitary, bathing and shower installations; keeping all areas always used by inmates fully clean[61]; requiring and facilitating personal hygiene; making available appropriate clothing and bedding, regular meals of nutritional value, water as needed and suitable exercise and sport.[62] Furthermore, negligence by the penal system in safeguarding the prisoners' health can be characterized by lack of compliance in procuring free healthcare, with similar standards of services as available in the community, organized "in close relationship to the general public health administration and in a way that ensures continuity of treatment and care, including for HIV, tuberculosis and other infectious diseases, as well as for drug dependence."[63] Moreover, the prison system could neglect the inmates' health needs by failing to have in place a healthcare service, with access to urgent care, entrusted with the evaluation and treatment of the physical and mental health problems of prisoners, through a multidisciplinary team including, dentists, psychiatrists and psychologists.[64] Further neglect in the healthcare of inmates could occur due to failure in providing initial and subsequent comprehensive medical assessments to identify, among other issues, the risk of suicide; infectious diseases or withdrawal symptoms; determining physical and mental fitness of the inmate to be assigned to a particular job, while undertaking all the appropriate individualized measures or treatment, preparing and maintaining complete medical files and preserving strict confidentiality and ethical standards.[65]

Neglect to Provide Prisoners with Rehabilitation and After-Release Care

Mistreatment of inmates by penal institutions can be manifested by a failure to provide prisoners with rehabilitation and after-release care through education, vocational training and work programs and other forms of assistance including those of a health, remedial, moral, spiritual, social, and sports-based nature.[66] In this context, penitential facilities could specifically neglect inmates by failing to provide them with appropriate and useful work, with industry organization and methods that resemble as closely as possible those of similar work outside of prisons, to maintain or increase their ability to earn an honest living after release, while preparing them for the conditions of normal occupational life.[67] Also, prison's neglect to provide inmates with rehabilitation and after release care can be exemplified by unavailability of programs offering development of inmate- family relations; education, vocational training, recreational and cultural activities as well as prison after release support including the procurement of documents, identification papers, suitable homes and work to go to, appropriate and adequate clothing and "sufficient means to reach their destination and maintain themselves in the period immediately following their release."[68]

Future Directions

There is a need to further determine the prevalence of different form of victimization affecting people living and working in prisons, their link to health risks, and strategies for their prevention. As such it is necessary to develop and implement:

- National cross-sectional studies to determine the prevalence of bullying and other forms of maltreatment affecting inmates and prison staff
- Longitudinal research to ascertain the association of bullying and other forms of victimization occurring among inmates or prison staff with psychosocial and health risks
- Research-based evidence programs for the prevention of bullying and other forms of maltreatment occurring in prisons
- Universal screening to ascertain exposure to victimization and associated health problems, occurring in prisons, among inmates or prison staff who are seen in any clinical setting, as part of a universal assessment to ascertain exposure to all forms of victimization (see Chapter 8)

The notion of the penal environment as a workplace should be further considered, and in this context special consideration should be given to the role of the prison healthcare service as focusing on occupational health,[69] invested with "full clinical independence" from the prison's leadership," and being employed and 'organized in close relationship to the public health administration."[64,70] In this role, the prison health system should determine the physical and fitness of the prisoners to work[71] and, conceivably may well be involved in monitoring that the protections for the workplace safety and health of inmates are being implemented, preferably in accordance to the workplace regulations put into effect by the government occupational health and safety agency, for workers outside the prison system. Along these lines we could advocate for government occupational and safety agencies around the world, to be able to regulate compliance with workplace health and safety within prisons.

Notes

1. The Government of Sweden. Arbetsmiljölagen, The Work Environment Act, Non-Official Translation. https://www.government.se/government-policy/labour-law-and-work-environment/19771160-work-environment-act-arbetsmiljolagen/. Accessed October 4, 2023.

2. Finland, Occupational Safety and Health Act, §27, §28. https://www.ilo.org/dyn/natlex/docs/ELECTRONIC/62320/60971/F1688833574/FIN62320%20English.pdf. Accessed May 2, 2022.
3. Ireland J. Distinguishing the perpetrators and victims of bullying behavior in a prison environment: a study of male and adult female prisoners. *Legal Criminol Psychol.* 2001:6(2):229–446.
4. Ireland J. *Direct and Indirect Prisoner behavior Checklist* (DIPC©). Preston, England: University of Central Lancashire; 1998. Cited in Ireland.[3]
5. Ireland JL. *Direct and Indirect Prisoner Behaviour Checklist—Revised* (DIPC-R). Preston, England: University of Central Lancashire; 2002.
6. Ireland JL. *Bullying among Prisoners: Evidence, Research, and Intervention Strategies.* Brunner-Routledge, Milton Park, Abingdon, Oxfordshire, UK, 2002.
7. Ireland J, ed. *Bullying among Prisoners: Innovations in Theory and Research.* William Publishing, Uffculme, Cullompton, Devon, UK; 2005.
8. Ireland JL, Ireland CA. Intra-group aggression among prisoners: bullying intensity and exploration of victim-perpetrator mutuality. *Aggress Behav.* 2008;34(1):76–87.
9. Ireland JL, Ireland CA. How do offenders define bullying? A study of adult, young and juvenile male offenders. *Legal Criminol Psychol.* 2003;8(2):159–173.
10. Ireland JL. Bullying behaviors among male and female prisoners: a study of adult and young offenders. *Aggress Behav.* 1999;25(3):161–178.
11. Ireland JL. *Bullying amongst Prisoners: A Study of Gender Differences, Pro Victim Attitudes and Empathy* [master's thesis]. Manchester, England: The Manchester Metropolitan University; 1997.. Cited in Ireland.[10]
12. Leddy J, O'Connell M. The prevalence, nature, and psychological correlates of bullying in Irish prisons. *Legal Criminol Psychol.* 2002;7(2):131–140.
13. Viljoen JL, O'Neill ML, Sidhu A. Bullying behaviors in female and male adolescent offenders: prevalence, types, and association with psychosocial adjustment. *Aggress Behav.* 2005;31(6):521–536.
14. Power KG, Dyson GP, Wozniak E. Bullying among Scottish young offenders: inmates' self-reported attitudes and behavior. *J Community Appl Soc Psychol.* 1997;7(3):209–218.
15. Ireland JL. Nature, extent, and causes of bullying among personality-disordered patients in a high-secure hospital. *Aggress Behav.* 2004;30(3):229–242.
16. Ireland JL. Official records of bullying incidents among young offenders: what can they tell us and how useful are they? *J Adolescence.* 2002;25(6):669–679.
17. Ireland JL. Psychological health and bullying behavior among adolescent prisoners: a study of young and juvenile offenders. *J Adolesc Health.* 2005;36(3):236–243.
18. Blaauw E, Winkel FW, Kerkhof AJ. Bullying and suicidal behavior in jails. *Crim Justice Behav.* 2001;28(3):279–299.
19. Vartia M, Hyyti J. Gender differences in workplace bullying among prison officers. *Eur J Work Organ Psychol.* 2002;11(1):113–126.
20. Beck A, Berzofsky M, Caspar R, Krebs C. Sexual victimization in prisons and jails reported by inmates, 2011–12. https://permanent.fdlp.gov/gpo45884/svpjri1112.pdf. Accessed August 2, 2022.
21. Caravaca-Sánchez F, Wolff N. Prevalence and predictors of sexual victimization among incarcerated men and women in Spanish prisons. *Crim Justice Behav.* 2016;43(8):977–991.
22. Wolff N, Blitz CL, Shi J. Rates of sexual victimization in prison for inmates with and without mental disorders. *Psychiatr Serv.* 2007;58(8):1087–1094. https://www.ncbi.nlm.nih.gov/pmc/articles/PMC2811043/pdf/nihms168251.pdf. Accessed August 2, 2022.

23. Wolff N, Shi J. Contextualization of physical and sexual assault in male prisons: incidents and their aftermath. *J Correct Health Care*. 2009;15(1):58–77.
24. Field MB, Davis E. *Victim, Perpetrator, and Incident Characteristics of Sexual Victimization of Youth in Juvenile Facilities, 2018—Statistical Tables*. Washington, DC: Bureau of Justice Statistics; 2020. https://bjs.ojp.gov/content/pub/pdf/vpicsvyjf18st.pdf. Accessed August 2, 2022.
25. Walsh K, Gonsalves VM, Scalora MJ, King S, Hardyman PL. Child maltreatment histories among female inmates reporting inmate on inmate sexual victimization in prison: the mediating role of emotion dysregulation. *J Interpers Violence*. 2012;27(3):492–512.
26. Gratz KL, Roemer L. Multidimensional assessment of emotion regulation and dysregulation: development, factor structure, and initial validation of the Difficulties in Emotion Regulation Scale. *J Psychopathol Behav Assess*. 2004;26:41–54. Cited by Walsh et al.[25]
27. Wolff N, Blitz CL, Shi J, Siegel J, Bachman R. Physical violence inside prisons: rates of victimization. *Crim Justice Behav*. 2007;34(5):588–599.
28. Sorensen JR, Cunningham MD, Vigen MP, Woods SO. Serious assaults on prison staff: a descriptive analysis. *J Crim Justice*. 2011;39(2):143–150.
29. Listwan SJ, Daigle LE, Hartman JL, Guastaferro WP. Poly-victimization risk in prison: the influence of individual and institutional factors. *J Interpers Violence*. 2014;29(13):2458–2481.
30. Caravaca-Sánchez F, Wolff N. Understanding polyvictimization in prison: Prevalence and predictors among men inmates in Spain. *J Interpers Violence*. 2021;36(7-8):3411–3437.
31. Steiner B, Ellison JM, Butler HD, Cain CM. The impact of inmate and prison characteristics on prisoner victimization. *Trauma Violence Abuse*. 2017;18(1):17–36.
32. McCorkle RC. Fear of victimization and symptoms of psychopathology among prison inmates. *J Offender Rehabil*. 1993;19(1-2):27–42.
33. Lennon MC. Sex differences in distress: the impact of gender and work roles. *J Health Soc Behav*. 1987:290–305. Cited by McCorkle.[32]
34. Campbell T, Kleinig J. Standard Minimum Rules for the Treatment of Prisoners. In: *Prisoners' Rights*. Milton Park, Abingdon, Oxfordshire, UK: Routledge; 2017:407–420. https://www.sivilombudet.no/wp-content/uploads/2019/02/UN_Standard_Minimum_Rules_for_the_Treatment_of_Prisoners.pdf. Accessed August 2, 2022.
35. United Nations Office on Drugs and Crime. The United Nations Standard Minimum Rules for the Treatment of Prisoners (the Nelson Mandela Rules). https://www.unodc.org/documents/justice-and-prison-reform/Nelson_Mandela_Rules-E-ebook.pdf. Accessed August 2, 2022.
36. United Nations Office on Drugs and Crime. The United Nations Standard Minimum Rules for the Treatment of Prisoners (the Nelson Mandela Rules), Rule 1 (page 2), Rule 43 (page 13), and Rule 47 (page 15). https://www.unodc.org/documents/justice-and-prison-reform/Nelson_Mandela_Rules-E-ebook.pdf. Accessed August 2, 2022.
37. United Nations Office on Drugs and Crime. The United Nations Standard Minimum Rules for the Treatment of Prisoners (the Nelson Mandela Rules), Rules 50–51 (page 16). https://www.unodc.org/documents/justice-and-prison-reform/Nelson_Mandela_Rules-E-ebook.pdf. Accessed August 2, 2022.
38. United Nations Office on Drugs and Crime. The United Nations Standard Minimum Rules for the Treatment of Prisoners (the Nelson Mandela Rules), Rules 97, 102, and 103 (pages 29–30). https://www.unodc.org/documents/justice-and-prison-reform/Nelson_Mandela_Rules-E-ebook.pdf. Accessed August 2, 2022.

39. United Nations Convention against Torture and Other Cruel, Inhuman, or Degrading Treatment or Punishment. Adopted by the General Assembly on December 10, 1984. https://www.ohchr.org/sites/default/files/cat.pdf. Accessed August 2, 2022.
40. Amnesty International. Torture. https://www.amnesty.org/en/what-we-do/torture/. Accessed August 2, 2022.
41. Modvig J, Jaranson JM. A global perspective of torture, political violence, and health. In: Wilson JP, Drozdek B, eds. *Broken Spirits: The Treatment of Traumatized Asylum Seekers, Refugees and War and Torture Victims*. Milton Park, Abingdon, Oxfordshire, UK: Routledge; 2004:33–52.
42. International Rehabilitation Council for Torture Victims (IRCT). Who We Are. https://irct.org/who-we-are/about-the-irct. Accessed August 2, 2022.
43. International Rehabilitation Council for Torture Victims (IRCT). Annual Report 2021. https://irct.org/wp-content/uploads/2022/08/IRCT_Annual_AuditReport_2021.pdf. Accessed October 4, 2023.
44. Kalt A, Hossain M, Kiss L, Zimmerman C. Asylum seekers, violence, and health: a systematic review of research in high-income host countries. *Am J Public Health*. 2013;103(3): e30–e42.
45. Piwowarczyk L. Asylum seekers seeking mental health services in the United States: clinical and legal implications. *J Nerv Ment Dis*. 2007;195(9):715–722. Cited by Kalt et al.[44]
46. Smith PS. The effects of solitary confinement on prison inmates: a brief history and review of the literature. *Crime Justice*. 2006;34(1):441–528.
47. Shalev S. *A Sourcebook on Solitary Confinement*. Available at SSRN 2177495. 2008. http://eprints.lse.ac.uk/24557/1/SolitaryConfinementSourcebookPrint.pdf. Accessed August 2, 2022.
48. Riveland C. *Supermax Prisons: Overview and General Considerations*. Washington, DC: National Institute of Corrections; 1999. https://www.prisonpolicy.org/scans/NIC_014937.pdf. Accessed August 2, 2022.
49. Haney C. Mental health issues in long-term solitary and "supermax" confinement. *Crime Delinq*. 2003;49(1):124–156. Cited by Arrigo BA, Bullock JL. The psychological effects of solitary confinement on prisoners in supermax units: reviewing what we know and recommending what should change. *Int J Offender Ther Comp Criminol*. 2008;52(6):622–640.
50. United Nations Office on Drugs and Crime. The United Nations Standard Minimum Rules for the Treatment of Prisoners (the Nelson Mandela Rules), Rule 11 (page 5). https://www.unodc.org/documents/justice-and-prison-reform/Nelson_Mandela_Rules-E-ebook.pdf. Accessed August 2, 2022.
51. United Nations Office on Drugs and Crime. The United Nations Standard Minimum Rules for the Treatment of Prisoners (the Nelson Mandela Rules), Rule 12 (page 5). https://www.unodc.org/documents/justice-and-prison-reform/Nelson_Mandela_Rules-E-ebook.pdf. Accessed August 2, 2022.
52. United Nations Office on Drugs and Crime. The United Nations Standard Minimum Rules for the Treatment of Prisoners (the Nelson Mandela Rules), Rule 67 (page 20). https://www.unodc.org/documents/justice-and-prison-reform/Nelson_Mandela_Rules-E-ebook.pdf. Accessed August 2, 2022.
53. United Nations Office on Drugs and Crime. The United Nations Standard Minimum Rules for the Treatment of Prisoners (the Nelson Mandela Rules), Rule 76 (page 23). https://www.unodc.org/documents/justice-and-prison-reform/Nelson_Mandela_Rules-E-ebook.pdf. Accessed August 2, 2022.

54. World Prison Brief. About the World Prison Brief. https://www.prisonstudies.org/about-us. Accessed August 2, 2022.
55. World Prison Brief. Highest to Lowest Occupancy Level (based on official capacity). https://www.prisonstudies.org/highest-to-lowest/occupancy-level?field_region_taxonomy_tid = All. Accessed August 2, 2022.
56. Ross T, Bulla J, Fontao MI. Space and well-being in high security environments. *Front Psychiatry*. 2022;13.
57. Rabe K. Prison structure, inmate mortality and suicide risk in Europe. *Int J Law Psychiatry*. 2012;35(3):222–230. Cited by Ross et al.[56]
58. Wolff H, Casillas A, Perneger T, et al. Self-harm and overcrowding among prisoners in Geneva, Switzerland. *Int J Prisoner Health*. 2016. Cited by Ross et al.[56]
59. United Nations Office on Drugs and Crime. The United Nations Standard Minimum Rules for the Treatment of Prisoners (the Nelson Mandela Rules), Rule 5 (page 3). https://www.unodc.org/documents/justice-and-prison-reform/Nelson_Mandela_Rules-E-ebook.pdf. Accessed August 2, 2022.
60. United Nations Office on Drugs and Crime. The United Nations Standard Minimum Rules for the Treatment of Prisoners (the Nelson Mandela Rules), Rule 14 (page 6). https://www.unodc.org/documents/justice-and-prison-reform/Nelson_Mandela_Rules-E-ebook.pdf. Accessed August 2, 2022.
61. United Nations Office on Drugs and Crime. The United Nations Standard Minimum Rules for the Treatment of Prisoners (the Nelson Mandela Rules), Rules 15–17 (page 5). https://www.unodc.org/documents/justice-and-prison-reform/Nelson_Mandela_Rules-E-ebook.pdf. Accessed August 2, 2022.
62. United Nations Office on Drugs and Crime. The United Nations Standard Minimum Rules for the Treatment of Prisoners (the Nelson Mandela Rules), Rules 18–23 (pages 6–7). https://www.unodc.org/documents/justice-and-prison-reform/Nelson_Mandela_Rules-E-ebook.pdf. Accessed August 2, 2022.
63. United Nations Office on Drugs and Crime. The United Nations Standard Minimum Rules for the Treatment of Prisoners (the Nelson Mandela Rules), Rule 24 (page 8). https://www.unodc.org/documents/justice-and-prison-reform/Nelson_Mandela_Rules-E-ebook.pdf. Accessed August 2, 2022.
64. United Nations Office on Drugs and Crime. The United Nations Standard Minimum Rules for the Treatment of Prisoners (the Nelson Mandela Rules), Rule 25 (page 8). https://www.unodc.org/documents/justice-and-prison-reform/Nelson_Mandela_Rules-E-ebook.pdf. Accessed August 2, 2022.
65. United Nations Office on Drugs and Crime. The United Nations Standard Minimum Rules for the Treatment of Prisoners (the Nelson Mandela Rules), Rules 26, 30, and 32 (pages 8–10). https://www.unodc.org/documents/justice-and-prison-reform/Nelson_Mandela_Rules-E-ebook.pdf. Accessed August 2, 2022.
66. United Nations Office on Drugs and Crime. The United Nations Standard Minimum Rules for the Treatment of Prisoners (the Nelson Mandela Rules), Rule 4 (page 3). https://www.unodc.org/documents/justice-and-prison-reform/Nelson_Mandela_Rules-E-ebook.pdf. Accessed August 2, 2022.
67. United Nations Office on Drugs and Crime. The United Nations Standard Minimum Rules for the Treatment of Prisoners (the Nelson Mandela Rules), Rules 96, 98, and 99 (page 29).

https://www.unodc.org/documents/justice-and-prison-reform/Nelson_Mandela_Rules-E-ebook.pdf. Accessed August 2, 2022.

68. United Nations Office on Drugs and Crime. The United Nations Standard Minimum Rules for the Treatment of Prisoners (the Nelson Mandela Rules), Rule 96 (page 29) and Rules 104–108 (page 31). https://www.unodc.org/documents/justice-and-prison-reform/Nelson_Mandela_Rules-E-ebook.pdf. Accessed August 2, 2022.
69. Montoya-Barthelemy A. The occupational health of prison inmates: an ignored population and an opportunity. *J Occup Environ Med.* 2019;61(2):e74–e76..
70. United Nations Office on Drugs and Crime. The United Nations Standard Minimum Rules for the Treatment of Prisoners (the Nelson Mandela Rules), Rule 27 (page 9). https://www.unodc.org/documents/justice-and-prison-reform/Nelson_Mandela_Rules-E-ebook.pdf. Accessed August 2, 2022.
71. United Nations Office on Drugs and Crime. The United Nations Standard Minimum Rules for the Treatment of Prisoners (the Nelson Mandela Rules), Rule 30(e) (page 10). https://www.unodc.org/documents/justice-and-prison-reform/Nelson_Mandela_Rules-E-ebook.pdf. Accessed August 2, 2022.

20
Witnessing Bullying and Other Forms of Maltreatment

What Is Known?

Most of the published studies concerning witnesses of bullying have focused on the factors contributing to their role in either protecting the victim; inspiring or encouraging the perpetrator or remaining a neutral or passive bystander.[1-12] In fact, some reports have advocated for a role of the bystander in bullying prevention strategies,[13-18] yet a limited amount of research has been given attention to the health risks associated with witnessing maltreatment.[19-24]

Types, Roles, and Social Dynamics of Bystanders to Bullying

Types and Roles

Bystanders to bullying have been classified by Salmivali et al.[25] in four groups, per group dynamics: the "assistant" or the bully's helper; the reinforcer who bolsters the bully's actions by laughing at the victim; the "outsider" who keeps away from the victimization and the "defender" who tries to stop the maltreatment and/or supports the victim.

Dynamic Factors Contributing to the Role of the Bystander

A considerable sum of research has concentrated on the factors contributing to the function of the bystander to bullying in either defending the victim, stimulating, or boosting the perpetrator or staying as a neutral or inactive witness.[1-12]

Empathy is the most regarded factor significantly associated with the role of the bystander in standing up for the victim.[1-7] Additional variables found to be strongly linked with the function of supporting a victim are "problem solving ability"[3] and "attitudes toward bullying"[3], while "concerns about being bullied"[3] is a significant dynamic correlated with being a "bully follower" or an "outsider" (neutral bystander).

Further elements which were found to be associated with an eyewitness' participation or lack of it, are "fear of retaliation,"[11] "moral disengagement," [5,7-9] conceptualized as "cognitive restructuring of inhumane conduct into a benign or worthy one by moral justification,"[26] and "social capital,"[10,12] exemplified by "resources and benefits gained from relationships and social interactions."[10]

Role of Bystanders in Bullying Prevention Strategies

Some studies have been in favor of supporting a task for the bystander in bullying prevention and intervention.[13-18] Almost two decades ago, Fonagy et al.[18] considered the contribution of the "audience of bystanders" as critical in either stimulating or ameliorating aggression and therefore contribute to create a peaceful learning environment through an anti-bullying program.

Stueve et al.[16] explored the difficulties preventing bystanders from taking positive actions and have advised for the identification of "norms, attitudes, and outcome expectancies that shape bystander behaviors to inform prevention efforts."[16]

Salmivalli et al.[13] clearly determined that the frequency of bullying in a classroom is negatively associated with bystanders' defending behaviors and positively linked with reinforcing actions, leading to their recommendations that bullying intervention strategies should, not only target the bully and the victim, but also "influence the bystanders, making them more likely to defend and support victimized peers and less likely to reinforce the bully."[13]

Witnessing School Bullying

Prevalence of Witnessing School Bullying

Some studies[27-29] conducted in countries of East Asia have shown that one-third of adolescent students witnessed incidents of bullying in the previous 2 to 12 months.

In 2016 Han et al.[27] led a survey to ascertain the prevalence of bullying among a national representative sample of 3,675 Chinese students from fourth grade through high school, showing that 29.9% of the participants witnessed incidents of school bullying, in the previous year.[27]

A survey conducted by Chen and Cheng[28] of 3,554 Taiwanese students in grades 7 to 12, has shown that 30% of the students surveyed indicated they witnessed at least two or three bullying events a month, in the previous six months.[28] Osuka et al.[29] ascertained the prevalence of "Ijime" (bullying) among 2,334 students, grade 4-9, in a middle size central city in central Japan, documenting that 32.8% of the students witnessed "some type of bullying act" in the previous two to three months.[29]

The notion that one-third of adolescents witnessed incidents of bullying has also been reported in Western Europe, as documented in a second analysis conducted by Callaghan et al.[30] of the 2013-2014 Health Behavior in School-aged Children survey, based on nationally representative sample of 7,522 Irish students age 12 to 18. This study[30] showed that 30.5% of participants reported having witnessed school bullying in the previous couple of months.

Yet, higher prevalence of students who have observers of bullying were reported in North America, as related by Bradshaw et al.[31] in a 2006 study based on a survey of 15,185 students attending elementary, middle, and high school in a large public school district in Maryland, USA. The results of the study[31] indicated that 71% of the students reported having witnessed bullying in the previous month.

A cross-sectional survey of 130 students in grades 6 to 8 in a public school in the northwest United States, conducted by Midgett and Doumas,[32] showed that 60.5% of the participants reported having witnessed bullying in the previous 30 days.[32]

A study led by Marraccini et al.[33] based on an online questionnaire administered to almost 340 US college students at a northeastern university, reported that almost 51% of the students have witnessed a professor or instructor bullying and almost 64% have seen a peer bullying in college.

Health Problems Linked to Witnessing School Bullying

Midgett and Doumas[32] have documented that being a bystander of bullying was significantly associated with higher levels of anxiety and depressive symptoms, even after controlling for frequency of being a victim or a perpetrator. The investigation[32] also provided evidence that students who were both victims and bystanders of bullying the depressive symptoms "may be particularly high due to co-victimization or re-victimization experienced when witnessing bullying."[32]

According to the research of Callaghan et al.,[30] students who witnessed others being bullied are significantly more likely to experience psychological symptoms (OR = 1.355), somatic symptoms (OR = 1.392) and low life satisfaction (OR = 1.268) than those who were not bystanders."[30]

A study conducted by Rivers et al.,[34] based on a representative sample of 2002 students attending state schools in the North of England, has established that witnessing victimization of peers is significantly associated with elevated scores of different aspects of psychopathology (somatic complaints; obsessive-compulsiveness; depression; anxiety; paranoid ideation), even after controlling for the effect of also being a victim or a perpetrator.[34] A report[20] based on this same study[36] has documented that student who witness bullying are more likely than those not involved in bullying in indicating "greater helplessness and potential suicidal ideation."[20]

The link between witnessing bullying and suicidal risk has been shown to be serially mediated by negative coping styles and depressive symptoms, in a 2018–2019 cross-sectional study led by Duan et al.[35] involving more than 12,000 secondary school students in Suzhou, China.

There is preliminary indication by Lambe et al.,[36] based on a cross-sectional study of Canadian sample of students who were witnesses of bullying, that bystander males who were involved in defending victims of bullying, were significantly more at risk of experiencing psychosocial difficulties (feeling sad, scared, angry, having sleeping difficulties, academic problems), as compared to boys who passively witnessed the bullying, without intervening on behalf of the victim.

Witnessing Cyberbullying

Prevalence of Witnessing Cyberbullying

A 2013-2014 survey[37] of a nationally representative sample of US youth, age 10-20-year-old, has documented that 80% of all the "in-person" or "technology related" peer harassment incident, experienced in the previous year, involved the presence of at least one bystander in addition to the victim and the harassing youth.

Lindfords et al.[38] led a study based on a self- administered questionnaire of more than 5500 adolescent Finns, reporting that 10% of males and 16% of females witnessed cyberbullying of their friends in the previous year.

A 2020 online survey of 1034 US children between the ages of 9 and 12, led by Patchin and Hinduja,[39] has revealed that almost 15% of them had seen cyberbullying at "any point in their lifetime."[39]

An online survey of 254 adults, conducted by Carter[40] established that 51.3% of the participants reported having been witnesses of cyberbullying on social media sites, and 31.4% indicated that knew others who have witnesses of cyberbullying.[40]

Doumas and Midgett,[41] using a survey[32] of 130 US middle school students, reported that 32.3% of those students surveyed witnessed cyberbullying, at least once, in the previous 30 days.[41]

A 2014 survey, led by Yoon et al.,[42] of more than 2900 10 th grade students in Los Angeles, California, has shown that 32.8% of those surveyed indicated that witnessed cyberbullying more than once in their lifetime but were never victims nor perpetrators.[42]

Health Problems Linked to Witnessing Cyberbullying

Doumas and Midgett[41] have documented that those students who witnessed cyberbullying in the previous month, experienced "significantly higher levels of depression ($P < .05$), anxiety ($P < .02$), and somatic symptoms ($P < .01$)"[41] than those who did not witnessed cyberbullying.

A one-year longitudinal study of 1,067 US students in grades 7 and 8 led by Wright et al.,[43] have shown a "positive association between being a bystander of cyberbullying and depression. and anxiety."[43] Also, "empathy moderated the positive relationship between bystander of cyberbullying and depression, but not for anxiety."[43]

Yoon et al.[42] conducted a longitudinal study to ascertain the association between participation in cyberbullying and substance use among adolescents, based on a one-year follow-up of most of the 2,900 high school students in Los Angeles, initially surveyed in 2014, as previously cited. The research[42] documented that students who at the beginning of the study reported to be exposed to cyberbullying only as bystanders or witnesses, 12 months later were found to have been at a significant risk, as compared to students not involved in cyberbullying, of abusing alcohol [adjusted OR (AOR) = 2.02]; cigarettes (AOR = 1.82); e-cigarettes (AOR = 2.05) and marijuana (AOR = 2.02).[42]

Witnessing Workplace Bullying

Prevalence of Witnessing Workplace Bullying

A 2010–2011 survey[44] administered to a nationally representative community-based sample of more than 1,500 adult Japanese residents has documented that almost 15% of the respondents witnessed workplace bullying during the previous 30 days. The subjective socioeconomic status of the employee, defined as "the individual's perception of his/her own position in the social hierarchy,"[45] was the only significantly variable associated with witnessing workplace bullying, after adjusting for gender, age, education, and household income.[44]

Ciby and Raya[46] have reviewed eight studies,[47-54] conducted in seven European countries[47-52,54] and the United States,[53] showing workers having witnessed bullying at the workplace at a prevalence ranging from 11%[48,53] to 43%[52] in the previous six months[48,49,51-53], or 30%[47] to 47%[54] in the previous year.[47,50,54]

Health Problems Linked to Witnessing Workplace Bullying

Considerable risk of depression (AOR = 1.69) has been found among bystanders to workplace bullying in a longitudinal study, led by Emdad et al.,[21] of more than 2500 Swedish workers. The frequency of women who witnessed workplace bullying and developed depressive symptoms, 18 months later was higher in comparison with men (33.3% and 16.4%, respectively), in spite that the number of men who were bystanders to bullying was larger compared to women[21].

A survey of almost 950 Finnish municipal employees, led by Vartia,[22] has documented that the employees who witnessed workplace bullying were at substantial risk (OR = 2.56) of experiencing mental stress reactions (feeling depressed, unusually tired, nervous, difficulties in falling asleep, staying awake at nights) as compared to colleagues who were not bullied[22].

Sprigg et al.[55] developed a study to ascertain the association between witnessing workplace bullying and work-related exhaustion, depression, and anxiety, in the context of availability of psychological working support acting as a buffer. The study[55] was based on an electronic survey administered to more than 3,600 employees of different industries in the United Kingdom, of whom only approximately 190 participants were available for a second survey six months later. The research[55] established that witnessing workplace bullying, as determined at point one of the study, was significantly associated with work related exhaustion, depression and anxiety experienced six months later, even after controlling for age, organizational tenure, and experience with bullying. Yet, the study[55] also demonstrated that "social support from coworkers significantly moderates the impact of witnessing bullying on emotional exhaustion and workplace depression, but not on anxiety,"[55] while "supportive supervisory style significantly buffered the impact of witnessing bullying on work-related depression and anxiety, but not on emotional exhaustion."[55]

Witnessing Victimization in the Family

Prevalence of Witnessing Victimization in the Family

Teicher and Vitaliano studied[56] 1,412 young adults' childhood history of witnessing violence towards, mother, father, and siblings. Their research has shown that 21% of the subjects reported seeing or hearing threats or assaults to their mother during childhood. Furthermore,

22% witnessed violence directed to their siblings, while 8% were aware of victimization perpetrated towards their father.

Hamby et al.[57] have examined the prevalence of exposure to family violence based on a data of the National Survey of Children's Exposure to Violence conducted from January to May 2008 through interviews of 4,549 US children and adolescents age 17 and younger. This research[57] has determined that, in the previous year, almost 6% to 7% of US youth was exposed to some form of physical assault or psychological/emotional violence between their parents, while 11% witnessed physical or psychological violence in the family.

The epidemiology of childhood witnessing domestic violence was studied by Gong et al.[58] through a 2019 survey of more than 3000 university students in Hunan Province, China, showing that 43% of them reported having witnessed domestic violence in childhood.

Health Problems Linked to Witnessing Victimization in the Family

Previously cited research led by Teicher and Vitaliano[56] documented that "witnessing threats or assaults to siblings was associated to a significant degree with ratings of depression, anxiety, somatization, anger-hostility, dissociation, and 'limbic irritability,'"[56] yet witnessing threats or assaults to mothers was not associated with symptoms while witnessing maltreatment of fathers was significantly associated with somatization.[56]

The effects of witnessing physical and psychological aggression in the family was investigated by Litrownik et al.[59] through a multisite prospective study of 682 children in different regions of the United States. The research[59] showed that witnessing family violence at age four, according to reports from both mother and children, predicted child problem behaviors at age 6, after controlling for mother reports of child problem behaviors on the Child Behavior Checklist[60] at age 4.[59]

The formerly mentioned epidemiological study by Gong et al.,[58] has documented that Chinese college students who reported having frequently (often or every day) witnessed domestic violence during their childhood, were significantly more at risk of attempting suicide or having higher scores in the Affective Lability Scale-18 (ALS-18)[61] instrument used to measure their emotional stability in terms of assessing shifts in anger, anxiety/depression, and depression/elation.[58]

Witnessing Victimization in the Community

An analysis by Finkelhor et al.[62] of data from the 2013 National Survey of Children's Exposure to Violence, involving a nationwide sample of 4000 US children and adolescents below age 18, has revealed that 18% of children and adolescents in the United States witnessed assault in their community in the previous year. This one-year prevalence widely varied by age group, ranging from almost 8% among children aged 2-5 years, to 33% among adolescents aged 14-17 years old. It is of note almost 58% of US adolescents age 14 to 17 witnessed assault in the community during their lifetime.

Health Problems Linked to Witnessing Victimization in the Community

The association between anxiety and depressive symptoms with witnessing violence was explored by Clark et al.[63] through a study based on the assessment 386 adult women living in urban neighborhoods in the northeastern United States. This research has documented, after controlling for marital status, education, age, and intimate partner violence, that those participants "who witnessed violent acts in their neighborhood were twice as likely to experience depressive and anxiety symptoms compared to women who did not witness community violence."[63]

Indirect Exposure to Distressing Events

The notion and effects of being indirectly exposed to traumatic circumstances through the personal narrative of the victim or via the verbal, written and or visual account provided in the media, has been explored by numerous studies.[64-92]

Indirect Exposure to a Distressing Event through a Victim's Narrative

Secondary exposure to victimization can be experienced by professionals "who frequently provide services to traumatized populations"[64] including mental health professionals[65-75]; lawyers and their staff[76-78] and police officers.[79-82]

The prevalence of Secondary Traumatic Stress (STS) among social workers was explored by Bride[65] through a survey of almost 300 master's-level social workers licensed in a southern state of the United States, by utilizing the Secondary Traumatic Stress Scale (STSS)[93] to ascertain the frequency of symptoms linked to STS resulting from working with traumatized populations.[65] This research[65] has documented that 77% of the participants indicated that occasionally or more frequently they worked with clients who dealt with traumatic issues. In this context, almost 41% of the social workers surveyed indicated that they experienced intrusive thoughts about their clients' traumatic events, while 19% suffered from psychological distress and 12% went through physiologic reactions in response to the intrusive thoughts.[65] Furthermore, at least 27% of the participants felt irritable and or have difficulties in concentration; and 15% had difficulties in recalling information pertaining to clients. Moreover, almost 25% of those surveyed experienced sleeping difficulties and emotional numbing while 14% felt hypervigilant and 5% to 6% reported disturbing dreams or "a sense of relieving the traumas reported by clients."[65]

Cieslak et al.[71] have conducted a detailed study of prevalence of secondary traumatic stress (STS) among a sample of 224 mental health providers working with military patients, while also investigating personal, work-related, and exposure-related correlates of STD. The research[71] showed that 19% of the providers met all the three core criteria for PTSD (intrusion/re-experiencing; avoidance and arousal. Intrusion was the most frequent (58%) symptom experienced by the providers, followed by arousal (35%) and avoidance (30%). A regression analysis demonstrated that providers' "personal history of trauma; complaints of having too many patients and more negative appraisals of the impact caused by and indirect exposure to trauma were correlates associated with higher frequency of STS symptoms."[71]

Indirect Exposure to Victimization through the Media

The nature and impact of indirect exposure to victimization through media reports have been underscored by several publications,[83-92,94] with some of them[85,86,88,94] focusing on the journalistic coverage of September 11, 2011 (9/11), terrorist attacks.

Schlenger et al.[94] examined psychological symptoms levels in the United States, within 1-2 months following the events of 9/11, through a study based on the survey of 2,271 adults, from households in New York City, Washington DC, and metropolitan areas. This study[94] has documented that during four to eight weeks after the 9/11 attack 11.6% of the population of the United States was experiencing "symptoms of clinically significant but nonspecific psychological distress" [94] based on the use of the 18-item version of the Brief Symptom Inventory (BSI 18).[95] We should notice that the frequency of symptoms of psychological distress in relation to indirect exposure to media, as documented by this study,[94] varied from 7.5% for individuals watching television less than 4 hours per day to 18% amid those who watched 12 or more hours of media daily.[94] Also, 4% of the participants experienced symptoms of probable PTSD, as assessed with the PTSD Checklist (PCL),[96] yet the rate of probable PTSD was as high as 10% among individuals who watched 12 or more hours of television.[94]

The association between indirect exposure though the media to the 2007 shooting massacre at the Virginia Polytechnic Institute (Virginia Tech) in Blacksburg, Virginia, and acute stress symptoms, was investigated by Fallahi and Lesik[84] through a survey of more tan 300 undergraduate and graduate students, attending a large state university in the Northeast of the United States, who were not directly involved in the Virginia Tech massacre, but who followed the case vicariously through the media. This study[84] has demonstrated that the number of hours that the participants reported having spent on TV viewing the news about the Virginia Tech case, in the few weeks after the event occurred, was significantly associated with the frequency of self-rated experience of acute stress symptoms. In this context, the probability of experiencing intrusive thoughts, sleep and appetite disturbance, fear and anger was of 9% for those students who viewed 10 hours of TV news of the case, yet the frequency of these symptoms was reported by 30% to 62% of the participants who were exposed to 40 hours of TV news coverage of the shooting.[84] Also, the study has documented that "for each hour watched of the Virginia Tech shootings, the odds of experiencing acute symptoms increased from 1.48 to 3.20 times, depending on the symptom."[84]

Future Directions

As we advance in efforts to detect, prevent, and treat morbidity associated with bullying, and other forms of maltreatment there will be a need to:

- Develop our understanding about the impact of witnessing victimization on the physical and emotional wellbeing of the bystander, through longitudinal studies

- Ascertain the influence of having been previously victimized as a risk factor associated with the impact of witnessing victimization
- Determine the effects of indirect exposure to victimization through the victim's account during friends' conversations or during a narrative by a group therapy member.
- Incorporate the role of witnessing bullying or other forms maltreatment in the spectrum of polyvictimization
- Include anamnesis about witnessing victimization as part of the clinical detection of morbidity related to bullying and other forms of victimization
- Consider preventing witnessing victimization during treatment of bullying related morbidity, to avoid re-victimization

Notes

1. Nickerson AB, Aloe AM, Livingston JA, Feeley TH. Measurement of the bystander intervention model for bullying and sexual harassment. *J Adolescence*. 2014;37(4):391–400.
2. Pozzoli T, Gini G, Thornberg R. Getting angry matters: going beyond perspective taking and empathic concern to understand bystanders' behavior in bullying. *J Adolescence*. 2017; 61:87–95..
3. Yang SA, Kim DH. Factors associated with bystander behaviors of Korean youth in school bullying situations: a cross-sectional study. *Medicine*. 2017;96(32):1–7. https://www.ncbi.nlm.nih.gov/pmc/articles/PMC5556233/pdf/medi-96-e7757.pdf. Accessed October 13, 2023.
4. Machackova H, Pfetsch J. Bystanders' responses to offline bullying and cyberbullying: the role of empathy and normative beliefs about aggression. *Scand J Psychol*. 2016;57(2):169–176..
5. Gini G, Albiero P, Benelli B, Altoe G. Determinants of adolescents' active defending and passive bystanding behavior in bullying. *J Adolescence*. 2008;31(1):93–105..
6. Lindegaard MR, Liebst LS, Bernasco W, et al. Consolation in the aftermath of robberies resembles post-aggression consolation in chimpanzees. *PLOS One*. 2017;12(5):e0177725.
7. Van Cleemput K, Vandebosch H, Pabian S. Personal characteristics and contextual factors that determine "helping," "joining in," and "doing nothing" when witnessing cyberbullying. *Aggress Behav*. 2014;40(5):383–396..
8. Thornberg R, Wänström L, Hong JS, Espelage DL. Classroom relationship qualities and social-cognitive correlates of defending and passive bystanding in school bullying in Sweden: a multilevel analysis. J Sch Psychol. 2017;63:49–62.
9. Howard AM, Landau S, Pryor JB. Peer bystanders to bullying: who wants to play with the victim? *J Abnorm Child Psychol*. 2014;42(2):265–276.
10. Jenkins LN, Fredrick SS. Social capital and bystander behavior in bullying: internalizing problems as a barrier to prosocial intervention. *J Youth Adolescence*. 2017;46(4):757–771..
11. Báez-León C, Moreno-Jiménez B, Aguirre-Camacho A, Olmos R. Factors influencing intention to help and helping behaviour in witnesses of bullying in nursing settings. *Nurs Inquiry*. 2016;23(4):358–367..
12. Evans CB, Smokowski PR. Negative bystander behavior in bullying dynamics: assessing the impact of social capital deprivation and anti-social capital. *Child Psychiatry Hum Dev*. 2017;48(1):120–135..
13. Salmivalli C, Voeten M, Poskiparta E. Bystanders matter: associations between reinforcing, defending, and the frequency of bullying behavior in classrooms. *J Clin Child Adolesc Psychol*. 2011;40(5):668–676.

14. Cook-Craig PG, Coker AL, Clear ER, et al. Challenge and opportunity in evaluating a diffusion-based active by-standing prevention program: Green Dot in high schools. *Violence Against Women*. 2014;20(10):1179–1202.
15. Potter SJ, Moynihan MM. Bringing in the bystander in-person prevention program to a US military installation: results from a pilot study. *Milit Med*. 2011;176(8):870–875.
16. Stueve A, Dash K, O'Donnell L, et al. Rethinking the bystander role in school violence prevention. *Health Promot Pract*. 2006;7(1):117–124.
17. Gini G, Pozzoli T, Borghi F, Franzoni L. The role of bystanders in students' perception of bullying and sense of safety. *J Sch Psychol*. 2008;46(6):617–638.
18. Fonagy P, Twemlow SW, Vernberg E, Sacco FC, Little TD. Creating a peaceful school learning environment: The impact of an antibullying program on educational attainment in elementary schools. *Med Sci Monitor*. 2005;11(7):CR317–CR325.
19. Rivers I. Morbidity among bystanders of bullying behavior at school: concepts, concerns, and clinical/research issues. *Int J Adolesc Med Health*. 2012;24(1):11–16.
20. Rivers I, Noret N. Potential suicide ideation and its association with observing bullying at school. *J Adolesc Health*. 2013;53(1):S32–S36.
21. Emdad R, Alipour A, Hagberg J, Jensen IB. The impact of bystanding to workplace bullying on symptoms of depression among women and men in industry in Sweden: an empirical and theoretical longitudinal study. *Int Arch Occup Environ Health*. 2013;86(6):709–716.
22. Vartia MA. Consequences of workplace bullying with respect to the well-being of its targets and the observers of bullying. *Scand J Work Environ Health*. 2001:63–69.
23. Hansen ÅM, Hogh A, Garde AH, Persson R. Workplace bullying and sleep difficulties: a 2-year follow-up study. *Int Arch Occup Environ Health*. 2014;87(3):285–294.
24. Werth JM, Nickerson AB, Aloe AM, Swearer SM. Bullying victimization and the social and emotional maladjustment of bystanders: a propensity score analysis. *J Sch Psychol*. 2015;53(4):295–308.
27. Han Z, Zhang G, Zhang H. School bullying in urban China: prevalence and correlation with school climate. *Int J Environ Res Public Health*. 2017;14(10):1116.
31. Bradshaw CP, Sawyer AL, O'Brennan LM. Bullying and peer victimization at school: perceptual differences between students and school staff. *Sch Psychol Rev*. 2007;36(3):361.
37. Jones LM, Mitchell KJ, Turner HA. Victim reports of bystander reactions to in-person and online peer harassment: a national survey of adolescents. *J Youth Adolescence*. 2015;44(12):2308–2320.
33. Marraccini ME, Weyandt LL, Rossi JS. College students' perceptions of professor/instructor bullying: questionnaire development and psychometric properties. *J Am Coll Health*. 2015;63(8):563–572.
38. Lindfors PL, Kaltiala-Heino R, Rimpelä AH. Cyberbullying among Finnish adolescents—a population-based study. *BMC Public Health*. 2012;12(1):1027.
44. Tsuno K, Kawakami N, Tsutsumi A, et al. Socioeconomic determinants of bullying in the workplace: a national representative sample in Japan. *PLOS One*. 2015;10(3):e0119435.
45. Jackman MR, Jackman RW. An interpretation of the relation between objective and subjective social status. *Am Sociol Rev*. 1973:569–582. Cited by Tsuno et al.[44]
56. Teicher MH, Vitaliano GD. Witnessing violence toward siblings: an understudied but potent form of early adversity. *PLOS One*. 2011;6(12):e28852.
62. Finkelhor D, Turner HA, Shattuck A, Hamby SL. Prevalence of childhood exposure to violence, crime, and abuse: results from the National Survey of Children's Exposure to Violence. *JAMA Pediatrics*. 2015;169(8):746–754.

25. Salmivalli C, Lagerspetz K, Björkqvist K, Österman K, Kaukiainen A. Bullying as a group process: participant roles and their relations to social status within the group. *Aggress Behav.* 1996;22(1):1–5. Cited by Rivers.[19]
26. Bandura A. Moral disengagement in the perpetration of inhumanities. *Pers Soc Psychol Rev.* 1999;3(3):193–209.
34. Rivers I, Poteat VP, Noret N, Ashurst N. Observing bullying at school: the mental health implications of witness status. *Sch Psychol Q.* 2009;24(4):211.
36. Lambe LJ, Hudson CC, Craig WM, Pepler DJ. Does defending come with a cost? Examining the psychosocial correlates of defending behaviour among bystanders of bullying in a Canadian sample. *Child Abuse Negl.* 2017;65:112–123.
28. Chen LM, Cheng YY. Prevalence of school bullying among secondary students in Taiwan: measurements with and without a specific definition of bullying. *Sch Psychol Int.* 2013;34(6):707–720.
29. Osuka Y, Nishimura T, Wakuta M, Takei N, Tsuchiya KJ. Reliability and validity of the Japan Ijime Scale and estimated prevalence of bullying among fourth through ninth graders: a large-scale school-based survey. *Psychiatry Clin Neurosci.* 2019;73(9):551–559.
32. Midgett A, Doumas DM. Witnessing bullying at school: the association between being a bystander and anxiety and depressive symptoms. *Sch Ment Health.* 2019;11(3):454–463.
30. Callaghan M, Kelly C, Molcho M. Bullying and bystander behaviour and health outcomes among adolescents in Ireland. *J Epidemiol Community Health.* 2019;73(5):416–421.
35. Duan S, Duan Z, Li R, et al. Bullying victimization, bullying witnessing, bullying perpetration and suicide risk among adolescents: a serial mediation analysis. *J Affective Disord.* 2020;273:274–279.
39. Patchin JW, Hinduja S. Cyberbullying among tweens in the United States: prevalence, impact, and helping behaviors. *J Early Adolescence.* 2022;42(3):414–430.
40. Carter MA. Third party observers witnessing cyber bullying on social media sites. *Procedia Soc Behav Sci.* 2013;84:1296–1309.
41. Doumas DM, Midgett A. Witnessing cyberbullying and internalizing symptoms among middle school students. *Eur J Invest Health Psychol Educ.* 2020;10(4):957–966.
43. Wright MF, Wachs S, Harper BD. The moderation of empathy in the longitudinal association between witnessing cyberbullying, depression, and anxiety. Cyberpsychology. 2018;12(4):6. https://cyberpsychology.eu/article/view/11419/10168. Accessed August 5, 2022.
42. Yoon Y, Lee JO, Cho J, et al. Association of cyberbullying involvement with subsequent substance use among adolescents. *J Adolesc Health.* 2019;65(5):613–620.
46. Ciby M, Raya RP. Workplace bullying: a review of the defining features, measurement methods and prevalence across continents. *IIM Kozhikode Society Manage Rev.* 2015;4(1):38–47.
47. Salin D. Prevalence and forms of bullying among business professionals: a comparison of two different strategies for measuring bullying. *Eur J Work Organ Psychol.* 2001;10(4):425–441. Cited by Ciby and Raya.[48]
48. Agervold M, Mikkelsen EG. Relationship between bullying, psychosocial work environment and individual stress reactions. *Work Stress.* 2004;18(4): 336–351. Cited by Ciby and Raya.[48]
49. Nielsen MB, Skogstad A, Matthiesen SB, et al. Prevalence of workplace bullying in Norway: comparisons across time and estimation methods. *Eur J Work Organ Psychol.* 2009;18(1):81–101. Cited by Ciby and Raya.[48]

50. Quine L. Workplace bullying in NHS community trust: staff questionnaire survey. *Br Med J.* 1999;318(7178):228–232. Cited by Ciby and Raya.[46]
51. Escartın J, Rodrıguez-Carballeira A, Zapf D, Porrua C, Martın-Pena J. Perceived severity of various bullying behaviours at work and the relevance of exposure to bullying. *Work Stress.* 2009;23(3):191–205. Cited by Ciby and Raya.[46]
52. Carter M, Thompson N, Crampton P, et al. Workplace bullying in the UK NHS: a questionnaire and interview study on prevalence, impact, and barriers to reporting. *BMJ Open.* 2013;3(6):e002628. Cited by Ciby and Raya.[46]
53. Lutgen-Sandvik P, Tracy SJ, Alberts JK. Burned by bullying in the American workplace: prevalence, perception, degree, and impact. *J Manage Stud.* 2007;44(6):837–862. Cited by Ciby and Raya.[46]
54. Bilgel N, Aytac S, Bayram N. Bullying in Turkish white-collar workers. *Occup Med.* 2006;56(4):226–231. Cited by Ciby and Raya.[46]
55. Sprigg CA, Niven K, Dawson J, Farley S, Armitage CJ. Witnessing workplace bullying and employee well-being: a two-wave field study. *J Occup Health Psychol.* 2019;24(2):286.
59. Litrownik AJ, Newton R, Hunter WM, English D, Everson MD. Exposure to family violence in young at-risk children: a longitudinal look at the effects of victimization and witnessed physical and psychological aggression. *J Fam Violence.* 2003;18(1):59–73.
60. Achenbach TM. *Manual for the Child Behavior Checklist.* Burlington, VT: Department of Psychiatry, University of Vermont; 1991. Cited by Litrownik et al.[59]
57. Hamby S, Finkelhor D, Turner H, Ormrod R. Children's Exposure to Intimate Partner Violence and Other Family Violence. 2011. https://biblioteca.cejamericas.org/bitstream/handle/2015/445/Childrens_Exposure_Intimate_Family_Violence.pdf?sequence = 1&isAllowed = y. Accessed August 29, 2022.
58. Gong J, Zhou L, Zhao L, Zhang S, Chen Z, Liu J. Epidemiology of childhood witnessing domestic violence and exploration of its relationships with affective lability and suicide attempts in Chinese young adults. *J Interpers Violence.* 2022:08862605211072221.
61. Oliver MN, Simons JS. The Affective Lability Scales: development of a short-form measure. *Pers Individ Differ.* 2004;37(6):1279–1288. Cited by Gong et al.[58]
63. Clark C, Ryan L, Kawachi I, Canner MJ, Berkman L, Wright RJ. Witnessing community violence in residential neighborhoods: a mental health hazard for urban women. *J Urban Health.* 2008;85(1):22–38.
64. May CL, Wisco BE. Defining trauma: how level of exposure and proximity affect risk for posttraumatic stress disorder. *Psychol Trauma Theory Res Pract.* 2016;8(2):233.
65. Bride BE. Prevalence of secondary traumatic stress among social workers. *Soc Work.* 2007;52:63–70. Cited by May and Wisco.[64]
66. Schauben LJ, Frazier PA. Vicarious trauma: the effects on female counselors of working with sexual violence survivors. *Psychol Women Q.* 1995;19:49–64. Cited by May and Wisco.[64]
67. Pearlman LA, Mac Ian PS. Vicarious traumatization: an empirical study of the effects of trauma work on trauma therapists. *Profess Psychol Res Pract.* 1995;26:558–565. Cited by May and Wisco.[64]
68. Ortlepp K, Friedman M. Prevalence and correlates of secondary traumatic stress in workplace lay trauma counselors. *J Trauma Stress.* 2002;15:213–222. Cited by May and Wisco.[64]
69. Elwood LS, Mott J, Lohr JM, Galovski TE. Secondary trauma symptoms in clinicians: a critical review of the construct, specificity, and implications for trauma-focused treatment. Clin Psychol Rev. 2011;31:25–36. Cited by May and Wisco.[64]

70. Shoji K, Bock J, Cieslak R, Zukowska K, Luszczynska A, Benight CC. Cultivating secondary traumatic growth among healthcare workers: the role of social support and self-efficacy. J Clin Psychol. 2014;70:831–846, Cited by May and Wisco.[64]
71. Cieslak R, Anderson V, Bock J, Moore BA, Peterson AL, Benight CC. Secondary traumatic stress among mental health providers working with the military: prevalence and its work-and exposure-related correlates. *J Nerv Ment Dis.* 2013;201(11):917.
72. Makadia R, Sabin-Farrell R, Turpin G. Indirect exposure to client trauma and the impact on trainee clinical psychologists: secondary traumatic stress or vicarious traumatization? *Clin Psychol Psychother.* 2017;24(5):1059–1068.
73. Badger K, Royse D, Craig C. Hospital social workers and indirect trauma exposure: an exploratory study of contributing factors. *Health Soc Work.* 2008;33(1):63–71.
74. Tarshis S, Baird SL. Addressing the indirect trauma of social work students in intimate partner violence (IPV) field placements: a framework for supervision. *Clin Soc Work J.* 2019;47(1):90–102.
75. Canfield J. Secondary traumatization, burnout, and vicarious traumatization: a review of the literature as it relates to therapists who treat trauma. *Smith Coll Stud Soc Work.* 2005;75(2):81–101.
76. Piwowarczyk L, Ignatius S, Crosby S, Grodin M, Heeren T, Sharma A. Secondary trauma in asylum lawyers. *Bender's Immigration Bull.* 2009;14(5):263–269.
77. Levin AP, Greisberg S. Vicarious trauma in attorneys. *Pace Law Rev.* 2003;24:245.
78. Levin AP, Albert L, Besser A, et al. Secondary traumatic stress in attorneys and their administrative support staff working with trauma-exposed clients. *J Nerv Ment Dis.* 2011;199:946–955. Cited by May and Wisco.[64]
79. Acquadro Maran D, Zito M, Colombo L. Secondary traumatic stress in Italian police officers: the role of job demands and job resources. *Front Psychol.* 2020;11:1435.
80. MacEachern AD, Jindal-Snape D, Jackson S. Child abuse investigation: police officers and secondary traumatic stress. *Int J Occup Safety Ergonomics.* 2011;17(4):329–339.
81. MacEachern AD, Dennis AA, Jackson S, Jindal-Snape D. Secondary traumatic stress: prevalence and symptomology amongst detective officers investigating child protection cases. *J Police Crim Psychol.* 2019;34(2):165–174.
82. Cronje JH, Vilakazi MJ. Secondary traumatic stress in police detective officers dealing with complainants of sexual crimes. *S Afr J Psychol.* 2020;50(4): 520–529.
83. Ben-Zur H, Gil S, Shamshins Y. The relationship between exposure to terror through the media, coping strategies and resources, and distress and secondary traumatization. *Int J Stress Manage.* 2012;19:132–150. Cited by May and Wisco.[64]
84. Fallahi CR, Lesik SA. The effects of vicarious exposure to the recent massacre at Virginia Tech. *Psychol Trauma Theory Res Pract.* 2009;1:220–230. Cited by May and Wisco.[64]
85. Schuster MA, Stein BD, Jaycox LH, et al. A national survey of stress reactions after the September 11, 2001, terrorist attacks. *N Engl J Med.* 2001;345(20):1507–1512. Cited by May and Wisco.[64]
86. Gil-Rivas V, Silver RC, Holman EA, McIntosh DN, Poulin M. Parental response and adolescent adjustment to the September 11, 2001, terrorist attacks. *J Trauma Stress.* 2007;20(6):1063–1068. Cited by May and Wisco.[64]
87. Slone M, Shoshani A. Indirect victimization from terrorism: a proposed post-exposure intervention. *J Ment Health Couns.* 2008;30(3):255–266.

88. Saylor C, DeRoma V, Swickert R. College students with previous exposure to crime report more PTSD after 9-11-2001. *Psychol Rep*. 2006;99(2):581–582.
89. Addington LA. Students' fear after Columbine: findings from a randomized experiment. *J Quant Criminol*. 2003;19(4):367–387.
90. Slone M, Shoshani A, Baumgarten-Katz I. The relation between actual exposure to political violence and preparatory intervention for exposure to media coverage of terrorism. *Anxiety Stress Coping*. 2008;21(3):243–261.
91. Pfefferbaum B, Pfefferbaum RL, North CS, Neas BR. Does television viewing satisfy criteria for exposure in posttraumatic stress disorder? *Psychiatry*. 2002;65(4):306–309.
92. Dougall AL, Hayward MC, Baum A. Media exposure to bioterrorism: stress and the anthrax attacks. *Psychiatry*. 2005;68(1):28–42.
93. Bride BE, Robinson MM, Yegidis B, Figley CR. Development and validation of the Secondary Traumatic Stress Scale. *Res Soc Work Pract*. 2004;14:27–35. Cited by Bride.[65]
94. Schlenger WE, Caddell JM, Ebert L, et al. Psychological reactions to terrorist attacks: findings from the National Study of Americans' Reactions to September 11. *JAMA*. 2002;288(5):581–588. Cited by Neria Y, Sullivan GM. Understanding the mental health effects of indirect exposure to mass trauma through the media. *JAMA*. 2011;306(12):1374–1375.
95. Derogatis LR. *Brief Symptom Inventory 18: Administration, Scoring, and Procedures Manual*. Minneapolis, MN: NCS Pearson; 2001. Cited by Schlenger et al.[94]
96. Weathers FW, Litz BT, Herman DS, Huska JA, Keane TM. The PTSD Checklist (PCL): reliability, validity, and diagnostic utility. Paper presented at: Annual Conference of the International Society for Traumatic Stress Studies; October 25, 1993; San Antonio, TX. Cited by Schlenger et al.[94]

Epilogue

Future Consideration of Sociopolitical Maltreatment

Future examination of the spectrum of maltreatment, as considered in this book, may include the notion of sociopolitical maltreatment by segments of society and or its leaders, as well as by other state nations. This concept would encompass all facets of physical, psychological, and relational mistreatment of an individual or groups of individuals because of social, economic, religious, or political beliefs, through rhetoric and or policies which can promote, cause, enable, or support violence, intimidation, harassment, defamation, disrespect, exclusion or neglect.

The study of sociopolitical victimization could include an examination of what is known about the nature, prevalence and health risks associated with, at least, the following issues:

- Violent attacks on unarmed civilians (i.e., terrorism, criminal violence, torture, capital punishment, police brutality, genocide)
- Slavery like practices (i.e., serfdom, forced labor, debt bondage, exploitation of migrant workers, trafficking in persons, forced or consensual marriages)
- Crimes against humanity (i.e., murder or extermination, enslavement, deportation, or forcible transfer of population, enforced disappearance of persons, persecution against any group on political, racial, national, ethnic, cultural, religious or gender)

The understanding and recognition of the significant health risks associated with this form of maltreatment would have significant implications in the development of immigration policies that call for the clinical assessment of prior victimization, among political refugees, to "ensure the provision of adequate health services and follow-up."[1]

Note

1.. Srabstein JC. The global implications of bullying and other forms of maltreatment, in the context of migratory trends and psychiatric resources. *Child Adolesc Psychiatr Clin*. 2015;24(4):799–810.

Index

Tables, figures, and boxes are indicated by *t*, *f*, and *b* following the page number

Abdelhamid, M., 300
abdominal pain, 47
ABI-10 (Academic Bullying Inventory), 372, 372*t*
abnormal weight gain, 49–50
absenteeism, 73
abuse
  adolescent dating victimization, 339–340
  among siblings, 265–268
  child, 272–277
  of consumers, 247–248
  by customers and patients, 244–245
  cyberdating, 340, 342
  of domestic workers, 278
  elder, 271–272
  parent, 270–272
  spouse, 268–270
abuse in the healthcare system (AHC), 247–248
Academic Bullying Inventory (ABI- 10), 372, 372*t*
academic performance, 73–74
accidental deaths, 90
acute stress disorder (ASD)
  onset/cause and duration, 134*t*
  psychopharmacology of, 139–141, 140*t*
  psychosocial risks or dysfunctions in, 134, 136*t*
  psychotherapy for, 141–143, 142*t*
  symptoms or conditions of, 134, 135*t*
  treatment of, 138–143, 140*t*, 142*t*
Adderley, C. R., 329, 330*t*
Adhia, A., 344
adjustment disorder
  onset/cause and duration, 134*t*
  psychosocial risks or dysfunctions in, 134, 136*t*
  symptoms or conditions of, 134, 135*t*
  treatment of, 138, 139*t*
adolescent dating victimization
  correlates of, 342–344
  cyberdating abuse, 340
  overview, 339
  prevalence of, 340–342
  prevention programs, 344–345, 345*t*
  teen dating relationships, prevalence of, 339
  victimization in dating relationships, 339–340
adolescent pregnancy, 76
adrenergic inhibitors, 140*t*
adverse childhood experiences, headaches and, 35–36
adverse social behavior, 237
after-release care for prisoners, 399–400
Agyemang, C., 329–330
AHC (abuse in the healthcare system), 247–248
Ahmer, S., 371
Al Ali, N. M., 212
Al-Bitar, Z. B., 14
alcohol abuse, 78–79, 380–381
Alexander, K., 355
Al-Harigy, L. M., 116
Alhusen, J. L., 50
Allison, S., 214
American Automobile Association Foundation for Traffic Safety, 328
American Psychiatric Association (APA) treatment guidelines, 138
Ammerman, B. A., 78
Anadria, D., 245
Anda, R., 36
Andershed, H., 314
Anderson, M., 87
antibullying laws. *See* legislative preventive initiatives
anticonvulsants, 140*t*
antipsychotics, 140*t*
antisocial behavior, 79
anxiety
  associated with bullying, 40–42
  cyberbullying and, 296
  neighborhood safety and, 322–323
  witnessing victimization in community and, 412
APA (American Psychiatric Association) treatment guidelines, 138
Apter, A. J., 323
Armiento, J., 77
Armour, C., 136–137
Arslan, S., 37
artificial intelligence, detecting school bullying with, 116
ASD. *See* acute stress disorder
Asfaw, A. G., 73
Asia, prevalence of cyberbullying in, 293, 294*t*
asthma, community violence and, 323
athletes, victimization among. *See* competitive sports, victimization in
Augustin, T., 323–324
Australia, 181, 293
autism spectrum disorder (ASD), 14, 264, 380

backache, 45–46
Bagley, C., 100
Bagley, E. J., 324
Baiden, P., 343
Baldwin, J. R., 30
Bang, Y. R., 85
Bannai, A., 235
Banyard, V. L., 341
Banzon-Librojo, L. A., 214

Barker, B., 75–76
Barlett, C. P., 295
Barlett and Gentile Cyberbullying Model, 295
barra bravas, 353
Barzilay, S., 85
Bar-Zomer, J., 264
Basoglu, M., 142*t*
Bauleo, M. F., 277
Beard, J. H., 321
Beaver, K. M., 38
Beck, N. I., 55
bedside manner, 246
Beehr, T. A., 238–239
behavioral-based therapy, 139*t*
Belfrage, H., 269–270
Benbenishty, R., 213
Benedek, D. M., 141
benzodiazepines, 140*t*
Berggren, A. W., 379
Berkowitz, R., 213
Bi, Y., 245
Bishop, V., 241
Bismarck, M. M., 248–249
Bjarnelind, S., 72
Bjorklund, W. L., 377
Bjørnseth, I., 353
Blaauw, E., 391
Blanco, V., 381
body shaming, 355
body weight and appearance, bullying related to, 14
Bohren, M. A., 246
Bonomi, A. E., 47
Bowes, L., 264
Bowles, L., 39, 42
Bowling, N. A., 238–239
Bowman, C. G., 325
Bradshaw, C. P., 407
brawls, physical aggression related to, 351–352
Brennenstuhl, S., 36
Brewer, N., 74
Bride, B. E., 412
broadcasting, 292
Broadhurst, R., 298–299
Bru, E., 47–48
Bruce, L. C., 42
Brunstein-Klomek, A., 76, 77, 264–265
Bryant, R. A., 137, 141
bullies, in school bullying, 212
bullying
  coverage in media and scientific literature of, 1, 2*f*
  legal definition of, 3
  medical concept of, 5–6
  notion across social settings, 5
  notion in public health domain, 3, 4*t*
  spectrum of maltreatment, 6–7
  understanding concept of, 1–2
bullying prevention plan, 145
bully/victim dual role, in school bullying, 212–213
burden on victim, 133
Burgess, A. W., 248
Butcher, K., 246
Buyuk, Y., 271
bystanders
  role in bullying prevention strategies, 407
  role in school bullying, 213
  types, roles, and social dynamics of, 406

Callaghan, M., 407, 408
Callahan, M. R., 343
Campbell, M., 370
Canada
  Family Violence Initiative, 181
  prevalence of cyberbullying in, 293
  workplace bullying in, 238
Capadoccia, M.C., 293
CAPTA (Child Abuse Prevention and Treatment Act), 272–273
Caravaca-Sanchez, F., 392, 395
cardiovascular disease (CVD), 51–52, 323–324
Carlisle, S. K., 325
Carr-Gregg, M., 116
Carroll, A. E., 100
carrying weapons, 74–75
Carter, M. A., 409
Carver, K., 339
Casey, P., 138
Catone, G., 54
Cavanaugh, C. E., 86–87
CBT (cognitive behavioral therapy), 139*t*, 141
Centers for Disease Control and Prevention (CDC), 3
CFAA (Computer Fraud and Abuse Act), 297–298
CFS (Cyber Friendly Schools) program, 103, 177, 297
Chan, K. L., 28*t*, 30
Chapell, M., 370
Chapman University Survey of American Fears (CASF), 322
Chard, K. M., 142*t*
Chaux, E., 215
Chen, L. M., 407
Chen, Y. Y., 72
Cheng, C., 300–301
Cheng, Y. Y., 407
child abuse or maltreatment, 272–277
Child Abuse Prevention and Treatment Act (CAPTA), 272–273
child fatalities linked to abuse and neglect, 275
childhood maltreatment
  abdominal pain and, 47
  anxiety and, 42
  back pain and, 46
  cardiovascular disease and, 52
  common pathophysiology for headaches and, 36–37
  corporal punishment laws, 174, 174*t*
  definitions of, 272–274
  depression and, 40
  detection of, 118–120
  diabetes and, 51
  dissociation and, 53
  domestic or family maltreatment prevention laws, 171–172, 171*t*, 172*t*, 173*t*

homicides and, 89–90
inflammation and, 49
injuries and, 55–56
nonsuicidal self-injury and, 77
poor academic performance and, 74
prevalence and correlates, 274–277
prevention, 105–106
psychotic symptoms and, 55
revictimization, 29
school dropout and, 75–76
sleep difficulties/nightmares and, 45
substance abuse and, 78–79
suicide attempts and, 78, 87
weight gain and, 50
child neglect, 273, 275
Christensen, J., 326
Chudal, R., 293, 294*t*
Ciby, M., 410
Cieslak, R., 412–413
CISA (Cybersecurity and Infrastructure Security Agency), U. S., 301
Clark, C., 52, 412
classroom environment, 215
Cleary, J. S., 378
clients
mistreatment by, 240–241
mistreatment of, 246–249
clinical detection of school bullying, 115–116
cognitive behavioral therapy (CBT), 139*t*, 141
cognitive processes, disruption in, 52–53
cognitive processing therapy (CPT), 141, 142*t*, 143
college students
bullying among, 370–371
bullying among healthcare students and professional trainees, 371–372
harassment and discrimination in colleges or universities, 378–379
hazing among, 375
health impact of victimization, 380–381
incivility among, 376–377, 377*t*
violence in colleges and universities, 379–380
Collins, C. L., 351
COMBAT program (Ghana), 180
community crime victimization, 319, 411–412
competitive sports, victimization in
definition of, 349
discrimination in sports, 356
emotional abuse in competitive sports, 354–356
neglect in sports, 356–357
overview, 349
physical aggression in sports, 350–353, 351*t*
prevalence of, 349–350
sexual violence in sports, 353–354
complex PTSD
association with bullying, 136
onset/cause and duration, 134*t*
psychological treatment of, 143
psychosocial risks or dysfunctions in, 134, 136*t*
symptoms or conditions of, 134, 135*t*
Computer Fraud and Abuse Act (CFAA), 297–298
Connelly, R. J., 377
Connolly, E. J., 38
ConRed Program, 103, 177, 297
Consortium for Street Children (CSC), 318
Constantino, J. N., 105
consumers
abuse of, 247–248
corporate victimization of, 249–250
fraud, 249
incivility of, 242–243, 243*t*
sabotage of, 247
Cook, P. J., 379
Copeland, W. E., 48
corporal punishment
laws regarding, 174, 174*t*
prevalence and correlates, 275–277
in schools, 218, 219*t*, 220*t*
corporate victimization
of consumers, 249–250
of employees, 240
Cortina, L. M., 376–377
Costa, D., 72
Costa, M. R., 314
Council of Europe's Cybercrime Treaty of 2001, 297, 298*t*
countries with prevention laws and initiatives
corporal punishment, 174*t*, 220*t*
cyberbullying, 167*t*, 176–177, 176*t*
dating violence, 178–179, 178*t*
domestic or family maltreatment, 171*t*
family violence, 181–182
harassment in streets and public areas, 175*t*
school bullying, 165*t*, 166*t*, 176–177, 176*t*
sexual violence, 179–181, 180*t*
sexual violence prevention programs, 180*t*
workplace bullying, 169*t*, 177–178
COVID- 19 pandemic, 275, 301
CPT (cognitive processing therapy), 141, 142*t*, 143
C-reactive protein (CRP) levels, 48–49
crime
cybercrime, 297–301
fear of, 320
gang violence, 316–317, 320
health impact of neighborhood safety, 322–324
perception of safety and, 319–320
victimization by strangers, 315–316
witnessing in community, 411–412
criminality, 79
Cripe, S. M., 36
Croall, H., 249–250
Crolley, L., 353
Cross, C., 341
Cross, D., 103
Cross, T., 352
Crow, R. B., 355
CRP (C-reactive protein) levels, 48–49
CSC (Consortium for Street Children), 318
Cuartas, J., 276
cultural distance, workplace bullying and, 17

customers
abuse by, 244–245
bullying by, 241
harassment by, 243–244
maltreatment between service providers and, 240–245
mistreatment by, 240–241
mistreatment of, 246–249
physical assault or violence by, 245
rudeness, incivility, or disrespect toward, 246
CVD (cardiovascular disease), 51–52, 323–324
cyberbullying
absenteeism and, 73
among adults, 294–295
among university students, 370, 380–381
anxiety and, 41
correlates of, 295
definition and nature of, 291–293, 292*t*
depression and, 38
detection of, 116
global prevalence of, 14–15, 15*t*
headaches and, 35
HRQoL and, 72–73
ill effects of, 296
national prevention strategies, 176–177, 176*t*
overview, 291
prevalence of, 293, 294*t*
prevention laws, 167, 167*t*, 168*t*, 169*t*
prevention of, 102–103, 296–297
sleep difficulties and, 43
stomachache and, 47
suicide attempts and, 77, 86
witnessing, 408–409
cybercrime
correlates of, 299–300
during the COVID- 19 pandemic, 301
definition of, 297–299, 298*t*
impact of, 300–301
prevalence of, 299
Cybercrime Treaty of 2001, Council of Europe, 297, 298*t*
cyberdating abuse, 340, 342
Cyber Friendly Schools (CFS) program, 103, 177, 297
Cybersecurity and Infrastructure Security Agency (CISA), U. S., 301
cyberspace, 291. *See also* cyberbullying; cybercrime
cybervictimization laws, 167, 167*t*, 168*t*
cyberviolence, 88
Cyclist Anger Expression Inventory, 328
cyclists, incivility toward and among, 328
Cyr, K., 28*t*

Danese, A., 49
dangerous driving, 327–328
Daniel, J. K., 245
Dantchev, S., 79
Daoud, N., 117–118
Date-e-Adolescence program, 179
Dating Matters: Strategies to Promote Healthy Teen Relationships (DM), 179
Dating SOS (SOS Namoro) intervention, 178
dating victimization
correlates of, 342–344
cyberdating abuse, 340
general discussion, 339–340
national prevention initiatives, 178–179, 178*t*
overview, 339
prevalence of, 340–342
prevention of, 103–105, 104*t*
prevention programs, 344–345, 345*t*
teen dating relationships, prevalence of, 339
dating violence victimization (DVV), 342–344
DDDI (Dula Dangerous Driving Index), 327
Debnam, K. J., 344
DeGue, S., 181
De Jongh, A., 143
De Kimpe, L., 299–300
De La Rue, L., 103–104, 104*t*
DelGreco, M., 326
delinquent youth groups, 316
Del Rey, R., 103
den Hamer, A. H., 295
dentofacial features, bullying related to, 14
de Oliveira, W. A., 14
depression
associated with bullying, 37–40
cyberbullying and, 296
intimate partner violence and, 269
neighborhood safety and, 322–323
sibling bullying and, 264–265
witnessing victimization in community and, 412
witnessing workplace bullying and, 410
detection
artificial intelligence to detect school bullying, 116
of child maltreatment, 118–120
clinical detection of school bullying, 115–116
of cyberbullying, 116
of intimate partner violence, 117–118
overview, 115
universal screening for exposure to victimization, 120–121
developmental conditions associated with bullying, 14
Devries, K. M., 269
diabetes, 50–51
diagnostic framework, treatment within, 134–136
Diesel, J. C., 50
di Leonardo, M., 325
direct aggressive behaviors, 3
Direct and Indirect Prisoner behavior Checklist (DIPC), 389–390
direct sanctions, 132, 133
direct self-injurious behavior (D-SIB), 76
discipline of children, 274, 275–277
discomfort in interacting with perpetrators, 133
discrimination
in colleges or universities, 378–379
perceived, 324
in sports, 356
in the streets, 324–325
disrespect toward customers or patients, 246

disruption in cognitive processes, 52–53
dissing, 292
dissociation, 53
distressing events, indirect exposure to, 412–413
Division of Violence Prevention (DVP), 180–181
DM (Dating Matters: Strategies to Promote Healthy Teen Relationships), 179
Doll, B., 215
domestic victimization. *See also* intimate partner violence; sibling bullying
  abuse among siblings, 265–268
  among parents, 268–270
  child abuse or maltreatment, 272–277
  maltreatment of domestic workers, 277–278, 279*t*
  maltreatment of parents by children, 270–272
  overview, 263
  prevention laws, 171–172, 171*t*, 172*t*, 173*t*
domestic workers, maltreatment of, 277–278, 279*t*
Domestic Workers Convention of 2011, International Labour Organization, 277
Dommes, A., 329
Dougé, N., 40
Doumas, D. M., 408, 409
driving, dangerous, 327–328
drug abuse, 78–79
D-SIB (direct self-injurious behavior), 76
Duan, S., 408
Due, P., 10, 41, 45–46
Duke, V., 353
Dula, C. S., 327, 327*t*
Dula Dangerous Driving Index (DDDI), 327
Dulin-Keita, A., 325
Duncan, R. D., 214
Dunn, E. C., 40
Dunne, M. P., 119
Dupper, D. R., 217
Duque, L. F., 319
Dutch detection of child maltreatment, 118
DVP (Division of Violence Prevention), 180–181
DVV (dating violence victimization), 342–344

ecological aspects of school bullying, 215
Economist Intelligent Unit, 319–320
educational stakeholders, maltreatment among, 221
Einarsen, S., 234, 239
elder abuse, 271–272
Elgar, F. J., 215
Ellaway, A., 323
Ellsworth, J. T., 317–318
El-Sheikh, M., 44
Emdad, R., 39, 410
EMDR (eye movement desensitization and reprocessing), 141, 142*t*
emotional abuse
  among siblings, 267
  of children, 273–274
  in competitive sports, 350, 354–356
  in dating relationships, 341
empathy, 213, 406
employer victimization of employees, 240
Engström, K., 90
Environmental Risk Longitudinal Twin Study, 30
Esselmont, C., 75
Estrada, A. X., 379
ethnicity
  discrimination in the streets, 324–325
  school bullying by, 12–13
EU Kids Online survey, 293, 294*t*
Europe
  prevalence of cyberbullying in, 293, 294*t*
  workplace bullying in, 236–237
European Agency for Safety and Health at Work (EU OSHA) report, 177
European Survey of Working Conditions (2005), 236–237
European Working Conditions Survey (2010), 16, 16*t*
Every Day Discrimination Scale, 324
Exner-Cortens, D., 342–343
exposure to distressing events, indirect, 412–413
eye movement desensitization and reprocessing (EMDR), 141, 142*t*

facial appearance, bullying related to, 14
Faergemann, C., 29
Fahy, A. E., 41, 296
Fallahi, C. R., 413
family. *See also* intimate partner violence; sibling bullying
  adolescent dating victimization and, 342
  maltreatment by children, 270–272
  parental occupation, bullying related to, 13, 15
  role in school bullying, 214–215
  victimization among parents, 268–270
Family for Safe Dates (FSD), 105
family violence
  national prevention initiatives, 181–182
  prevention laws, 171–172, 171*t*, 172*t*, 173*t*
  witnessing victimization in, 410–411
Family Violence Initiative (Canada), 181
Family Violence Prevention and Services Program (FVPSA Program), 181–182
fans and physical aggression in sports, 352
Fanslow, J. L., 55, 269
Fattori, A., 72
Feagin, J. R., 324
fear
  of crime, 320
  of gangs, 320
  of prison victimization, 395
  of terrorism, 322
Federal Bureau of Investigation (FBI) 2020 Internet Crime Report, 299
Fedina, L., 379
Feinstein, B. A., 38
Fekkes, M., 47
Feltner, C., 117
Ferguson, C. J., 276
fibromyalgia, 47–48
Fields, S. K., 352
fights, physical, 75, 315, 351–352

Finkelhor, D., 27, 28, 28t, 266, 272, 411
Finnish Occupational Safety and Health Act, 220
flaming, 292
Flin, R., 328
Flury, M., 268
Fnais, N., 378
Fonagy, P., 217, 407
Fonseca-Machado, M. D., 42
football hooliganism, 352–353
Ford, J. D., 30
Ford, R., 297
foreign-born youth, school bullying and, 12–13
Forjuoh, S. N., 56
Forman-Hoffman, V., 141, 143
Forshee, V. A., 105, 343
Forsyth, A., 323
Foshee, V. A., 342
foul play, physical aggression related to, 350–351, 351t
Fried, E. I., 146
Frisén, A., 72
Frosdick, S., 353
Fruhen, L. S., 328
Frumkin, M., 146
FSD (Family for Safe Dates), 105
Fu, K. W., 296
FVPSA Program (Family Violence Prevention and
Services Program), 181–182

Gaetz, S., 318
Gágyor, I., 371
Galea, S., 321
Galeazzi, G. M., 244
Gallagher, B., 218
Gambrill, E., 329
Gámez-Guadix, M., 38
gang violence, 316–317, 320
GAO (Government Accountability Office)
report, 376
Gao, W., 39
Gartlehner, G., 141
Gartrell, N., 248
Gatti, U., 316
Gelaye, B., 45
Geller, E. S., 327, 327t
gender nonconformity and school bullying, 12
General Well-Being Scale (GWB), 395
Gentile, D. A., 295
Geoffroy, M. C., 86
Gershoff, E. T., 218, 276–277
Gibson, W., 291
Gilchrist, G., 39–40
Gilkey, D. P., 46
Gillen, P. A., 105
Gillies, D., 143
Gini, G., 35
Glambek, M., 46
global prevalence of bullying
cyberbullying, 14–15, 15t
developmental conditions associated with
bullying, 14
overview, 10
physical characteristics linked to bullying, 14
school bullying, 10–13, 11t
workplace bullying, 16–17, 16t
Global School-based Student Health Survey (GSHS),
3, 4t, 10, 11t
Global Status Report on Violence Prevention 2014, 176
Goldman-Mellor, S., 322–323
Gong, J., 411
Gong, Z., 41
González-Cabrera, J., 72–73
Gordon, S., 297
Government Accountability Office (GAO)
report, 376
grandparents, maltreatment by grandchildren, 272
Greiner, T., 138
Grogan Kaylor, A., 276–277
GSHS (Global School-based Student Health Survey),
3, 4t, 10, 11t
Guillen, P. A., 250
Gullander, M., 39
GWB (General Well-Being Scale), 395

hacking, 292
Hale, R., 214–215
Hamby, S., 344, 411
Han, Z., 407
Haney, C., 397–398
Hansen, Å. M., 44
happy slapping, 292
harassment
in colleges or universities, 378–379
of domestic workers, 278
in military training, 379
street, 325–326
in streets and public areas, laws preventing, 174–
175, 175t
Harris, L. C., 247
hazing
among military trainees, 376
among university students, 375
definition of, 91n.9
in sports, 355
of university students, 381
headaches, 35–37
HEADSS evaluation, 116
Health Behavior in School-aged Children
(HBSC) survey
cyberbullying, 14–15, 15t, 293
description of bullying in, 3, 4t
overview, 56n.2
school bullying, 10, 11t, 212
youth participation in street fights, 315
healthcare
abuse by patients, 244–245
bullying by patients, 241
harassment by patients, 243–244
mistreatment by patients, 240–241
mistreatment of patients, 246–249
physical assault or violence by patients, 245

rudeness, incivility, or disrespect toward patients, 246
sexual misconduct in, 248–249
students, victimization of, 371–372, 378
health impact
abdominal pain, 47
anxiety, 42
back pain, 46
cardiovascular disease, 52
corporal punishment laws, 174
of cyberbullying, 296
depression, 40
diabetes, 51
headaches, 36–37
inflammation, 49
injuries, 55–56
musculoskeletal pain/fibromyalgia, 47–48
of neighborhood safety, 322–324
nonsuicidal self-injury, 77
of polyvictimization, 29–30
of prison victimization, 391
of revictimization, 30
sleep difficulties/nightmares, 45
spouse abuse and, 269
substance abuse, 78–79
of victimization in tertiary education or military training, 380–381
weight gain, 50
of witnessing cyberbullying, 409
of witnessing school bullying, 408
of witnessing victimization in community, 412
of witnessing victimization in family, 411
of witnessing workplace bullying, 410
health intervention to stop ongoing bullying, 143–146
health-related quality of life (HRQoL), 71–73
Hébert, M., 341
Heide, K. M., 266
higher education, victimization in. *See* tertiary education, victimization in
Hinduja, S., 291, 409
Ho, F. K., 52
Hoel, H., 241
Hoertel, N., 87
Högberg, G., 142*t*
Holmwall, C. M., 243*t*
Holshausen, K., 55
Holstein, B. E., 10
home, victimization at. *See* domestic victimization
homeless people, 317–318
homicide
adolescent dating victimization and, 344
cyberviolence and, 88
intimate partner, 89, 269–270
maltreatment and, 89–90
parricide, 271
school violence and, 87–88, 88*t*
sibling, 266
of unsheltered adults, 318
workplace violence and, 88–89
Hong, J. S., 270
household, definition of, 279n.1
HRQoL (health-related quality of life), 71–73
Huang, H., 213
Huang, J. H., 72
Huemer, J., 141
Hulette, A. C., 53
Hyyti, J., 392

ICAST (ISPCAN Child Abuse Screening Tool), 119–120
ICVS (International Crime Victims Survey), 319
identity theft, 292
idiographic models, 146
ILO (International Labour Organization), 177–178
Ilola, A. M., 35
Ilse, R., 241
impersonation, 292
inattention, school bullying and, 52–53
incivility
of consumers, 242–243, 243*t*
in neighborhood, 326–327
pedestrian safety and, 328–329
in tertiary education, 376–377, 377*t*
toward and among cyclists, 328
toward customers or patients, 246
income inequality, school bullying and, 215
Incredible Years, The, 105
indirect aggressive behaviors, 3
indirect exposure to distressing events, 412–413
inflammation, 48–49
injuries
adolescent dating victimization, 344
associated with bullying, 55–56, 90
intimate partner violence and, 269
physical aggression in sports, 350–353, 351*t*
inmates, prison
bullying among, 389–391
inmate-on-staff assaults, 394
mistreatment by prison system, 396–400
physical aggression in prisons, 393–394
polyvictimization, 394–395
predictors of victimization, 395
sexual abuse in prisons, 392–393
insomnia, 43–45
interacting with perpetrators, discomfort in, 133
International Crime Victims Survey (ICVS), 319
International Labour Organization (ILO), 177–178, 277
International Rehabilitation Council for Torture Victims (IRCT), 397
Internet. *See also* cyberbullying
cybercrime, 297–301
cyberviolence, 88
pro-self-harm web sites, impact of exposure to, 76
StopBullying.gov, 176*t*
interventions. *See also* prevention
health intervention to stop ongoing bullying, 143–146
overview, 132
to prevent further victimization, 132–133

intimate partner violence (IPV). *See also* adolescent dating victimization
anxiety and, 42
back pain and, 46
cardiovascular disease and, 52
dating violence prevention, 103–105, 104*t*
definition of, 268
depression and, 39–40
detection of, 117–118
diabetes and, 50
headaches and, 36
health risks, 269
homicide, 269–270
homicides, 89
HRQoL and, 72
inflammation and, 49
injuries and, 55
national dating violence prevention initiatives, 178–179, 178*t*
poor academic performance and, 74
prevalence and correlates, 268–269
prevention laws, 171–172, 171*t*, 172*t*, 173*t*
psychotic experiences and, 54
school dropout and, 75
sleep difficulties/nightmares and, 44
stomachache and, 47
suicidal behaviors and, 86–87
suicide attempts and, 77–78
weight gain and, 49–50
intrusive memories, 53
IPV. *See* intimate partner violence
IRCT (International Rehabilitation Council for Torture Victims), 397
Ireland, C. A., 390
Ireland, J. L., 389, 390, 391
irritability, 37
ISPCAN Child Abuse Screening Tool (ICAST), 119–120

Jacobsen, D. P., 48
Jadambaa, A., 293
Jaranson, J. M., 397
Jenaro, C., 293
Jewkes, R., 217
Johns, M. M., 14
Juel, K., 235
Jung, Y. E., 296
Juvenile Victimization Questionnaire (JVQ), 27, 28

Kahn, L. M., 356
Kahnn, L., 87
Kalt, A., 397
Karatas, H., 371–372
Kärnä, A., 102
Kasen, S., 215
Kashikar-Zuck, S., 48
Katz, C. M., 320
Keashly, L., 373
Kerr, G., 350, 355
Kerr, G. E., 354–355
Kessler, R. C., 324
Khoury-Kassabri, M., 217
Kim, S., 296
Kimerling, R., 29, 30, 380
King, K. A., 100
KiVa Antibullying Program, 102, 103, 176, 216, 297
Kivimäki, M., 38, 48, 51
Klein, L. B., 378
Klomek, A. B., 85
Knoll, J., 218
Kochenderfer-Ladd, B., 213
Kõiv, K., 372
Konda, S., 88
Konijn, E. A., 295
Kowalski, R. M., 291–292
Krienert, J. L., 266, 267, 271
Kubiszewski, V., 43
Kveton, P., 373

Ladd, G. W., 213
Låftman, S. B., 13
Lam, L. T., 295
Lambe, L. J., 408
Lasiter, S., 377
Law 5659 (Paraguay), 174
Lawoko, S., 117–118
Lazarov, A., 137
Le, M. T., 28*t*
Leahy, T., 353–354
Leddy, J., 390
legal definition of bullying, 3
legislative preventive initiatives
corporal punishment, 174, 174*t*
cyberbullying and cybervictimization, 167, 167*t*, 168*t*, 169*t*
domestic or family maltreatment, 171–172, 171*t*, 172*t*, 173*t*
future, 182–183
harassment in streets and public areas, 174–175, 175*t*
overview, 164
school bullying, 164, 165*t*, 166*t*
workplace bullying, 167–168, 169*t*, 170*t*
Lehti, V., 76
Leisner, S., 46
Lemieux, F., 321
Lenzi, M., 214
Lereyra, S. T., 43, 212, 214
lesbian, gay, bisexual, and transgender (LGBT) youth, 12, 15
Lesik, S. A., 413
Levan, S., 2
Lewis, J. M., 352
Leymann, H., 234
Li, J., 35, 43
Li, L., 51
Li, X., 328–329
Li, Y. L., 245
Lights 4Violence, 178
Lind, M. J., 45
Lindfords, P. L., 409

Listwan, S. J., 394
Litrownik, A. J., 411
Liu, L., 276
Logan, L. S., 325
Lowe, S. R., 321
Ludemir, A. B., 39
Lundy, C. J., 220–221
Luukkonen, A. H., 78, 85

Macintosh, E. W., 355
Madden, D. J., 245
Magerøy, N., 374
Makarem, N. N., 240
Malhotra, R., 277
maltreatment, spectrum of, 6–7
Mandelli, L., 40
Mannava, P., 248
Manocha, R., 116
MAOIs (monoamine oxidase inhibitors), 140*t*
Mapayi, B., 42
Marks, S., 353–354
Marraccini, M. E., 370, 408
Marracho, P., 350
Marsil, D. F., 378–379
Martin, S. L., 378
Mason, S. M., 49–50
mass shootings, 321, 413
Mathews, H., 314
Mavranezouli, I., 143
Mayes, S. D., 14
Maynard, B. R., 13
McBride, O., 137
McCabe, A., 354
McCabe, R. E., 41
McCorkle, R. C., 395
McCrea, R., 320
McIvor, R. J., 244
McNamara, C. L., 378–379
Media Heroes program, 102–103, 177, 296–297
media reports
  bullying-related mortality in, 84–85
  coverage of bullying, 1, 2*f*
  indirect exposure to victimization through, 413
mediation, 132, 133
medical concept of bullying, 5–6
medical students, victimization of, 371–372, 378
Menéndez, C. K., 88
mental health. *See also* anxiety; depression
  adolescent dating victimization and, 342–343
  bullying and psychiatric disorders, 14
  cyberbullying and, 296
  dissociation, 53
  intrusive memories, 53
  irritability, 37
  neighborhood safety and, 322–323
  nonsuicidal self-injury, 77
  polyvictimization and, 30
  of prison inmates, 399
  psychotic symptoms, 55
  sibling bullying and, 264–265
  sleep difficulties/nightmares, 45
  suicide attempts, 78, 87
  of witnessing school bullying, 408
Mercy, J. A., 270
Meriläinen, M., 372, 373
Messias, E., 86
method of shared concern, 132, 133
Midgett, A., 408, 409
Miedema, B. B., 244
migraines, 35–37
military training
  bullying in, 374–375
  harassment in, 379
  hazing in, 376
  sexual victimization in, 380
Miller, W. B., 316
Mills, L. D., 268
Min, J. Y., 46
Minkkinen, J., 76
mobbing. *See* workplace bullying
Modvig, J., 397
monoamine oxidase inhibitors (MAOIs), 140*t*
Monson, C. M., 142*t*
Monteith, S., 301
Moor, A., 179
morbidity associated with bullying
  abnormal weight gain, 49–50
  anxiety, 40–42
  backache, 45–46
  cardiovascular disease, 51–52
  clinical vignette, 34
  depression, 37–40
  diabetes, 50–51
  disruption in cognitive processes, 52–53
  headaches, 35–37
  inflammation, 48–49
  injuries, 55–56
  insomnia, 43–45
  intrusive memories, 53
  irritability, 37
  musculoskeletal pain/fibromyalgia, 47–48
  overview, 34–35
  psychotic symptoms, 53–55
  stomachache or abdominal pain, 47
  symptom-targeted treatment, 146
  tertiary prevention, 164
  treatment within diagnostic framework, 134, 135*t*
Morill, M., 266
mortality. *See also* homicide
  accidental or other unnatural deaths, 90
  information derived from news reports, 84–85
  overview, 84
  suicide, 85–87, 269
Moulden, H. M., 217–218
Mundy, L. K., 73
Muñoz-Fernández, N., 179
musculoskeletal pain, 47–48

Nabe-Nielsen, K., 44
Nansel, T. R., 74, 75

narratives of victims, indirect exposure through, 412–413
National Cyber Security Centre (NCSC), U. K., 301
National Health Interview Survey (2010), 237
National Inmate Survey, 392
National Plan (Australia), 181
national prevention initiatives
 corporal punishment laws, 174, 174*t*
 cyberbullying and cybervictimization laws, 167, 167*t*, 168*t*, 169*t*
 for dating violence, 178–179, 178*t*
 domestic or family maltreatment laws, 171–172, 171*t*, 172*t*, 173*t*
 for family violence, 181–182
 future legislative initiatives, 182–183
 overview, 164
 for school bullying and cyberbullying, 176–177, 176*t*
 school bullying laws, 164, 165*t*, 166*t*
 for sexual violence, 179–181, 180*t*
 street and public harassment laws, 174–175, 175*t*
 for workplace bullying, 177–178
 workplace bullying laws, 167–168, 169*t*, 170*t*
National Study of Student Hazing, U.S., 375
National Survey of Children's Health, 2016, 319
NCSC (National Cyber Security Centre), U. K., 301
neglect
 child, 273, 275
 of inmates, 398, 399–400
 in sports, 356–357
neighborhood, maltreatment in
 aggression/violence in the streets, 315
 dangerous driving and road rage, 327–328
 discrimination in the streets, 324–325
 fear of crime, 320
 fear of gangs, 320
 fears of terrorism, 322
 gang violence, 316–317
 health impact of, 322–324
 impact of mass shootings, 321
 incivility and pedestrian safety, 328–329
 incivility in neighborhood, 326–327
 incivility toward and among cyclists, 328
 neighborhood bullying, 314
 neighborhood crime and perception of safety, 319–320
 nuisances, 329–330, 330*t*
 overview, 314, 331*t*
 people living in the streets, 317–318
 street children, 318
 street harassment, 325–326
 victimization by strangers, 315–316
 witnessing, 411–412
Neilipovitz, D., 241
Nelson Mandela Rules, 396
Netterstrøm, B., 235
network analysis of symptom structure, 136–137, 146
Newton, R., 353
Newton, T. L., 49
New Zealand Family Violence Clearinghouse (NZFVC), 182
Nhundu, T. J., 217
Niedhammer, I., 44
Nielsen, M. B., 239
nightmares, 43–45
Nimal, R., 356
9/11 terrorist attacks, 413
nonsuicidal self-injury (NSSI), 77
nuisances in neighborhood, 329–330, 330*t*

O'Connell, M., 390
O'Donnell, M. L., 138
Ogbonna, E., 247
O'Grady, B., 318
Olweus, D., 2, 100, 211–212
Olweus Bullying Prevention Program (OBPP), 102, 176, 216
Onat, I., 322
Ongoing Violence Assessment Tool (OVAT), 117
oppressive coercive behavior, 374
Osuka, Y., 407
outing, 293
OVAT (Ongoing Violence Assessment Tool), 117
overcrowding of prisons, 398–399
overwork
 maltreatment of domestic workers, 277
 in school workplace, 220–221, 221*b*
 workplace bullying, 235–236

Pabian, S., 41
Pallitto, C. C., 269
Paolucci, E. O., 276
Papini, S., 137
Paquin, G. W., 329
Paraguay, corporal punishment law in, 174
parents
 adolescent dating victimization and, 342
 maltreatment by children, 270–272
 parental occupation, bullying related to, 13, 15
 role in school bullying, 214–215
 victimization among, 268–270
Park, J. H., 85
parricide, 271
participants in school bullying, roles of, 211–215
Paschall, M. J., 276
Patchin, J. W., 291, 409
patients
 abuse by, 244–245
 bullying by, 241
 harassment by, 243–244
 mistreatment by, 240–241
 mistreatment of, 246–249
 physical assault or violence by, 245
 rudeness, incivility, or disrespect toward, 246
Patrick, D. L., 72
Paul, R. J., 352
Pavey, A. R., 269
PE (prolonged exposure) therapy, 141, 142*t*

Peck, J. H., 266
pedestrian safety, incivility and, 328–329
peer victimization
  anxiety and, 40–41
  depression and, 38
  HRQoL and, 71–72
  poor academic performance and, 73–74
  psychotic symptoms and, 53–54
  sleep difficulties/nightmares and, 43
  suicide attempts and, 77
Pelletier, M. E., 213
Peltzer, K., 77–78
Pengpid, S., 77–78
people living in the streets, 317–318
perceived discrimination, 324
perception of safety, neighborhood crime and, 319–320
Percy-Smith, B., 314
Pereda, N., 28*t*
Perez, D. J., 325
perinatal risks, in intimate partner violence, 269
perpetrators, discomfort in interacting with, 133
Pershing, J. L., 376
personal security index, 319–320
Peruvian sexual harassment law, 175, 175*t*
Petrov, M. E., 45
Petrovic, A. B., 238
Peyton, R. P., 55
Pfeffer, R. D., 14
Phillips, T., 326
physical characteristics linked to bullying, 14
physical fights, 75, 315, 351–352
physical punishment, 274, 275–277
physical victimization
  adolescent dating victimization, 340–341
  aggression/violence in the streets, 315
  among siblings, 265–266
  of children, 273, 274–275
  by customers or patients, 245
  gang violence, 316–317
  people living in the streets, 317–318
  in prisons, 393–394
  in sports, 350–353, 351*t*
  against sports officials, 352
  by strangers, 315–316
  at work, 236, 237
Piazza T., 35
Pillemer, K., 272
Pinto-Cortez, C., 28*t*
Polling, C., 322
polyvictimization
  composite clinical vignette, 25–27
  definition and epidemiology of, 27–28, 28*t*
  health impact of, 29–30
  overview, 25
  in prisons, 394–395
postsecondary education, victimization in. *See* tertiary education, victimization in
posttraumatic stress disorder (PTSD)
  intrusive memories, 53
  network analysis of symptom structure, 137
  onset/cause and duration, 134*t*
  psychopharmacology of, 139–141, 140*t*
  psychosocial risks or dysfunctions in, 134, 136*t*
  psychotherapy for, 141–143, 142*t*
  symptoms or conditions of, 134, 135*t*
  treatment of, 138–143, 140*t*, 142*t*
Power, K. G., 391
Prakash, R., 75
prazosin, 140
pregnancy, adolescent, 76
prevalence
  of adolescent dating victimization, 340–342
  of child abuse or maltreatment, 274–275
  of cyberbullying, 14–15, 15*t*, 293, 294*t*
  of cybercrime, 299
  developmental conditions associated with peer victimization, 14
  of maltreatment of parents by children, 270–271
  overview, 10
  physical characteristics linked to bullying, 14
  of prison victimization, 390
  of school bullying, 10–13, 11*t*, 216
  of sibling bullying, 264
  of victimization among parents, 268–269
  of victimization in competitive sports, 349–350
  of witnessing cyberbullying, 408–409
  of witnessing school bullying, 407
  of witnessing victimization in community, 411
  of witnessing victimization in family, 410–411
  of witnessing workplace bullying, 409–410
  of workplace bullying, 16–17, 16*t*
prevention
  of child maltreatment, 105–106
  of cyberbullying, 102–103, 296–297
  of dating violence, 103–105, 104*t*, 344–345, 345*t*
  interventions to prevent further victimization, 132–133
  overview, 100
  role of bystanders in bullying prevention strategies, 407
  of school bullying, 100–102, 216
  of workplace bullying, 105, 250
prevention laws
  corporal punishment, 174, 174*t*
  cyberbullying and cybervictimization, 167, 167*t*, 168*t*, 169*t*
  domestic or family maltreatment, 171–172, 171*t*, 172*t*, 173*t*
  future, 182–183
  harassment in streets and public areas, 174–175, 175*t*
  overview, 164
  school bullying, 164, 165*t*, 166*t*
  workplace bullying, 167–168, 169*t*, 170*t*
PREVNET, 177
primary prevention
  of domestic or family abuse, 172
  of school bullying, 164, 165*t*
  of workplace victimization, 168

prison victimization
  bullying among prison inmates, 389–391
  bullying among prison officers, 392
  fear of, 395
  mistreatment of inmates by prison system, 396–400
  neglect of inmates, 398, 399–400
  overcrowding, 398–399
  overview, 5, 389
  physical aggression in prisons, 393–394
  polyvictimization, 394–395
  predictors of, 395
  sexual abuse in prisons, 392–393
  solitary confinement, 397–398
  torture of inmates, 396–397
Pritchard, C., 100
professional trainees, bullying among, 371–372
prolonged exposure (PE) therapy, 141, 142*t*
property abuse, sibling, 267–268
pro-self-harm web sites, impact of exposure to, 76
psychiatric disorders
  bullying related to, 14
  polyvictimization and, 30
  sibling bullying and, 264–265
psychodynamic psychotherapy, 139*t*, 141
psychological abuse
  adolescent dating victimization, 340, 341
  among siblings, 267, 267*t*
psychological effects
  adolescent dating victimization and, 342–343
  of cyberbullying, 296
  neighborhood safety and, 322–323
  of witnessing school bullying, 408
psychopharmacology, 139–141, 139*t*, 140*t*
psychosocial impact of headaches, 37
psychosocial problems
  absenteeism, 73
  adolescent pregnancy, 76
  carrying weapons, 74–75
  criminality, 79
  overview, 71
  physical fights, 75
  poor academic performance, 73–74
  poor health-related quality of life, 71–73
  school dropout, 75–76
  self-injurious behavior, 76–77
  substance abuse, 78–79
  suicide attempts, 77–78
  treatment within diagnostic framework, 134, 136*t*
psychotherapy, 139*t*, 141–143, 142*t*
psychotic disorders
  associated with bullying, 53–55
  sibling bullying and, 265
PTSD. *See* posttraumatic stress disorder
public areas, laws preventing harassment in, 174–175, 175*t*
public health domain, notion of bullying in, 3, 4*t*
Pyrooz, D. C., 316

quality of life (QoL), 71

Rabe, K., 398
race
  discrimination in sports, 356
  discrimination in the streets, 324–325
  school bullying by, 12–13
ragging, 91n.10, 375
rape
  in colleges and universities, 379
  in military training, 380
  prevention programs, 179
  by teachers, 217
Rasberry, C. N., 73
Rauer, A. J., 44
Raya, R. P., 410
rehabilitation for prisoners, 399–400
Rehan, W., 42
Rehling, D. L., 377
Resick, P. A., 142*t*
residence area, bullying related to, 13, 15
restorative practice, 132
revictimization
  composite clinical vignette, 25–27
  definition and epidemiology of, 28–29
  health impact of, 30
  overview, 25
Rhoads, J. M., 235
Rigby, K., 100, 101
risk behaviors
  absenteeism, 73
  adolescent pregnancy, 76
  carrying weapons, 74–75
  criminality, 79
  overview, 71
  physical fights, 75
  poor academic performance, 73–74
  poor health-related quality of life, 71–73
  school dropout, 75–76
  self-injurious behavior, 76–77
  substance abuse, 78–79
  suicide attempts, 77–78
  treatment within diagnostic framework, 134, 136*t*
Rivers, I., 408
road rage, 327–328
Robinson, E. M., 55, 269
Rodriguez-Muñoz, A., 42
Romito, P., 44
Rosenstein, J. E., 379
Rospenda, K. M., 380
Ross, T., 398
Rothbaum, B. O., 142*t*
Rothman, E. F., 380
rudeness toward customers or patients, 246
Runyan, D. K., 119
Russell, D., 40
Russell, K. N., 344–345, 345*t*
Rying, M., 269–270

sabotage of consumers, 247
SAD (social anxiety disorder), 42
Sadeh, A., 45
Safe Dates Project, 104–105, 104*t*

safety in neighborhood. *See* neighborhood, maltreatment in
Salmivalli, C., 213, 406, 407
Salmon, G., 41
Saltzman, L. E., 270
Sampasa-Kanyinga, H., 86
Sampson, R. J., 315
Sanchez, S. E., 44
sanctions, 132, 133
Sansone, R. A., 242
Sanz-Barbero, B., 75
Sasson, G., 295
Sasson, H., 295
Schlenger, W. E., 413
Schnurr, P. P., 142*t*
Schønning, V., 45
school absenteeism, 73
school bullying
  absenteeism and, 73
  adolescent pregnancy and, 76
  anxiety and, 40–41
  by area of residence, 13
  artificial intelligence, detecting with, 116
  backache and, 45–46
  bullies, 212
  bully/victim dual role, 212–213
  bystanders, role of, 213
  clinical detection of, 115–116
  criminality and, 79
  depression and, 38
  dissociation and, 53
  ecological aspects of, 215
  family, role of, 214–215
  gender nonconformity and, 12
  global prevalence of, 10–13, 11*t*
  headaches and, 35
  inattention and, 52–53
  inflammation and, 48–49
  injuries and, 55
  interventions to prevent further victimization, 132–133
  irritability linked to, 37
  maltreatment among educational stakeholders, 221
  musculoskeletal pain/fibromyalgia and, 47–48
  national prevention strategies, 176–177, 176*t*
  overview, 211
  overwork in school workplace, 220–221, 221*b*
  by parental occupation/socioeconomic status, 13
  participants' roles, 211–215
  physical fights and, 75
  prevalence of, 216
  prevention laws, 3, 164, 165*t*, 166*t*
  prevention of, 100–102, 216
  by race, ethnicity, or being foreign-born, 12–13
  school corporal punishment, 218, 219*t*, 220*t*
  school violence and homicide, 87–88, 88*t*
  stomachache and, 47
  stressful circumstances affecting school stakeholders, 221, 222*t*
  substance abuse and, 78
  teachers, role of, 213–214
  teachers as victims of bullying, 216
  teachers' mistreatment of students, 216–218
  victims of, 212
  weapon-carrying and, 74–75
  weight gain and, 49
  witnessing, 407–408
school climate, 215
school corporal punishment, 218, 219*t*, 220*t*
school dropout, 75–76
school hygiene, 220–221
Schreier, A., 53–54
scientific literature, bullying in, 1, 2*f*
Scott, R. A., 318
screening
  for child maltreatment, 118–120
  for IPV, 117–118
  for school bullying, 115–116
secondary prevention
  of domestic or family abuse, 172
  of school bullying, 164, 166*t*
  of workplace victimization, 168
secondary traumatic stress (STS), 412–413
Second Step: Student Success Through Prevention (SS-SSTP), 176
selective serotonin reuptake inhibitors (SSRIs), 139–140, 140*t*
self-injurious behavior, 76–77
Selkie, E. M., 38, 380–381
Semenya, S. W., 12
September 11, 2011 (9/11) terrorist attacks, 413
serotonin-norepinephrine reuptake inhibitors (SNRIs), 140
service providers, maltreatment between customers and, 240–245
service sabotage, 247
SES (socioeconomic status), 13
Sesar, K., 53
sexual harassment
  in military training, 379, 380
  prevention laws, 174–175, 175*t*
  in sports, 353–354
  in street, 325–326
  of university students, 378
  at work, 236, 237, 243–244
sexual victimization
  adolescent dating victimization, 340, 341
  among siblings, 266–267
  of children, 273
  in colleges and universities, 379
  in health care, 248–249
  in military training, 380
  national prevention initiatives, 179–181, 180*t*
  in prisons, 392–393
  in sports, 350, 353–354
  substance abuse and, 78–79
  by teachers, 217–218
Sha, R., 54
Shamu, S., 39
Shareck, M., 323
shared concern, method of, 132, 133
Sharpe, C., 316

Shi, J., 393, 394
Shield, M., 244–245
Shields, E. W., Jr., 351
Shields, M., 78–79
Shields, M. E., 51
Shumba, A., 217
sibling bullying
  abuse among siblings, 265–268
  antisocial behavior or criminality and, 79
  anxiety and, 42
  definition of, 263
  depression and, 39
  homicide, 266
  overview, 263
  prevalence and correlates, 264
  psychiatric risks and, 264–265
Silverman, B. C., 246
Simon, R. I., 249
Singham, T., 52–53
Sinkkonen, H. M., 370–371
Sinyor, M., 85
SL (supervised learning), 116
Slee, P., 101
sleep difficulties, 43–45, 324
sleep paralysis, 45
Smart, R. G., 327–328
Smith, K., 342
Smith, M. D., 352
Smith, P., 326
Smith, P. K., 2, 132–133
smoking, 323
SMRs (Standard Minimum Rules for the Treatment of Prisoners), U.N., 396
SNRIs (serotonin-norepinephrine reuptake inhibitors), 140
Snyder, J. A., 380
social anxiety disorder (SAD), 42
social conditions, school bullying and, 215
social regard, 246
social settings, notion of bullying across, 5
socioeconomic status (SES), 13
sociopolitical victimization, 421
Sodl, J. F., 381
solitary confinement, 397–398
Sommovigo, V., 242–243
Sorensen, J. R., 394
Sosa-Rubi, S. G., 179
SOS Namoro (Dating SOS) intervention, 178
Sourander, A., 47, 79, 296
Spaaij, R., 352
spectator violence in sports, 352
spectrum of maltreatment, 6–7
Spiller, T. R., 137
sports, victimization in
  definition of, 349
  discrimination in sports, 356
  emotional abuse in competitive sports, 354–356
  neglect in sports, 356–357
  overview, 349
  physical aggression in sports, 350–353, 351*t*
  prevalence of, 349–350
  sexual violence in sports, 353–354
sports officials, physical violence against, 352
spouse abuse, 268–270
Sprigg, C. A., 410
SPUTOVAMO screening test, 118
Srabstein, J., 35, 37, 115
Srivastava, S. K., 299
SSRIs (selective serotonin reuptake inhibitors), 139–140, 140*t*
SS-SSTP (Second Step: Student Success Through Prevention), 176
stalking, 244, 340, 378–379, 381
Standard Minimum Rules for the Treatment of Prisoners (SMRs), U.N., 396
Stanyon, D., 54
Stein, D. J., 140
Steiner, B., 395
Steiner, R. J., 73
Stephens, A. N., 328
Steps to Respect (STR), 176
Sternthal, M. J., 323
Stirling, A. E., 349, 354–355, 356–357
Stöckl, H., 89
Stoltenborgh, M., 274
stomachache, 47
StopBullying.gov, 176–177
stopping ongoing bullying, intervention for, 143–146, 164
STR (Steps to Respect), 176
strangers, victimization by, 315–316
Straus, M. A., 276
Strauss, C. V., 381
street children, 318
streets
  dangerous driving and road rage, 327–328
  discrimination in, 324–325
  fear of crime, 320
  fear of gangs, 320
  fears of terrorism, 322
  gang violence, 316–317
  harassment in, 325–326
  harassment prevention laws, 174–175, 175*t*
  incivility and pedestrian safety, 328–329
  incivility in neighborhood, 326–327
  incivility toward and among cyclists, 328
  neighborhood bullying, 314
  neighborhood crime and perception of safety, 319–320
  neighborhood safety, health impact of, 322–324
  people living in, 317–318
  street children, 318
  victimization by strangers, 315–316
  violence in, 315
strengthening the victim, method of, 132, 133
stress and/or harmful events, disorders specifically linked with, 136
stressful circumstances affecting school stakeholders, 221, 222*t*
structural network, analysis of trauma symptoms as part of, 136–137

STS (secondary traumatic stress), 412–413
Stueve, A., 407
substance abuse, 78–79, 380–381
suicide, 85–87, 269
suicide attempts, 77–78, 85–86
suicide risk, 343
supervised learning (SL), 116
support group method, 132, 133
Sutin, A. R., 49
Swahn, M. H., 344
Swanberg, K., 247–248
Swedish Work Environment Act, 220
Sweeten, G., 316
symptomics, 136–137
symptom-targeted treatment, 146
Szabo, A., 353

Takaki, J., 39
Takizawa, R., 48–49
Tamakoshi, A., 235
Tang, C. S., 378
teachers
  maltreatment among educational stakeholders, 221
  mistreatment of students, 216–218
  overwork in school workplace, 220–221, 221*b*
  role in school bullying, 213–214
  school corporal punishment, 218, 219*t*, 220*t*
  sexual abuse by, 217–218
  stressful circumstances affecting, 221, 222*t*
  as victims of bullying, 216
teams, workplace bullying among, 239
Teen Choices program, 345
teen dating victimization. *See* adolescent dating victimization
Teeuw, A. H., 118
Teicher, M. H., 410–411
Temple, J. R., 342
terrorism, 322, 413
tertiary education, victimization in
  bullying among college/university students, 370–371
  bullying among healthcare students and professional trainees, 371–372
  bullying among university staff, 372–373
  bullying in military training, 374–375
  harassment and discrimination, 378–379
  harassment in military training, 379
  hazing among military trainees, 376
  hazing among university students, 375
  health impact of, 380–381
  incivility, 376–377, 377*t*
  overview, 370
  sexual victimization in military training, 380
  violence in colleges and universities, 379–380
tertiary prevention
  of domestic or family abuse, 172, 173*t*
  of school bullying, 164
  of workplace victimization, 168, 170*t*
Tesarz, J., 46
Tharp, A. T., 344
Thompson, F., 132–133
Tiesman, H. M., 89
Tietjen, G. E., 36
Timm, A., 372
Tippet, N., 264
Tochigi, M., 43
Tonmyr, L., 78–79
top–toe inspection (TTI), 118
torture of inmates, 396–397
Toseeb, U., 264
trauma symptoms
  network analysis of symptom structure, 136–137, 146
  polyvictimization and, 29–30
treatment
  of adjustment disorder, 138, 139*t*
  of ASD and PTSD, 138–143, 140*t*, 142*t*
  within diagnostic framework, 134–136
  disorders specifically linked with stress and/or harmful events, 136
  network analysis of symptom structure, 136–137
  overview, 132, 133–134
  symptom-targeted, 143–146
trickery, 293
tricyclic antidepressants, 140*t*
Triple P, 105
Troop-Gordon, W., 213
Truman, A., 244
TTI (top–toe inspection), 118
Tucker, C. J., 263, 264, 266, 267
Turchik, J. A., 380
Turner, H. A., 29–30
Twemlow, S. W., 216, 217

UNICEF, 318
United States
  prevalence of cyberbullying in, 293
  workplace bullying in, 237
universal screening
  for child maltreatment, 118
  for exposure to victimization, 120–121
  for IPV, 117
university academic or administrative staff, bullying among, 372–373
university students
  bullying among, 370–371
  bullying among healthcare students and professional trainees, 371–372
  harassment and discrimination, 378–379
  hazing among, 375
  health impact of victimization, 380–381
  incivility among, 376–377, 377*t*
  violence in colleges and universities, 379–380
unnatural deaths, 90
unsheltered homeless, victimization of, 317–318
US Child Maltreatment Report, 274

Vaara, J. P., 374
Vaithianathan, R., 55–56
Van Cleemput, K., 103
Vandebosch, H., 41

van der Kolk, B. A., 142*t*
van Dulmen, M. H., 343
van Geel, M., 43, 74
van Konijnenburg, E. M., 118
van Tilburg, M. A., 47
Van Winkle, E., 379
Vartia, M., 392, 410
venlafaxine, 140
victim narratives, indirect exposure through, 412–413
victims, of school bullying, 212
Viennese Social Competence (VISC) training, 176
Vignoli, M., 48
Viljoen, J. L., 390–391
Vincent-Höper, S., 243–244
Violato, C., 276
violent discipline of children, 274, 275–277
Virginia Tech shootings, 413
virus writing, 293
VISC (Viennese Social Competence) training, 176
Vitaliano, G. D., 410–411
Vives-Cases, C., 46
Vreeman, R. C., 100
Vveinhardt, J., 349–350

Waalen, J., 117
wages, delayed payment or nonpayment of, 277
Waldron, J. J., 355
Walsh, A. L., 246
Walsh, J. A., 266, 267, 271
Walsh, K., 393
Wang, M., 276
Wang, M. J., 295
Wang, W., 74
WAST (Woman Abuse Screening Tool), 117
Wathen, C. N., 117
Watters, D. A., 351
W-CBT (work-focused CBT), 139*t*
weapons, carrying, 74–75
weight, body, 49–50, 323
Wensley, K., 370
Wheeler, A. R., 239
Whitted, K. S., 217
WHO (World Health Organization), 272, 273
Widom, C. S., 29
Wilinsky, C. L., 354
Wilkins, K., 244–245
Wilkins-Shumer, A., 71–72
Williford, A., 103
Wilson, E., 355
Wilson, N. L., 243*t*
Wilson, S. M., 380
witnessing victimization
  among university students, 370, 381
  cyberbullying, 408–409
  family victimization, 410–411
  indirect exposure to distressing events, 412–413
  overview, 406
  role of bystanders in bullying prevention strategies, 407
  school bullying, 407–408
  types, roles, and social dynamics of bystanders, 406
  victimization in community, 411–412
  workplace bullying, 409–410
Wolfe, D. A., 178
Wolfe, J., 277
Wölfer, R., 102
Wolff, H., 398–399
Wolff, N., 392, 393, 394, 395
Wolitzky-Taylor, K. B., 343
Wolke, D., 43, 79, 263, 264
Woman Abuse Screening Tool (WAST), 117
Wong, J. Y., 275
Woodford, M. R., 381
work-focused CBT (W-CBT), 139*t*
"Working without bullying," campaign, 177
workplace bullying
  absenteeism and, 73
  among members of working teams, 239
  among prison officers, 392
  antecedents and consequences of, 238–239
  anxiety and, 42
  backache and, 46
  in Canada, 238
  cardiovascular disease and, 51–52
  corporate or employer victimization of employees, 240
  corporate victimization of consumers, 249–250
  cultural distance and, 17
  depression and, 38–39
  diabetes and, 50
  epidemiology of, 236–238
  in Europe, 236–237
  examples not specific to work environment, 236, 236*t*
  examples specific to work environment, 235–236, 235*t*
  global prevalence of, 16–17, 16*t*
  headaches and, 35–36
  homicide and, 88–89
  HRQoL and, 72
  maltreatment between customers and service providers, 240–245
  maltreatment of domestic workers, 277–278
  measuring, 238
  mistreatment of customers, clients, or patients, 246–249
  musculoskeletal pain/fibromyalgia and, 48
  national prevention initiatives, 177–178
  overview, 5, 234
  overwork in schools, 220–221, 221*b*
  prevention, 105, 250
  prevention laws, 167–168, 169*t*, 170*t*
  sleep difficulties and, 43–44

in United States, 237
university faculty members, 372–373
witnessing, 409–410
World Health Organization (WHO), 272, 273
Wright, M. F., 409

Xing, X., 276
Xu, T., 50, 51–52

Yamasaki, S., 54
Ybarra, M. L., 88
Ye, L., 116
Yimgang, D. P., 322
Yoo, T., 43–44
Yoon, Y., 409
youth gangs, 316
youth participation in street fights, 315
Youth Relationships Project (YRP), 178
Youth Risk Behavior Surveillance System (YRBSS), 10, 15
Youth Risk Behavior Survey (YRBS), 340–341

Zaborskis, A., 77
Zabrodska, K., 373
Zogby Analytics, 16
Zolotor, A., 74, 119–120
Zottis, G. A., 214
Zweig, J. M., 340